HEALTH
POLITICS
AND POLICY

0-8273-4555-0

Health Politics and Policy

2nd edition

Theodor J. Litman, Ph.D.
Professor, Division of Health Services
Administration
University of Minnesota
Minneapolis, Minnesota

Leonard S. Robins, Ph.D.
Professor, Public Administration
Program
Roosevelt University
Chicago, Illinois

 DELMAR PUBLISHERS INC.®

NOTICE TO THE READER

Delmar Staff

Executive Editor: Barbara E. Norwitz   Project Editor: Christopher Chien
Developmental Editor: Marjorie A. Bruce   Production Supervisor: Helen Yackel
Managing Editor: Susan Simpfenderfer   Design Coordinator: Susan C. Mathews

For information address Delmar Publishers Inc.
2 Computer Drive West, Box 15–015
Albany, New York 12212

Printed in the United States of America
Published simultaneously in Canada
by Nelson Canada,
a division of The Thomson Corporation

10   9   8   7   6   5   4   3   2   1

Library of Congress Cataloging-in-Publication Data:

Health politics and policy / [edited by] Theodor J. Litman, Leonard S. Robins.—2nd ed.
    p.   cm.
    Includes bibliographical references.
    Includes index.
    ISBN 0-8273-4555-0
    1.   Medical policy—United States. 2. Medical care—Political aspects—United States. 3. Public health—Political aspects—United States. 4. United States—Politics and government—1945–
I. Litman, Theodor J. II. Robins, Leonard S.
    [DNLM: 1. Health Policy—United States. 2. Politics—United States. WA 540 AA1 H48]
RA395.A3H4257 1991
362.1'0973—dc20
DNLM/DLC
for Library of Congress   90-13984
                                                                                              CIP

Introduction to the Series

This Series in Health Services is now in its second decade of providing top quality teaching materials to the health administration/public health field. Each year has witnessed further strengthening of the market position of each of the principal books in the Series, also reflecting the continued excellence of the products. Each author, book editor, and contributor to the Series has helped build what is widely recognized as the top textbook and issues collection of books available in this field today.

But we have achieved only a beginning. Everyone involved in the Series is committed to further expansion of the scope, technical excellence, and usability of the Series. Our goal is to do more for you, the reader. We will add new books in important areas, seek out more excellent authors, and increase the physical attributes of the book to make them easier for you to use.

We thank everyone, the authors and users in particular, who have made this Series so successful and so widely used. And we promise that this second decade will be dedicated to further expansion of the Series, and to enhancement of the books it contains to provide still greater value to you, our constituency.

Stephen J. Williams
Series Editor

Delmar Series in Health Services Administration

__ Stephen J. Williams, Sc.D., Series Editor

Introduction to Health Services, third edition
Stephen J. Williams and Paul R. Torrens, Editors

Health Care Economics, third edition
Paul J. Feldstein

Health Care Management: A Text in Organization Theory and Behavior, second edition
Stephen M. Shortell and Arnold D. Kaluzny, Editors

Ambulatory Care, Management, second edition
Austin Ross, Stephen J. Williams, and Eldon L. Schafer, Editors

Health Politics and Policy, second edition
Theodor J. Litman and Leonard S. Robins, Editors

Strategic Management of Human Resources in Health Services Organizations
Myron D. Fottler, S. Robert Hernandez, and Charles L. Joiner, Editors

Contributors

Odin W. Anderson, Ph.D.
Professor
University of Wisconsin
Madison, Wisconsin
Professor Emeritus
University of Chicago
Chicago, Illinois

Charles H. Backstrom, Ph.D.
Professor
Department of Political Science
University of Minnesota
Minneapolis, Minnesota

Roger M. Battistella, Ph.D.
Professor
Health Policy and Management
Sloan Program in Health Services
   Administration
Department of Human Service Studies
College of Human Ecology
Cornell University
Ithaca, New York

James W. Begun, Ph.D.
Professor
Department of Health Administration
Virginia Commonwealth University
Richmond, Virginia

William P. Brandon, Ph.D.
Professor
Department of Political Science
Seton Hall University
South Orange, New Jersey

Robert J. Buchanan, Ph.D.
Assistant Professor
Sloan Program in Health Services
   Administration
Department of Human Service Studies
College of Human Ecology
Cornell University
Ithaca, New York

Tom Christoffel, J.D.
Professor
School of Public Health
University of Illinois
Chicago, Illinois

Richard C. Elling, Ph.D.
Associate Professor and Director
Graduate Program in Public Administration
Department of Political Science
Wayne State University
Detroit, Michigan

Robert G. Evans, Ph.D.
Professor
Department of Economics
University of British Columbia
Vancouver, British Columbia
Canada

David Falcone, Ph.D., MHA
Associate Professor
Departmentof Health Administration
Associate Director
Long Term Care Resources Program
Center for the Study of Aging
Duke University
Durham, North Carolina

Paul J. Feldstein, Ph.D.
Professor and
FHP Foundation
Distinguished Chair in Health Care Management
Graduate School of Management
University of California—Irvine
Irvine, California

Irene Fraser, Ph.D.
Project Manager
Division of Health Policy
American Hospital Association
Chicago, Illinois

Lynn Cook Hartwig, Dr.P.H.
Director, Center for Community Health
Health and Human Services Division
University of Southern Mississippi
Hattiesburg, Mississippi

Bette S. Hill, Ph.D.
Assistant Professor
Department of Political Science
University of Akron
Akron, Ohio

Katherine A. Hinckley, Ph.D.
Associate Professor
Department of Political Science
University of Akron
Akron, Ohio

William W. Lammers, Ph.D.
Professor
Department of Political Science
Senior Research Associate
Ethel Percy Andrus Gerontology Center
University of Southern California
Los Angeles, California

Donald W. Light, Ph.D.
Professor
Health and Mental Health Policy
University of Medicine and Dentistry of New
  Jersey
Camden, New Jersey

Debra J. Lipson, M.H.S.A.
Assistant Director
Department of Programs and Policies
The Children's Defense Fund
Washington, D.C.

Theodor J. Litman, Ph.D.
Professor
Division of Health Services Administration
School of Public Health
University of Minnesota
Minneapolis, Minnesota

James A. Morone, Ph.D.
Associate Professor
Department of Political Science
Brown University
Providence, Rhode Island

Paul E. Pezza, Ph.D.
Assistant Professor
Program in Health Policy and Management
Providence College
Providence, Rhode Island

Mitchell F. Rice, Ph.D.
Professor
Public Administration Institute
Louisiana State University
Baton Rouge, Louisiana

Leonard S. Robins, Ph.D.
Professor
Public Administration Program
Roosevelt University
Chicago, Illinois

David A. Rochefort, Ph.D.
Associate Professor
Department of Political Science and Public
  Administration
Northeastern University
Boston, Massachusetts

Camilla Stivers, Ph.D.
Member of the Faculty
Graduate School of Public Administration
Evergreen State College
Olympia, Washington

Frank J. Thompson, Ph.D.
Professor and Dean
College of Public Affairs and Policy
Nelson A. Rockefeller Graduate School of Pub-
  lic Affairs
State University of New York
Albany, New York

Mylon Winn, Ph.D.
Assistant Professor
Department of Political Science
Miami University
Oxford, Ohio

Contents

List of Tables

Foreword

In 1974, with a recent Ph.D. in Political Science but no formal education or experience in health care whatsoever, I was offered an Assistant Professorship at a leading School of Public Health. I had no formal credentials, but neither, at that time, did many others, so I guess that from the School's perspective I was as qualified as most.

It is now nearly twenty years since then, but the study of health policy and health politics has burgeoned enormously, as the voluminous Bibliography to this edition of *Health Politics and Policy* well attests. And while conventional academic taxonomies may still not adequately account for those laboring in this increasingly fruitful vineyard, there is now a recognizable field with at least 27 identifiable practitioners—the authors represented in this fine volume.

At least this once, more importantly, the academic output appears consonant with the operational realities. For while the process was certainly far advanced even in those dim, dark, long-ago days of 1974, by now the interpenetration of the health care and political/policy systems is so thorough and so pervasive that one cannot operate effectively in either sphere without an adequate understanding of the other. And as the share of national resources devoted to health services has continually increased, most dramatically but not uniquely in the United States, the centrality of the political/policy system to health care, and of health care to the political/policy system, has become ever more apparent.

Not so long ago, we interlopers from the sphere of public policy routinely encountered a sort of puzzled hostility from health professionals who wondered who had granted us license to meddle in their territory. Physicians and other health professionals viewed their sphere of professional activity as solely their own, immune from intervention by the rest of society. As any political scientist should have been able to predict, however, no enterprise which derives so large an amount of money from public sources can long remain immune to public scrutiny and governmental intervention. In professions where training is so heavily subsidized by public sources, where hospitals derive more than half of their operating revenues from government programs and most of their capital from tax-subsidized sources, and where even physician incomes are derived, on average, approximately 30 percent from government, the surprising thing about the extent of government involvement is how long it took to develop.

I've often been amused to note how quickly many physicians, nurses, and other health care professionals, once dragged willy-nilly into the political fray, come not only to enjoy it but to be quite good at it. Unfortunately, this sometimes reinforces their learned instincts

Conversely, it's hard to conceive how even the most zealous ideologues of the Reagan years could imagine dealing effectively with the health system's many acknowledged problems without a strong government role. Indeed, much of what passed for "pro-competition" or "pro-market" strategies in the '80s, such as Medicare's Prospective Payment System, was transparently government regulation under another name. And the American Medical Association, to take only the most extreme example in terms of professional representation, not only no longer automatically opposes government intervention in health care matters, but even actively seeks it in such areas as the institutionalization of professional peer review, medical malpractice tort reform, and protection from the abuses of private utilization review firms.

As we enter the 1990s, the problems of the American health care system, and of the public policies that so profoundly dominate that system, appear almost overwhelming. A large and ever-increasing proportion of the population, because they lack health insurance or for other reasons, are effectively denied access to needed services. Costs continue to grow substantially more quickly than the economy as a whole, consuming an ever larger share of national resources, taxpayer dollars, and corporate profits. Yet critically important providers of health services, especially in inner cities and rural areas, are dying of economic thirst in the middle of this ocean of expenditures. We have far more hospitals, and probably far more physicians, than we really need, yet at the same time there exists a critical undersupply of primary care, mental health services, and other long-term care for the chronically ill.

If we are to solve any of these problems, let alone all, public policy will be the critical instrument, and political forces will determine policy outcomes. The agenda is long, complex, and formidable. If a more thorough and systematic comprehension of the issues and problems is a necessary precondition for designing effective solutions, Litman's and Robins' book constitutes an extremely valuable resource.

Bruce C. Vladeck
President
United Hospital Fund
New York, New York

Preface

A short time before his untimely death from cancer, former Vice President Hubert H. Humphrey noted that the moral test of a government—and, we would add, a nation—is how it treats those who are in the dawn of life, its children; those who are in the twilight of life, its aged; and those who are in the shadow of life, its sick, needy, and handicapped. For a government (society), he went on to observe, that can neither educate its children, care and sustain its elderly, nor provide hope and meet the needs of its infirmed sick, its poor, and disabled, is a government without compassion and a nation, we would argue, without a soul.

The resolution of such issues, more often than not, tends to be a political one, arrived at in the political arena as part of a political process. It is toward understanding the process and the context within which such decisions are made vis-á-vis health and health care that this book is addressed. It is intended to provide interested students and faculty in the health sciences, government, and public administration with a comprehensive analytical overview of the politics of health. Through an examination of the historical and contemporary involvement of government and politics in the organization, financing, and delivery of health care both here and abroad, it attempts to underscore the important role political factors play in the development of health policy.

The first edition of this book was written at the onset of the Reagan Presidency. A number of leading academicians and practitioners in the field were invited to prepare original expositions on the politics of health and health care. In the ensuing years, the U.S. health care system has seen many dramatic changes, the most important of which have been: 1) the growing advocacy of free market competition as the solution to the problems of financing and the delivery of services; 2) the introduction, paradoxically, by the Reagan Administration of the most intrusive regulatory control over the health care system in the nation's history with the adoption of DRG based prospective payment to hospitals under Medicare; and 3) the limitation that the nation's fiscal and budgetary policies have placed on the Federal government's potential for initiatives in health and health care.

In light of the above, a number of substantive changes have been made in the organization and content of this second edition in order to give readers a greater insight into the role of the governmental process in health policy. While some chapters were retained and updated, notably those by Litman, Anderson, Battistella and Begun, Falcone and Hartwig, Thompson, Elling and Robins, and Feldstein, several new authors were also commissioned: Light; Lammers; Lipson; and Stivers, and/or topics added, e.g., Law (Christoffel); Public Opinion (Rochefort and Pezza); Health Interest Groups (Hill and Hinckley); Health Care Reform (Morone); Finance (Evans); Access to Services (Fraser); Black Health Care (Rice and Winn);

The Aged and Long Term Care (Brandon) and AIDS (Robins and Backstrom). As a result, the volume has been expanded from sixteen to twenty chapters, with over half of the contributions new to this edition.

The content of the book is organized around four major themes. Following Theodor Litman's introductory overview and sociopolitical analysis of the relationship of government and health (Chapter 1), the remainder of Part One seeks to place health politics and policy in perspective. In Chapter 2, for instance, Odin Anderson traces the history and development of the U.S. health services enterprise over the course of the past 100 years. This is then followed by Donald Light's analysis of the historical and contemporary forces that have led and now shape the restructuring of the American health care system. Finally, Part One concludes with a review by Roger Battistella, James Begun, and Robert Buchanan of the major ideological influences that have governed the health policy debate in this country.

In Part Two, our focus shifts to an exploration of health policy and the political structure, beginning with William Lammers' examination of the strengths and limitations of Presidential leadership in health policy. In their chapter, David Falcone and Lynn Hartwig focus on the increased impact of budget constraints and the relative unimportance of Congressional structure and process in determining health policy outcomes. Tom Christoffel then explores the theoretical and potential role that law and the courts can play in health policy. This is followed by Frank Thompson's exposition on the implementation process and the effect politics and bureaucracy may have in shaping health policy. Debra Lipson then examines the role that the states have and continue to play in health policy making and the organization, financing, and delivery of health services. The section concludes with a review by Richard Elling and Leonard Robins of the forms of intergovernmental assistance including the Reagan Health Block Grants.

Part Three examines the role of interest groups and public opinion in health policy. Paul Feldstein leads off the section by providing a theoretical framework for explaining the legislative positions taken by health provider groups. Taking a somewhat different tack, Bette Hill and Katherine Hinckley analyze the political behavior of health interest groups and their impact on health legislation. Finally, David Rochefort and Paul Pezza explore the influence and relationship of public opinion on health policy.

Health policy and the political process provide the focus of Part Four. The section begins with a consideration of the politics of health care reform by James Morone. Then, noting that the politics of health care finance is dominated by the inevitable conflict between those who pay for care and those who are paid, Robert Evans concludes in Chapter 15 that the failure of cost control efforts in the United States may be attributed to the nation's failure to develop effective mechanisms for negotiations with providers. The dual problems of inadequate access to health care and the growing number of the uninsured are examined by Irene Fraser, while the crisis of black health is the subject of the chapter by Mitchell Rice and Mylon Winn. In a somewhat different vein, the health care issues affecting the elderly are discussed by William Brandon within the context of the politics of the aged and the aging support system. Then, drawing from her experience as Associate Director of the Institute of Medicine's study on The Future of Public Health, Camilla Stivers traces the field's relative ineffectiveness in influencing health policy to its lack of political sophistication. The final essay by Leonard Robins and Charles Backstrom deals with the politics of perhaps the most serious and far-reaching public health policy problem in recent history—AIDS.

The volume then concludes with an Epilogue and a chronology of capsule highlights of the involvement of government in health and health care in the United States, followed by an extensive research bibliography.

Finally, a compilation such as this represents the efforts of a number of persons. In addition to our contributors, a special note of gratitude and appreciation is owed the Division of Health Services Administration, School of Public Health at the University of Minnesota and our secretary, Beth Freund, without whose assistance the final preparation of this book would not have been possible.

Theodor J. Litman
Leonard S. Robins

Part One

Health Politics and Policy In Perspective

Chapter 1

Government and Health:

The Political Aspects of Health Care —A Sociopolitical Overview

Theodor J. Litman

When the Eighty-ninth Congress adjourned in 1966, its record of legislative accomplishments made it the most health-minded Congress in U.S. history.[1] Not only had more national health legislation been enacted into law during its first session than had been passed in both sessions of all Congresses in the past decade, but it had appropriated more money for health in the last two years of its term than its predecessors had in the previous 168 years. Never before had one session of Congress produced legislation of such far-reaching implications for the health, education, and socioeconomic welfare of the American people than had been enacted in 1965 (Gardner et al. 1967). So extensive was the legislative activity in terms of the number and scope of health actions taken that one observer depicted the period as a turning point in health law (Forgotson 1967).

As far as health care financing was concerned, the issue no longer was one of public versus private enterprise. According to Anne Somers, that issue had seemingly been settled in favor of the nation's or the United State's unique pluralistic health care economy with its programmatic amalgamation of public and private activities. What had changed was the nature of the mix,

[1]A total of 15 pieces of legislation that had direct and far-reaching impact on health services were enacted: the most publicized were. Medicare and Medicaid, Titles XVIII and XIX of the 1965 amendments to the Social Security Act. Others included PL 89–239 Heart Disease, Cancer and Stroke amendments of 1965 (Regional Medical Program); PL 89–74 Drug Abuse Control amendments of 1965; PL 89–92 Federal Cigarette and Labeling and Advertising Act; PL 89–105 Mental Retardation Facilities and Community Mental Health Centers Construction Act amendments of 1965; PL 89–109 Community Health Services Extension amendments of 1965; PL 89–115 Health Research Facilities amendments of 1965; PL 89–234 Water Quality Act of 1965; PL 89–272 The Clean Air Act amendments and Solid Waste Disposal Act of 1965; PL 89–290 Health Professions Educational Assistance amendments of 1965; PL 89–292 Medical Library Assistance Act of 1965; PL 89–4 The Appalachian Regional Development Act; PL 89–73 The Older Americans Act; PL 89–333 The Vocational Rehabilitation Act amendments of 1965; PL 89–117 The Housing and Urban Development Act of 1965. A sixteenth bill, PL 89–749, Comprehensive Health Planning, was passed in 1966.

which seemed to lean markedly in favor of the public sector (Somers 1966). Moreover, with the passage of the National Planning and Resources Development Act (PL 93–641) in 1974 (Rubel 1975), the question of the federal government's right to interfere in the private practice of medicine appeared to be decided, for all intents and purposes, in favor of government.

The role of the federal government in the organization, financing and delivery of health care services in the United States at mid-decade seemed assured, and the prospects for adoption of some form of national health insurance seemed imminent, if not a foregone conclusion.

But if the federal initiatives in health during that period had been seen by many as a sociopolitical watershed in which the powers and machinery of government were mobilized to improve access to services, to further distributive justice and equity, and to redress social and economic wrongs (Fein 1980), times and circumstances changed. The heady optimism and faith in the unbridled growth and intervention of the federal establishment soon gave way to suspicion, distrust, and disillusionment with government programs. Thus, in spite of a number of notable accomplishments—such as demonstrated gains in access to care and in health status among the poor and the elderly (Mooney 1977), greater rationalization of the health planning process, and increased production of health personnel—skepticism and dissatisfaction with such initiatives began to grow in the face of rising costs, economic stagflation, limited revenues, diminished financial resources, programmatic cutbacks, indifferent if not hostile central administration, and bureaucratic insensitivity to the infringement of federal policies, directives, and regulations on state and local prerogatives, culminating in the Reagan election in 1980.

The response was sudden and pointed. The new chief executive, who had ridden to victory on a promise to get government off the backs of the American people, moved quickly and decisively. Within six months of taking office, through the deft and imaginative use of the budgetary process and with the support of a group of conservative Democrats (known as the Boll Weevils) who were ideologically closer to the Republican party than their own, the president succeeded in gaining congressional approval of a package of budget cuts that repealed and modified scores of programs that had become integral parts of the nation's social and economic fabric, while he was seeking to reverse the federal expansion of the last half-century and reduce the size and scope of government.

As he left office eight years later, the impact his administration had on the nation's health care system was judged by some to be greater than any of his predecessors since Lyndon Johnson. In contrast with the expansionist policies of Johnson's Great Society, however, the Reagan years were marked by a reductionist effort to cut health care costs and shift responsibility for many programs from the federal government to the states and private sector (Sorian 1989). According to Rabe (1987), the Reagan strategy to defederalize health care in the United States followed three general lines of attack: 1) Decentralization, i.e., the transfer of authority to the states by the dismantling of existing federal categorical programs and consolidation of others into block grants; 2) Deregulation, through the abolition or weakening of regulations, appointment to leadership positions of individuals who were opposed or unsympathetic to the basic mission or purpose of certain bureaus or agencies, as well as a reduction in funding, and 3) Redistribution, i.e., proposed reductions in or elimination of, direct forms of government assistance to individuals through entitlement programs, such as Medicare.

The results, as several authors in this volume note, were mixed. Moreover, despite the President's espousal of and commitment to the concept of minimalist government, honed and sharpened during his term as governor of the State of California, the Reagan years were marked by major entreaties, both in policy and practice, which called for extensive government intrusion into the privacy of the home (e.g., abortion and family planning), the workplace (e.g., mandatory drug testing), as well as medical practice, including the physician-patient relationships itself (e.g., DRG-based prospective payment).

And so, at the dawn of a new decade, it remains to be seen whether the activities and the events of the Reagan presidency constitute a major shift in sociopolitical thought in this country, vis-à-vis the relationship of government to the individual and his or her health care, as many pundits have suggested, or whether they were merely an aberrational interlude in the nation's continuing flirtation with the adoption of some form of universal health insurance. Suffice it to say that the answer is likely to lie in an understanding of the peculiar nature and role government and politics play in American life, with the decision reached being the product of a deliberative political process.

Government and Health in the United States

A number of years ago, the noted British social historian T.H. Marshall observed that no modern government could disdain responsibility for the health of its people nor would it wish to do so. Policies, he noted, differ not so much in the aims pursued as in the methods adopted in pursuit of them (Marshall 1965). But although the notion of a national system of health services has long been a well-established fact in much of the rest of the world, it has been slow to take hold in the United States. Since the first governmental system of health care was established in Germany under Bismarck in 1883, the provision of health and medical care to an entire population on a nationwide basis through some form of national health service or insurance mechanism has been adopted in nearly half of the world's sovereign nations, including most of those in Western Europe. On the whole, this development has generally come about through an evolutionary rather than revolutionary process, a function of the social, cultural, political, and economic fabrics of the various countries involved. In most cases, government programs for the financing of health care services have evolved as part of a broader system of social benefits. To a large extent, each nation's health care system is a reflection of its own particular legacy of traditions, organization, and institutions, and the American experience has been no exception (Litman and Robins 1971). Thus, to understand where the United States is and may be heading, it is necessary to know something of the past and the nature of the governmental system.

The United States System of Government

As most students of government are aware, ours is a limited system of federalism predicated on the notion of representative government with an emphasis on minority rights, majority rule, and the preservation of individual liberty. Historically, the American conception of freedom has taken the guise of rights to be protected from restraint, rather than duties to be performed, and a suspicion of established authority. Thus, largely in response to government oppression experienced in Europe, the framers of the Constitution provided an extensive system of checks and balances upon the federal establishment. Although Madison and others recognized the need for national supremacy—earlier attempts to rest sovereignty in the state or colonial legislatures as called for under the original Articles of Confederation had proven unsuccessful—they were also aware of the need for protection from the arbitrary use of power by the national government. To pit sovereignty against sovereignty, however, was seen as a formula for disaster.

The solution was outlined in Federalist Paper No. 5:

> In the compound republic of America, the power surrendered by the peoples, is first divided between two distinct governments, and then the portion allotted to each, subdivided among distinct and separate departments. Hence a double security arises to the rights of the people. The different governments will control each other at the same time that each will be controlled by itself.

As set forth under Article I, Section 8 of the Constitution, the relationship between the states and the federal government was fairly well drawn, with the federal government given certain prescribed delegated powers, other powers reserved for the states, and still others left to be exercised jointly.[2]

---

[2]Significantly, the Constitution did not specify the functions and powers of the states, nor were the lines between national and state powers precisely drawn. Consequently, in order to maintain supremacy of the national government over the constituent states in any conflict of authority, the original framers took the following steps: (1) They included a supremacy clause in the Constitution that made the Constitution, federal laws, and treaties of the United States binding on the judges in all states; (2) they required all state officers and judges to take an

But the framers were also farsighted and realized that the United States was bound to change over time. As a result, the Constitution was envisioned to be a flexible document, confined neither in time nor place. Thus, the role of government in American life has evolved over the past 200 years or so in large part through judicial interpretation and response to executive initiatives and legislative action.

Federalism and the Constitutional Relationship between the National Government and the States

The question of the proper role of government in general, as well as the relative distribution of powers among the national, state, and local governments in particular, has been the subject of prolonged philosophical debate in the United States, with the line in any given controversy ultimately drawn by the courts. Such deliberations have ranged from Marshall's Doctrine of National Supremacy (*McCulloch v. Maryland*)[3] to the Doctrine of Dual Federalism of the Taney court (*Cooley v. Board of Wardens*),[4] with the states having concurrent powers in those matters considered to be truly local in character, to the Coop-

erative Federalism of the Cardozo court (Steward Machine Company case)[5] to the concept of Creative Federalism under President Johnson[6] and the New Federalism[7] and new New Federalism of the Nixon and Reagan administrations.

Before the 1930s, both federal and state legislation in the field of social welfare were invalidated by the courts on the basis of the due process clause.[8] In 1937, however, the Supreme Court reversed itself (*West Coast Hotel Company v. Parrish*) and repudiated the old doctrine that the due process could be used to crush social welfare legislation. Nevertheless, it was Marshall's interpretation of the commerce clause and the supremacy of the central government that served as the basis for much of the legislative initiatives of the New Deal (Roosevelt), the Fair Deal (Truman), the New Frontier (Kennedy), and the New Society (Johnson).

State-Federal Regulations

The role of the states in the U.S. political system has changed dramatically over the past 200 years as events and trends have altered the fiscal, functional, and political balance within the federal system and rekindled debate over the proper division of powers and responsibilities among the constituent units (Advisory Commission on Intergovernmental Relations 1980; Stenberg 1980).

The expansion of the federal government's role in U.S. life has been neither an historical accident nor an altogether noxious historical legacy, but has come about for good historical reasons (Ken-

---

oath to support the U.S. Constitution including the supremacy clause; (3) they provided for a national guarantee of a republican form of government in each state, which implied the right of the national government to intervene in state governments; and (4) they provided for judicial review of state legislative acts in federal courts. Finally, no state was permitted to nullify or obstruct the acts of the national government (Anderson, 1955).

[3]Chief Justice John Marshall proclaimed that the U.S. government was one of enumerated powers derived from those specifically delegated to it by the Constitution; that is, Article I, Section 8 sets forth seventeen enumerated powers, plus those implied from the "necessary and proper clause." Later, in Gibbons v. Ogden, Marshall held that Congress's power over commerce was plenary, absolute, and complete, subject to no limitations except that expressly stated by the Constitution. The power to regulate was the power to prescribe rules by which commerce was governed.

[4]This doctrine upheld state action in interstate commerce via the state's police powers. Within the powers reserved by the Tenth Amendment, the states were sovereign, with final determination of the scope of state powers to rest with the national judiciary. Taney allowed for concurrent regulation by the state while acknowledging both state and national government powers. It permitted state action where the federal government failed to act.

[5]This case envisioned cooperation between the two levels of government.

[6]The expression was used by President Johnson in 1964 in a speech given in Ann Arbor, Michigan, and referred to an improved system of federal relations with state and local governments in connection with the transfer of federal funds for a variety of programs and purposes to local governments. It had been used earlier in conjunction with state and federal sharing arrangements such as federal grants-in-aid, interstate compacts and revenue sharing under the Eisenhower administration.

[7]This term is epitomized in the use of block grants.

[8]For example, *Lochner v. New York* (attempted state restrictions on working hours). *Adkins v. Children's Hospital* (minimum wage law) *Hamner v. Dagenhardt* (attempt to restrict child labor in manufacturing).

nedy 1981). The Constitutional Convention of 1787, for example, was called largely to cure the crippling chaos of decentralized government under the old Articles of Confederation. In his well-known Federalist Paper No. 10, Madison argued that a federal government, presiding over the large and disparate polity, would be proof against "faction" or the monopoly of political power by a small group. A corollary is that only the central government, by virtue of its aloofness from local passions, is equipped to lift the nation above the petty parochialisms and prejudices of local interests (Kennedy 1981).

Over the course of the past two decades, however, notably under both the Nixon and Reagan administrations, increasing interest has been expressed in the importance of the relations among the various levels of government. At issue has been how large the federal government's role should be in its relations with its state and local counterparts. The answer has been caught up in philosophical differences that separate not only Democrats from Republicans but also conservatives from liberals within each party (Congressional Quarterly 1972).

Beginning under Roosevelt's New Deal and continuing under the Democratic administrations of the sixties, a fairly broad agreement was reached in Congress that the federal government should play an active role in areas traditionally within the province of state and local governments, particularly regulation where state laws were either nonexistent or failed to conform to one another. There was also broad agreement that the federal government should have a role in providing financial assistance to states and localities for a variety of purposes, such as fighting poverty, pollution control, local law enforcement, and housing. The issue was no longer legitimacy of whether the federal government should be involved in such areas but rather how it should go about assisting the state and local governments (Congressional Quarterly 1972).

Traditionally, federal assistance has been in the form of categorical grants-in-aid made to a variety of governmental and other public and private entities for specific purposes. Such grants-in-aid enable state and local governments to preserve their autonomy within a framework of federal assistance to assure minimum levels of services regardless of income inequities among states and localities, and to help achieve national objectives that states and localities may be unwilling or unable to pursue as well as stimulate, through federal matching, increased investment of state and local funds. Moreover, since federal taxes are generally more progressive than their state and local counterparts, federal grants help reduce interstate inequities both in the level of government services and the tax burden. As a matter of fact, one of the major reasons for the proliferation of categorical grants programs was that not only could the federal government tap far more revenue sources than the states and localities, but also the latter officials could not or would not provide funds to deal with certain problems (Congressional Quarterly 1972).

On the other side of the coin, the expansion of federal power at the expense of state and local government is inherent in such revenue-sharing mechanisms, leading to federal domination or control. It was in reaction to just such concerns, as well as the trend toward centralization of government authority in Washington, D.C., that the concept of block grants was developed. Block grants, which are federal payments to states or local governments for specified purposes such as health, education, or law enforcement, have been pushed by Republicans in Congress and the executive branch since the 1960s as a way of returning federal decision making to state and local officials. In contrast to categorical grants, which can only be used for specific programs directed by Congress, block grants allow state or local officials to make the decisions on how the money is used within the general program area (Congressional Quarterly 1981).

The New Federalism

The debate continued with President Reagan's efforts to return many government programs to the states. However his proposal, although clothed in the mantle of the "New Federalism," represented less a sorting out of functions among the various levels of government than opposition of fiscal conservatives to large-scale public sector spending on particular domestic activities regardless of the level of government

(Falkson 1976).[9] Moreover, although the Reagan proposal to return power and responsibilities to the states was viewed by some as a watershed in the history of U.S. federalism, critics saw the president's New Federalism and Economic Recovery Act as a device to reduce federal expenditures for key domestic activities, and as an abandonment of the national commitments to certain costly social programs, involving the transfer of responsibility to the states and their political subdivisions without adequate funding (Stavisky 1981).

And, as Nexon (1987 80) observed, "with no specific services provided by the federal government, no clearly identifiable needs to which funds were targeted, and no constituency for the funds beyond state health officials," the Administration hoped that not only would Congressional interest in the block grant program be small but that the "life of the new blocks would be short."

Such criticisms aside, however, the president's initiative in this area, like that of his predecessor, Nixon, was directed at a number of real and purported deficiencies associated with the federal government's expanded domestic role in the sixties and seventies. Among these were:

1. The inefficiency, complexity, and inequity of categorical grants
2. The vesting of policymaking and control in quasiindependent agencies, unaccountable to any constituency, that is, the voters, nor responsive to local needs and priorities, that is, local health service agencies (HSAs)
3. The distortion of state and local priorities through the stifling of local initiative and taxing ability, forcing local governments to structure themselves around categorical programs rather than their own needs
4. The imposition and enforcement of stereo-

typed, inflexible solutions for local recipients by federal bureaucrats, out of touch and unaccountable to the public
5. Maldistribution of federal funds to those who master the grants application procedure rather than those who have the greatest need (Penchansky and Axelson 1974; Richardson 1973)

The Reagan proposal also seemed to strike a responsive chord with the American public. Although the public was concerned about the impact of such a program on their state and local taxes, and the ability of states and cities to serve the needs of the disadvantaged through block grants, as well as uneasy about the complexity of transferring responsibility from the federal to the state governments, an October 18, 1981 Gallup Poll revealed initial public support, at least in principle, for the President's overture (Gallup 1981).

As states and local units of government were forced to struggle with the need to provide more human services in the face of ever-diminishing financial resources, proposals to return such functions to their control, without a commensurate transfer of funds, tended to lose much of their aura and appeal, and the debate over the proper role of government in U.S. life continues (Elling and Robins Chapter 10).

Representative Government, Interest Group Politics, and the Legislative Process

The political process in the United States revolves around two complementary but at times conflicting themes—the notions of participatory democracy and of representative government. To many, the quintessence of the U.S. governmental system is found in Madison's Federalist Paper No.10:

> Extend the sphere, and you take in a greater variety of parties and interests, you make it less probable that a majority of the whole will have a common motive to invade the rights of other citizens or if such common motive exists, it will be more difficult for all who feel it to discover their own strengths and to act in unison with each other.

---

[9]The New Federalism proposed by President Reagan should not be confused with that advocated under the Nixon administration a decade or so earlier. The latter embodied a broad spectrum of sociopolitical philosophies advocated by people who shared a common background of experience in state and local government, as well as federal service, and a common belief in the need for reforming the structure of domestic policymaking and program implementation. Although both the new federalists and fiscal conservatives are generally concerned about growth of federal power, only the latter has sought total cessation of public sector spending on social programs (Falkson 1976).

From this flows the electoral system of "single-member" districts, a citizen congress composed of members elected on the basis of state and local areas, and a theory of public interest representation. The framers of the Constitution carefully set forth a tripartite structure of government involving an intricate system of checks and balances and a separation of powers among the three branches—the legislative, executive, and judicial.

Legislative Process

The power of Congress to legislate is defined in Article I, Section 1 of the Constitution. In addition to writing federal laws, Congress has the power to conduct investigations; monitor federal agencies; impeach federal officials (including the president); declare war; approve treaties; raise or lower federal taxes; appropriate money; and approve appointments to federal agencies, the judiciary, and the armed forces. It may also override a presidential veto with a two-thirds majority vote in each chamber.

The legislative process, however, is a slow and deliberate one, especially in the case of controversial issues. A wide diversity of political views and regional interests, coupled with political caution, serve to deter change. As a result, Congress is more prone to following trends than creating them (Fuchs and Hoadley 1987, 215; Sheler 1985 46).

Committee System.   At the heart of the legislative process is the congressional committee system that has existed in the House and Senate since 1789 and allows for a division of work as well as an orderly consideration of legislation. There are about 19 Senate and 23 House standing committees plus a host of special, select, and *adhoc* committees and subcommittees (136 in the House and 107 in the Senate).

Committee assignments are allocated on the basis of seniority and in proportion to the representation of the party's membership in each chamber. Members generally want to be on committees related to their personal interests and backgrounds and the economic interests of their districts or state. Some committees, however, are more powerful than others. Among the latter

are the Senate and House Appropriations Committees that control the flow of money to programs authorized by other committees, the Senate Finance and House Ways and Means Committees that consider tax legislation, and the House and Senate Budget Committees that establish national priorities through the preparation of the national budget.

Health and the Committee Structure.[11]   Although the word "health" does not appear in the official title of any congressional committee, at least 14 committees and subcommittees in the House and 24 in the Senate have been identified as having some direct or oversight responsibility in health (Lewis 1976). Of these, six committees—three in the House and three in the Senate—control much of the legislative activity in Congress. The House committees are as follows:

Ways and Means Committee has the power to tax and was the launching pad for much of the health financing legislation passed in the sixties and early seventies under the chairmanship of Representative Wilbur Mills (Dem., Ark.). In addition to sole jurisdiction over Medicare Part A, it shares jurisdiction over Medicare Part B with the Energy and Commerce Committee.

Committee on Energy and Commerce (formerly the Committee on Interstate and Foreign Commerce) and its *Subcommittee on Health and the Environment* have jurisdiction over Medicaid, matters of public health, mental health, health personnel, health maintenance organizations, food and drugs, the Clean Air Act, Consumer Protection Safety Commission, health planning, biomedical research, and health protection.

Committee on Appropriations and its *Subcommittees on Labor, Health and Human Services, and Education* allocate and distribute federal funds

---

[11]Whereas 25 years ago, one could be rest assured that any major piece of health legislation would bear the clear imprint of Congressman Wilbur Mills (Dem., Ark.), chairman of the powerful House Ways and Means Committee, and to a lesser degree Senator Russell Long (Dem., La.), then Chairman of the Senate Finace Committee, with the congressional reforms of the seventies, the attendant diffusion of responsibility for health legislation over several committees in both Houses, and the weakening of the committee chairs and party leadership, not only is such determination far less certain today, but so too is the prospect of successful passage of legislation on the floor in unaltered form.

for individual health programs. The Senate committees are:

Committee on Labor and Human Resources has jurisdiction over most health bills referred to it, including health planning, health maintenance organizations, health personnel, mental health legislation, for example, Community Mental Health Centers Act. This committee formerly included a subcommittee on Health and Scientific Research, which was used by its chairman, Senator Kennedy (Dem., Mass.), as a forum for debate on national health insurance. When the full committee came under Republican control in the 1980s, the subcommittee was abolished.

Committee on Finance and Subcommittee on Health, like the Ways and Means Committee in the House, the Senate Finance Committee has jurisdiction over taxes and revenues, including matters related to Social Security, Medicare, Medicaid, national health insurance, and child health and is responsible for many of the Medicare and Medicaid amendments, such as Professional Services Review Organizations (PSROs), prospective reimbursement, and controlling hospital and nursing home costs.

In 1989, ostensibly in an effort to ease its heavy workload and keep all its members happy, the Finance Committee decided to split its health subcommittee in two, with responsibility for Medicaid policy and the problems of making health insurance available to the uninsured assumed by the subcommittee on Health for Families and the Uninsured, and oversight of Medicare and the search for ways to cover the high cost of long term nursing home care to be dealt with by the subcommittee on Medicare and Long Term Care.

Committee on Appropriations and Subcommittees on Labor, Health and Human Services, and Education, like their counterparts in the House, allocate and distribute federal funds for individual health programs.

It has been estimated that although the tax committees (House Ways and Means and Senate Finance) have jurisdiction over only 15 percent of all health programs' legislation, they control about 70 percent of all federal health dollars expended. The two principal authorizing committees, on the other hand—the House Committee on Energy and Commerce and the Senate Committee on Labor and Human Resources—review

approximately 70 percent of all federal health program legislation but directly affect only 15 percent of the total health dollars (Schmidt 1980).

Once considered stable legislative bodies, with long tenure for members and a committee seniority system that ensured enduring power to multiterm members, especially committee chairs, the House and Senate in recent years have been plagued by high membership and staff turnover, overlapping jurisdictions, and changes in rules that have significantly increased the independence of individual members at the expense of party discipline, institutional accountability, and legislative efficiency.

Of particular concern, as far as it affects the development of congressional policy on health and medicine, has been the high turnover rate among members and their aides who have had a special interest or involvement in these areas. Between 1977 and 1981, for example, while the turnover rate among members in both houses of Congress approximated 40 percent, and for their aides, nearly 90 percent, membership changes in the six key committees and subcommittees that deal with most health legislation were massive, that is, 66 percent, and nearly 90 percent for their staff. Moreover, of the 435 representatives and 100 senators who had voted on the Medicare and Medicaid legislation sixteen years earlier, only sixty-eight (13 percent) of the former and thirteen (13 percent) of the latter still remained in office in 1981. Similarly, a survey of the personal aides and professional staffs serving the six legislative committees that organized and funded these programs and continue to have jurisdiction over them revealed not a single staff member remains who had played a significant role during that period (Grupenhoff 1982).[12] In the absence of experienced staff, there is no institutional memory. As a result, Congress has been left with

---

[12]A similar concern has been voiced by Levine (1984) at the state level, where continuing budget crises, inadequate compensation, competition from the private sector, the rise of single issue politics, and legislative burnout have eroded the legislative and bureaucratic infrastructure of state government at the very time the federal government has proposed returning to them more responsibility for the implementation of human service programs. While such turnover may provide a means of bringing new ideas and people into government, new members are largely the least effective and poorly informed (Hanson 1987).

a huge vacuum in terms of knowledge and expertise in such matters at the very time it must grapple with major administration initiatives designed to alter greatly these and related programs.

Role of the Executive Branch.   Despite Congress' predominant role in the legislative process, the executive branch is not without its resources. In addition to proposing, lobbying, and vetoing legislation, it can effectively thwart, if not emasculate, legislative intent by withholding or rescinding funds through the Office of Management and Budget (OMB)[13] and/or weaken enforcement by nominating or not nominating agency heads or appointing persons unsympathetic or antagonistic to direct the program involved.[14]

Interest Group Politics and Health

The efforts of organized interest groups to influence government policy in the United States are an inherent part of the political process and, in large measure, rest on First Amendment guarantees of free speech and the people's right to petition government for a redress of grievances. The increasing complexity of modern life and the attendant increase in the role of government in the everyday lives of its citizens has tended to heighten such organizational activity as part of the political process. Thus, as power has moved toward the federal government, there has been a proliferation in interest group activity (in both number and variety) at the national level. Each year hundreds of such organized interest groups attempt to wield considerable influence over government policy, constituting what has been referred to as the Washington Lobby[15] (*Congressional Quarterly* 1972; also see Drew 1967; Felicetti 1975; Hixson 1976; Milbrath 1964; Redman 1974)

In their efforts to gain results, such organizations, often directed by professionals in the art of government, tend to direct their focus at key points in the decision-making and policy implementation process. If unsuccessful in Congress, for example, a group may continue to pursue its aims in the agency charged with responsibility for its execution. The legislative game, then, does not end with congressional passage of a bill and its subsequent signature; rather, the entire thrust of a piece of legislation may be muted, if not reversed, in the writing of the regulations and/or administration of the act.

In addition to attempting to influence the views of individual representatives and senators or key members of the executive branch on specific issues, many organized interest groups take an active part in the elective process itself, contributing large sums of money to the campaign coffers of individual candidates as well as those of the political parties themselves (in many cases hedging their bets by contributing to the candidates on both sides of the political aisle). In the last few years, in fact, considerable concern has been raised over single-issue interest groups and their power to wield a disproportionate influence on the legislative elective process through the creation of lavishly funded political action committees (*Congressional Quarterly* 1972).

While traditionally interest group activity in the United States has involved groups of individuals representing similar economic or social interest, e.g. labor unions, business, farmers, etc., as the federal government broadened its sphere of activities, a new type of pressure group developed—the coalition of diverse economic and so-

---

[13]The OMB has been likened to a shadow government (Downey 1975). Just as Congress has relied on the power of the purse strings to wend its will, so too has the OMB, especially under the directorship of David Stockman in the Reagan administration. Stockman, through his deft use and mastery of the budgetary process, was far more powerful and had a much greater impact on public policy, although less publicly accountable, in his role of director of OMB than in his former role as Congressman from Michigan, where he was but one voice among 535. (see *Congressional Quarterly* 1986.)

[14]The latter was epitomized by the controversy in the Reagan administration over the management of the so-called superfund and the Environmental Protection Agency (EPA) under the direction of Anne Gorsuch-Burford. Burford, who resigned her position under fire in March 1983, had earned a reputation as a staunch opponent of environment protection laws while she was a member of the Colorado state legislature before appointment to head the EPA.

---

[15]Especially noteworthy in the area of health was the role played by Mary Lasker (Drew 1967; Redman 1974). An equally if not more important influence on government is that wielded by the large think tanks such as The Brookings Institution. American Enterprise Institute for Public Policy Research, the Urban Institute and the Rand Corporation (Guttman 1976: Federation of American Hospitals 1979).

cial interests brought together by concerns over a single issue (*Congressional Quarterly* 1988). Moreover, in the case of highly charged political controversies, given the heightened nature of the rhetoric and the euphemistic characterization of the opposing sides, it is often difficult to discern the players without a score card as this excerpt of a letter, written by then Surgeon General C. Everett Koop, that accompanied his report to the President on the health effects of abortion on women, clearly attests:

> It is difficult to label the opposing groups in the abortion controversy. Those against abortion call themselves pro-life. On the other hand, those who are not pro-life say they are not pro-abortion; rather, they refer to themselves as pro-choice and are supportive of women's right to choose abortion.
>
> It is true that some who are pro-choice are personally opposed to abortion. It is not clear to them where the lines should be drawn between the rights of the fetus and the rights of the mother. So the pro-choice forces are not monolithic.
>
> Nor are the pro-life forces monolithic. Many ardent pro-life individuals who are dedicated to preserving the life of the fetus do not consider contraception to be ethically, morally, or religiously wrong. But others in the pro-life camp do; indeed, some equate contraception with abortion (as quoted in Shannon 1989).

For the most part, however, interest groups tend to gear their operations to the power structure and procedures of Congress, with much of their efforts directed at the committee system. It has been estimated, for example, that about 90 percent of all legislation passed on the floor of either house was passed in the form previously reported by the committee having jurisdiction over it (*Congressional Quarterly* 1972).

The power of committees to draw and prevent legislation as well as determine its nature makes them an inviting target for interest group activity. The Washington Lobby, for example, goes to great lengths to keep abreast of government developments that might have a bearing on the interest of its membership. It makes sure to know and watch the work of committees important to its interests, establish and maintain working relationships with key committee members and their staff, stay informed on potential or actual legisla-

tive developments, and provide testing and submit prepared statements setting forth its organization's view before the committee (*Congressional Quarterly* 1972).

On the whole, a group's power to influence legislation rests as much, if not more, on the size of its membership, the financial and personnel resources it can bring to bear on an issue, the astuteness of its representatives, and its political acumen and skills, as it does on the soundness or righteousness of the ideas or positions it expounds (*Congressional Quarterly* 1988). As one observer has noted, "The majority of the American people are not members of special interest groups and hence are much less articulate on particular issues than are the interested minority whose affiliation with some active organization gives them a greater political leverage" (George B. Galloway, as quoted in *Congressional Quarterly* 1972 4).

Falik (1975) has argued that the power potential of health as a political issue is circumscribed by the equivocal nature of interest group politics. Although the politicization of health issues helps stimulate public debate, educate the public, and broaden the population base for affirmative legislative action on national health matters, it is equally true that political gamesmanship tends to give disproportionate advantage to those groups that are effectively organized for lobbying. In the health field, this has largely been representative of the medical-educational complex, that is, health professional schools, organized medicine, hospital industry, and third party payors (Falik 1975; Health Policy Advisory Center 1968). Such vested interest group activity manifests itself in the currying of the support of elected officials in both the legislative and executive branch by representatives of major provider groups in order to gain protection and funding of their favorite programs. For example, a *Health-Week* survey of Federal Election Commission reports revealed that contributions by Political Action Committees (PACs) affiliated with major health care companies and their professional and trade associations to presidential candidates, members of key Congressional committees and challengers during the 1987–88 election campaign totaled more than $6.1 million (Kimball and Ready 1988).

Historically, the most formidable organized interest group in health has been the American Medical Association (AMA), which, year in and year out, is one of the United States' richest and most profligate sources of campaign funding and legislative lobbying.[16] (Pressman 1984) In addition to its long and expensive campaigns against "socialized medicine" and government interference in the practice of medicine (Carter 1958; Harris 1967; Hyde and Wolff 1954; Means 1953), the AMA gained a certain degree of notoriety when it successfully blocked the appointment of Dr. John Knowles, director of Massachusetts General Hospital, to the position of assistant secretary, Health, Education and Welfare, for health and scientific affairs in the Nixon administration because of what were considered to be his overly liberal views (*Congressional Quarterly* 1972). Although its power has waned over the past two decades, the organization remains a potent force in health politics (see Fackelman 1989, as well as Hill and Hinckley in this volume).

Participatory Democracy and Health

Public involvement in the determination of health policy in this country has not been confined to organized interest group activity alone, but has taken other forms as well, e.g., community participation, initiative, and referendum.[17] While community participation represents an extension of our democratic heritage and has been seen as a means to perfect the democratic process (Burke 1968), initiative and referendum constitute a basic right accorded at the state and local level for the exercise of direct public control over legislation (Roemer 1965).

Community Participation and Health.   Historically, participation of the public in the making of health policy decisions was subsumed in the involvement of the community power structure in institutional governance—a pluralistic, class-based system. A series of classic studies (Elling and Lee 1966); Belknap and Steinle 1963; Holloway et al. 1963) has described the relationship between community influentials and voluntary and official health and welfare institutions and its impact on organizational decision making (Elling 1968; also see Section 8.4 of the bibliography at the end of this book). More recently, Riska and Taylor (1978) have noted that not only are such board members recruited from a very narrow segment of the population, but also they share a narrow view of health policy that may be at variance with that of those whom they purport to serve, that is, their consumers.

The opportunity for full community or citizen participation in the determination of health policy was institutionalized under the provisions of the model cities (PL 88–164) and health planning legislation (PL 89–749) of the Johnson administration. The movement toward broader participation in human service decision making, including health, has been attributed to diverse factors such as dissatisfaction with professional dominance in the area and a growing recognition of the political nature of decision making regardless of professional input (Silver 1973). Not surprisingly, the application of the concept has resulted in a collision between what Geiger (1969) has termed "community insistence and professional resistance" and has led in some cases, unfortunately, to a politicalization of the health care delivery system over the issue of who truly represents the community and what "participation" and "community" really mean (Geiger; Bellin 1969, 1970; Brandon 1977; Gordon 1969; Moore 1971; Thompson 1974; and Feingold 1973).

Initiative and Referendum.   Finally, a note should be added concerning the use of initiative and referendum in health. Unfortunately, the experience of the scientific communities with such extralegislative devices has been anything but

---

[16]During the 1988 Congressional Campaign, AMPAC, the AMA's political action committee, raised over $4.8 million, placing it behind the Teamsters Union and the National Association of Realtors among all the nation's PACs that year (Meyer 1988a). Of the $3.6 million spent by AMPAC on primary and general Congressional elections, $2.1 million went for traditional direct contributions to candidate, $800,000 for independent campaign expenditures, i.e., independent of the candidate's own campaign apparatus, and $615,000 for election research and campaign volunteer training. In contrast with its unsuccessful 1986 strategy which sought to "knock off" unfriendly incumbents—notably Representative Fortney "Pete" Stark (Dem., CA)—no incumbents were ticketed by AMPAC for defeat in 1988 (Meyer 1988b).

[17]The initiative is an electoral device that empowers the people to propose legislation; the referendum is an electoral mechanism that accords the people the power to approve or reject legislation enacted by their representatives (Roemer 1965).

promising. The submission of health issues to public referendum, for example, has produced mixed, if not discouraging, results. By far the most extensively studied case has been that related to the fluoridation of water. Of the 600 referenda held on the issue during the 1950s and 1960s, despite widespread endorsement by the health care community, over 60 percent were rejected (Crain et al. 1968, see also Section 8.5 of the bibliography at the end of this book). Moreover, recent efforts with such campaigns have produced equally dismal results. Of about nineteen referenda held on the issue in the United States in the first six months of 1980, seventeen were defeated (Isman 1981).

Although a number of reasons have been offered to explain the failure of such proposals at the hands of voters, including ignorance, voter apathy, a growing distrust of government, and the health care establishment (Isman 1981; Marmor et al 1960; Gamson 1961), suffice it to conclude the following:

> The submission of controversial health-related issues for voter approval is risky and should be entered into with great caution.
>
> Reliance on the rationality of the voter, the persuasiveness of scientific evidence, the righteousness of the issues, the prestige of the health professions, and the implausability of the charges of the opposition is presumptuous at best, if not self-defeating.
>
> The successful undertaking of such an endeavor requires considerable political skills, extensive knowledge of the community, and mobilization of broad-based, communitywide support.

The Growth of the Government's Role in Health and Health Care in the United States

Evolution not Revolution

It has long been a truism of U.S. political life that government is only permitted to do that which private institutions either cannot do or are unwilling to do. The basic economic justification

for government intervention, Blumstein and Zubkoff (1973) note, is as a remedy for some market failure. In essence, the traditional basis for government involvement has been a remedial one, when, for whatever reason, the market does not achieve an efficient allocation of resources.

In the area of health and welfare, such a view was perhaps best expressed by a 1965 U.S. Chamber of Commerce Task Force on Economic Growth and Opportunity recommendation on the role of government: "Government programs should be used to help the sick, disabled and aged only if voluntary and private means—truly tried and tested—cannot adequately meet society's needs" (United States Chamber of Commerce 1965).[18]

A related corollary to the above would add that with the exception of those powers delegated to it by the Constitution, the growth of the federal government's involvement has generally come about in those areas in which the states have also been found wanting. The Interstate Commerce Act of 1887, for instance, was passed only after the states had failed to control the spiraling interstate railroad networks, and enactment of the New Deal came after four years of economic collapse that found the states broke, with only seventeen having old age pension plans, most which were woefully underfunded (Kennedy 1981).

The expansion of government or public intervention in health and health care in the United States has essentially been one of evolution rather than revolution, a function of social, economic, and political forces as well as judicial interpretation.

Constitutional Base

The bases for government involvement in health and health care at the state and federal levels rest on quite different constitutional principles. In the case of the states, this has been

---

[18]Stevens (1982), for example, has noted that government hospitals in the United States were established only where community need was self-evident and private efforts were unavailable, for example, to safeguard merchant seamen, protect the general public from infectious and contagious diseases, isolate and treat the mentally ill, and provide care and shelter to the poor (Stevens 1982).

through the police powers[19] to "enact and enforce laws to protect the health, safety . . . and general welfare" of the public. The states, for example, have rather broad, comprehensive legal authority to regulate or affect virtually every aspect of the health care system within their boundaries (Grad 1973; Wing 1976). Such intervention, even by compulsion as in the case of immunization against communicable diseases, has been sustained by the courts [*Jacobson v. Massachusetts*, 197 U.S 11 (1905)] even in the face of a constitutional challenge to its abridgement of the exercise of First Amendment rights to the free expression of religion (Blumstein and Zubkoff 1973).[20]

Federal involvement, on the other hand, has rested upon judicial interpretation of the Welfare Clause and, in the case of drugs and medications, the Commerce Clause,[21] which has been honed and expanded over the past forty years. Historically, for example, the definition of commerce has varied widely and Congress' power in this area has vacillated between restricted regulation and a broad grant of power, subject to judicial interpretation. In periods such as 1880 to 1936, for example, when business has been dominant, the courts have tended to keep government under close reign through a narrow interpretation öf the Commerce Clause. On the other hand, in periods in which the government is paramount, such as the past forty years, the court has given a rather broad interpretation to the word "commerce."

Historical Development

Over the course of the past 200 years, the role of government in the organization, financing and delivery of health care services in the United States has evolved from that of a highly constricted provider of services and protector of public health to that of a major financial underwriter of an essentially private enterprise whose policies and procedures have increasingly encroached on the autonomy and prerogatives of the providers of care, as he who pays the piper calls the tune.

Although extensive and, at times, seemingly pervasive, such growth has come about neither capriciously nor because legislators or bureaucrats have had any great desire to interfere in this area of endeavor, but rather because the parties primarily involved—the providers (with the notable exception of organized medicine), consumers, insurance carriers, and politicians—realized and came to recognize the need for assistance and government involvement.

Government's role in health and medical care in the United States has thus evolved over time.[22] In the early days of the republic, for example, there were few organized government health programs at either the state or national level (Lee 1968). There were no state health departments. Foreign quarantine was the responsibility of each port. Programs for communicable disease control and environmental sanitation were the responsibility of local government. Government intervention in health generally was confined to protecting society from the common risks, such as epidemic disease, and to meeting the essential needs of the poor and the destitute—a heritage from the Elizabethan poor laws. This was coupled with support provided by religious and other charitable agencies, fraternal societies, lodges, and clubs organized by immigrant groups (Falk 1967b).

For the most part, the federal government's role in matters of health could be characterized as paternalistic, custodial, and, most of all, minimal, consisting essentially of responsibility for the care and treatment of merchant seamen and members of the armed forces—past, present, and future (Falk 1967b). As a matter of fact, the

---

[19]The police power of the state is much broader than that of any power of the national government. It is a power that was reserved to the states and never given up by them.

[20]Compulsory fluoridation of water extends the concept of permissible infringement of personal freedom to include protection against a noncommunicable, non-life-threatening condition.

[21]The Congress shall have power to regulate commerce with foreign nations, and among the several States, and with the Indian tribes."

[22]In addition to the specific sources cited, we have also drawn on the following references: Falk 1967; Foltz and Brown 1975; Foltz 1975; Jackson 1969; Clarke 1980; Rosen 1974; Mustard 1945; Russell and Burke 1978. For a more detailed capsule outline of the key social, political, and legislative developments that underscored the evolution of the government's role in health and health care in the United States, see Appendix 2.

first major involvement of the national government with illness and the provision of medical care for other than the military services began with the Marine Hospital Service Act in 1798 to provide for sick or disabled seamen.[23] Later this was extended to include American Indians who were held in protective custody on reservations as wards of the state. Out of this developed the Indian Health Service, which in 1976 was the object of a major resolution of the Alaska Medical Society calling for its dissolution as inimical to the private practice of medicine.

Through much of early U.S. history, health and medical care was considered essentially a private and personal matter—a pattern that continued relatively unchanged for almost 80 years. It remained as such until the 1920s when, with the passage of the Sheppard-Towner Act on Maternity and Infancy in 1921, the federal role in health and medical affairs began to take on its modern form. This act established the first continuing program of federal grants-in-aid to state health agencies for the direct provision of services to individuals, the forerunner of the present-day maternal and child health program. The act, however, largely through the action of the AMA, was allowed to die in 1929 (Schlesinger 1967; Chapman and Talmadge 1970, 1971).

The enactment of the Social Security Act in 1935, which marked the beginning of the U.S. system of social welfare, provided the next major development in the growth of the federal involvement in matters of health. From this legislation two concepts of social welfare emerged: (1) social insurance for the working population, that is, unemployment insurance, workers compensation, and guaranteed retirement benefits; and (2) public assistance, that is, direct financial aid provided by the states for those unable to work.

Although not intended as a medical insurance program for recipients of categorical assistance (considered too costly and neither the time nor the place by President Roosevelt), this precedent-setting law provided for federal grants to the states for public health, maternal and child

health, and services for crippled children, as well as for public assistance for the aged, blind, and families with dependent children.

It is interesting to note, however, that while initially invoked and promoted on largely humanitarian grounds, the passage of many pieces of social health legislation, ostensibly those dealing with occupational safety and rehabilitation, rested essentially on utilitarian or pragmatic grounds, that is, returning people to the work force and investing in the future—a reflection of our reliance and belief in the Protestant ethic.

In 1950, the program was extended to include the permanently disabled, and in 1960, a more generous, open-ended federal-state program of medical assistance for the elderly—the Kerr-Mills Act—was enacted. The latter, a conservative response to the more extensive and liberal-backed King-Anderson Medical Care for the Elderly Bill supported by President Kennedy, was a forerunner of the Medicaid law (Filerman 1962).

The passage of the Hill-Burton Construction Act in 1946, which provided federal assistance to the hospitals whose physical plants had grown increasingly warn and obsolescent following the depression and World War II, served as a prototype for federal involvement in health care. In addition to establishing the principles of local initiative, state review, and federal support sharing, it also called for, via congressional mandate, at least the first vestiges of planning, that is, a state plan. Federal support was further extended to medical education and research in the 1950s and early 1960s, often over the bitter opposition of organized medicine (Anderson 1966; 1968a; Carter 1958; Harris 1967; Hyde and Wolff 1954; Rayack 1967).

It remained, however, for the Eighty-ninth Congress under the Johnson administration to bring the federal role in health care to full fruition with the passage in 1965–1966 of legislation providing for the establishment of regional medical programs, comprehensive health planning, extensive aid to medical and other related health profession education, and Titles XVIII and XIX of amendments to the Social Security Act of 1965—Medicare and Medicaid.

Certainly the sleeper here was the Medicaid bill, which was an extension and purported improvement of the earlier Kerr-Mills program and, like its predecessor, relied on the existing welfare

---

[23]It is interesting to note that the origin of most of the major national health care systems in the world can be traced to the assumption by government of the responsibility for the medical care of merchant seamen and the maritime trades that were considered crucial to the lifeblood of the nation, dependent as they were on import-export trade (Straus 1950, 1965).

system. The Medicaid bill was quickly and hastily passed as part of a political compromise to appease conservatives; thus, its architects neither delineated clear goals nor came to grips with the problems inherent in the entire welfare system—particularly the determination of eligibility, which was left to the states. Moreover, as Medicaid began, policymakers had little if any sense of the potential costs of the program nor the impact of pumping vast sums of federal dollars into the private medical market (Friedman 1977a, b; Davis 1974, 1975a, b, 1976a, b, 1977; Lewis et al. 1976; Stevens and Stevens 1970; Stevens and Stevens 1974; Weikel and Leamond 1976).

Like the Kerr-Mills program before it, Medicaid tended to epitomize the problems inherent in reliance on the states and a states' rights approach to resolving broad social programs. In attempting to retain state autonomy and decision making under the program, for example, the rich states tended to get richer whereas the poor states either took no action or had minimal participation in the program. Moreover, despite the offer of federal assistance, many states, especially in the South, either were unwilling or unable to expend the funds. As a result, there was a considerable lack of uniformity both between and within states, which became even further exacerbated in the face of a decline in the economy. Thus, a number of states encountered excessive costs brought on by an explosion of claimants as a result of the 1970 recession and were forced to cut back severely on their programs or, as was the case of New Mexico, pull out of the program altogether.

In addition, in return for the preservation of local control and the determination of local needs, such programs were subjected to the petty political jealousies and idiosyncratic administrative behavior of local welfare officials and county boards. Moreover, like much of President Johnson's War on Poverty and the welfare system itself, Medicaid proved to be an administrative nightmare. In contrast to Medicare, which had the advantage of being a completely new program administered solely at the federal level by a well-established and accepted entity in the Department of Health, Education and Welfare, using the private sector and the insurance industry as fiscal intermediaries, a major debate soon arose as to whether Medicaid was an income-maintenance or health service program and whether it should be administered by the welfare administration or the Public Health Service—a debate finally resolved in favor of welfare.

Growing concern on the part of the federal and state governments over the administration of the program led to the enactment of several provisions to improve its management. These included the establishment of federal guidelines requiring that the states review on a continuing basis the cost, administration, and quality of the health care services rendered under their programs, including stricter standards to ensure quality care and periodic review of nursing home use.

In 1967, Congress mandated expansion of the program to include early and periodic screening diagnosis and treatment of children and youth under the age of 21 eligible for Medicaid. As a result, not only was the health of low-income children considered a major program priority, but the states were expected to administer and the federal government to oversee a program for the direct provision of health care services (Foltz and Brown 1975; Foltz 1975).

Continued disenchantment with the program was reflected in the 1972 amendments to the Social Security Act that called for the withholding of federal funds from states that failed to implement the utilization review and Early and Periodic Screening, Diagnosis, and Treatment (EPSDT) programs mandated by Congress as well as the establishment of PSROs to provide a comprehensive and ongoing review of services rendered under Medicaid and Medicare to determine their medical necessity. This was later followed by repeated efforts under the Nixon, Ford, Carter, and Reagan administrations to constrain costs by reducing services and transferring more of the financial burden back to providers and their patients.

But if the actions of the 89th Congress mark the high point of government entreaties in the field of health and health care in this country, followed by continuous and persistent attempts over the course of the next twenty-five years by successive Republican administrations to modify, slow down or reverse the thrust of such efforts, as the nation enters the last decade of this century, the role of government in this formerly private endeavor remains pervasive and far reaching (albeit centering primarily on controlling costs) and calls for the adoption of some form of nation-wide, universal coverage to redress the problems of access and quality are once again being heard throughout the land (*The Nations Health* 1989).

Nature of the Government Role in Health and Health Care in the United States

Both traditionally and historically, responsibility for the medical care of recipients of public assistance, veterans with service-connected disabilities, and other special populations such as Indians and the armed forces and for public health in the United States has rested with government, whereas responsibility for the cost of facility construction and health personnel training has been shared among various levels of government and the private sector. The provision of direct personal health services, on the other hand, is and has been essentially a private endeavor.

According to Falk (1967a), government intervention in the U.S. health care system has tended to embrace the following features:

1. Financial underwriting in order to assure the availability to all in the population through either contributory insurance (e.g., Medicare), general tax revenues (e.g., Medicaid), or both

2. The development and establishment of various standards and procedures to safeguard the quality of services financed through public funds

3. The provision of services wherever possible through nongovernmental practitioners and institutions

4. Extension toward comprehensiveness in publically financed services

5. Direct financial support for the modernization, construction, and equipment of health care facilities and for the education and training of needed personnel

Similarly, Brown (1989 2), in an insightful

piece prepared for the Ford Foundation, has noted that the federal government in this country as well as central governments in many comparable countries, intervene in the health care system with four objectives in mind and rely on four main policy strategies to achieve them. For instance, in addition to 1) efforts to influence the supply of health care services and resources via subsidized grants and assistance to providers and institutions, government may seek to: (2) influence the demand for health care among all or part of its population—usually through the financing of a health insurance program created under public auspices; (3) alter the organization of the health care system by building new structures to serve special population groups, e.g., the VA health care system and the National Health Service Corps, or advance some larger goal such as improving access to care or contain costs through adoption or support of HMOs; and (4) influence the behavior of providers with respect to the use, price and quality of services, as well as the size, location and equipment of facilities through major regulatory programs such as peer review organizations, health systems agencies and prospective payment.

The ownership, financing, and operation of the health services system in this country, Anderson (1968a, 1968b) has observed, is diffused, with a wide dispersion of sources of funds and decision-making units. It is a pluralistic system in which the public and private sectors find themselves in what he has termed "uneasy equilibrium" with the various sectors negotiating with and accommodating one another.[24] As a matter of fact, the coexistence within the U.S. health care system of a wide variety of providers, organizational forms, and funding sources has been viewed by many as a positive attribute that contributes to the rapid diffusion of new technology, the enhancement of quality of care, and the capacity of the system to innovate and adapt to change (National Center for Health Services Research 1977).

The flow of government funds to voluntary

---

[24]In contrast to many of its European counterparts, much of the health care delivery system in the United States is in the private sector. As a result, government is forced to bargain because it neither owns the facilities nor hires the personnel (Anderson 1968b). The request in early 1983 by the Reagan administration for hospitals to reserve beds for use in a possible nuclear attack is a case in point.

hospitals has a long and venerable history in the United States. According to Stevens (1982), state funding of voluntary general hospitals prior to the depression was generally on a selective, ad hoc, individualized basis, often in response to specific requests from influential local groups. Government aid to hospitals at the local level, on the other hand, was determined by a combination of local political conditions, common sense, the strength of local interest groups, and the taxing structures of the respective states. This "distinctive American practice" as Goldwater (1909) termed it, that is, the appropriation of public funds for the support of hospitals managed by private benevolent corporations, is attributed by Stevens (1982) to the lack of distinction that has existed between "public and private" functions in the development of U.S. charitable institutions.

Federal Role

As indicated earlier, the federal role in health throughout much of U.S. history has tended to be a constrained one, limited to crisis intervention (Falk 1967a), the control and prevention of disease in public health. Typically, as Blumstein and Zubkoff (1973) have noted, federal intervention in the health area has been on an ad hoc basis without an overall plan, a formulation of objectives, or theoretical underpining. Moreover, in the absence of any specific formulation, national health policy in the United States has been more or less an amorphous set of health goals, derived by various means within the federal structure (Finch 1970), with little overall concordance or coordination.

Health Policy at the Federal Level

For the most part, the legislative initiatives in health at the federal level over the course of the past twenty years, as Battistella, Begun, and Buchanan remind us in Chapter 4, rested on a set of assumptions and presumptions, many of which were well meaning and seemed to embrace the conventional wisdom of the period but have proven to be overly optimistic, idealistic, or unfounded.

To a large extent, according to Brown (1978), federal health care policy in the United States has tended to embrace two essentially antithetical models or approaches that are "nurtured in tension." Thus, while "mainstream" equalizing programs continue to receive strong public support, they are challenged by a set of federal proposals based largely on "revisionist" premises concerning constraints on supply and demand for services. As a result, U.S. health care policy has tended to be discontinuous, inconsistent, and, at times, contradictory. Brown goes on to note that by avoiding hard choices and by reconciling in public policy such seemingly contradictory models, we have tended to institutionalize our ambivalence, while preserving the claims of equality of medical services on one hand and delimiting its scope on the other.

Role of the States

In contrast to their federal counterparts, whose influence over health stems in large measure from enormous fiscal power, the states have rather broad, comprehensive legal authority for a wide variety of programs. As a result, their role in health has taken a number of forms: (1) financial support for the care and treatment of the poor and chronically disabled, including the primary responsibility for the administration of the federal and state Medicaid program; (2) quality assurance and oversight of health care practitioners and facilities, for example, state licensure and regulation; (3) regulation of health care costs and insurance carriers;[25] (4) health personnel training, that is, states provide the major share of the cost for the training of health care professionals; and (5) authorization of local government health services (Clarke 1980).[26]

Similarly, although historically the power of the governor has been limited, a throwback to the colonists' distrust of the royal governor in the

---

[25]In 1981, 8 states had adopted programs to regulate hospital costs directly, 7 had enacted some type of comprehensive health insurance legislation, and 18 had sought tighter standards for the sale of Medigap health insurance policies to the elderly (Clarke 1980; Merritt 1981b).

[26]Local governments ultimately derive their powers from the states.

area of public taxation, the states' chief executive appears to exert considerable influence in determining health policy via the power of appointment. A recent review of the statutory authority governing public health decision making in the 50 states, for instance, (Gilbert et al. 1983; Gossert and Miller 1973) found the governor responsible for the appointment of about 91 percent of the 427 positions on the states' board of health. In 11 states, the members of the board sit at the pleasure of the governor. Moreover, turnover among state health officials has been reported as "brisk" with about 60 percent of them being replaced every 2 years (Association of State and Territorial Health Officials 1981).

State Expenditures for Health

State spending and responsibility in health have traditionally been directed toward broad public health activities, institutional care of the mentally ill, and the purchase of health care services for the economically disadvantaged. During the past 35 years, state spending in health and other human services has been increasingly shaped by federal prescriptions and initiatives, including a variety of apportionment formulas and project grants. As a matter of fact, a familiar characteristic of the U.S. federal system is that many of the programs that carry out national policies are created and operated by the states under rules established by federal legislation and regulations. Moreover, variable methods of federal funding related to purpose, budgetary limits, formulas, and duration impose similar variability on the states' application of funds to the counties (Kramer 1972; Davidson 1978).

Like their federal counterparts, state expenditures for health are provided through direct provision of services and indirect purchase of services and have been the subject of considerable political debate over the scope, cost, level of funding, and appropriateness of such expenditures. For all this costs money, and the funds may not be readily available in times of economic recession. Thus, while many states found themselves with expanding treasuries during the late 1960s and early 1970s, fueled by inflation and aided and abetted by increased federal revenue sharing and a thriving economy, in the face

of a serious economic downturn nationally, declining state revenues, reduced federal aid, rising costs, a heightened demand for health and welfare services, threatened taxpayer revolts, and bulging budget deficits,[27] they were forced to cut back greatly on their programs and allow more and more of the burden to fall back on their local counterparts, a pattern that may well be repeated in the 1990s (Sheler 1989).

The Impact of Federal Initiatives in Health on States and Localities

Finally, although the evidence on the extent of the impact of federal initiatives on state and local priorities in health is limited, the key to understanding the ways in which federal aid influences state health goals and programmatic activities appears to lie in the political environment of the state. A study of six states and four public health programs, for example (Buntz et al. 1978) found that although federal programs facilitate rather than inhibit the attainment of state health goals, federal influence tends to be secondary to that of the state's political environment. A federal program, they note, may elevate an issue to the states' active policy agenda but need not necessarily lead to formulation of a state policy or goals unless interests within the state are receptive. Moreover, the federal influence on state health policy appears to be both state and program specific, reinforcing changes supported at the state level and altering state goals at the margin. Such changes in state goals, however, are likely to occur only when the political environments of states are receptive to change. For although the federal government has the power to force states to pay attention to certain national goals, it cannot force them to shift their goals in any fundamental way nor to accept those goals as legitimate.

According to Lehman (1987), a major effect of the Reagan Administration's policies on state

---

[27]Unlike the federal government, states are prevented by law from operating with a budget deficit. In the first part of 1983, 40 states reportedly had experienced budget problems as a result of the recession, and, in the case of California, government was forced to issue scripts, that is, IOUs, to creditors until a mutually acceptable budget balancing bill could be worked out between California's governor and the legislature.

and local governments was the creation of a fiscal environment that forced state and local officials to rely more on their own—at times, inadequate—resources. This came about in several ways. First, federal aid as a percentage of total state-local outlays dropped from 25 percent in 1981 to around 19 percent in 1987, reversing a twenty-year trend from the 1950s to 1978. Second, in contrast to the practice under previous administrations, the federal government did not provide compensatory aid to states and localities hard hit by the economic downturn of the 1980s. As a result, many states created so-called rainy day funds to protect themselves should their state economies suffer a serious downturn. Third, the Reagan administration continued the traditional federal policy towards the poorest states, i.e, no special aids, forcing many to let programs formerly paid for by the federal government die. Finally, Reagan, like his predecessors, and with the help of Congress, increased the number of federally mandated but underfunded programs, requiring state and local governments to deliver more services in such areas as mental health and drug treatment, without additional funds to pay for them.

Public and Private Financing of Health Care in the United States

Although initial consideration of the adoption of some form of national health insurance in the United States occurred at about the same time as in Europe—at the turn of the century—and in reaction to similar forces—industrialization, urbanization, the demise of the extended family, and employment practices and policies that heightened the threat of work-related injuries and disease as well as unemployment—unlike Europe, the implementation of social security in the United States came through selected income maintenance programs and the preservation of the voluntary sector (Blanpain 1978).

Moreover, whereas in Europe, national health insurance was built on a universal consensus that health care is a right, such protection in the United States has essentially revolved around work-related insurance in the private sector, leaving government a gap-filling role and from 10 to 15 percent of the population without any such coverage. All of this led Brown (1989 p. 51) to observe that "in the United States, health care is a fringe benefit for most of the population, an entitlement qualified by categorical criteria for many, a matter of chance and charity for some."

Thus, the provision of third-party health insurance coverage in the United States developed primarily on a voluntary basis through Blue Cross-Blue Shield and the commercial insurance industry. The attendant mixture of approaches resulted in a complex pattern of health care financing in which (1) the employed are predominantly covered by voluntary insurance provided through contributions made by their employers and themselves; (2) the aged are insured through a combination of coverages financed out of Social Security tax revenues and voluntary insurance for physician and supplementary coverage; (3) the health care of the poor is covered through Medicaid via federal, state, and local revenues; and (4) special population groups such as veterans, merchant seamen, Indians, members of the armed forces, Congress, and the executive branch have coverage provided directly by the federal government (National Center for Health Services Research 1977).

According to Kramer (1972), private health insurance primarily has been a collection of payments mechanism that supports and reinforces existing patterns of health services. Government spending for health, on the other hand, has been largely confined to filling the gap in the private sector, that is, environmental protection, preventive services, communicable disease control, care for special groups, institutional care for the mentally and chronically ill, provision of medical care to the poor, and support for research and training. The high cost of public medical care programs, Kramer reminds us, owes its genesis to the unique division of risk taking and responsibility between the public and private sector that has thrust upon government the cost of caring for those segments of the population with the highest incidence of illness and greatest need for care, that is, the aged, poor, mentally ill, retarded, chronically ill, and disabled.

Finally, the use of fiscal stimuli through grants-in-aid, the commitment of major financing programs to retrospective reimbursement of costs on a fee-for-service basis, and reliance on peer review for quality assurance reflect a preference for the achievement of public objectives through strategies that offer inducements, persuasion, and positive rewards to providers for compliance rather than impose penalties or costs for failure to comply (National Center for Health Services 1977; Anderson 1968b). Such strategies, however, have been inherently expansive, tending to minimize the need for deliberative allocative choices by increasing the flow of resources into the health care system. Once costs rise and revenues become short, such choices no longer can be put off and questions of constraint and costs are raised.

Government Financing of Personnel Training: The Case of Medical Education

Before the enactment of the Health Professions Educational Assistance Act in 1963, the financing of graduate education in general and health professions in particular was traditionally within the purview of state government, students, and/or their families. The provision of direct financial aid from the federal government to medical schools in the 1960s and early 1970s to encourage biomedical research and expanded enrollments, bypassing the more traditional intergovernmental transfer approach to funding aid, has been depicted by Millman (1980) as "private federalism."

At the state level, medical education tends to be addressed in the context of higher education, rather than as part of health policy, and in response to state and local needs, rather than to those of the nation as a whole, whereas the opposite is true of federal endeavors. As the federal government has assumed an increasing role in the financial support of biomedical research and physician training—to the point where any given medical condition from prickly heat to cancer had its own congressional advocate for federal funding—an unduly large proportion of such support tended to be diverted from a focus on primary care to research and specialty training, distorting the teaching function of the educational institutions and perverting the long-standing reliance of public institutions on the largess of the state legislatures. So entwined had medical school financing become with the federal funding for research and training that the state

legislators and policy-makers ended up on the outside looking in (Rogatz et al. 1970; Bloom and Martin 1976). But if medical school dependence upon federal financial support had become manifest over a twenty-five-year period, there was a point beyond which medical faculties were unwilling to go. This was reached in the late 1970s when, in return for continued federal funding under the Health Professions Educational Assistance Act, 1976 (PL 94–484), Congress mandated that medical schools provide training for United States students studying abroad (US FMS). Following the lead of two private institutions, Yale and Northwestern, and one state, Indiana, U.S. medical schools, citing the abridgement of the right of educational institutions to determine their own admission policy, announced their refusal to go along with such a directive even if it cost them the price of federal support. In the face of such oppositions, Congress "blinked," and the requirement was withdrawn.

The heyday of federal funding of health personnel training, however, appears to have been reached. So active and effective were such efforts that by the end of the last decade, the nation found itself with potentially more physicians and hospital beds than it needed. As a result, beginning in the mid-1970s and escalating rapidly during the Reagan administration, federal goals have moved from a position: of fostering a larger supply of health professionals to reducing sharply tax-based support for this purpose, leaving health professional schools and their students caught in the squeeze of rising educational costs, declining federal support, and reduced state revenues (Lewin and Derzon 1981). Such action, however, may have the salutary effect of making medical schools and their faculties more responsive to state needs, and, as Lewin and Derzon (1981) note, this may be the case. In contrast to the ebb and flow of federal funding, for example, they found state support for health professions education has grown steadily, that is, at an average annual rate in excess of 10 percent for each profession, from 1974 to 1980, with most such funding directed toward public institutions.

Problem of Cost Versus Services in Government Programs

The amount of money that a nation spends for its health services, as Anderson and Newhauser

(1969) noted, tends to be a product primarily of a political process arrived at by implicit and explicit public policy decisions within the body politic. An equally appropriate maxim, however, is that whatever government giveth, it can taketh away. In other words, although public programs often initially are enacted on essentially altruistic grounds, for example, increased accessibility to health care services by removing financial barriers to care while defraying costs over a wide segment of the public, once this is done and the costs that originally were borne by patients, their families, and/or the private sector and are now assumed by government rise, there is a strong tendency on the part of the latter to cut back on its commitment by reducing coverage and increasing the amount paid by those who use the services.

Thus, as costs rise, the tendency is to cut back on the coverage especially if the constituency being served is not a very powerful or influential one, such as the poor, the socially and economically disadvantaged and, up to the 1960s, the elderly.[28] For as commendable and needy as service may be and as legitimate as government involvement is, the question ultimately gets down to a fundamental economic one: the cost of the service given the limited funds (however defined)available for it.

Therefore, beginning in the latter part of the 1960s and early 1970s, the federal government and the states, confronted by escalating costs and depleted resources, began to cut back on the Medicare and Medicaid programs. Thus, in contrast to when the dual programs were first enacted and the primary policy concern was increased access to health care services for more U.S. citizens, ostensibly the aged and economically disadvantaged, the programs were so successful that the budget soon became incapable of containing them. As a result, the policy has taken a 180-degree turn, going, in David Mechanic's (1986) terms, from one of advocacy to allocation, and greater restriction and control,

with adverse effects on access and quality of care, in many cases proving to be "penny cheap and pound foolish" (Roemer et al. 1975).

Case of Medicaid. This conflict between costs and services has been especially true of the Medicaid program, whose expenditures tend to be particularly susceptible to the forces of unemployment and inflation. For not only does the size of its clientele, that is, recipients of public assistance and "the medically indigent," vary with the level of unemployment, but the services it renders are purchased in the general medical marketplace and are susceptible to the impact of inflation. In addition, the negative effect of reduced tax receipts on state and local revenues as a result of a national economic recession tends to place both levels of government in a whipsaw as the demand for services on them rises because of heightened unemployment while their capacity to pay for them diminishes.

Not all states, however, experience the impact of the burden equally. Since the federal contribution to Medicaid expenditures depends on its per capita income relative to the national average 2 years earlier, the federal share is relatively insensitive to the distribution of the burden of the recession among the states as well as the mobility of welfare recipients between and within states (Davis 1974, 1975, 1976b).

At any rate, in the face of declining economic circumstances and reduced revenues, a substantial growth in the use of inpatient hospital, nursing home, and intermediate care facilities; a loss of general revenue-sharing monies; continued medical care price inflation; and state and local tax limitations, cutbacks in the program have generally taken a variety of forms, such as those listed below, as our admonition of costs versus services tends to prevail:[29]

---

[28]Historically, considered politically impotent by politicians and political scientists alike, the aged, stimulated by their success in the battle over Medicare, have become an extremely potent electoral force in U.S. political life, heightened by their proclivity to vote. In contrast with their younger counterparts, those under 25 years of age, elderly voters consistently exhibit higher rates of electoral participation (see Donahue and Tibbits 1962).

[29]In 1981, over half of the states reported significant budget problems with their Medicaid programs. In many cases, Medicaid was the most expensive item in the state's budget, consuming 10 to 15 percent of state general funds. Even more alarming to the states, however, was the fact that the program's costs were rising faster than state revenues. Some 21 states reported either increases in current copayments on some optional services or new copayment requirements on optional services. Almost half the states were considering significant changes in provider reimbursements ranging from decreasing or freezing payment levels for physicians to restructuring nursing home reimbursement formulas. Reduction or elimination of some group from further eligibility was proposed in 14 states (Merritt 1981).

1. Reductions in the levels of eligibility, usually by lowering the income ceiling thereby cutting down the number of potential recipients. In the case of the medically indigent, states had wide discretion in their determination of eligibility.

2. Placing limitations on the types and amount of services covered, that is, what and how much. This has generally taken the form of limitations on inpatient hospital services, that is, number of days per spell of illness and/or per year, cutbacks on optional services (other than those specifically mandated under the law), and reduction in services to the medically indigent.

3. Reductions in the amount of reimbursement; placement of ceilings on maximal allowable profit; suspension of payments to providers, that is, physicians, hospitals, and nursing homes, sometimes arbitrarily determined; and, after the services have been rendered, leaving the patients to pay out-of-pocket, if they could, or the provider to absorb the cost—all of which has created considerable bitterness between patients and providers, as well as providers and government. In fact, a major criticism levied at the program by physician and health care institutions has been its inadequate reimbursement and excessive red tape. This led many providers to opt out of the program—leaving recipient patients to fend for themselves, avoid care, rely on an increasingly limited number of overworked private practitioners who would see them or on the services of notorious "Medicaid mills," seek care from the hard-pressed public hospitals, or to make up the loss of income by excess visits, overuse of diagnostic lab work, and various forms of creative billing (Fever Chart 1976).

4. The establishment of requirements for prior authorization or approval before treatment could be rendered as well as restrictions on where services could be obtained.

5. The use of deductibles and copayment provisions in order to force recipients to share in the cost of the services by increasing their out-of-pocket expenses which in turn, it has been argued, not only discourages use but

helps offset or reduce the cost to government.[30]

6. Imposition of restrictions on the sources of care beneficiaries may go to those which afford the lowest cost to government, including the adoption of managed care arrangements.

Case of Medicare. The situation has been much the same with the federally run Medicare program as the government has sought to recoup or reduce its costs, while reneging on its promises. Thus, beginning with the Nixon and Ford and continuing under the Carter, Reagan and Bush administrations, attempts have been made to reduce the costs of the program by placing curbs on provider reimbursement while making the elderly assume more of the costs themselves by increasing the size of the deductible, the amount of copayment required, and the premium for Part B, Supplementary Physician Coverage (e.g., from an initial $3.00 per month in 1966 to $24.80 in 1988 and a projected $50.00 or more by mid-decade), culminating in a proposal by the Reagan administration in early 1983 that called for the imposition of "means test" on program beneficiaries.[31] Such provisions not

[30]Such political—economic rhetoric and, perhaps, conventional wisdom aside, experience with such cost-sharing measures in the private sector, at least as far as inpatient hospital care is concerned, has proven to be far less cost effective in reducing costs while often denying care for those most in need, delaying the need of more extensive services when such patients are ultimately admitted (*Blue Cross Perspectives* 1972). Moreover, such devices focus primarily on the patients rather than the physicians who, through both their gate-keeping and decision-making roles, constitute the primary generators of costs in the institution. The reluctance, on the other hand, of politicians and government officials to impose controls on health care providers is a function of the essentially private character of the U.S. health care system. Thus, drafters of the Medicare and Medicaid legislation were wary of placing onerous restrictions on providers lest they withhold their services or fail to participate in the programs, fearing a possible replication of Canada's experience with a physicians' boycott in Saskatchewan (Tollefson 1964). As a result, reliance was placed on the good faith of the medical profession and the provision of financial incentives to hospitals and third-party carriers for cooperation (Feingold 1966; Marmor 1970; Skidmore 1970).

[31]In contrast to the infamous requirement of a pauper's oath to determine eligibility under the old Kerr-Mills program in the early 1960s, which was considered to be particularly demeaning by the elderly, most of whom had lived through the depression and had taken pride in their independence and unwillingness to accept charity, the Reagan proposal sought to reduce

only are a perversion of the original intent of the Medicare legislation, that is, to relieve the elderly of the fear and heavy financial burden of the high cost of health and medical care while allowing them to retain their sense of dignity through the mechanism of social insurance, but these provisions operate in direct contradistinction to the recommendations of almost every government and nongovernment advisory group and study commission appointed to look at the program since its inception, including the 1971 and 1981 White House Conferences on Aging.

Such arguments aside, however, in the face of a growing budget deficit and rising health care costs, the movement came to full fruition with the passage of the catastrophic health insurance bill in 1988 which for the first time required that the cost of the program be borne by the recipients themselves through the imposition of a self-financing provision tied to a progressive tax structure, with income to be used as a determinant of the level of payment rather than as a basis of eligibility. But while perhaps justifiable on economic grounds, permitting an expansion of the Medicare Program and and an extension of benefits without an adverse effect on the federal budget, it evoked an immediate negative response from many of the nation's middle and upper income elderly who beseeched their elective representatives with demands to repeal the act, rescind its income-related payment features and return the benefits to entitlement status.

Finally, while all such cost-containment measures may well make public officials and their statistics look good,[32] they offer little solace to those who, in many cases through no fault of their own, are in need of care but are ineligible to receive it. Moreover, shifting the cost of such services to those who use them neither solves the problem nor removes the burden, but merely shifts it back to those least able to bear it.

Thus, given the central focus cost containment has come to assume in government health and social programs, the ultimate question the United States must come to grips with is how much deterrence because of cost is both tolerable and permissible and in what areas. Again, it is the constituency with the least political power—the poor and socially disadvantaged—who are the most likely to feel the brunt of such cuts.

A Case for a Federal Presence in Health and Health Care

The growth in the federal government's role in health and health care in the United States has not been without its problems and negative consequences, such as escalating costs, bureaucratic inflexibility, excessive regulation, red tape and paper work, arbitrary and, at times, conflicting public directives, inconsistent enforcement of rules and regulations, fraud and abuse, inadequate reimbursement schedules, arbitrary denial of claims, insensitivity to local needs, consumer and provider dissatisfaction, and charges that such efforts tend to promote dependence rather than work. The arguments for decentralizing such programs are all too familiar: The federal government has grown too large, intrusive, and paternalistic; it is too impersonal, distant, and unresponsive; state and local governments are closer to the people and more familiar with local needs and, therefore, more accessible and accountable to the public and better able to develop responsive programs than are federal agencies (Fein 1980).

Such problems and criticisms aside, the reason for a national endeavor in this area is not only that more funds are available and collectible at the federal level, but also and more importantly, there is an implied national commitment to action and resolution of the problem.[33] Illness and disease, for example, simply do not recognize jurisdictional boundaries and are nationwide in scope. Chronic disease, alcoholism and drug

---

the payment of benefits to the more affluent by placing an upper income limit on eligibility. The eventual result, however, would be the same, that is, the conversion of the program from an earned entitlement available to all to an income-based benefit program limited to just some.

[32]To some, the "cheapest program" of all is the one in which no expenditures are made even though the cost of doing nothing ultimately may be higher.

---

[33]Nevertheless, as Clarke and others have aptly observed, although federal health policy may constitute a national consensus to do something, the actual implementation of such policy is often dependent on the influence of the "political environment" of the states (Clarke 1981; Buntz, et al. 1978; Altenstetter and Bjorkman 1978).

abuse, hypertension and stroke are as much a threat to the suburban as the inner-city population. Moreover, worldwide transportation and communication systems make a disease anywhere a potential problem everywhere, as exemplified by the various versions of the Asian flu in the 1970s. Thus, although health and human service programs may well be more administratively amenable to state and local control, the latter's track record in this area has been anything but impressive.

While the states, with the prompting of the U.S. Supreme Court in the early 1960s, have tended to improve greatly the administrative and legislative structures that were the object of allegations of incompetence and insensitivity to the needs of the socially and economically disadvantaged just a generation ago, they still possess a number of inherent weaknesses that severely deter their ability to assume a more extensive role in the organization, financing, and delivery of health and human services. In addition to being unequal in financial ability, states differ widely in their needs for services and financial capacity to provide them. As a result, they are vulnerable to interstate competition as to which state can provide the lowest amount of services to the fewest numbers in order to offer or maintain the most attractive business tax climate. Although innovative and at times ahead of their national counterparts, state action tends to be piecemeal and lacking in uniformity. Moreover, state regulation of nursing homes, health insurance, pollution control, and so on, has often proved to be weak, episodic, and susceptible to industry capture. Finally, states tend to be parochial in their outlook and ready to pursue and preserve their own self-image in competition with other states in regard to population, industry, and the welfare burden; which leads to serious inequities in the assumption and delivery of services.

A similar situation exists at the local level. Often plagued by antiquated administrative structures, a lack of legal authority, insufficient financial resources, and a dearth of qualified personnel, local efforts frequently have been susceptible to petty conflicts of interests such as rural-urban or urban-suburban differences, racial and economic discrimination, and lack of uniformity in the provision of services or the requirements for eligibility. In some southern and rural counties, county welfare officials in the 1960s and 1970s waged deliberate campaigns to encourage families on relief to go to the more industrialized states or cities of the Northeast and Midwest where welfare payments were higher—even providing one-way tickets so as to reduce their own expenditures for welfare.

Many county officials, moreover, prefer local determination in deciding who should get benefits, regardless of the provisions of the law vis-à-vis eligibility. Some years ago (1968) at a joint meeting on legislative affairs put on by Minnesota's health and welfare departments, a county commissioner from one of the state's southern rural areas was heard to say how he liked to know who was on welfare and determine for himself whether they *really* belonged there and needed what they claimed. "You know, when you live out there, you kind of get to know who should and shouldn't be on the [welfare] rolls." Federal or state rules and regulations aside, his role, as he perceived it, was that of a self-proclaimed judge and jury.

Similarly, many county boards, in the face of angry taxpayers and disgruntled voters (the taxpayer's revolt), tend to be particularly tightfisted with regard to expenditures for such services, often with self-defeating results. Several years ago, for example, an orthopedic patient at the Kenny Rehabilitation Institute in the Twin Cities would have been able to return home and lead a fairly productive life if the county had agreed to purchase a wheelchair. The country refused to do so, however, on grounds that such an expenditure was a luxury, resulting in a medically unnecessary and prolonged high-cost hospital stay at the county's expense.

Finally, the heavy reliance of local government on the property tax makes the provision of such services extremely difficult. This is especially so in view of the regressive nature of the tax as well as the fact that those who tend to benefit the most from such services or use them disproportionately more are the very ones—the poor and the elderly—who are the hardest hit by the tax and most resistant to increases in it, even to pay for the very services they rely or depend on.

And so, given that many of our problems of health and health care are not restricted to or confined by city, county, township, or state lines and can effectively be resolved only on a broader geographic basis, we have tended to opt for a more global approach. As Anderson (1955) and others have noted, when problems tend to be national in scope, they call for national solutions. And over time, it has been the federal rather than constituent states who have had to act—sometimes alone, sometimes with the aid of the states, and sometimes in the aid of states. It has done so, moreover, consonant with the values and structure of the U.S. social, political, and economic system.

Conclusion

The growth in government's involvement in health has been an evolutionary one, a response to changes in times and circumstances. Over the past 40 years, there have been major shifts in the role and posture of the federal government in the organization, financing, and delivery of health care services and its relationship with the states in which the following have occurred:

1. The traditional federal role of sharing the cost of health care gradually has been expanded to include programs of care purchased by the government itself as well as the use of federal funding to initiate and develop new forms of delivery, for example, neighborhood health centers and health maintenance organizations (HMOs) (Penchansky and Axelson 1974).
2. An increased use of categorical and project grants in health found the federal government involved in the budget funding of local programs and bypassing local governments considered unresponsive to the needs of the poor (Penchansky and Axelson 1974).
3. The federal focus has shifted from encouraging the expansion of state programs to assuring their integrity and from concern over improving access to services to control over their costs with both patients and providers often caught in the middle.

The progression in such involvement has been a slow and steady one, a function of the nature of the nation's political process and social and economic systems. Incrementalism, rather than fundamental changes in the structure of the

health care delivery system, has been the hallmark of federal policies (Falik 1975). What has evolved then, as Anderson (1968a) has aptly observed, has been a partnership—sometimes rather tenuous and strained—between government (federal and state) and the voluntary system, working together, not as rivals but as partners—not necessarily equally or smoothly, but as partners nevertheless.

In light of the experience of the United States and other countries over the past half century or so with various government entreaties in health and health care, what lessons can be learned? The following are suggested for future consideration.

1. Reform of the health care system in the United States is likely to be incremental, a compromise involving the resolution of a number of competing interests.
2. All modern national health care systems, predicated as they are on sophisticated technology, are inherently costly (Anderson and Newhauser 1969).
3. All third-party coverage, whether private or public, such as Medicare and Medicaid, contributes to inflation (Davis 1974).
4. Open-ended reimbursement to providers on the basis of cost is inflationary, whereas unrealistic or picayune controls tend to be self-defeating, leading providers to opt out of the system and leaving recipients a limited range of choices of care.
5. There is a significant positive correlation between a country's national income per capita and the share of that income devoted to health care (Evans 1986, 587).
6. An open-ended system of health care financing invites uncontrolled expenditure growth. The provision of "a la carte" financing in which each service component, i.e., hospital, physician, nursing home and home health care, is purchased separately from the same or different providers, and in which each provider is then paid for each service, is inherently inflationary, since vendors have a financial incentive to maximize the use of their services and thereby increase their own revenues, regardless of budgetary constraints on individual pa-

tients or the overall health care system (Waters and Tierney 1984, 1251).

7. A conflict between cost and services is inherent in government programs.

8. Equality in financing is not sufficient to guarantee equal access to medical care (Davis 1974).

9. Utilitarianism, that is, "put people back to work" and "get them off the welfare rolls and onto the tax-paying rolls," rather than humanitarianism and altruism, is the underlying motive for the ultimate adoption of most government human services programs.

10. The maintenance of separate financing systems under a pluralistic system of health care financing leads to cost-shifting—with each source of payment, public and private, seeking to protect itself at the expense of others by shifting costs to someone else. Such cost shifting may be minimized and financial responsibility for care fixed and apportioned through the adoption of an all payors system (Waters and Tierney 1984).

11. Government efforts to reduce expenditures for health services programs by transferring their costs, without appropriate financial safeguards, to lesser levels of government or recipients of services does not effectively reduce the overall costs of the services but merely shifts the financial burden to those least able to bear it while depriving those most in need.

12. While rising costs appear to be independent of type of ownership, source of funding, method of payment or organization of delivery systems (Anderson 1976), the ability to control such costs is not. For not only do industrialized, western nations with the greatest degree of government funding and administration of health services have the most extensive population coverage and the lowest administrative costs, but those in which the central government plays a major role in financing health services via general central taxation tend to have the greatest success in controlling health care expenditures (Navarro 1985).

13. National programs require consideration of regional and local problems and needs.

14. Regional variations and the diversity and voluntary-private nature of the health care enterprise makes the imposition of national fee schedules, reimbursement formulas, and facility guidelines difficult, if not impossible, to achieve.

15. States vary in their fiscal capacity and political willingness to organize and underwrite care, with often those in greatest need, the least able, i.e., in terms of fiscal resources, and least willing to do so. The same may be said at the local level.

16. While well meaning and innovative, private charity may supplement and complement, but not substitute for, government programs. For not only are the needs too large and the resources too few, but the likelihood of their being reproducible on a large scale is questionable (Fein 1988).

17. Employment related benefit programs, unless subsidized by government directly or indirectly, e.g., via tax credits, are unlikely to attain universal coverage due to the inability or unwillingness of small employers (i.e., less than 100 employees) to offer such benefits because of uncertainty over those firms' fiscal stability and viability, significant start-up and potential termination costs associated with pension plans, and disproportionately high administrative costs.

18. Although any government system is likely ultimately to impose restrictions on the autonomy and prerogatives of providers, in a society such as the United States, where the private sector is dominant, such controls can neither be arbitrary nor capricious but should seek the cooperation of professional interests and the use of financial incentives and rewards.

19. Protection against the financial burden of health and medical care is impossible without the placement of a ceiling on the patient's financial responsibility. Unless the family is guaranteed that its share of the cost of care will not exceed some reasonable fraction of income, the goal of preventing or protecting against the financial

burden of health care services cannot be achieved (Davis 1974). But while what that level of income or ceiling is or should be is open to debate, it should be noted that artificial financial barriers or income cutoffs tend to be highly susceptible to the tyranny of inflation; that is, as dollar amounts soar, real value and purchasing power decline.

20. The use of administrative and regulatory conrols, such as Medicare's former requirement of a three-day hospital stay before a patient may be authorized to be admitted to a nursing home, second opinion requirements, inadequate reimbursement to providers, reduction of the tax deduction for health and medical expenditures, and elimination of deductibility for health insurance premiums, rather than civil or criminal penalties, tend to be misdirected, self-defeating, and ultimately ineffective.

21. Programs covering only poor people must be carefully designed so as to avoid adverse incentives and inequities in which some people receive substantial assistance and others equally in need or deserving, that is, the near or working poor, receive nothing or practically nothing.

22. Assumptions that the elderly are protected against the cost of longterm care by Medicare are ill-founded and in error. The only government-provided protection the elderly have against the cost of long-term chronic illness is Medicaid—a welfare program.

23. Government health care programs predicated on the virtues of competition and the free marketplace and a preferred single delivery system ignore the fact that one of the major sources for the high cost of hospital care in the United States has been the virtually unfettered, costly competition between health institutions for staff, equipment, and so on, which results in a duplication of services and minimizes the value of a diverse pluralistic system of delivery and the variable needs and demands of consumers as well as providers.

24. Despite claims to the contrary, there is no historical proof of the superiority of either government regulation or market competition in achieving optimal performance of the health care system (Schramm 1986).

25. Legislative intent may often be thwarted, if not obviated, by the Executive branch through the appointment of unsympathetic or even antithetic administrators, delay or failure to promulgate enabling regulations, issuance of contradictory orders, failure to spend or rescind appropriated funds, e.g., OSHA, Environmental Protection, the Super-Fund, Family Planning and Abortion, under the Nixon and Reagan administrations.

26. While governments are generally adept at creating and distributing benefits, whether in the form of direct subsidies or services, they are often woefully inexperienced and lack the political will to reduce or eliminate such benefits and services, particularly if they affect politically important constituencies eg. entitlement programs such as Medicare and Social Security and the aged (Rabe 1987, 40; Light 1985).

27. Whatever the future role of government in health in the United States is to be, it will be the product of a deliberative decision made in the political arena and will likely embrace the unique features of the nation's social, political, economic, and health care system.

That some of these may seem contradictory is a reflection of the complexity involved in such endeavors in meshing the needs of the disparate parts of a pluralistic society such as ours, predicated and reliant as it is on the private sector for the provision of health care services.

Health Politics and Political Science[34]

There has been considerable speculation—if not actual sharp intellectual debate—over the years among political scientists specializing in the study of the politics of health as to whether there is something analytically unique *from a political science perspective* about health politics

---

[34]This section was coauthored by Leonard Robins.

other than its subject matter. We would tend to concur with Falcone (1980–1981) that the politics of health is not *theoretically* different from the politics of other policy areas, such as defense, welfare, and education. In doing so, however, we wish to stress that insightful political understanding of various policy areas requires not simply general political insight coupled with specialized substantive expertise, but also requires that the specific political implications of the substantive issues in various policy areas be carefully analyzed and understood as well. Thus, there are aspects of health politics that, while individually not unique, need to be presented in overview form to help the reader understand developments in the various areas of health politics discussed by the contributors to this volume.

Health politics, for example, is usually conducted in a favorable political climate. The notion of health is a popular one: The public, for good or ill, remains convinced of the efficacy of medicine in promoting and maintaining it and believes that future medical advances guarantee less sickness and longer life. This results in strong popular support for spending money in all fields of health: public health, biomedical research, and especially medical care services. The only important constraint is, obviously, budgetary; that is, people do not want their taxes raised or the budgets unbalanced, which would hurt the economy.

Other fields are not so fortunate when they enter the political arena. Welfare spending, for example, is not merely opposed because of possible adverse tax or spending consequences, but there are important segments of the public that oppose welfare spending *in principle*. They believe that it is worse than doing nothing, because it encourages laziness and dependency on the part of those receiving welfare.

It would be a mistake, however, to assume that all health policies have the same type of politics. Lowi (1964), for example, describes three major patterns of political conflict that are said to be associated with three different types of public policies—distributive, regulative, and redistributive.[35] Elaborating on Lowi's typology, Marmor

(1973) has noted that considerable effort has been expended by political scientists in recent years trying to specify the ways by which different issues are raised, disputed, coped with, and, at times, "solved."

It is clear that actual policies are never as distinct as Lowi's typology suggests. All public programs redistribute resources, but most are not primarily attempts to do so. Likewise, all government programs depend on an ultimate capacity to regulate the conduct of citizens, but most do not make such regulation their prime object. And almost all government programs involve the distribution of goods and services among different groups, though the question of which county or which social class should receive them is not always salient.

Given the debate surrounding Lowi's and other's attempts to identify policy arenas and the politics associated with them precisely, no one typology can be presented as being definitive. It is important, however, to recognize that the politics of obtaining funds for biomedical research is not the same as the politics of drug regulation and that neither is the same as the politics of national health insurance.

That different policies may be associated with somewhat different political processes is now relatively commonly accepted by political scientists. Before the work of Lowi, however, this was not generally well recognized, and this failure constituted one of the major reasons for the relative inattention political scientists have given to health. Although the vast majority of political scientists were very concerned with public policy *as citizens*, they did not feel that public policy was their concern *as political scientists*. They felt that their proper concerns as political scientists were the political and governmental *processes* that produce policy—not public policy itself. Political scientists' interest in public policy dramatically heightened, however, when, to use research terminology, it came to be increasingly accepted that public policy was, in certain circumstances and for appropriate purposes, an important independent variable in the study of political phenomena as well as the traditional dependent variable to be explained.

---

[35]Distributive policies that parcel out public benefits to interested parties provoke a stable alliance of diverse groups that seek portions of the pork barrel. Regulative policies, which constrain the relationships among competing groups and persons, provide incentives for shifting coalitions, pluralistic competition, and the standard forms of compromise. Redistributive policies, on the other hand, reallocate benefits and burdens among broad socioeconomic population groups and foster polarized and enduring conflict in which large national pressure groups play central roles (Lowi 1964).

What remains unexplained, however, is why health has received relatively little attention in political science as a policy domain in comparison with other fields such as education, law enforcement, and defense. Despite both its practical implications and potential theoretical relevance, the politics of health has been a generally neglected area of inquiry among political scientists. In contrast with their counterparts in sociology and economics, the latter—with the notable exceptions of Garceau's (1941) classic pioneering exposition on the political life of the AMA, Eckstein's (1960) landmark analysis of pressure group politics in the British Medical Association, and Glaser's (1960) penetrating look at doctors and politics—have evidenced little interest or involvement in the study of health politics.

The minimal role political science has played in the development of the study of health politics appears to be the result of a variety of factors. Weller (1977), for example, has attributed the discipline's limited contributions to its relatively narrow focus, concentrating on too few groups or too narrow a set of issues, that is, the physician and the medical profession; an overreliance on case studies confined to either a particular group, issue, or piece of legislation; a disciplinary boundary problem over whose purview health policy belongs, that is, political science, public administration, social welfare, or something else; the complex nature of the health field; and the belief on the part of some political scientists, at least, that the pressure group approach exhausts the possibilities for the political analysis of health.

In addition, the general paucity of available research support for the study of such "politically sensitive" subject matter and the historically "private" character of health care delivery in the United States have come into play. In the case of the latter, although it can persuasively be argued that politics occurs in nearly all endeavors in life, political scientists have traditionally and still primarily do emphasize those political phenomena that essentially relate to government. Thus, whereas the vast bulk of taxing, spending, and employment in the fields of education, law enforcement, and defense have been in the public sector, that for health, at least up to the 1960s, was ostensibly a private endeavor and as such held little fascination or interest for political scientists.

With the passage of Medicare and Medicaid, along with the other legislative initiatives noted earlier, the degree of public involvement in health has changed dramatically. And although the politics of health may never become as important to political science as, for example, medical sociology is to sociology or health economics is to economics, there is reason to believe that it will assume a far greater research significance than it has had within the discipline as political scientists give increasing attention to the politics of public policy in general and that of health in particular.

But if political science has been found wanting as far as its contribution to the politics of health is concerned, the field of health and medical care has been equally remiss in its lack of knowledge and understanding of the political environments within which it operates. Ignorance or neglect of political factors in the organization, financing, and delivery of health care services omits a critical element in the potential resolution of health care problems. For, like it or not, as Kaufman (1966) has succinctly observed, health and health care have become so deeply enmeshed in the body politic that in order to achieve success within it, there is a need for health care administrators and practitioners to learn to understand it, adjust to it, and turn it to their advantage.

Toward this end, such developments as:

1. The formation of the Committee on Health Politics in the early 1970s by a group of interested faculty members in programs in hospital and health services administration.
2. The introduction of courses and seminars on the politics of health in programs in health administration, schools of public health, and nursing and other health professional schools.
3. The establishment of the *Journal of Health Politics, Policy, and Law.*
4. The publication of Marmor and Durham's (1982) penetrating exploration of the role and limits of the application of political science to the field of health and health care.
5. The publication of the recent special issue on "Health Care in the United States: Access, Costs, and Quality" in *PS* (Hoadley 1987).
6. The recognition by the Institute of Medicare's Committee for the Study of the Future of Public Health (1988) of the need to in-

crease that professions awareness, knowledge, understanding, and facility to use, and work within, the political arena.

These are all steps in the right direction and would seem to bode well for the future.

REFERENCES

Advisory Commission on Intergovernmental Relations. 1980. *The Federal Role in the Federal System: The Dynamics of Growth.* Washington, D.C.:Advisory Commission on Intergovernmental Relations.

Altenstetter, Christa and James Bjorkman. 1978. *State Health Politics and Impacts: The Politics of Implementation.* Washington, D.C. University Press of America.

Anderson, Odin W. 1966. Compulsory medical care insurance, 1910–1950. *Medicare: Policy and Politics.* Edited by Eugene Feingold, San Francisco:Chandler Publishing Co.

Anderson, Odin W. 1968a. *The Uneasy Equilibrium, Private and Public Financing of Health Services in the U.S. 1875–1965.* New Haven: College and University Press.

Anderson, Odin W. 1968b. Health Services in a Land of Plenty. William R. Ewald Jr., ed. *Environment and Policy: The Next Fifty Years.* Bloomington:Indiana University Press 59–102. Also *Health Administration Perspectives No. A7.* Chicago:University of Chicago Center for Health Administration Studies, Graduate School of Business.

Anderson, Odin W. 1976. All Health Care Systems Struggle Against Rising Cost. *Hospitals* 50:(October 1), 97–102.

Anderson, Odin W. and Duncan Newhauser. 1969. Rising costs are inherent in modern health care. *Hospitals* 43:February 16, 50–52.

Anderson, William A. 1955. *Nations and States: Rivals or Partners.* Minneapolis:University of Minnesota Press.

Association of State and Territorial Health Officials. 1981. *Internal Newsletter.* Washington, D.C.

Belknap, Ivan and John G. Steinle. 1963. *The Community and Its Hospitals: A Comparative Analysis.* Syracuse:Syracuse University Press.

Bellin, Lowell E. 1969. Medicaid in New York: Utopianism and bare knuckles public health. *American Journal of Public Health* 59:820–825.

Bellin, Lowell E. 1970. The New Left and American Public Health—Attempted Radicalization of the American Public Health Association Through Dialectic. *American Journal of Public Health* 60:973–981.

Blanpain, Jan with Luc Delesie and Herman Nys. 1978. *National Health Insurance and Health Resources. The European Experience.* Cambridge:Harvard University Press.

Bloom, Bernard S. and Samuel P. Martin. 1976. The role of the federal government in financing health and medical services, *Journal of Medical Education* 51:161–169.

Blue Cross Perspectives. 1972. 7, 3:1–5.

Blumstein, James W. and Michael Zubkoff. 1973. Perspectives on Government Policy in the Health Sector. *Milbank Memorial Fund Quarterly* 51:395–431.

Bowler, M. Kenneth. 1987. Changing politics of federal health insurance programs. *PS* 20:(Spring) 202–211.

Brandon, William. 1977. Politics, administration and conflict in neighborhood health center. *Journal of Health Politics, Policy and Law* 2:79–99.

Brown, Lawrence D. 1989. *Health Policy in the United States: Issues and Options.* Occasional paper 4, New York:Ford Foundation.

Brown, Lawrence D. 1978. The scope and limits of equality as a normative guide to federal health care policy. *Public Policy* 26:481–532. Also *Brookings Institution General Series Reprint No. 350.* Washington, D.C.:The Brookings Institution, 1977.

Buntz, C. Gregory, Theodore F. Macaluso and Jay Allen Azarow. 1978. Federal influence on state health policy. *Journal of Health Politics, Policy and Law* 3:71–78.

Burke, Edmund. 1968. Citizen participation strategies. *Journal of the American Institute of Planners* 34:287.

Carter, Richard. 1958. *The Doctor Business.* New York: Doubleday and Co.

Chapman, Carleton B. and John M. Talmadge. 1970. Historical and political background of federal health care legislation. *Law and Contemporary Problems* 35:334–347.

Chapman, Carleton B. and John M. Talmadge. 1971. The evolution of the right to health concept in the united states. *The Pharos* 34:(January) 30–51.

Clarke, Gary J. 1980. State government: Where the action is, *The Nation's Health* (April):16.

Clarke, Gary J. 1981. The role of the states in the delivery of health services. *American Journal of Public Health* 71:(Supplement) 59–69.

Congressional Quarterly. 1971. Background. *Congressional Quarterly Almanac.* Washington, D.C.:Congressional Quarterly, Inc 698:2-A.

Congressional Quarterly. 1972. Lobbies: The Washington lobby: A continuing struggle to influence government policy. *Congressional Quarterly Guide. Current American Government.* Washington, D.C.: Congressional Quarterly, Inc. 1–4.

Congressional Quarterly. 1981. Block grants: an old Republican idea. *Congressional Quarterly* (March 14):449.

Congressional Quarterly. 1982. Reconciliation's long-term consequences in question as Reagan signs massive bill. (Spring):55–60.

Congressional Quarterly. 1986. Budget office evolves into key policy maker. *Congressional Quarterly Almanac.* Washington, D.C.:Congressional Quarterly, Inc. (Spring):7–11.

Congressional Quarterly. 1988. Lobbies. The Washington lobby: A continuing effort to influence government policy. *Congressional Quarterly Almanac.* (Spring):83–87.

Crain, Robert L., Elihu Katz and Donald B. Rosenthal. 1968. *The Politics of Community Conflict—The Fluoridation Decision.* Indianapolis:Bobbs-Merrill Co.

Davidson, Stephen M. 1978. Variations in state Medicaid programs. *Journal of Health Politics, Policy and Law* 3:54–70.

Davis, Karen. 1976a. Medicaid payments and utilization of medical services by the poor. *Inquiry* 13:127–135.

Davis, Karen. 1976b. Achievements and problems of Medicaid. *Public Health Reports* 91:309–316. Also *Brookings Institution General Series Report* No. 318, 1977.

Davis, Karen. 1975a. Equal treatment and unequal benefits: The Medicare program. *Milbank, Memorial Fund Quarterly/Health and Society.* 53:449–488. Also *Brookings Institution General Series Report* No. 317, 1974.

Davis, Karen. 1975b. National health insurance. Benefits, Costs and Consequences. Washington, D.C.:The Brookings Institution.

Davis, Karen. 1974. Lessons of Medicare and Medicaid for National Health Insurance. *Brookings Institution General Series Report* No. 295. Washington, D.C.:The Brookings Institution.

Donahue, Wilma and Clark Tibbits, eds. 1962. *Politics of Age.* Ann Arbor:Division of Gerontology, University of Michigan. 36–47, 48–59, 63–74.

Downey, Gregg W. 1975. OMB, the secret of the secret agency. *Modern Health Care* (September):23–27.

Drew, Elizabeth. 1967. The health syndicate—Washington's noble conspirators. *Atlantic Monthly* 220 (December):75–82.

Eckstein, Harry. 1960. *Pressure Group Politics: The Case of the British Medical Association.* Palo Alto:Stanford University Press.

Elling, Ray H. and Ollie Lee. 1966. Formal connections of community leadership to health systems. *Milbank Memorial Fund Quarterly* 44 (Part 1, July):294–306.

Elling, Ray H. 1968. The shifting power structure in health. *Milbank Memorial Fund Quarterly* 46:119–144.

Evans, Robert G. 1986. Finding the Levers, Finding the Courage: Lessons from Cost Containment in North America. *Journal of Health Politics, Policy and Law* 11:587.

Fackelmann, Kathy A. 1988. AMA's identity crisis. *Medicine and Health Perspectives* (October) 24.

Falcone, David. 1980–81. Health policy analysis: Some reflections on the state of the art. *Policy Studies Journal* 9: (Special No. 1):188–197.

Falik, Marilyn. 1975. Health as a political issue: The national foci. *Health Politics, A Quarterly Bulletin* 5 (Summer):12–17.

Falk, Isidore S. 1967a. Medical care in a university teaching program for hospital administration. *Medical Care* 5:6.

Falk, Isidore S. 1967b. Medical care and social policy. *Medical Care in Transition,* PHS Publication No. 1128, 3:269–274.

Falk, Isidore S. 1977. National health insurance for the United States. *Public Health Reports* 92:399–406.

Falkson, Joseph. 1976. Minor skirmish in a monumental struggle: HEW's analysis of mental health services. *Policy Analysis* 2:93–119.

Federation of American Hospitals. 1979. Brookings and AEI: Testing grounds for 'shadow cabinets,' and policy ideas. *Review* 12:29–33.

Fein, Rashi. 1980. Social and economic attitudes shaping American health policy, *Milbank Memorial Fund Quarterly/Health and Society* 8:349–385.

Fein, Rashi. 1988. Toward adequate health care. Why we need national health insurance. *Dissent* (Winter):98–104.

Feingold, Eugene. 1966. *Medicare: Policy and Politics.* San Francisco:Chandler Publishing Co.

Feingold, Eugene. 1973. Citizen participation: A review of the issues. *The Citizenry and the Hospital* 1973 Duke Forum, Duke University, Durham: 8–16.

Feldstein, Paul J. 1977. *Health Associations and the Demand for Legislation: The Political Economy of Health Care.* Cambridge:Ballinger Publishing Co.

Felicetti, Daniel A. 1975. *Mental Health and Retardation Politics: The Mind Lobbies in Congress.* Lexington, MA.:Lexington Books.

Fever chart. 1976. *American Medical Association News,* March 22,

Filerman, Gary L. 1962. The legislative campaign for the passage of a medical care for the aged bill. Master's thesis, University of Minnesota.

Finch, Robert. 1970. Testimony given before the United States Congress Senate committee on government operations. *The Federal Role in Health* (The Ribicoff Report) Senate Report No. 809. Washington D.C.:U.S. Government Printing Office, 224.

Foltz, Anne-Marie. 1975. The development of ambiguous federal policy; Early and periodic screening diagnosis and treatment. (EPSDT). *Milbank Memorial Fund Quarterly/Health and Society* 53:35–64.

Foltz, Anne-Marie and Donna Brown. 1975. State response to federal policy: Children, EPSDT and the Medicaid muddle. *Medical Care* 13:630–642.

Forgotson, Edward H. 1967. 1965: The turning point in health law—1966 Reflections. *American Journal of Public Health* 57:934–946.

Friedman, Emily. 1977a. Medicaid: The promise path. *Hospitals* (August 16):51–56.

Friedman, Emily. 1977b. The problems and promises of Medicaid, *Hospitals* 51 (Series April–November).

Fuchs, Beth C. and John F. Hoadley. 1987. Reflections from inside the beltway: How Congress and the President Grapple with Health Policy, *PS* 20 (Spring):212–220.

Gallop, George. 1981. Gallup poll: Transfer of power to states favored. *Minneapolis Tribune* (October 18):26A.

Gamson, William A. 1961. Social science aspects of fluoridation, A Summary of Research. *Health Education Journal* 19:159–169.

Garceau, Oliver. 1941. *The Political Life of the American Medical Association.* Cambridge: Harvard University Press.

Gardner, John W., Wilbur J. Cohen and Ralph K. Huitt. 1967. *1965: Year of Legislative Achievements in Health, Education and Welfare, Health Education and Welfare Indicators* April 1965–February 1966 (Reprint). Washington, D.C.:U.S. Government Printing Office, iv.

Geiger, H. Jack. 1969. Community control—or community conflict? *NTRDA Bulletin* (November) Reprint.

Gilbert, Benjamin, Merry-K Moos and C. Arden Miller. 1983. State-level decision making for public health: The status of boards of health. *Journal of Public Health Policy* 3:51–63.

Ginsburg, Paul B. and Larry M. Manheim. 1973. Insurance, copayment and health services utilization: A critical review. *Journal of Economics of Business* 25:142–153.

Glaser, William A. 1960, Doctors and politics. *American Journal of Sociology* 66:230–245.

Goldwater, S.S. 1909. The appropriations of public funds for the partial support of voluntary hospitals in the United States and Canada. *Transactions of the American Hospital Association* 11:242–294.

Gordon, Geoffrey, B. 1969. The politics of community medical projects: A conflict analysis. *Medical Care* 7:973–981.

Gossert, Daniel J. and C. Arden Miller. 1973. State boards of health, their members and commit-

tments. *American Journal of Public Health* 63:486–493.

Grad, Frank. 1973. *Public Health Manual.* American Public Health Association, 3rd edition. Washington, D.C.

Grupenhoff, John T. 1982. The Congress: Turnover rates of members and staff who deal with medicine/health/biomedical research issues. *Communications* No. 1. Science and Health Communications Group.

Guttman, Daniel and Barry Wittner. 1976. *The Shadow Government: The Government's Multi-Billing Dollar Giveaway of its Decision-Making Powers to Private Management Consultants, Experts and Think Tanks.* New York:Pantheon Books.

Hanson, Royce. 1987. Lawmaker turnover rate hurts. *Minnesota Journal* (July 21):9.

Harris, Richard. 1967, *A Sacred Trust.* New York:New American Library.

Health Policy Advisory Center, Institute for Policy Studies. 1968. Medical empires: Who controls? *Health-PAC Bulletin* 1 (November–December):3–6.

Hixson, Joseph. 1976. *The Patchwork Mouse: Politics and Intrigue in the Campaign to Conquer Cancer.* New York:Anchor-Doubleday.

Hoadley, John F. 1987. Health care in the United States: Access, costs, and quality *PS* 20:197–241.

Hodgson, Godfrey. 1973. The politics of American health care. *The Atlantic* 232 (October):45–61.

Holloway, Robert G., Jay H. Artis and Walter E. Freeman. 1963. The participation patterns of 'economic influentials' and their control of a hospital board of trustees. *Journal of Health and Human Behavior* 4:88–98.

Hyde, David R. and Payson Wolff. 1954. The American Medical Association: Power, purpose and politics in organized medicine. *Yale Law Journal* 63:938–1022.

Institute of Medicine Committee for the Study of the Future of Public Health. 1988. *The Future of Public Health.* Washington, D.C.: 4, 5, 14, 119, 120, 154, 155.

Isman, Robert. 1981. Fluoridation: Strategies for success. *American Journal of Public Health* 71:717–721.

Jackson, Charles A. 1969. State laws on compulsory immunization in the United States. *Public Heath Reports* 84:787–794.

Kaufman, Herbert. 1966. The political ingredient of public health services: A neglected area of research. *Milbank Memorial Fund Quarterly* 44:13–34.

Kennedy, David M. 1981. The federal role: It's still necessary. *Minneapolis Star and Tribune:* (editorial page).

Kimball, Merit C. and Tinker Ready. 1988. Health industry donates more than $6 million to legislators, Survey Finds. *Health Week.* (October 31).

Kramer, C. 1972. Fragmented financing of health care. *Medical Care Review* 29:878–943.

Lee, Philip R. 1968. Role of the federal government in health and medical affairs. *New England Journal of Medicine* 279:1139–1147.

Lehman, Tom. 1987. "Federalism Under Reagan, Has Anything Changed?" *Humphrey Institute News,* 10:25–26.

Levine, Peter B. 1984. "An Overview of the State Role in the United States Health Scene," pp. 194–230, *Health Politics and Policy,* edited by Theodor J. Litman and Leonard S. Robins, New York: John Wiley and Sons (1st edition).

Lewin, Lawrence S. and Robert A. Derzon. 1981. "Health Professions Education: State Responsibilities Under the New Federalism," *Health Affairs,* 1:69–85.

Lewis, Charles. 1976a. Medicare, *A Right to Health. The Problem of Access to Primary Medical Care,* edited by Charles Lewis, Rashi Fein and David Mechanic 144–164. New York:John Wiley & Sons.

Lewis, Charles. 1976b. Medicaid. *A Right to Health. The Problem of Access to Primary Medical Care,* edited by Charles Lewis, Rashi Fein and David Mechanic 165–187. New York:John Wiley & Sons.

Lewis, Charles, Rashi Fein and David Mechanic, eds. 1976. *A Right to Health. The Problem of Access to Primary Medical Care.* New York: John Wiley & Sons.

Lewis, Ted, Jr. 1974. The incredible machine. How it grew. *Prism* (January) 17.

Light, Paul. 1985. *Artful Work: The Politics of Social Security Reform.* New York:Random House.

Litman, Theodor J. and Leonard Robins. 1971. Comparative analysis of health care systems: A sociopolitical approach. *Social Science and Medicine* 5:573–581.

Lowi, Theodore. 1964. American business, public policy, case studies, and political theory. *World Politics.* 16:677–715.

Marmor, Judd, Viola W. Bernard and Perry Ottenberg. 1960. Psychodynamics of group opposition to health programs. *American Journal of Orthopsychiatry* 30:330–345.

Marmor, Theodore R. 1973. *The Politics of Medicare.* London and Chicago: Aldine Publishing Co.

Marmor, Theodore R. and Andrew B. Dunham. 1982. Political science and health. *From Social Sciences Approaches to Health Services Research,* edited by Thomas Choi and Jay N. Greenberg 54–80. Ann Arbor:Health Administration Press.

Marshall, T.H. 1965. *Social Policy in the Twentieth Century.* Hutchinson University Library.

Means, James Howard. 1953. *Doctors, People and Government.* Boston: Little, Brown and Co.

Mechanic, David. 1986. *From Advocacy to Allocation: The Evolving American Health Care System.* New York:The Free Press.

Merritt, Richard. 1981a. State health reports. *The Nation's Health* (January):5.

Merritt, Richard. 1981b. *1981 IHPP Survey,* Washington, D.C.:Intergovernmental Health Policy Project.

Meyer, Harris. 1988a. AMPAC nixes incumbent challenges in independent congressional bids. *American Medical News* (October 21):2.

Meyer, Harris. 1988b. Congressional handicapping: AMPAC back 92 percent of winners. *American Medical News* (November 18):3.

Milbrath, Lester W. 1964. *The Washington Lobbyists.* Chicago:Rand McNally.

Millman, Michael L. 1980. *Politics and the Expanding Physician Supply.* Montclair, N.J.:Allanheld, Osmun and Co.

Mooney, Anne. 1977. The great society and health: Policies for narrowing the gaps in health status between the poor and the nonpoor. *Medical Care* 15:611–619.

Moore, Mary L. 1971. The role of hostility and militancy in indigenous community health groups. *American Journal of Public Health* 61:922–930.

Mustard, Harry S. 1945. *Government in Public Health.* Boston:Commonwealth Fund.

National Center for Health Services Research. 1977. *Controlling the Cost of Health Care.* NCHSR Policy Research Report 1970–1977, DHEW Pub. No. (HRA) 77–3182. Hyattsville, MD:National Center for Health Services Research.

The Nation's Health. 1978. Common cause: Money talks on health issues (December):5.

The Nation's Health. 1989a. New interest in a U.S. health plan but little movement in washington (February):1.

The Nation's Health. 1989b. Congress facing catastrophic fallout; other issues (February):5.

Navarro, Vicente. 1985. The public private mix in the funding and delivery of health services: An international survey. *American Journal of Public Health* 75:1318–1320.

Nexon, David. 1987. The politics of congressional health policy in the second half of the 1980s. *Medical Care Review* 44:65–88.

Penchansky, Roy and Elizabeth Axelson. 1974. Old values, new federalism, and program evaluation. *Medical Care* 12:893–905.

Pressman, Steven. 1984. Physicians' lobbying machine showing some signs of wear. *Congressional Quarterly Weekly Report* 42:77–81.

Rabe, Barry G. 1987. The Refederalization of American Health Care. *Medical Care Review* 44:37–63.

Rayack, Elton. 1967. The American Medical Association and the development of voluntary insurance. Parts 1, 2. *Social and Economic Administration* (April):3–25; (July):29–55.

Redman, Eric. 1974. *The Dance of Legislation.* New York:Simon & Schuster.

Richardson, Elliot L. 1973. The maze of social programs. *Washington Post and Times Herald* 96:3C, as reported in *Medical Care Review* 30:147.

Riska, Elaine and James A. Taylor. 1978. Consumer attitudes toward health policy and knowledge about health legislation. *Journal of Health Politics, Policy and Law* 3:112–123.

Roemer, Milton I. 1945. Government's role in medicine: A brief historical survey. *Bulletin of the History of Medicine* 18:145–168.

Roemer, Milton I., Carl E. Hopkins, Lockwood Carr and Foline Gartside. 1975. Copayments for ambulatory care: Penny-wise and pound foolish. *Medical Care* 13:457–466. (See also comments by Chen, pp. 958–63; Dyckman, pp. 968–69, and authors' response pp. 963–64.)

Roemer, Ruth. 1965. Water fluoridation: Public health responsibility and the democratic Process. *American Journal of Public Health* 55:1337–1348.

Rogatz, Peter, Robert Bruner and Donald Meyers. 1970. Health services working conference, Farleigh Dickinson University. Farleigh Dickinson University:19–46.

Rosen, George. 1974. *From Medical Police to Social Medicine.* New York: Science History Publications, Neale Watson.

Rubel, Eugene. 1975. Health planning act seen as declaration of federal role in health care system. *American Medical News* (July 7):14.

Russell, Louise B. and Carol S. Burke. 1978. The political economy of federal health programs in the United States: An historical review. *International Journal of Health Services* 8:55–77.

Schlesinger, Edward R. 1967. The Sheppard-Towner era—A prototype case study in federal-state relations. *American Journal of Public Health* 57:1034–1070.

Schmidt, Terry L. 1980. The congressional process. An overview of how a bill becomes a law. *Group Practice Journal* 29 (January):9–29.

Schramm, Carl J. 1986. Revisiting the competition/regulation debate in healthcare cost containment. *Inquiry* 23:236–242.

Shannon, Iris. 1989. President's column. *The Nation's Health* (March 12):2.

Sheler, Jeffery L. 1985. Congress proud protection of its independence. *U.S. News and World Report* (January 28):43–47.

Sheler, Jefferey L. 1989. States and cited facing the

budget music. *U.S. News and world Report* May 29:29.

Silver, George A. 1973. Participation and health resource allocation. *International Journal of Health Services* 3:117.

Sisk, Jane E., Peter McMenamin, Gloria Ruby and Ellen S. Smith. 1987. An analysis of methods to reform Medicare payment for physician services. *Inquiry* 24:36–47.

Skidmore, Max J. 1970. *Medicare and the American Rhetoric of Reconciliation.* Tuscaloosa: University of Alabama Press.

Somers, Anne R. 1966. Some basic determinants of medical care and health policy. An overview of trends and issues. *Health Services Research* 1:193–208.

Sorian, Richard. 1989. A Reagan retrospective. *Medicine and Health Perspectives.* (January 16).

Stavisky, Leonard P. 1981. State legislatures and the new federalism (book reviews). *Public Administration Review* 41:701.

Stenberg, Carl W. 1980. Federalism in transition: 1959–79, Advisory Commission on Intergovernmental Relations. *Intergovernmental Perspective* (Winter):4–9.

Stevens, Robert and Rosemary Stevens. 1974. *Welfare Medicine in America: A Case Study of Medicaid.* New York:Free Press.

Stevens, Rosemary and Robert Stevens. 1970. Medicaid: Anatomy of a dilemma. *Law and Contemporary Problems* 1970:348–425.

Stevens, Rosemary. 1982. A poor sort of memory: Voluntary hospitals and government before the depression. *Milbank Memorial Fund Quarterly/Health and Society* 60:551–584.

Straus, Robert. 1950. *Medical Care for Seaman: The Development of Public Medical Services in the United States.* New Haven:Yale University Press.

Straus, Robert. 1965. Social change and the rehabilitation concept. *Sociology and Rehabilitation,* edited by Marvin B. Sussman. Washington, D.C.:American Sociological Association, 1–34.

Thompson, Theodis. 1974. *The Politics of Pacification: The Case of Consumer Participation in Community Health Organizations.* Washington, D.C.:Howard University Institute for Urban Affairs and Research.

Tollefson, E.A. 1964. *Bitter Medicine. The Saskatchewan Medicare Feud.* Saskatoon, Saskatchewan: Modern Press.

United States Chamber of Commerce. 1965. 1965 Task Force on Economic Growth and Opportunity Report. *Poverty, the Sick, Disabled and Aged.* Washington, D.C.:U.S. Chamber of Commerce.

Waters, William J. and John T. Tierney. 1984. Hard

lessons learned. *New England Journal of Medicine* 311:1251–1252.

Weikel, M. Keith and Nancy A. Leamond. 1976. A decade of Medicaid. *Public Health Reports* 91:303–308.

Weller, G.R. 1977. From pressure group politics to medical-industrial complex. The development of approaches to the politics of health. *Journal of Health Politics, Policy and Law* 1:444–470.

Wing, Kenneth R. 1976. *The Law and the Public's Health.* St. Louis:C. V. Mosby.

Chapter 2

Health Services in the United States:

A Growth Enterprise for a Hundred Years

▓ Odin W. Anderson ▓

In the United States, growth in the health services enterprise is nothing new. It has been growing relative to gross national product (GNP) and the consumer price index (CPI) for a long time. The issue, however, has become the pace of the expenditure increase, particularly after 1960 when it accelerated. Personal health services have been embedded in an essentially private sector of the U.S. economy, a mixture of non-profit and profit enterprises with gradually increasing government support and intervention. The concept of intervention is used as part of political jargon. It implies that government intrudes in an otherwise normal situation. This mixture has changed over the years primarily with regard to sources of funding for day-to-day operations and to some degree capital financing. Social and political values in the United States have manifested a great deal of ambiguity as to the responsibilities of citizens as free-standing individuals for their own health care and the extent to which they enter into collective solutions through government. Collective solutions through community fund drives for hospital construction, for example, have had a long history and easy acceptance. But collective solutions, even through some form of private health insurance, have been adopted cautiously. Early acceptance of life and fire insurance, predictable contingencies, were not regarded as applicable to illnesses and their costs until the 1930s. In general, insurance was considered a normal and prudent means for Americans to protect their own solvency. Medical care for the poor, on the other hand, was regarded as a responsibility of the *noblesse oblige* of the physician and the charitable tradition of the hospital, buttressed in part by local government funding and the compassion of philanthropic organizations.

Development of the United States Personal Health Services System

It may be helpful to present briefly the major stages of development of the personal health services system in the United States, including a brief mention of public health and mental hospitals, which preceded and then paralleled the growth of personal health services. The development of personal health services in the United States can be divided into three fairly distinct periods, each with its own characteristics, revealing the evolution of an exceedingly complex and expensive enterprise. These periods are (1) the development of the health services organizational structure, physical facilities, and personnel infrastructure and methods of paying for the services before health insurance during the years 1875 to 1930; (2) the emergence of voluntary health insurance as a means for people to pay for the costs of health services as these became increasingly costly during the years 1930 to 1965; and (3) the application of constraints on the health services in order to manage and direct the pace of rising expenditures and assure greater equality of access and more equitable distribution of facilities and personnel, which began in 1965 and will continue indefinitely.[1]

The Period 1875–1930

It took over fifty years for the modern personal health services delivery system to evolve from a general-practice-centered to a specialty- and hospital-centered enterprise. In 1875, physicians and, to some extent, pharmacists were the sole dispensers of professionally recognized health services, two professions with long and prestigious traditions. On the periphery were recognized and unrecognized midwives who, by the turn of the century, were beginning to be replaced by physicians. A great deal of reliance was placed on home medication. The general hospital as it is known today was nonexistent. The poorhouses and almshouses were institutions for taking care of the destitute and the destitute ill who had no families to which to turn. Illnesses were treated mainly in patients' homes and physicians' offices. Physicians and pharmacists were, as they still are, largely private entrepreneurs presumably working within a code of eth-

---

[1]These stages have been presented in detail in (Anderson 1985). In this chapter the last stage is brought up-to-date since 1980.

ics, standards, and services not strictly of a profit-making enterprise but undoubtedly influenced by the laissez-faire atmosphere that characterized the United States in the latter nineteenth-century. There were then as many physicians in relation to the population as there are now. They made a living by treating patients for fees and received very little income from government and philanthropic sources. No other country has been able to support as many physicians from private fee-for-service patients as has the United States. The same was true for pharmacists who eventually established the familiar corner drug store because income from prescriptions alone was not sufficient. There were too many pharmacists because physicians frequently did their own dispensing from the relatively simple materia medica of the period. Private practice and fee-for-service became firmly embedded in the American medical practice tradition.

Two specific medical-technical discoveries sparked the creation of the modern hospital system—antisepsis and anesthesia. Antisepsis made surgery safe from infections, and anesthesia made it relatively painless. Since most surgery had to be performed in a hospital setting, surgery was the medical specialty that initiated growth of the modern hospital. Hospital treatment of medical patients followed in some volume by the turn of the century. (Births in the hospital, however, did not grow to any great volume until the later 1920s.) All this meant, of course, that the health care industry was needing more and more money compared to other goods and services and the gross national product. New money was needed for capital financing of hospitals and for the great increase in surgical procedures. By 1875, surgical procedures had become highly developed in the charity hospitals of the great cities of Europe and on the East Coast of the United States by trial and error on charity patients who were the sole source of "clinical material." But with the advent of anesthesia and antisepsis, the middle and upper classes, who would not have used the historically famous hospitals began to seek the services of surgeons who, in turn, sought hospital admitting privileges. By 1900 there were 4000 general hospitals in the United States, compared to only a few score in 1875.

The hospitals were established mostly by voluntary community boards and church bodies. The latter had a long history of caring for the sick poor, and this tradition was transformed into the modern general hospital. The capital funds came from the multi-millionaires and the many lesser millionaires who came forth with the tremendous industrial development following the Civil War. These new millionaires were essentially Calvinists who believed that their material rewards for hard work and prudence should be used in part for the good of the community. A fortuitous and appropriate object of their *noblesse oblige* was the emerging medical-technical infrastructure. Only a small minority of general hospitals was built by the municipalities for the poor. The voluntary hospitals, through their charitable and nonprofit charters, were obliged to provide care for the poor who sought help, but by and large they constituted a minority of the patients. The burgeoning U.S. economy enabled the hospitals to obtain capital funds from philanthropy and daily operating funds from pay patients. The physician, particularly those who expected to be surgeons, made deals with the hospitals to admit their private patients who paid both the hospital charges and the surgeon's fees. In turn, the surgeons were provided a free workshop in which they provided free care for the poor, an ideal symbiotic arrangement for both hospitals and surgeons.

The United States has had a long tradition of voluntary self-help on a community level, and the voluntary hospitals have been a prime example of this tradition. The family nurturance functions found expression in the voluntary hospital when the home became unequal to the technical demands and setting of increasingly high technology medicine.

The hospitals were thus able to survive and prosper (i.e., with respectable deficits) by serving the large and growing middle class for a fee. Approximately two-thirds of the hospital income came from fees paid by private patients, and one-third came from philanthropy, public funds, and other charities for the poor. It is significant that the general hospitals in the United States were the only hospitals in any country that could survive on income from private patients. Consequently, this country was able to mount a personal health delivery system for private patients, and the poor became a residual of this system. Just the opposite was true in Europe where the paying patients were a residual.

By the turn of the century, the self-supporting element of the U.S. population was at times finding it difficult to pay for hospital care. As a spokesman for the American Hospital Association observed, the poor got free care, the rich could afford it, but the cost of hospital care was getting out of the reach of the Third Estate, the broad middle-income class. The political answer surfaced in sixteen states between 1916 and 1920 when an attempt was made to pass legislation for some form of compulsory health insurance for workers. A model bill was formulated by the American Association for Labor Legislation (AALL) made up of social reformers from the ranks of academic economists, social workers, sociologists, and a few sympathetic physicians. The American Medical Association (AMA) also set up a study commission to investigate the problem of high costs of health services.

But nothing came of it. There was no real grass roots political support. The broad middle-income groups were not sufficiently aroused. The trade unions were indifferent and, in fact, Samuel Gompers, the head of the American Federation of Labor (AFL), was actively hostile. Moreover, labor distrusted government for its persistent injunctions against strikes. Then World War I intervened, and it was discovered that compulsory health insurance was invented in Germany in 1883 under Bismarck, thus discrediting it for the United States. The AMA and the drug and insurance companies went on the offensive with tremendous propagandistic fanfare and won easily because the proponents had no political base. Thus, it was not until the 1930s that the Third Estate, that is, the middle class, found some relief from the high cost of health care through the establishment of voluntary health insurance plans sponsored by the hospitals and medical societies.

Dentists paralleled physicians as private entrepreneurs earning their living from fees from private patients. Since the public perceptions of dental health were then rather primitive, the services of dentists were hardly in great demand. Dentists also benefited greatly from the appearance of anesthesia and antisepsis. In fact, a dentist was the first health professional to use ether for extractions, thus ushering in anesthesiology.

The source of health personnel—physicians, dentists, and nurses—was multifold. During the nineteenth century most of the physicians came from apprenticeship arrangements with practicing physicians and so-called diploma mills established by practicing physicians to train many students at a time in rather primitive arrangements. Later, private and public universities established medical schools related to the basic sciences. Dentists went through a similar proprietary educational period, and eventually dental schools became established in universities. Nurses, on the other hand, were trained by hospitals that, in return, obtained an inexpensive supply of labor. Eventually, as medical science advanced, other types of health personnel, such as laboratory technicians, began to appear.

All this took money, which became available with the growth of the economy as the surplus among other priorities poured into personal health services in increasing volume, as it has to this day. Personal health services were a wanted service and, up to the 1930s, the people of the United States bought it without help of government or private insurance. By the 1930s the personal health services infrastructure was in place as we know it today: voluntary hospitals, privately practicing physicians and dentists, and private pharmacies. But many changes were to take place later external to this structure, chiefly sources of funding, as well as planning and regulation, and competition.

Public health services and mental hospitals, have not been a wanted service in the same sense as those of a more personal or individual nature. They have evolved for a variety of other reasons. Before 1875, cities and counties began to establish health departments when their water supplies became contaminated from the effluents filling up in cities resulting in sporadic cholera epidemics. Later, when communicable diseases in children could be controlled through immunization and pasteurization, health departments took on an additional function based on bacteriology and epidemiology. Public health nursing for mothers and infants emerged with the addition of public health training to the education of registered nurses. Public health, however, separated itself early from the private practice of medicine. Although public health officers were usually required to be physicians, they did not practice medicine. They were administrators and dealt with groups, while clinicians dealt with individuals.

The building of mental hospitals—usually out of the cities and in the country—began before the development of personal health services. They were, and continue to be more or less separate from personal health services. Mental hospitals are largely publicly owned and operated. Like public health departments, they are not a wanted service, as revealed in the amount of their funding from taxes in relation to the magnitude of the problem. Personal health services through sheer demand and popularity corner the great portion of available funding. This was the state of affairs at the end of the period 1875–1930, and it continues today.

In contrast with the above, the prominence of the voluntary hospital system was determined by hospital owners, the medical profession, and philanthropy. Government, except by licensure and standards, did nothing to direct the system. The general public presumably approved the structure to date because they used and paid for the system in increasing numbers. The government provided an indirect source of operating subsidy, however, by permitting the hospitals to be tax-exempt enterprises. In addition, capital gifts to hospitals were tax-exempt and interest free. Thus emerged the mixed health services economy, a reflection of the mixed nature of the U.S. economy as a whole.

And so, stimulated by the enormous dynamics of medical science, technology, and money, the acute disease oriented personal health services system in the 1930s was poised for an even more dynamic expansion on top of the one that emerged since 1875. Public health departments and mental hospitals, on the other hand, barely held their own.

The Period 1930–1965

Whereas the period from 1875 to 1930 witnessed the development of the health service infrastructure, the period from 1930 to 1965 was mainly characterized by the emergence of the third party to pay for the day-to-day operating expenses of this imposing edifice.

In the early 1930s, consumer incomes fell drastically, causing hospital admission rates and payments from private patients to drop as well. Both hospitals and the Third Estate, as well as the poor, became hard pressed. The Great Depression was upon the United States. The 1930s saw the start of the hospital-sponsored prepayment plans, eventually known as Blue Cross. Although such plans would have undoubtedly come about without the Great Depression, their development was likely hastened by it. Hospital stays had become relatively costly and lent themselves to the application of the insurance principle. A relatively predictable number of people would incur hospital expenses. Concurrently and separately, because the hospitals and physician services were two separate interests and enterprises, prepayment plans for physician services in the hospital, mainly surgery, began to appear in the latter 1930s as well. These plans were sponsored by state medical societies and later became known as Blue Shield plans. Again, surgical care, which was relatively costly, lent itself to the insurance principle.

Government continued its health services for the poor through the states, and eventually a shared program between the federal government and the states emerged. During the early formulation of the Social Security Act in 1935, health insurance was considered but not included. The architects of the act who were interested in old age pensions and unemployment compensation feared that health insurance would be so controversial as to jeopardize the income maintenance intent of the act. Health care reformers pressed for the inclusion of health insurance, but when this became known, the AMA raised such a storm that it was not included in the bill that finally went to the Congress. As was the case from 1916 to 1920, there was no adequate grass roots support for national health insurance, and the AMA once again had an easy victory.

During the 1940s and into World War II, private insurance companies discovered on the basis of the experience of the Blue Cross and Blue Shield plans that hospital care and surgery were insurable and their costs could be predicted. Congress gave the voluntary plans a shot in the arm by decreeing during the wartime control on wages that health insurance—and pensions—were fringe benefits that need not be regarded as in-creases in wages. This was an example of government encouragement of the private sector, since the portion paid by the employers was tax exempt as a business expense, in other words an indirect public subsidy. Further, signing up for fringe benefits on the part of employees became a condition of employment, an acceptable form of compulsion, whereas direct compulsion in a government program was regarded as interfering with individual freedom. Thus, voluntary health insurance received a tremendous stimulus as employers began increasingly to assume a greater share of the premiums and health insurance became part of collective bargaining. In the meantime, bills on national health insurance were moved to the back burner of the congressional kitchen stove from 1937 to 1952, the year Truman (a strong supporter of government health care) ended his presidency. The failure to enact national health insurance was a great disappointment to him.

Under the conditions described, the Blue Cross and Blue Shield plans and private insurance companies were spectacularly successful in enrolling employee groups in the major industries, so that by 1952 over one-half of the U.S. population was covered by some form of health insurance, mainly hospital care and physician services in the hospital. With the election of President Eisenhower, the first Republican president since 1932, the venomous controversy over voluntary versus government health insurance subsided only to reemerge a few years later in the form of health insurance for the aged. For the rest of the population, voluntary health insurance plans were left with a clear field to demonstrate that they could solve the public's problems.

The salient point in this third-party development was that the existing infrastructure of health services that had emerged since 1875 and had stabilized by 1930 was taken as a given and that the voluntary insurance agencies and the government were concerned mainly with paying its charges. In the case of hospitals, the concept was charges or costs. Physicians were paid by voluntary health insurance by a generously negotiated fee schedule with Blue Shield plans and no negotiations at all with private insurance companies, because there were no contracts with them. In retrospect, these reimbursement methods seem administratively irresponsible. but for people who lived through those times, money flowed freely in a rapidly expanding economy. Further, the public was exhorted to "see your doctor early." Visits to physicians and admissions to hospitals increased dramatically from the latter 1930s to the 1960s. For example, hospitals admissions increased from 90 per 1000 population per year to 145; the proportion of the population who saw a physician in one year increased from 39 to 65 percent. The supply of hospital beds and physicians increased but less in relation to the demand. The physician became increasingly busy and prosperous. The hospital occupancy increased.

To add to the stock of hospitals and beds, particularly in rural areas, Congress in 1946 passed the Hospital Construction Act (Hill-Burton) supported by a cross section of interests such as the American Hospital Association, the American Medical Association, and labor organizations, ordinarily in conflict over government health insurance. This act was designed as a one-shot grant to hospitals—public and voluntary—for start-up costs that were to be matched by the hospitals. For the first time, each state took an inventory of its hospital supply, and the grants were made to hospitals within the framework of a loosely knit plan. The act supplied around 25 percent of the capital expenditures for hospitals that, in turn, generated a considerable sum of money from private and public services, but mainly private.

The main object of the act was to buttress the voluntary hospital, with the public hospital being a relatively minor partner and regarded as spillover from the mainstream of the hospital system. The old sources of capital funds from philanthropy and community fund drives were drying up. Thus, the act came at a very opportune time and provides another example of government support being condoned to assist the private nonprofit sector. The voluntary hospital is obviously an integral part of U.S. local community life, mixing the private and public sectors.

By the early 1950s, an era of expansion had been assured, with funding for the day-to-day operation of the hospital and physicians' services provided essentially from private sources and that for the supply of hospital beds, physicians, and other personnel from public and private sources. The general economy and the health

services economy benefitting from the affluence being created was also in full swing. The existing health services infrastructure continued to be accepted as a given. Within the relatively private and nonprofit nature of the U.S. health services economy, however, there was a development that concerned itself directly with restructuring the delivery of physicians' services and, indirectly, hospital care. This was the emergence of group practice prepayment plans that attempted to replace the solo practice and fee-for-service type of medical delivery by engaging a range of specialists on a salary, providing a full range of physician services from curative to preventive, and serving a known population. The Kaiser Permanente plans were established in the West and the Health Insurance Plan of Greater New York (HIP) in the East. In cities such as Washington, D.C., Seattle, St. Louis, and Minneapolis-St. Paul, similar programs were established more or less on a consumer-cooperative basis. Initially, the opposition on the part of the medical profession to these new arrangements was fierce. Gradually, however, such programs began to take their place in the spectrum of health services delivery types and, in some areas, became regarded as options in labor-management negotiations for health services fringe benefits. Their influence, however, appeared to be out of proportion to their numbers—involving about 4 percent of the population—nevertheless, they soon became reference points for quality health services at a "reasonable" price. It seems that only in the U.S. context, with the organization of private medical group practice giants such as Mayo, Lahey, Crile, and Ochsner plus many lesser ones, was the diversity of delivery types possible. Physicians in the United States have an entrepreneurial propensity with ability to raise capital unlike any other country. The private group practice concept, which lived on fees, undoubtedly inspired the group practice prepayment concept that lived on premiums divided among physicians for salaries.

The proponents of national health insurance, having failed in their efforts from the 1930s to the early 1950s, began to look for another approach, and they found it in the aged. Although voluntary health insurance was doing a reasonably adequate job for the mainstream employed segment of the population—at least enough to dampen agitation for universal health insurance—the aged became a burden on the voluntary health insurance and the broad middle-income segment of the population. Again the Third Estate made itself felt.

Toward the end of the period from 1930 to 1965, the private engine of finance was aided and abetted by the public engine of finance with the passage of Medicare for the aged and Medicaid for the poor in 1965. Medicare was a federal program, and Medicaid was a shared federal-state program, as it still is. Medicare took the costs of the care of the aged off the backs of voluntary health insurance and families with ailing elderly relatives. Medicaid assuaged the national conscience regarding the poor and eased the pressure on the shaky revenue structure of the states. The states, however, still had to raise more money to match the federal portion. By then, private and nonprofit insurance agencies were supplying 42 percent of the charges of day-to-day operations of the hospitals and 30 percent of physicians' services, and government was paying for 38 percent of the hospital charges and 6 percent of the physicians services, mainly surgery. The stage was set for spectacular increase in both price and use. There were no built-in controls on cost. The health services enterprise had become accustomed to being paid what it asked, and the funding sources did not demur either. From 1950 to 1965, expenditures as a percent of gross national product rose from 4.6 to 5.9. Expenditures per capita for all services rose from $78 to $198 without accounting for inflation, which was quite moderate during that period. The private insurance agencies and the government teamed up, as it were, to assure a health service where cost would be of no consequence.

Concurrently, the proportion of people 65 years of age and over was increasing, particularly those 75 years and older. Ineluctably associated with aging are chronic illness and disability and increasing helplessness, overtaxing family financial resources for their elderly. By the 1950s, the expenditure for nursing homes had become a visible portion of the national medical dollar. Only a small portion of this cost, however, could be afforded by direct-pay patients. Public medical assistance for the indigent in nursing homes became a prime source for funding day-to-day operations, which was later buttressed greatly by the Medicaid Act of 1965. True to the U.S. tradition, the market for nursing homes was met largely by the private sector, both profit and nonprofit, with standards set by the states along with the federal Medicaid and Medicare programs. Since the government was incapable or unwilling to supply nursing home beds in sufficient quantity to meet the demand and need, it bought services from the private sector. As with general hospitals, government paid most of what the nursing homes were charging in an affluent economy. Resistance, however, began to appear in the third and last period of development.

The Period From 1965 Onward

It was not until the latter 1960s that there began to be general concern by the big buyers of services—government, employers, and labor unions, as well as insurance and prepayment agencies—with the rising expenditure for personal health services, usually referred to as escalating or spiraling costs. Particularly alarming was the pace of the increase, with costs rising faster than those for the economy as a whole as reflected in the consumer price index. The general public was mainly interested in keeping reimbursements to providers and insurance premiums low. Hospital expenditures were rising at the dizzying pace of 15 percent annually. Expenditures for physicians' services were close behind. Providers said the increase in expenditures was justified in large part because of improved services and increased use as well as rising labor costs in a labor-intensive enterprise. While no one knew what was an appropriate level of expenditures, there seemed to be general agreement that the contemporary level of expenditures was too high. The theories of costs and expenditures were as primitive as this level of thinking. It should be noted that the phenomenon of rising costs of health services is not peculiar to the comparatively open and pluralistic U.S. system. The same phenomenon appears in all industrialized countries regardless of funding sources, ownership, and organizational structures. Personal health services are very popular everywhere. In the United States, health services exploded with no obvious potential checks, at the time, other than what premiums and taxes would bear. Systems abroad also exploded, but they were a part of implicit, if not explicit, political decisions. Budget caps were at least potentially possible given the political will.

This period was thus characterized by an intense concern with how to manage the health service enterprise so that buyers would know what they are buying and providers would know what they are selling. The wide-open era of simply paying what the providers asked was seriously questioned. The payment mechanism was to be used to manage the system rather than act as a mere paying agency. Three methods to do so were to emerge, largely in the following order: monitoring of physician decision making in hospitals, control of hospital beds, and control of hospital reimbursement rates.

Attempts at rationalization of personal health services were expressed mainly in the group practice prepayment plans described previously, but they were not simply a means of saving money but one of providing high-quality and comprehensive services efficiently and conveniently. It seemed that saving money was a secondary, although acknowledged, consideration. Likewise, the scores of hospital planning councils that were established in the major cities and sponsored by local hospitals and funded in large part by the Department of Health, Education and Welfare (now the Department of Health and Human Services) were aimed less at saving money as much as at systematizing hospital relationships and cooperation on a local level. Gross duplication of services and equipment, such as cobalt bombs across the street from each other or maternity beds in all hospitals, in the face of a declining birth rate were the objects of attention and interhospital discussions. The council concept was intended to serve as an information clearinghouse on the hospital situation in local areas, the presumption being that the hospitals would recognize their mutual self-interest and survival. These councils may have had other effects, but evidence showed that the reduction in the duplication of services or stabilization of the bed supply was not among them.

The seeming lack of success of the hospital council concept led to establishment of the federal Comprehensive Health Planning (CHP) program that incorporated many of the hospital planning councils as agents of the state and was directed at facility planning. A concurrent federal endeavor, also through the states, was the Regional Medical Program (RMP) that aimed at the delivery of services for heart disease, cancer, stroke, and related diseases. It attempted to relate practicing physicians to medical schools and major medical centers whereby they could benefit from the latest knowledge concerning these diseases and refer patients more rapidly. Saving money was not a primary concern; rather, it was hoped that physicians' services might be better integrated and improve quality. Again, both CHP and RMP failed to accomplish the hardly explicit objectives set for the programs.

In the meantime, expenditures increased apace; the internal and external dynamics of this tremendous growth enterprise was indeed awesome. Two prestigious government commissions, one on hospital effectiveness (1968) followed by one on Medicaid or medical care for the poor (1970) were appointed, with the vague charge to consider the entire delivery structure and its problems. The tone in both reports was confusion and frustration, as well there might be. They were ambiguous toward planning and distressed by the prospect of further government intervention, although helpless to suggest anything else. The Medicaid report, however, did begin to refer to competition between delivery options as a means of containing rising expenditures.

More specific attempts at containing expenditures, however, were expressed in the Medicare Act and also applied to Medicaid. In the Medicare Act there was mandated by law the creation of utilization review of physicians' decisions as to length of stay in hospitals, that is, direct monitoring of professional decision making. From the medical profession's viewpoint this was a radical step.

At the state level, legislature after legislature began to pass laws calling for issuance of certificates of need for hospital beds. The building of new hospitals or the expansion or renovation of old hospitals had to be approved by a state planning agency, a control on supply. Also, in state after state, legislation began to be passed to regulate hospital rate setting, a control on price.

In addition, as an outgrowth of the utilization review mandate in 1965, Congress passed a law requiring utilization review of hospital care, that is, physician decision making on an areawide basis by committees (professional standards review organization) made up of physicians. To cap all these developments Congress passed the National Health Resources Planning Act (PL 93-641) in 1974 mandating the creation of over 200 health planning areas administered by health service agencies (HSAs) whose board of governors were to be comprised of a majority of consumers. Consumers were to be appointed by racial, ethnic, income, and area criteria. The health services agencies were to pass on the appropriateness of hospital construction, distribution, and renovation and the purchasing policies of hospitals regarding expensive equipment such as computed tomography (CT) scanners. Further, the health service agencies were to measure health needs in their areas in a master plan according to federal guidelines to be passed up to counterpart state and federal agencies for review. Congressional intent was to place need determination and control of facility construction at the local level. Needs, as determined by health service agencies, would then be submitted to upper levels of state and federal governments. Upper levels of government could then react in terms of their funds and priorities and work out compromises. Congress and perhaps the bureaucracy were exceedingly chary of imposing a blueprint on the states and local areas, preferring to set up fairly loose guidelines for discussion. It was apparently Congress' intent to put a planning apparatus in place before the enactment of some form of national health insurance so as to have a framework in which to implement such legislation and to have a handle on costs and the direction of the development of the personal health services. Certificate of need and rate control, although state level functions. were in effect turned over to the health service agencies for decision. The state appeared to respect health service agencies' decisions, and both state and federal governments could withhold payment from hospitals that did not comply. Even so, the planning apparatus did not have a firm place in national political policy, and the Reagan administration abolished it altogether in 1983. The states, of course, were free to continue supporting the health service agencies using state funds but few did so.

The latest approach now being presented—old as a concept but relatively new in terms of government support to contain the cost escalation—is the Health Maintenance Organization (HMO). Health Maintenance Organizations embody several types of prepayment plans that attempt to monitor physician decision making, set a fixed premium for comprehensive services, to serve a known population, and offer voluntary enrollment. These plans have shown that they use hospital services less than the mainstream fee-for-service system and hence tend to cost less. The free enterprise competition concept is thus being carried over to health services delivery by encouraging choice of plans among employed groups with the hope that price competition between options will slow the rise in health service costs.

In the meantime, despite Professional Standards Review Organization (PSRO), certificate of need, rate review, second opinion, and planning, the personal health services economy still grows, expenditures continue to rise, and attempts to manage the system do not seem to have much effect. Between 1965 and 1980, the percentage of the gross national product devoted to health services increased from 6.2 to 9.5. The per capita expenditure increased from $217 to $1078. The ultimate weapon, of course, is for the big buyers of services to refuse to provide more money—in short, institute budget caps—but the pluralistic nature of the funding sources makes this method difficult even though the government is now the source of 40 percent of all expenditures for personal health services.

Current Observations

The period of Management and Control continued at an increasingly intensive pace after the Reagan Administration took over in 1980. The trend toward encouraging competition between options offered by the employer heightened. The HMO concept and its varieties have garnered about 12 percent of the market nationally, although there are local area market penetrations as high as 50 percent as in the Minneapolis St. Paul area with a market of two million people.

Employers are becoming even more cost conscious as their contributions to health insurance fringe benefits for their employees press harder on their profit margins in a sluggish economy. The federal and state governments are putting the financial screws on the providers through both Medicare and Medicaid. While the former relies mainly on payroll taxes and the latter on general revenue, both are politically volatile. This is particularly true of Medicaid because of its sole reliance on general revenue. The entire political thrust of American governments is to shun general revenue sources because increased expenditures should not be reflected in government budgets. The presumably least painful source of revenues, in terms of direct taxes for private sector insurance, or any new venture such as the employed uninsured, is the employers.

During the Reagan Administration, in a period of retrenchment, two issues became politically viable; that is, they became worthwhile for the politicians to pay attention to on the part of their constituents: (1) the original limitations of Medicare to cover "catastrophic costs" of long-term acute care, and (2) the 38 million or so people in this country who have no health insurance whatsoever. In addition, a simmering issue has been long-term care in nursing homes and home care, particularly the former, which is covered in large part by Medicaid. Coverage by Medicaid requires a means test and divestiture of assets to conform more or less to a poverty level concept. For those who have hardly any assets at all, they have nothing to give up. Increasingly, however, middle income persons with assets have had to "spend down" to the level of eligibility required by Medicaid and declare themselves destitute in order to qualify for benefits. As a result, this self-reliant and self-supporting middle income group has sought changes in Medicaid that would allow them to retain a higher percentage of their assets in order for them to remain eligible for the program.

While the concept of incrementalism in the liberal-democratic political process is a given, like gravity, the extreme slicing up of the American population until everyone is covered by some program or criterion is incrementalism with a vengeance. All other countries with universal coverage have gone through the usual stages of starting with the workers and then covering more large segments such as white collar workers, farmers, and the self-employed. But the United States is carrying this salami–slicing technique to a high degree of absurd refinement because of our extreme reluctance to rely more on general revenues as a source of funding social programs.

Although the eight years of the Reagan administration were marked by competition between delivery systems, retrenchment of financing for Medicare and Medicaid, and the slicing off of small problem segments of the population for health insurance, I do not necessarily attribute to that administration the policies that have emerged and are being implemented. For these policies were both latent and manifest in the American political consciousness before Reagan. Moreover, during Reagan's second term both houses of Congress were controlled by Democrats. The philosophy of limited government financial responsibility lies deep in the American body politic quite independent of political party positions, although the Reagan administration has given greater expression to these policies.

The concrete expression of the move toward health insurance for the uninsured was the adoption of legislation in Massachusetts where employers of firms above a certain number of employees are mandated to cover the uninsured employees in their firms. Also, employers are taxed so that the state can cover other categories of uninsured such as the unemployed and the self-employed. Similar programs have been considered in many other states. Nationally, Congress passed and then later repealed a "super" catastrophe bill to supplement the mini-catastrophe coverage of the original Medicare Act. Held for a future time was consideration of long-term care for the chronically ill in nursing homes to back up Medicaid and modification of the means test so as not to make heretofore self-sufficient elderly destitute because of nursing home costs.

A major financial method to control hospital costs for Medicare was the implementation of prospective pricing using Diagnostic Related Groups (DRG's). Under this system which became effective in 1983, each admission is assigned a maximum cost for in-hospital services, in short a budget cap for each diagnosis rather than a global budget cap for the hospital. If the length of stay is exceeded according to the national criterion, the hospital (or patient) loses money; if the length of stay is shorter, the hospital makes money. As could be anticipated, there were allegations of premature discharge including testimonies before congressional committees. Tension between the advocates for the elderly such as the American Association of Retired Persons (AARP) and the Health Care Financing Administration (HCFA) increased. Some hospitals made money and some lost money. Since 1983 HCFA has been monitoring this control method to shake out the hospitals that are making or losing money.

Congress and the administration have been squeezing the private hospital sector and the physicians financially because it is felt that the system was "fat," with the objective to reduce this fat and thus reduce costs, hoping the result would be a leaner and more efficient enterprise. While the usual litany accompanying this objective was, of course, " without eroding the quality of care," the available quality measures are so crude that it will take quite a reduction in costs before results can be measured by mortality rates, convenience and comfort.

There is so much "fat" in the system that the governments are loading on to the private sector the responsibility for serving the uninsured and the indigent in a period when the providers are supposed to compete with each other for markets and lowest possible prices. In a number of states, hospitals are even taxed on their inpatient income to cover the costs of uninsured and indigent care, a curious philosophy in which a public responsibility is being pushed on the private sector.

The financial pressures on hospitals and reduced occupancy have resulted in a large minority of hospitals if not a majority to merge in various ways from cooperative agreements to outright ownership of chains of hospitals. Hospitals are retailing exercise and life style change classes, nutrition classes, screening for various diseases,and so on in order to survive. These are worthy enough endeavors in themselves, and they do not cost the government or insurance companies anything. Finally, this is the only country which is contracting its hospital bed supply without government regulation directly, but by reducing the admissions and length of stay, that is, the demand. Thus hospitals cannot "blame" regulatory and planning agencies, but only the impersonal "invisible hand" of classical economics.

In this connection it is clear that this country has shifted completely from social planning as attempted by the National Health Planning and Resources Development Act, (PL 93–641) in 1974, and discarded as ineffective by 1983, ineffective in that neither the Congress or the people were enthusiastic about the philosophy. What was taking place concurrently, and now in full swing, is corporate planning by large medical complexes testing the perimeters of their respective "turfs," a process which seems to be congenial to the American entrepreneurial style.

Despite all these financial control measures, the trend of rising expenditures persists at an unacceptable rate as regarded by the funding sources, and has recently (1987–88) accelerated again as measured by the premiums charged by insurance companies and HMO's. Employers are digging in their heels by various devices: turning to self-insurance, requiring increased deductibles and coinsurance, and offering employees choices of selecting varying benefit packages at varying prices to fit their needs at any given age group. This pernicious practice fragments the entire health services benefit structure so that some groups in the population have lower or higher costs depending on their age composition and employment situation. This practice then distorts the balance of access and referral to the entire spectrum of personal health service components because of financial considerations. A comprehensive health service and health insurance system, public or private, facilitates an appropriate choice of services not unduly influenced by whether or not particular services are covered by insurance. As the benefit package becomes increasingly fragmented leaving "unpopular" illnesses such as alcoholism, chemical dependency, and VD uncovered by insurance, these increasing residuals are thrown into the dustbins of inadequate public programs, thus pressuring governments to enlarge their programs and increase taxes, a trend which the private sector and competition was supposed to prevent in the first place. Even HMOs whose original concept was open access to all services with little or no charge at time of service have been forced into offering custom made benefit packages for special markets of employees.

As seen by past experience and future projections as well as comparisons with other countries the upward trend of expenditures for personal health services is inevitable, given reasonably equitable access, continuing innovations in technology, and the aging of the population. Further, the public places a high priority on personal health services.

In a very short period, then, say, five years or less, a whole host of issues have come to the fore in this country with attempts at cost retrenchment and methods to control it like HMOs and competition. Simultaneously, the health services enterprise is literally reeling under very intractable problems, a selected list of which are elaborated on below.

Malpractice Costs

The cost of malpractice insurance is burdening providers who are already pressured to lower or control costs. The American public is the most litigious population in the world. I hypothesize that the basic reason for this lies in an increasingly impersonal system rather than in general low-quality practice. In the face of high population mobility, competition encourages easy shifting from medical plan to medical plan.

Bioethical Issues

Bio-ethical issues are now on the front pages of newspapers every day. A pluralistic ethnic and religious society finds it difficult to come to some workable resolution on the issues of abortion, and the keeping of both infants and adults alive by means of sophisticated, high technology clinical procedures. While vital organ transplants—hearts, lungs, kidneys, livers—are becoming increasingly clinically feasible, there is a continuous shortage of organs. Organ procurement agencies locally and nationally are working hard to induce the population to donate organs from dead or living bodies—or from bodies which are near death. Although it is difficult enough to procure organs for next of kin, people are being asked to donate body parts to total strangers. States have made provisions for space on drivers' licenses for owners to sign their names giving permission to ambulance staffs and the police to transport a dead body found in an automobile accident as soon as possible to the nearest hospital in order to retrieve viable body parts for patients waiting for them.

Supply of Personnel

There is an imminent surplus of physicians whose very presence may increase national expenditures for medical care, because the market for physicians is sufficiently elastic that their services will be sought. A possible solution is to make the opportunities to practice so tight that a certain excess of physicians may have no place to practice. In contrast, there is a shortage of nurses, and means are being sought to increase their supply, raise wages, or rationalize the entire various levels of caring staff so that highly qualified nurses will be doing more highly technical tasks. During the last 50 years or so there have been cycles of perceived surpluses and shortages of both physicians and nurses, indicating the primitive nature of our criteria for determining adequate supply of health personnel.

Provider Competition

The very important and apparently generally accepted concept of competition between various types of HMOs and the mainstream fee-for-service system trying to cope with its relatively new competitors is not well understood. Employers are complaining that HMOs are not lowering costs as anticipated while premiums are continuing to rise. There are no standards as to what is a "reasonable" premium or level of expenditures. Economists who promote price competition do not really understand the nature of the health services market as compared with other goods and services. They are mystified by the continuing rise in expenditures and premiums. It is likely that health services are not regarded by the public as a commodity like automobiles and refrigerators, but health services have become a basic need and right, regardless of cost.

Long time students of the health field, like Eli Ginzberg are raising the question, after ten years or so of experience, whether competition results in a continuous destabilization of a very complex enterprise which requires trust as the major variable to function.

I forsee the possibility of prices between various types of delivery systems in competition becoming quite similar because of the inherent extensiveness of the health services and the insistent demands for them. Competition will then have to be based on convenience of access, and quality as perceived by the public (I.e., were the receptionists, physicians, and nurses pleasant?).

There is a prevailing view that the traditional mainstream fee-for-service-insurance and open choice of physicians will disappear as the HMO concept and its varieties cover more and more of the population. Some estimates of such coverage are as high as 65 percent of the population on a national average, and even higher in metropolitan areas. These estimates may be right depending on the definition of the fee-for-service concept. The traditionally wide-open system of "unmanaged care" and reimbursing physicians on the basis of usual, customary, and reasonable fees, as well as retroactive reimbursement of hospitals, is a thing of the past, but the tenacity of the fee-for-service, open choice style, should not be underestimated in a country with the free enterprise, consumer choice characteristics of the United States. As more and more Americans experience the constrictions imposed on them by limited choice and closed delivery systems as represented by the, say, staff and group model HMOs, an appreciably large minority will be selecting more open systems like the Independent Practice Associations (IPA), the medical professions response to the competition of the closed system models; that is, if, and it might be a big if, the professions can group themselves in a not necessarily self-serving manner, to deliver an open choice system at a cost approximating the cost of the closed system models. It should be remembered that the closed systems may be reaching the bottom line of cost control as discounts from providers are harder to negotiate because the latter need to survive too.

It would seem that a tiered system of various types of HMOs from staff to IPA models will emerge to serve various segments of the population on an income class basis analogous to the great variety of automobiles from Ford Escorts to Mercedes which all get you there with various degrees of comfort, convenience, and style. So, there might well develop three levels of delivery systems - basic, middle class, and luxury. The basic level would provide reasonably good access to primary care, for the full range of illnesses, with general practitioners as gatekeepers, and quick access to hospitals for acute and emergency care. There might be, however, hemming and hawing on the part of the primary physicians to facilitate quick access or access at all for elective surgery and for medical conditions, treatment for which can be delayed to see how they turn out. This is the United Kingdom model, the most equitable system in the world, and has evolved almost without deliberate plan but in ingenious response to low budgets. The middle class plan would have both reasonably good access to primary care, open access to all physicians, no gatekeepers, little negotiation for access for elective conditions, and quick access to hospitals for acute and emergency care. Finally, for the luxury level, everything is provided, albeit, naturally, at a price. Is such a system equitable? In a pure sense, of course not, but it may be *just,* in that life and health on the lowest level are not jeopardized. Such a system is simply not as comfortable and convenient. It would seem that comfort and convenience cannot be provided equally. This would be too expensive.

Will this country in time have universal health insurance? Arguably, the trend toward complete coverage is clear and is gaining political momentum. The providers, among others, want to unburden themselves of the uninsured who are unable to pay. There is even some semblance of bad conscience in the body politic, that believes that it is grossly unfair and callous to have anyone in the country exposed to high expenditures for medical care or no care at all.

What will evolve then in the coming years is a pattern of segments of the population, all with health insurance, but with different programs, budgets, and sources of funding. These will include the currently uninsured employed and unemployed, the poor, the elderly, and the employed. A day will come when the country will suddenly discover that we have universal health insurance, but not on the pattern of other countries that do not differentiate their population to this extreme degree, and that have funding mainly from public sources. Consolidation and coordination may come in time, as this patchwork quilt reveals its unmanageable complexity.

REFERENCES

American Medical Association. 1960. *The Story of America's Medical Schools.* Chicago:The American Medical Association.

Andersen, Ronald, Joanna Lion and Odin W. Anderson. 1976. *Two Decades of Health Services: Social Survey Trends in Use and Expenditure.* Cambridge: Ballinger.

Anderson, Odin W. 1968. *The Uneasy Equilibrium; Private and Public Financing of Health Services in the United States, 1875–1965.* New Haven:College and University Press.

Anderson, Odin W. 1972. *Health Care: Can There Be Equity? The United States, Sweden and England.* New York:John Wiley & Sons.

Anderson, Odin W. 1976. *Blue Cross Since 1929; Accountability and the Public Trust.* Boston:Ballinger.

Anderson, Odin W. 1985. *The American Health Services: A Growth Enterprise Since 1875.* Ann Arbor: Health Administration Press.

Anderson, Odin W. 1988. The fragmentation of the medical profession. *Minnesota Medicine* 71:20–21.

Asgis, Alfred J. 1941. *Professional Dentistry in American Society: A Historical and Social Approach to Dental Progress.* New York:Clinical Press.

Boorstin, Daniel J. 1953. *The Genius of American Politics.* Chicago:University of Chicago Press.

Burrow, James A.M.A. 1963. *Voice of American Medicine.* Baltimore:Johns Hopkins Press.

Campion, Frank D. 1984. *The AMA and U.S. Health Policy Since 1940.* Chicago:Chicago Review Press.

Carter, Richard. 1961. *The Gentle Legions.* Garden City, N.Y.:Doubleday.

Committee on the Costs of Medical Care. 1933. *The Final Report of the Committee,* adopted October 21, 1932. No. 26. Chicago:University of Chicago Press.

Committee on the Grading of Nursing Schools. 1928. *Nurses, Patients, and Pocketbooks. Report of a Study of the Economics of Nursing.* New York:The Committee.

Connery, Robert H. et al. 1968. *The Politics of Mental Health: Organizing a Community Mental Health in Metropolitan Areas.* New York:Columbia University Press.

Corwin, E. A. L. 1946. *The American Hospital.* New York:Commonwealth Fund.

Dahl, Robert A. 1967. *Pluralist Democracy in the United States—Conflict and Consent.* Chicago:Rand McNally.

Davis, Karen and Cathy Schoen. 1978. *Health and the War on Poverty; a Ten-year Appraisal.* Washington, D.C.:The Brookings Institution.

Davis, Michael M. and Andrew R. Warner. 1918. *Dispensaries: Their Management and Development.* New York:Macmillan.

Dietrick, John E. and Robert C. Berson. 1953. *Medical Schools in the United States at Mid-Century.* New York:McGraw-Hill.

Duffy, John. 1976. *The Healers, the Rise of the Medical Establishment.* New York:McGraw-Hill.

Enthoven, Alain C. 1980. *Health Plan: The Only Practical Solution to the Soaring Cost of Medical Care.* Reading, Mass.:Addison-Wesley Publishing Co.

Falk, I. J., Margaret Klem and Nathan Sinai. 1933. *The Incidence of Illness and the Receipt and Cost of Medical Care Among Representative Families: Experiences in Twelve Consecutive Months During 1928–31.* Committee on the Costs of Medical Care. No. 26. Chicago:University of Chicago Press.

Falkson, Joseph L. 1980. *HMO's and the Politics of Health System Reform.* Chicago:American Hospital Association.

Flexner, Abraham. 1910. *Medical Education in the United States and Canada; A Report to the Carnegie Foundation for the Advancement of Teaching.* Bulletin No. 4. New York:Carnegie Foundation.

Gibson, Robert M. and Marjorie Smith Mueller. 1976. National health expenditures, fiscal year, 1976. *Social Security Bulletin* 40:2–22.

Ginzberg, Eli. 1986. The destabilization of health care. *New England Journal of Medicine* 315:757.

Gunn, Selskar M. and Philip S. Platt. 1945. *Voluntary Health Agencies: An Interpretative Study.* New York:Ronald Press.

Health Care Financing Administration, Office of the Actuary, Division of National Cost Estimates. 1987. National health expenditures, 1986–2000. *Health Care Financing Review* 8:1–36.

Jamieson, Elizabeth M. and Mary F. Sewall. 1954. *Trends in Nursing History; Their Relationship to World Events.* 4th ed. Philadelphia:W. B. Saunders Co.

Lowi, Theodore. 1969. *The End of Liberalism: Ideology, Policy, and the Crisis of Public Authority.* New York: W. W. Norton.

Luft, Harold S. 1981. *Health Maintenance Organizations; Dimensions and Performance.* New York:Wiley.

Marmor, Theodore R. and Jan S. Marmor. 1970. *The Politics of Medicare.* London:Routledge and Kegan Paul.

Means, James Howard. 1953. *Doctors, People, and Government.* Boston:Little Brown.

Mustard, Harry S. 1941. *Government in Public Health.* New York:Commonwealth Fund.

The President's Commission on the Health Needs of the Nation. 1952. *Building American Health* Vol. 1. Washington, D.C.:Government Printing Office.

Roberts, Mary M. 1954. *American Nursing: History and Interpretation.* New York:Macmillan.

Rosen, George. 1958. *A History of Public Health.* New York:M. D. Publications.

Shryock, Richard H. 1948. *The Development of Modern Medicine.* London:Gollancz.

Shryock, Richard H. 1960. *Medicine and Society in America 1660–1860.* New York:New York University Press.

Sinai, Nathan and Odin W. Anderson. 1948. *E.M.I.C., A Study of Administrative Experience,* Research Series No. 3. Ann Arbor:University of Michigan School of Public Health.

Sonnedecker, Glenn, Revision of Kremers and Urdang. 1976. *History of Pharmacy* 4th ed. Philadelphia: J. B. Lippincott.

Stern, Bernard. 1945. *American Medical Practice in the Perspective of a Century.* New York:Commonwealth Fund.

The Truman memoirs. 1956. *Life* Vol. XL:104.

Williams, Ralph C. 1951. *The United States Public Health Services, 1798–1950.* Bethesda, Md.:Commissioned Officers Association, U.S. Public Health Services.

Witte, Edwin E. 1962. *The Development of the Social Security Act.* Madison:University of Wisconsin Press.

Chapter 3

The Restructuring of the American Health Care System

▓ Donald W. Light ▓

The American health care system, one of society's largest and most influential institutions, is undergoing profound cultural and structural changes because large buyers of services are wresting partial control from providers in order to restrain escalating costs.[1] Major corporations and state health programs have awakened from the habit of passively paying medical bills and are aggressively pursuing ways to stop medical costs from continuing to rise at about twice the general rate of inflation. Government health programs, especially Medicare and Medicaid but also those of the Veterans Administration, the armed services, and federal employee benefit programs, are under constant pressure from Congress to keep costs down.

These large purchasers are buying medical services in volume at wholesale prices and even dictating terms, a radical change from the long-held custom of individuals paying for their care retail on a case-by-case basis. Institutional buyers want to know what they are getting for their money, a simple question that has threatened the autonomy of physicians and hospitals to the core because the answers require detailed data, close scrutiny, and ultimately outside judgment of whether the services are worth their cost. The nature of insurance is being changed as buyers and insurers shift the risk of costs to patients and providers. Increasingly, the fiduciary relation between doctor and patient is stressed, perhaps even tainted, by competition for business and prepayment, whereas before it was compromised by paying doctors every time they did a procedure.

These fundamental changes—and the resistance to them—are easier to describe than to analyze. Our purpose here is to provide readers

[1]This essay is based on a policy research project to analyze the restructuring of American health care and its consequences for society. Support is gratefully acknowledged from The Twentieth Century Fund. I also wish to thank Howard Freeman, Sol Levine, Odin Anderson, Peter Conrad and Renee Fox for their suggestions and critical remarks.

with a framework for understanding the reconstruction of the American health care system going on today. Central to that framework is new historical research showing that corporations and other institutional buyers were setting terms and contracting wholesale for medical services around 1900 as part of industrialization at that time. As a result, physicians were providing medical services for a fixed annual fee (capitation) or according to a discount fee schedule like today's preferred provider organizations. These buyers' markets were vigorously opposed through legal, economic, and political pressure by medical societies and were suppressed until the late 1970s when institutional buyers once again reasserted themselves.

Early Corporate Health Care

During the nineteenth century, the corporate practice of medicine began in the railroad, mining, and lumber industries, where remote locations, high accident rates, and the growth of lawsuits by injured workers called for some corporate form of health care. These industries contracted for medical services on a retainer basis or on salary; some even owned hospitals and dispensaries for their workers. In the textile industry this included establishing comprehensive medical services in the mill towns. Thousands of doctors were involved in these contracts or worked on salary (Williams 1932; Selleck with Whittaker 1962).

By the end of the nineteenth century, however, more and more businesses with none of these special needs also began to contract on a competitive basis for the health care of their employees. For example, the Michigan State Medical Society reported in 1907 that many companies (of no particular size or reputation) were contracting for the health care of their employees (Langford et al. 1907). The Plate Glass Factory contracted with physicians and hospitals for all medical and surgical care of its employees and families for $1.00 a month apiece. The Michigan Alkali Company did the same but did not include family members. Several other companies had contracts for the treatment of accidents and injuries. Commercial insurance companies of the day also got involved, putting together packages of services for a flat amount per person per year (capitation) or for a discounted fee schedule.

More widespread than early corporate health care plans were comprehensive health care medical services, offered for a flat subscription price per year to members of the fraternal orders that had proliferated rapidly during the same period. The national and regional orders of the Eagles, the Foresters, the Moose, the Orioles as well as other national or regional fraternal associations, offered medical care at deeply discounted prices through their local lodges (Ferguson 1937; Gist 1940). Various reports from medical societies and commissions in Louisiana, Rhode Island, California, and New York attest to the prevalence of such plans and of contract practice, as competitive health care was then called. "[T]he growth of contract practice has been so amazingly great during the last twenty-five years as almost to preclude belief," reported a committee of physicians in 1916. "Practically all of the large cities are fairly honeycombed with lodges, steadily increasing in number, with a constantly growing membership" (Woodruff 1916).

The government also became heavily involved in organized buying near the turn of the century. Most of the more comprehensive reports on contract practice describe municipal, county, and state agencies putting out for bid service contracts for the poor, for prisoners, and for civil employees. At the federal level, the armed services and Coast Guard had long contracted for medical services at wholesale prices (Burrow 1971; Richardson 1945).

In response to these developments, more and more physicians were offering medical services at discount fees or for a low capitation fee. This greatly threatened independent practitioners, who were already facing keen competition from the glut of doctors being trained at proprietary medical schools, and from other kinds of providers such as homeopaths, osteopaths, naturalists, and chiropractors. Equally threatening to professional status, the institutions or organizations writing these contracts set the conditions under which medicine should be practiced.

Suppressing Contract Medicine

To battle contract medicine, county and state medical societies took a number of actions. They conducted studies and reported on the terrible conditions under which contract physicians worked. Strangely enough, however, the few times that remarks were published by physicians doing contract work, they said they liked the guaranteed income rather than having a quarter of their patients (on average) not pay their bills. They remarked on how they learned to handle hypochondriacs and other abusers of free medical care, and they pointed out that contract medicine provided an excellent way to build up a private practice. Societies were also forced to acknowledge that a sizable proportion of their members actively bid for contracts and did contract work. (Langford et al. 1907; Lytle 1909; *Bulletin* 1909; Haley 1911; Woodruff 1916).

To those leading this campaign, however, complicity appears to have been a good reason to redouble their efforts and save their colleagues from their own bad judgment. Some societies drew up lists of physicians known to practice contract medicine in order to embarrass them. Others drew up "honor rolls" of members who promised to swear off competitive contracts. Society committee members would ferret out recalcitrant colleagues and make group visits to pressure them to abandon contract practice. Some societies threatened expulsion or censure to members who did not cooperate in stamping out price-competitive medicine (Burrow 1971).

These pressures worked much more effectively than they had in the nineteenth century, because medical societies succeeded in getting hospitals not to grant privileges to any physician who was not a member in good standing. The hospital had established itself as the center of modern medicine and professional status (Stevens 1989). Therefore the granting of staff privileges became a powerful control mechanism. Malpractice insurance and other professional needs were contingent on membership too. More broadly, the success of practice depended on good relations with one's colleagues.

Although organized medicine never eliminated competitive contracts entirely, it greatly reduced their number. Fraternal orders did not want to cause a row with doctors and shifted coverage to partial payments for wages lost and medical bills rather than contracted services. Reimbursement allowed doctors to set their own fees and eliminated any middlemen setting the terms of service. Several court decisions supported the profession's opposition to the corporate practice of medicine, even though its legal basis was (and is) weak (Rosoff 1986–7). In a number of states, the medical profession persuaded legislators to pass legislation prohibiting the corporate practice of medicine or the practice of medicine by organizations run by nonphysicians. They also got other laws passed against the organized practice of medicine for profit. Medical societies, meanwhile, dusted off their old fee schedules and raised their prices to a professionally respectable level (Schwartz 1965; Burrow 1971; Rosen 1983; Starr 1982).

The goal of these and other efforts to gain control over the practice of medicine has never been to eliminate competition entirely but rather to keep outsiders (i.e., consumers and buyers) from setting terms, especially price. Guilds secured a monopoly over a domain and then let members compete freely within it (Weber 1968). By the 1920s, the medical profession had contracts confined to a few industries with special needs, to group purchasing of services for the poor and the military, and to a few maverick experiments on the periphery of medicine (Williams 1932).

Making Insurance Provider-Friendly

Although organized medicine had successfully opposed national health insurance, unpaid bills during the Great Depression made subscriptions and forms of prepayment appealing. Groups of physicians, county and even state medical societies, individual hospitals, employers, and employee groups all began to experiment with prepaid contracts again. Although the American Medical Association remained adamantly opposed to any such arrangement, especially if it placed a middleman between doctor and patient, the American Hospital Association listened more sympathetically to the plight of member hospitals. Many could not meet payroll and had "payless days." An unknown but probably large percentage of them started to sell hospital days to one group or another on a monthly prepaid basis of fifty cents per member or a dollar per family (Leland 1932; Williams 1932; Schwartz 1965; Stevens 1971; Rayack 1967; Sigmond 1989; Greenberg 1978). Again the profession and now the hospital industry faced the threat of competition pitting one provider against another.

Out of this turbulence emerged the insurance scheme that came to be known as Blue Cross. Although Justin Ford Kimball is usually credited with having the genius to find the solution because of his dynamic charisma and travels throughout the country advocating his hospital prepayment plan, in fact Kimball's Baylor University Hospital was not the first to implement such a plan (it was Grinnell Hospital in 1917). Moreover, he advocated competing hospital plans and opposed middlemen as the insurance administrators for multi-hospital plans. Instead, it was the soft-spoken, self-effacing Quaker, C. Rufus Rorem, and a small group of colleagues who realized that a prepaid hospital plan would have to include many or all of the hospitals in an area so that the doctor and the patient could have free choice.

On other basics, Kimball and Rorem seemed to agree: the plan should be non-profit and not include doctors' services so as to avoid opposition from the AMA. They also understood that they were selling the middle class access to semi-private services (not necessarily semi-private rooms) instead of ward services if they went to the hospital unable to pay. The genius of Rorem's vision lay in persuading state legislatures that in lieu of the sizable reserves required of insurance plans, hospitals could substitute guaranteed services. Indeed, the trick of early multi-hospital plan administrators was to negotiate a contract of payments with hospitals for their services that lay within the limits of the $.50/1.00 per month that subscribers were willing to pay in.

Because prepaid hospital plans freed up the patient's purse to pay doctors' fees, and because noncompetitive plans avoided the awkward problem of a doctor being affiliated with one hospital but the patient having a subscription to another, local physicians and medical societies backed Rorem's approach. Although many hospitals had at least one prepaid contract with a group, the idea quickly spread as a form of insurance that provided the working and middle classes with free choice and semi-private services (Rorem 1940; Reed 1947; Rayack 1967).

From a comparative and historical point of view, Blue Cross is notable for covering only hospital services and, at that, only for groups of workers who could afford the premium. More comprehensive and cost-effective alternatives, like prepaid group practice, did not receive professional support and were passed over. Moreover, the special enabling legislation passed in many states to circumvent insurance laws required that hospital administrators, trustees and physicians hold the majority of seats on the Board. Even though there was tension and even conflict between Blue Cross plans and member hospitals in negotiating how much the plans could pay, Blue Cross was from the start provider-friendly insurance focused on what the profession valued most: specialized care and surgery in the "temple of medicine." When the AMA and state and local medical societies decided a few years later that prepaid hospital plans were an idea worth imitating, they made Blue Shield even more provider-friendly by emphasizing payment for services rather than service contracts and leaving the physician free to bill as much as desired. By the 1950s, Blue Cross and Blue Shield had become provider-controlled vehicles for pass-through insurance (Goldberg and Greenberg 1978; Law 1974).

Instituting health insurance along professional lines and defeating prior efforts to legislate national forms of social insurance completed what is called "the health service infrastructure (Anderson 1990). The nature of that infrastructure is outlined in Figure 3–1 and can best be characterized as a professionally driven health care system. At the heart of that system is the goal of providing the best possible clinical care to every sick patient wherever physicians choose to practice. Complementary goals include developing scientific medicine to its highest level and protecting the autonomy of physicians.

These goals, worthy in their own right, led to excesses and distortions that by the 1970s resulted in widespread discontent and revolt by consumers and buyers. For example, professional goals emphasize state-of-the-art clinical interventions and specialization rather than primary care and prevention. Costs rise sharply, especially if reimbursed by provider-controlled insurance. The right of doctors to practice what they want and where they want leads at the system level to fragmentation and undeserved areas. An integrated delivery system that serves rural and inner city patients as well as others

Ideal Type of a Professional Health Care System

Inherent Values and Goals	To provide the best possible clinical care to every sick patient where physicians choose to practice. To develop scientific medicine to its highest level. To protect the autonomy of physicians and keep the state or others from controlling the health care system. To increase the power and wealth of the profession. To generate enthusiasm and admiration for the medical profession.
Organization	A loose federation, administratively collegial and decentralized. Emphasis on acute, high-tech intervention and specialty care. Organized around clinical cases and doctors' preferences. Organized around hospitals and private offices. Weak ties with other social institutions. Services and recruitment follow the stratification of the society.
Key Institutions	Physicians' associations Autonomous physicians and hospitals. Medical schools as the wellspring of professional advance, prestige, and legitimation.
Power	Profession the sole power. Uses state powers to enhance its own. Protests state interferences. Protests, boycotts all competing models of care.
Finance and Cost	Private payments, by individual or through private insurance plans. Doctors' share of costs more than in mutual aid model.
Image of the individual	A private individual. Chooses how to live and when to use the medical system.
Division of Labor	Hierarchical. Centered on physicians, especially specialists.

FIGURE 3–1

Source: POLITICAL VALUES AND HEALTH CARE: THE GERMAN EXPERIENCE, by Donald W. Light and Alexander Schuller, Copyright 1986 by MIT Press. Reprinted by permission.

would require a loss of professional autonomy. As Figure 3–1 indicates, the resulting system consists of a loose federation of local offices and hospitals organized around physicians' preferences, with weak ties to other sectors such as the schools or the workplace. Power centers on professional associations, which use the legal powers of the state to enhance their position but protest state interference in the practice of medicine. The American system differs from its counterpart in many other countries by the relative weakness of the state (Larkin 1983; Willis 1983; Coburn Torrence and Kaufert 1983; Wilsford 1987). While the medical profession in those countries faced many similar issues of legitimacy and control and used similar tactics, they worked with the state in matters of organization and financing.

Creating a Haven for Capitalism

An ironic consequence of the American case is that the medical profession created protected markets where capitalism could flourish and eventually exert control over the profession itself. Although today we think of this happening with health care corporations, the earliest and perhaps most important case is the pharmaceutical industry (Burrow 1963; Rorem and Fischelis 1932; Caplan 1981). As early as 1906, the AMA mounted a vigorous campaign against nostrums and patent medicine.

Joined by druggists who were also feeling the competition from patent medicine manufacturers, the AMA and some state medical societies sought to cordon off and control sale of those drugs whose recipes were revealed, tested, and approved by the AMA. They succeeded and in effect created a protected professional market. Given that the profession opposed any state participation and that capitalism constituted the "natural" economic environment of the nation, it was inevitable that 'ethical' drug companies (that is, in conformity with AMA ethics) experienced tremendous growth and profits. What the profession did not anticipate is that these companies would soon influence professional judgment and make many facets of professional life dependent on them (Goldfinger 1987; Lexchin 1987; Mintz 1967).

Corporations have flourished in every other protected medical market—hospital supply, hospital construction, medical devices, laboratories, and insurance—until the only large sector left untouched was medical service itself. The profession somehow thought that it could allow corporations to dominate every other sector without being touched themselves. Meanwhile, their professional judgments and decisions were being commercialized in numerous ways: by how insurance policies were written, by what medical devices were promoted, by how supplies were packaged, by what new lab tests were made available, by which company sponsored a professional presentation, and by which salesmen they saw.

Finally, by the 1960s the only sector that had not been corporatized was medical care itself. Yet in creating a protected domain where physicians could order what they wanted and have someone pay the bill, the profession had created an ideal environment for medical service corporations to flourish as well. With the passage of Medicare and Medicaid providing coverage for the age group that used hospitals and nursing homes the most, for-profit hospital and nursing home chains flourished. Soon all kinds of other medical service corporations sprang up. This development greatly disturbed the medical profession. Leading physicians saw these corporations as alien invaders who threatened everything they stood for (Relman 1980), and indeed many observers still do not realize that the rise of corporate *providers* was an integral part of the system which the profession put in place.

The Revolt of Institutional Buyers

During the 1960s and '70s, all the tendencies we have described of the professionally driven health care system increased. Finally, corporate buyers, other employers, and legislators became alarmed at the sharp rise in medical expenses and a number of related problems. The 1970s opened with a burst of criticisms against unnecessary surgery, excessive drug prescriptions, inefficient hospitals, too many specialists who did not care about the patient as a person, the lack of primary care, and the neglect of the poor despite Medicaid. From every sector of society arose cries for national health insurance and a total revamping of what was seen as a chaotic, wasteful-system (*Fortune* 1970; Greenberg 1971; Ehren-reich 1971; Bodenheimer, Cummings, and Harding 1972; Kennedy 1972; Ribicoff 1972). Numerous proposals for national health insurance came before Congress, but each differed enough from the next that in the end no one proposal garnered enough support to pass (Davis 1975).

During this period, Congress as the buyer behind Medicare passed several bills to control costs through regulation. Congress focused on planning (HSAs), regionalizing expensive facilities and equipment (CONs), and reviewing physicians' orders (PSROs). These and similar measures, however, lacked the powers of enforcement, and they had loopholes which health care administrators and consultants quickly learned to exploit. By the end of the 1970s, policy makers concluded that "regulation doesn't work." It would have been more accurate, however, to conclude that weak and partial regulation does not work. The seventies ended with health care costing about three times what it had in 1970 and consuming 9.5 percent of GNP rather than 7.5 percent.

During the 1980s, institutional buyers went into open revolt against the professionally driven system under the banner of "competition." The one competitive buyer's action begun during the 1970s (by President Nixon) was to promote health maintenance organizations (HMOs) as the ideal counter-system that integrated all levels of care under one management. Moreover, because the HMOs receive a flat amount per member per month for their entire budgets, they would manage all aspects of health care in a cost-effective manner. At the time, HMOs delivered all health care for 10–40 percent less money than fee-for-service providers and hospitals, and the HMO Act of 1973 required employers to offer HMOs as an alternative to regular health insurance (Falkson 1983). Although HMOs ran into many complications, they set a precedent for offering competitive plans, and during the 1980s employers greatly expanded the choices. In fact, one strategy taken by some employers has been to limit their contribution to benefits and then let employees choose the mix they want. This "cafeteria plan" approach gives employees a great deal of choice, while it allows institutional buyers to limit the relentless increase in contributions to benefits. Employees think they are getting more when over the long run they may get less.

Beginning in the 1970s, HMOs and employers both pressed for amendments and changes in administrative rules that would allow HMOs to be more competitive. One can see a gradual relaxing of requirements right on through the 1980s to allow HMOs to respond to a wide array of market demands by employers. In addition, PPOs (preferred provider organizations) were invented to provide still more alternatives and flexibility. Essentially, a PPO is any group of providers who agree to discounted fees in return for an employer giving employees incentives to use them. Whatever the employer covers through health insurance applies to treatment by a PPO, but if the employees choose another physician, they pay anything billed above the coverage level.

Through the 1980s, the boundaries between PPOs and HMOs began to blur. On one hand, some PPOs agreed to capitated payments. On the other hand, some HMOs did not provide comprehensive care but were targeted to certain types of medical service. The basic point, however, is that health care changed from a sellers' (i.e., providers') market to a buyers' market. Flexing their fiscal muscles, buyers from Medicare on down to mid-sized companies in local markets were telling providers what services they wanted and what prices they thought were reasonable. The buyers' market was greatly aided by a surplus of sellers, that is, by an excess number of hospital beds and an increase in physicians that greatly exceeded population growth.

The goals, values and policies of institutional buyers is summarized in Figure 3–2. Buyers aim to dismantle and reshape the laws, customs, and institutions put in place over the past several decades by the medical profession so that buyer choice and competition can take place. No longer is there the sacred trust in physicians that prevailed in the 1950s. Doctors were ordering too many tests, prescribing too many drugs, performing too much surgery, and bouncing too many patients from specialists to specialist. Buyers found that neither they nor their insurance companies knew how their money was being spent or what they were getting for it. Quality and accountability became chief concerns. Buyers also want integrated care, and by putting con-

Dimensions of Change in American Health Care

FROM	TO
Provider dominance (a system run and shaped by doctors)	Buyer dominance (an effort to dismantle and reshape the laws, customs, and institutions established by organized medicine to allow buyer choice and competition
Sacred trust in doctors	Distrust of doctors' values, decisions, even competence
Quality assured by medical profession as high (but uneven and unattended)	Quality a major focus of systematic review
"Nonprofit" guild monopoly	Competition for profit (even among nonprofit organizations)
Cottage industry structure	Corporate industry structure
Specialization and subspecialization	Primary care and prevention, with minimal referrals to specialists.
Hospital as the "temple of healing"	Home and office as equal centers of care
Fragmentation of services as a byproduct of preserving physicians' autonomy	Coordination of services to minimize error and reduce unnecessary and inappropriate services and costs (slow in coming)
Payment of costs incurred by doctors' decisions	Fixed prepayment, with demand for a detailed account of decisions and of their efficacy
Cross-subsidization of the poor by the more affluent, of low-tech and service departments by hi-tech departments	Cross-subsidization seen as "cost shifting," a suspect maneuver that imposes hidden charges on buyers

FIGURE 3–2

Source: Light, Donald W. (1988).

tracts out for bid that cover a sizable number of people, they have prompted providers to restructure into forms that offer co-ordinated care. Large group practices, joint ventures between hospitals and physician groups, managed care systems, and consortia of all kinds have grown.

Tightening prices and especially fixed prices have forced providers to rethink their basic relationship to the market. They have combined into purchasing groups in order to purchase supplies at minimal costs in large volume. They have established internal monitoring systems to weed out or re-educate those providers who run up expenses with too many tests or procedures. And some have changed the way they pay providers so that there are incentives to keep costs down.

Because buyers want to know what they are getting for their money, it does not take long for them to demand detailed accounts of what services are being rendered at what cost. To most people's surprise, providers often do not know what their services cost nor even have good data on the services rendered. These data are inherently intrusive; they lead to buyer control and monitoring systems. The battle over control of data is fierce.

Even more significant, the demand for accountability is shifting from measuring inputs (supplies, equipment, facilities, and medical procedures) to outcomes (whose patients get better faster and cheaper). It is not unreasonable to predict that soon those hospitals, medical teams, or physicians whose outcomes are substandard will either lose business or be subject to retraining.

Many professional customs and beliefs are being shaken and altered by buyers who question their clinical necessity or financial worth. For example, the variations in how physicians treat the same problems range in cost from threefold to sixfold after controlling for type of disorder, its prevalence, and demographic characteristics of the population (Wennberg 1984). This and related examples make buyers wonder about the cost of physician autonomy. Still, however, little remains known about what goes into these great variations in practice style.

Medicare and the Power of Buyer Dominance

No institutional buyer has done more to restructure the American health care system than Medicare and the administrators of HCFA (the Health Care Financing Administration). Behind them, as the taxpayers' agent, Congress has steadfastly pressed to find ways to keep Medicare expenses from rising so fast that they bankrupt the Medicare Trust Fund. From the mid-1970s on, HCFA sponsored a wide range of research projects and experiments in payment schemes, competitive delivery systems, and methods for monitoring costs.

No research project, however, has had more impact than the one at Yale University to design a system for managing hospital costs by diagnostic group. Used first in the late seventies at the state level in New Jersey as a way to pay hospitals, HCFA adopted a stricter version of this system for hospital payment under Medicare in 1983. Called the prospective payment system (PPS), it seemed the answer to Medicare's problems: when a patient was admitted, Medicare knew in advance that they would pay a fixed amount unless it was an unusually expensive case.

PPS has had a tremendous impact on the hospital industry and on the health care system in general. Although it actually contains incentives to admit more patients because a hospital receives a payment for each admission, admissions actually declined. Hospital administrators were so concerned about PPS that they cut staff, reduced inventory, and had briefing sessions with physicians. As a result, profits (or surpluses) in the mid-eighties reached an all-time high, but the era of dehospitalization had begun. Congress responded by authorizing very small increases in PPS payments for each of the following years and did not give the hospitals an increase as large as overall medical inflation until 1989. Profits and surpluses quickly dropped to razor-thin levels, and many hospitals ran deficits. Admissions and length of stay continued to decline. In addition, peer review had been greatly strengthened so that the newly restructured Peer Review Organizations contracted with the government for specific target reductions in surgical and other procedures.

Unshackling Competition

Besides strong buyer action, the health care system was challenged by price competition, which had been suppressed since the turn of the century. In a landmark case involving the issuance of a fee schedule by the Virginia Bar Association, the United States Supreme Court ruled for the first time that "learned professions" were not exempt from antitrust laws (*Goldfarb* 1975). The Court even dismissed the argument that the fee schedule had been approved by the Supreme Court of Virginia and was therefore exempt as a state action. It was price-fixing, plain and simple. Within months the Federal Trade Commission began gathering evidence against medical societies and several specialty societies for restricting advertisement by members and restraining price competition (Pollard 1981). Soon the dominance of hospital administrators on Blue Cross and physicians on Blue Shield boards came under scrutiny. Laws which the medical profession had put through against the corporate practice of medicine and against prepaid health care plans came under attack. In short, the entire structure of legal protections against competitors began to crumble (Havighurst 1980; Weller 1985; Gee 1989). Moreover, many states began to pass new laws in the late 1970s and 1980s to facilitate the creation of HMOs and PPOs.

If one believes that shifts in the law usually reflect shifts in the body politic, and especially in priorities of major interest groups, then the *Goldfarb* case and several other key cases reviewed by the Supreme Court or other senior courts must be seen as part of the profession's fall from grace and the rise of institutional buyers (Havighurst 1980).

These major court decisions also reflect the almost sacred status which competition holds in American culture. The assumption in most textbooks and conversations is that competition fosters not only high quality at the lowest price, but also efficiency, productivity, democracy, and liberty. One does not hear about the cases of competition producing dislocation, waste, higher prices, inefficiency, deception, or inferior quality. The Supreme Court captured the competition ethos when it wrote:

> The Sherman act was designed to be a comprehensive charter of economic liberty aimed at preserving free and unfettered competition as the rule of trade. It rests on the premise that the unrestrained interaction of competitive forces will yield the best allocation of our economic resources, the lowest prices, the highest quality and the greatest material progress, while at the same time providing an environment conducive to the preservation of our democratic political and social institutions. (356 U.S. 4 1958)

Evidence for competition doing all these things in health care is scant.

In addition, buyer dominance conflicts with competition as a strategy for keeping costs in line. Strong restraining actions by monopoly *buyers* are as anti-competitive as are restraining actions by monopoly sellers, even though the buyers may say they are fostering competition. The Reagan administration, for example, talked about PPS being competitive, but it was basically price-fixing on a grand scale. And it worked, as far as it went.

In 1989, Congress adopted legislation calling for a major revision of Medicare's physician payment system. Key provisions of the multifaceted approach included: limits on balanced billing, establishment of a value performance system and the phasing in over a five-year period of a national, resource-based, relative value fee schedule. But while this may be enlightened policy because it redresses the payment imbalance between time spent with the patient and the performance of technical procedures, and while it may work, it is not competition. From a competitive point of view, buyers and sellers coming together to design jointly an efficient, cheap delivery system is conspiracy. Setting maximum ceilings on fees is price-fixing just as much as setting minimum fees. Given all the difficulties in creating competitive conditions in health care, a competition strategy may destroy whatever professional altruism there once was, commercialize medical care for the sick, and induce providers to play elaborate games in the marketplace without saving much money. Is it buyer dominance we want or competition? And if the answer is competition, are we ready to favor competition when the market becomes again a sellers' market, as the baby-boom generation becomes old?

Conclusions

This new interpretation of how the American health care system developed illustrates the degree to which its legal, institutional, and economic features were built to minimize price competition and cost containment by institutional buyers. These features haven't changed. Medical schools still train each student cohort and provide leadership for the entire profession in state-of-the-art clinical medicine, subspecialization, and new technology—the core values of the professional model and a chief cause of escalating costs (Light 1989). Licensing and certification rules form a battlement around this core of the professionally driven health care system. By the end of the 1980s, after twenty years of efforts to restrain the rise of medical expenses using partial forms of regulation and competition, the pace of increase has not slowed. Physicians and the incentives of the payment system they designed remain largely in place, outcries from the profession notwithstanding.

Although many of the laws which organized medicine put in place to prevent competitive medicine have recently been removed or changed, in many states the corporate practice of medicine is still illegal (Rosoff 1986-7).These laws have just not been invoked—so far. But pressure to do so may mount as a growing number of talented, ambitious, and debt-laden doctors begin practice each year at a rate two and a half times the rate of physicians who stop practicing.

Most important, the public still wants the best medical care possible and may sue if dissatisfied. A court decision in 1986 from the Second Appellate District Court in Los Angeles also makes the third party (i.e., the buyer/insurer) liable for omitted services (*Wickline v. Medi-Cal in Medical Benefits* 1986). Thus a reasonable prediction is that the revolt of institutional buyers will significantly increase accountability at all levels and integrate services to reflect more fully consumers' needs, but providers will still control many parts of the system, and not much money may be saved (Light 1984). Instead, we may see a profound restructuring of the American health system towards ambulatory and home care spanning a wide spectrum of clinical services, organized in "efficient" corporate forms that nonetheless produce a great deal of administrative expense and unnecessary investment in the name of choice and efficiency.

REFERENCES

Bodenheimer, Tom, Steve Cummings and Elizabeth Harding, eds. 1972. *Billions for Bandaids.* San Francisco:Medical Committee for Human Rights.

Bulletin of the American Academy of Medicine. 1909. X(1): special section 587–631.

Burrow, James G. 1963. *A.M.A: Voice of American Medicine.* Baltimore:The Johns Hopkins University Press.

Burrow, James G. 1971. *Organized Medicine in the Progressive Era: The Move Toward Monopoly.* Baltimore:The Johns Hopkins University Press.

Caplan, Ronald L. 1981. Pasturized patients and profits: The changing nature of self-care in American medicine. Ph.D. diss. Department of Economics, University of Massachusetts, Amherst.

Coburn, D., G. M. Torrance and J. Kaufert. 1983. Medical dominance in Canada in historical perspective: Rise and fall of medicine? *International Journal of Health Services* 13:407–432.

Davis, Karen. 1975. *National Health Insurance: Benefits, Costs, and Consequences.* Washington, D.C.:The Brookings Institution.

Ehrenreich, Barbara & John Ehrenreich. 1971. *The American Health Empire: Power, Profits and Politics.* New York:Vintage.

Falkson, Joseph L. 1980. *HMOs and the Politics of Health System Reform.* Chicago:American Hospital Association and Robert J. Brady Co.

Ferguson, Charles W. 1937. *Fifty Million Brothers: A Panorama of American Lodges and Clubs.* New York:Farrar & Rinehart.

Fortune. January 1970. Special issue: Our ailing medical system.

Gee, M. Elizabeth. 1989. FTC antitrust actions in health care services. Washington, D.C.:Federal Trade Commission, typescript.

Gist, Noel P. 1940. Secret societies: A cultural study of fraternalism in the United States. *The University of Missouri Studies* XV(4):entire issue.

Goldberg, Lawrence G. and Warren Greenberg. 1978. The emergence of physician-sponsored health insurance: A historical perspective." In *Competition* in the Health Care Sector: Past, Present, and Future, edited by Warren Greenberg Germantown, MD.:Aspen Systems.

Goldfarb v. Virginia State Bar 95 S. Ct. 2004 (1975).

Goldfinger, Stephen E. 1987. A Matter of Influence. New England Journal of Medicine 316:1408–9.

Greenberg, Selig. 1971. The Quality of Mercy: A Report on the Critical Condition of Hospital and Medical Care in America. New York:Antheneum.

Haley, Edward E. et al. 1911. The evils of the contract system. New York State Journal of Medicine 11:394–6.

Havighurst, Clark C. 1980. Anti-trust enforcement in the medical services industry: What does it all mean? Milbank Memorial Fund Quarterly 58:89–123.

Kennedy, Edward. 1972. In Critical Condition. New York: Simon & Schuster.

Langford, T. S., A. S. Kimball, H. B. Garner, E. H. Flynn, T. E. DeGurse. 1907. Report of the committee on contract practice. Journal of the Michigan State Medical Society VI:377–380.

Larkin, Gerald. 1983. Occupational Monopoly and Modern Medicine. London:Tavistock.

Leland, Roscoe G. 1932. Contract Practice. Chicago: American Medical Association.

Lexchin, Joel. 1987. Pharmaceutical promotion in Canada: Convince them or confuse them." International Journal of Health Services 17:77–89.

Light, Donald W. 1984. Overstated gains in the war on health costs. The New York Times, August 6, 1984:30.

Light, Donald W. 1988. Toward a new sociology of medical education. Journal of Health and Social Behavior 29:307–322.

Light, Donald W. and Alexander Schuller. 1986. Political Values and Health Care: The German Experience. Cambridge, MA:MIT Press.

Lytle, Albert T. 1915. Contract medicine—An economic study. New York State Journal of Medicine 15:103–6.

Medical Benefits. 1986. Payers can be held liable for care limits. (October) 15:3.

Mintz, M. 1967. By Prescription Only, 2nd ed. revised. Boston:Houghton Mifflin.

Pollard, Michael R. 1981. The essential role of antitrust in a competitive market for health Services. Milbank Memorial Fund Quarterly 59:256–268.

Rayack, Elton. 1967. Professional Power and American Medicine: The Economics of the American Medical Association. Cleveland:World Publications Co.

Reed, Louis. 1947. Blue Cross and Medical Service Plans. Washington:Federal Security Agency.

Relman, Arnold S. 1980. The New Medical-Industrial Complex. The New England Journal of Medicine 303 (17):963–970.

Ribicoff, Abraham with Paul Danaceau. 1972. The American Medical Machine. New York:Saturday Review Press.

Richardson, J.T. 1945. The origins and development of group hospitalization in the United States, 1890–1940. The University of Missouri Studies XX:entire issue.

Rorem, C. Rufus. 1940. Non-profit Hospital Service Plans. Chicago:Commission on Hospital Service.

Rorem, C. Rufus and Robert P. Fischelis. 1932. The Costs of Medicine. Chicago:University of Chicago Press.

Rosen, George. 1983. The Structure of American Medical Practice 1875–1941. Philadelphia:University of Pennsylvania Press.

Rosoff, Arnold J. 1986–7. The business of medicine: Problems with the corporate practice of medicine doctrine. Cumberland Law Review 17:485–503.

Schwartz, Jerome L. 1965. Early history of prepaid medical care plans. Bulletin of the History of Medicine 39:450–475.

Selleck, Henry B. with Alfred H. Whittaker. 1962. Occupational Health in America. Detroit:Wayne State University Press.

Sigmond, Robert M. 1989. Oral History Interview (spring).

Starr, Paul. 1982. The Social Transformation of American Medicine. New York:Basic Books.

Stevens, Rosemary. 1971. American Medicine and the Public Interest. New Haven:Yale University Press.

Stevens, Rosemary. 1989. In Sickness and in Wealth. New York:Basic Books.

Vogel, Morris. 1980. The Invention of the Modern Hospital. Chicago:University of Chicago Press.

Warner, John Harley. 1986. Therapeutic Perspectives: Practice, Knowledge and Identity in America 1820–1885. Cambridge, MA:Harvard University Press.

Weber, Max. 1968. Economy and Society: An Outline of Interpretive Sociology. Edited by Guenther Roth and Claus Wittich, New York:Beminster Press.

Weller, Charles D. 1983. The primacy of standard antitrust Analysis in Health Care. Toledo Law Review 14:609–637.

Wennberg, John. 1984. Dealing with medical practice variations: A proposal for action. Health Affairs 3:6–32.

Williams, Pierce. 1932. The Purchase of Medical Care Through Fixed Periodic Payments. New York: National Bureau of Economic Research.

Willis, Evan 1983. Medical Dominance: The Division of Labour in Australian Health Care. Sydney:Allen and Unwin.

Wilsford, David, 1987. The cohesion and fragmentation of organized medicine in France and the United

States. *Journal of Health Politics, Policy and Law* 12:481–504.

Woodruff, John V. 1916. Contract practice. *New York State Journal of Medicine* 16:507–511.

Chapter 4

The Political Economy of Health Services:

A Review of Major Ideological Influences

Roger M. Battistella

James W. Begun

Robert J. Buchanan

The attention now commanded by health policy in the national political affairs of the United States is warranted by the enormously strategic position that health services occupy in the general economy, and by public aspirations for the good life. It is also a reflection of the requirements for accountability that have accompanied the increased dependence of consumers and providers on public financing.

Due to developments such as the aging of the population, the growing importance of diseases that require lengthier and costlier forms of treatment, and the rising demands for equity in the distribution and quality of publicly funded services, government is under constant pressure to increase the size of health outlays. This pressure is occurring, however, at a time of severe macroeconomic disturbances stemming from the financial burden of servicing massive accumulations of public and private debt, the difficulty of maintaining economic superiority in an increasingly global economy, and the threatened gradual decline in living standards due to disincentives for savings and economically productive long-term investments. Additional disturbances stem from the diversion of national resources to military spending and from the ascendancy of political ideology wary of growth in the size of central government and federal spending for social programs.

Since resource scarcity first attracted serious national attention in the early 1970s, following a lengthy post-World War II prosperity in which affluence was popularly assumed to have become a permanent condition of American life, efficiency has emerged as the solution of choice to the dilemma of how to do more without spending more. Disagreement over means, however, produced a welter of confusing and contradictory initiatives, running the gamut from command planning and regulation to market competition, in which failure was the single constant. Frustration over the inability to contain costs has fueled doubts about the value of health spending and concentrated policy more sharply on organizational and financial modifications for improving health-services quality and targeting government spending on the truly needy. (Battistella and Buchanan 1987).

The dissatisfaction and skepticism accompanying the succession of failures to control expenditures obscures recognition of some remarkable health policy achievements that began in the 1960s. These include the virtual elimination of the hospital and physicians' services utilization gap between upper- and low-income people; the modernization and technological upgrading of the nation's hospitals; the return to the community of many physically and mentally disabled persons previously destined to spend their lives in oppressive institutional settings; the correction of aggregate deficiencies in the supply of health personnel; and the improved protection of the aged and low-income groups against the high cost of medical services. Whether attributable to health services or other causes, a notable increase in life expectancy also has benefited. U.S. citizens (Roemer 1980a). Another largely unrecognized achievement has been the progress made in converting the organizational and managerial profile of health services from turn-of-the-century handcraft to modern industrial-corporate lines (Battistella and Weil 1986).

Against this backdrop of mixed and confused events, the political-economic examination of health services in the United States is undertaken. Political-economic inquiry involves the study of changes in economic relationships and the composition of political power within a framework of superordinate values regarding what is fair and just. In the ensuing analysis, health policy is presented largely as the outcome of the interplay of political and economic orientations whose influence has varied over time. For convenience, these orientations have been organized under four principal headings: the normative approach, the rationalist approach, the neoconservative approach, and the neo-Marxist approach. After a description of each of these four ideological approaches is presented, their significance in the evolution of postwar national health policy is discussed and the prospects for continuing equity gains are assessed in the light of the increased economic drive for efficiency and cost containment.

The Normative Approach

The predominant approach to health services in the United States until recently has been normative in character. That is to say, individuals and groups have sought to influence the role of government in the health services field mainly on the basis of strong convictions about what is or ought to be highly valued. Disagreement has arisen over the extent to which government programs depart from goals perceived to be important (Donabedian 1973).

At the core of policy disputes one can usually discern the influence of the enlightenment philosophers (Locke, Hobbes, Montesquieu, and Rousseau in particular), whose perspectives on human nature and the function of government gave justification to American independence and inspired the formulation of human rights guaranteed in the U.S. Constitution. Among the more important concepts associated with this school of thought are individual freedom, equality, compassion, fraternalism, and the malevolence or benevolence of power.

Normative positions on general philosophical issues are often used in the classification of political parties and actions of government. Individuals and groups believing that human nature, though mixed, is essentially good or perfectible, that human intelligence is superior to natural forces in problem solving, and that government is largely an instrument for the advancement of individual and community welfare are classified as liberal. Individuals and groups taking a less sanguine view of human nature and exhibiting a distrust of power, especially in government, are usually classified as conservative. These value differences are the source of most controversies over the direction and control of health services.

The normative approach to health services emerges clearly in the uncompleted saga of national health insurance in the United States. Armed with the knowledge of precedents of governmental intervention in Germany and England, under conditions of widespread unemployment and medical needs similar to those then prevailing in the United States, reformers at the turn of the century unsuccessfully sought to humanize many of the demeaning aspects of charity and welfare medicine institutionalized in practices derived from Elizabethan Poor law. In doing so, they endeavored to establish the principle that health services ought to be provided as a right on the basis of medical need regardless of ability to pay (Davis 1975).

After nearly 50 years of ceaseless but unfulfilled striving, these efforts were rewarded partially with the passage of Medicare in 1965, which established a compulsory program of hospital benefits for retired and disabled workers along with a voluntary program of physicians' benefits for the aged. Treatment of end-stage renal disease for all age groups was included in 1972. At the same time, reformers succeeded in vastly enlarging the influence of the federal government in the operation of state and local public assistance programs, in eliminating some of the harsher features of eligibility tests, and in broadening the reach of welfare medical programs beyond the indigent to include the working poor. Most of these gains were incorporated in the Medicaid program (Fein 1986).

Marked by sharp ideological divisions, the battle for national health insurance swirled around the issue of whether access to health care was a privilege or a right. Arrayed on the side of privilege were the professional interest groups, the American Medical Association (AMA), the American Hospital Association (AHA), and the American Dental Association (ADA). They feared restrictions on their freedom to pursue unrestricted economic rewards, their autonomy in clinical decision making, and their powers for self-regulation and governance. Their cause was championed by political, commercial, and manufacturing organizations, such as the National Association of Manufacturers, the Chamber of Commerce, and the Young Americans for Freedom, which tended to regard themselves as custodians of competitive market values (Bowler 1978).

Both sides of the national health insurance issue received considerable support from academic economists. Competitive market economists, led by Milton Friedman (1962), maintained, both then and now, that medical care is a private good in that the benefits accrue to the individual rather than society. The implications for groups outside the labor force through no fault of their own, retirees and the permanently and totally disabled, were frequently obscured in abstract polemics exalting the competitive market as an instrument for maximizing individual freedom and economic efficiency (Lindsay 1980).

Because competitive market proponents consider medical care to be much like economic goods and services in general, they, to the consternation of many of their allies in the medical profession, assert that restricting the practice of medicine to licensed doctors of medicine is an abridgement of market efficiency and an enticement to abuse. This is the logical result of their belief that human nature is incorrigibly acquisitive and selfish. Conservative economists are prepared to make only the slightest allowance for negative health care externalities endangering the welfare of others connected to environmental pollution, and such lifestyle hazards as smoking and alcohol and drug abuse. To the fullest extent practical, they prefer market incentives (taxes and fines) rather than publicly administered programs to safeguard community well-being (Fein 1980).

On the other hand, economists immersed in the sociopolitical history of medicine stress the vulnerability of the sick to exploitation in the marketplace due to the special dimension of anguish in illness and other constraints on consumer rationality. The professional status of medicine is seen as an instrument for community integration as well as the enrichment of individual welfare. Economists holding that health care is a right typically argue that spending for maternal and child health services and the working-age population is a good investment in economic growth.

Perhaps the best recognized defense of the special character of health service is that prepared by Kenneth Arrow (1963), who concluded that health services are based largely on non-market relationships that substantially curtail the relevance of competition theory. Sociologists opposed to using the market to ration health services, on the other hand, tend to underscore the moral and utilitarian aspects of health services. The late Talcott Parsons (1951), for example, was foremost among his colleagues in the scholarly defense of the idea that health care is a social good.

Shortcomings of the Normative Approach

The normative approach to health policy prevailed up to the mid-1960s. Since then it has fallen into disfavor. Critics deride the normative approach for being "value laden," for being overly disputatious and rhetorical, and for using data to buttress policy preferences rather than scientific aims (Battistella 1972a).

The accusation in brief is that normative analysis tends to simplify the issues and portrays antagonists in hues of good and evil. For example, organized medicine, led by the AMA, often was pictured by reformers as a reactionary monolith, whereas groups favoring reforms in the organization and financing of solo fee-for-service medicine were stereotyped by status-quo adherents as disciples of subversive socialist and communist teachings. Likewise, progress in the implementation of welfare state principles was characterized as well-intentioned but impractical foolishness or, conversely, as tangible proof of the innately noble affinity of human nature for altruism and justice (Battistella and Wheeler 1978). Amidst such ideological sparring, impulses to enlist government in campaigns against poverty invited denunciation of such involvement as disguised paternalism that does more to perpetuate dependency on public programs than to advance responsibility and independence among the disadvantaged.

Criticism of the normative approach, however, is not without fault either. It is seldom dispassionate, since it originates from interests advocating a purportedly superior alternative. Also, the handicaps under which the normative approach functioned were rarely acknowledged. One such handicap that invited appeals to emotion rather than reason was the shortage of reliable data to guide decision making. For example, nationwide registration of births did not occur until 1933. Reliable information on the populations's need for health services was not available until passage of the National Health Survey Act of 1956, which provided for a continuing survey and special studies of sickness and disability in the nation. Later improvements produced an explosion in the amount of information on the cost effectiveness of new technologies and the quality and economy of services given by providers. Finally,

considerable progress has been made in the co-ordination of intergovernmental statistical reporting systems and in the disaggregation of data for subnational health services planning, monitoring and evaluation (Jonas 1981).

The fact that proponents of social justice in the availability of health services typically are characterized as misguided idealists or worse, in contrast to proponents of free enterprise medicine who often are viewed more favorably, mirrors a powerful attachment to private market values in U.S. culture. The emotional power of this belief system poses a barrier to impartial study and discussion. In the past, organized hospital and medical interests opposing reforms adroitly deflected criticism by ensconcing themselves behind rhetorical bulwarks in defense of free enterprise (Harris 1966).

Free enterprise values have successfully withstood the postwar advance of welfare state services. Notwithstanding a substantial increase in public spending following passage of Medicare and Medicaid in the mid-1960s, the nation's health sector remains predominantly private. Public outlays for example, represent only about two-fifths of total health spending, in marked contrast to other highly industrialized free market nations in Western Europe where the public share averages nearly four-fifths of all health expenditures (Schieber and Poullier 1987). The United States, moreover, remains the only major industrial power without a comprehensive national health insurance program (Simanis 1980). Finally, the situation in the health sector closely resembles that of the economy as a whole, where government spending accounts for only about 37 percent of the gross national product (GNP). In many other highly developed western and northern European countries on the other hand, the amount of national wealth commanded by government runs between 48 and 63 percent (Organization for Economic Co-Operation and Development 1987).

Growth of Government Intervention in the Health Sector

Although the United States is less a welfare state than other highly industrialized market economies, substantial changes have occurred in the political economy of health services. The enshrinement of free market values in national folklore and in medical politics masks a slow but steady advance of governmental intervention. From the Great Depression to the present, the perception of health services has changed from a private good to a public good, with the result that the U.S. government is now involved with health services in a big way.

Paradoxically, some of the greatest pressures for increased public financing and regulation have come from decisions taken to buttress and preserve the private features of U.S. health services (Ebenstein et al. 1970). The collapse of the national economy in the decade before World War II not only strained the ability of state and local government to continue vital public health services, but also it signaled financial ruin for voluntary hospitals deprived of patient revenues and philanthropic funds. In both cases, the federal government intervened to lend the necessary assistance.

A wartime ruling by the Supreme Court that relaxed wage and price controls to allow labor unions to bargain for health insurance and other fringe benefits helped restore the flow of provider revenues from private-paying patients. However, access to capital remained a problem. At the behest of the American Hospital Association, the government enacted the Hospital Survey and Construction Act of 1946, popularly known as the Hill-Burton Program, to discourage harmful competition among hospitals within the same service area and to subsidize the construction of new beds in medically underserved areas (Commission on Hospital Care 1947). As the economy unexpectedly prospered after the war, the federal program became established as a principal source of money for plant modernization and expansion.

Widespread doubt, however, over the ability of unfettered free markets to allocate scarce capital efficiently, subsequently led the states and federal governments in the 1960s and 1970s to limit new construction, plant modernization, and major technology acquisitions to hospitals complying with certificate-of-need criteria (CON) set by planning agencies. Notwithstanding the political unpopularity of compulsory planning among health providers and eventual withdrawal of fed-

eral funding, CON programs continue to play a role in capital allocation, largely as a check against the costly overlap and duplication invited by unregulated competition. (Another Upset for Health Planning 1987).

Public subsidies also were instrumental to overcoming shortages of health professionals. From 1965 to 1985, the number of medical schools grew from 84 to 127, and since 1970, when efforts to expand the number of physicians began to take hold, the number of active physicians has grown by nearly 67 percent. That the principal worry today is one of oversupply (Ginzberg 1985; Clare et al. 1987) reflects the success of this endeavor. These subsidies were the product of supply-side economic thinking. The supposition was that once deficiencies due to inadequate productive capacity and to the barrier effects of high tuition costs were corrected, market forces would result in a redistribution of physicians from medically overserved to underserved areas and from specialties in which there was an oversupply, to those requiring more practitioners. Much to the chagrin of unregulated market adherents, however, this did not happen.

Whereas the unexpected expansion of the postwar economy made it possible to enrich the package of private health insurance benefits provided to enrollees, competition between profit-making and nonprofit-making carriers resulted in the erosion of arrangements designed to bring insurance within the financial reach of many low-income and high-risk individuals. Unlike community rating in which everyone paid the same regardless of health status, experience rating methods favored by commercial carriers assigned premiums such that the groups most in need of protection (the sickest people) were required to pay the most. As it became harder for aged and low-income people to be insured privately, there was a corresponding resurgence of the hospital bad debt problem and political agitation from population groups deprived of access to private care. The enactment of Medicare and Medicaid was an accommodation to these strains pursued in the context of prevailing free-enterprise values (Harris 1966).

The popular retrospective interpretation of Medicare and Medicaid as economic and administrative failures underscores an important lesson from U.S. health policy—the design of publicly funded medical care programs is influenced less by dictates for efficiency than by cultural tradition and political philosophy. Other highly developed countries choosing to finance health services centrally under a unified system of planning and administration have achieved far greater results in raising health standards while spending considerably less of their gross national product (Roemer 1980b).

The mammoth capital requirement of biomedical research was another important force in drawing the federal government more deeply into the health services field. The perception that scientific medicine had reached the takeoff stage, and that the conquest of many dreaded diseases was imminent, fueled a veritable explosion of federal support after World War II. Beginning with the creation of the National Cancer Institute in 1937, the number of federally sponsored national research centers has multiplied to the point where the National Institutes of Health is a conglomerate of specialized research institutes with an annual operating budget of nearly $4 billion (Rushmer 1980; Ginzberg 1985).

Further intervention followed in the wake of the revelation that orthodox supply and demand relationships do not work well in the health sector. Experience revealed that subsidies to expand supply and productivity did not function as predicted by economic theory. Increasing the supply of physicians and hospital beds and the introduction of sophisticated technology failed to lower prices and redistribute services more evenly. To the contrary, they compounded problems of costs and maldistribution. For reasons largely accepted as peculiar to the health field, it was concluded that supply created its own demand (Fein 1980).

Passage of the Comprehensive Health Planning Act of 1966 and its farther-reaching successor, the National Health Planning and Resources Development Act of 1974, limited the unilateral powers of hospitals to expand and modernize and restricted new hospitals in their choice of location. Enactment of the Professional Standards Review Organization Program in 1972 constrained the freedom of physicians with respect to the admission of patients to hospitals and lengths of stay, and opened clinical decisions to compulsory scrutiny by medical peers. Finally, the provision of federal incentives for the spread of prepaid group practice vis-a-vis the Health Maintenance Organization Act of 1973 struck at the heart of free enterprise medicine by challenging the viability of solo fee-for-service practice.

Rationalist Approach

Although the factors responsible are in dispute, the dominant presence of government in the health sector nevertheless was an established fact before the 1960s ended—if not as a percentage of total spending, then certainly in terms of fiscal leverage and the growth of planning and regulatory activities.

Against a backdrop of sharp controversy throughout the 1970s over the appropriateness of a larger federal presence in the health sector, the simultaneous escalation of previously modest and unconnected rates of inflation and unemployment spurred broad agreement on the need to constrain health spending. Inaction was rejected as too costly, because annual price increases for hospital and health services historically had been growing at twice the rate of increase as for consumer goods and services in general. For reasons yet undetermined, Medicare and Medicaid caused the gap to widen (Council on Wage and Price Stability 1976). Demands to contain health costs were amplified and a general conviction emerged that some form of national health insurance was inevitable (U.S. Department of Health, Education and Welfare 1976).

Higher unemployment compounded the strains on government budgets. Loss of wages and private health insurance among the unemployed expanded the size of the population eligible to receive Medicaid coverage and public assistance. Less apparent were the social costs of prolonged unemployment. Subject to different lead times, the combination of physical deprivation and emotional-mental stress was documented to be highly correlated with higher rates of suicide, homicide, criminal activities, infant mortality, cardiovascular disease, cirrhosis, and mental hospital admissions (U.S. Joint Economic Committee 1980b). Another unanticipated consequence of recession was the inducement for financially-squeezed states to shift welfare costs to the federal government. Creative accounting practices and program restructuring were commonly used by the states to maximize the federal contribution in shared-financial-responsibility services (Bulgaro and Webb 1980).

Additional financial concerns stemmed from the growth in spending for other social welfare services which together with health spending accounted for roughly one-half of the federal budget. While some observers celebrated this as an irrefutable signal of the triumph of welfare-state principles, others fretted about the demise of conservative economic and political values. Still others became apprehensive about the implications of changes in the composition of the federal budget for productivity and for the ability to generate savings sufficient to finance investments in economic growth necessary to pay for social services (Janowitz 1976).

The political and economic tensions accumulating during this period from the activism of government and the ascendancy of welfare-state principles helped to provoke the reaction against the normative approach to policy decision making. Although conflict among overtly competing values helped to define issues and solutions, there often was a steep price to pay in terms of legislative paralysis. Additionally, the unwillingness to compromise and cooperate obstructed sound public administration and program evaluation. These shortcomings prompted interest in alternatives for expediting decision making (Battistella and Smith 1974). The sheer magnitude of health outlays, moreover, stirred curiosity about the returns to society. In combination with mounting concerns over the share of national wealth consumed by government, these concerns prompted efforts to quantify the costs and benefits of government programs (Battistella and Smith 1974).

Increased political conflict due to a slowing of economic growth on the one hand and rising demands for more and better services on the other propelled the emergence of techniques for depoliticizing decision making. In the prevailing zero-sum decision making environment, elected officials, typically harried by the complaints of unhappy constituents and job insecurity, were predisposed to welcome the introduction of purportedly objective and value-free decision-making methods which diffused responsibility for unpopular decisions. Because these methods

characteristically involve an economic or technical means-end orientation in which the calculation of self-interest is synonymous with rational behavior, this form of decision making is described in the policy-analysis literature as the rationalist approach[1] (Smith 1978).

Resisted at first by health professionals socialized in the venerable code of medical ethics that rejects the placement of a monetary value on health and life, the rationalist approach ultimately prevailed, and skepticism concerning the application of quantitative methods became more the exception than the rule (Smith 1978). Familiarity with cost-benefit analysis, systems analysis, program budgeting, zero-based budgeting, and other quantitative techniques, especially in the areas of accounting and finance, became widely established as evidence of managerial competence.

The significance of the rationalist approach extends beyond the introduction of decision-making techniques. It encompasses belief in the efficiency of centralized administration, economies of scale, and scientific management and planning principles. These principles comprise the management paradigm of big business. In searching for efficiency and effectiveness, health professionals intuitively look to big business and industry in the hope that the latter's presumably superior management methods can be transferred (Battistella and Chester 1972; Battistella 1985).

Unlike the image of clarity and conciseness as-

---

[1]Use of the label "rationalist" to identify this school of thought is not meant to imply that the approach is more "rational" than the normative approach (or, for that matter, the neomarxist and neoconservative perspectives introduced later in this chapter.) Both approaches are rational since they make the same use of reason, are subject to the same rules of logic, and are ultimately subject to the same test of how closely they match reality. The distinction is that one approach (the normative) starts with certain overt beliefs about what should be based on philosophical convictions. In purporting to deal solely with what can be measured, the other approach (rationalist) conceals from view the behavioral assumptions underlying quantitative methods. In point of fact, both are value laden, since both are based on beliefs about how people should behave. The term "rationalist" is used because of its prominence in the field of policy analysis and to highlight the political implications of allegedly objective-quantitative methods. Another choice would have been to substitute the work "empirical" for "rationalist." The authors are indebted to Edmund D. Pellegrino for his suggestion to clarify the reasons for choosing the "rationalist" label.

sociated with decision making in the private sector, the term "scientific management" is somewhat vague. Among believers in competition, scientific management achieves cost control and efficiency payoffs from market discipline and the application of quantitative methods in cost accounting, finance, marketing, and production. Among non- believers, however, the purpose of these methods is to escape market discipline through the substitution of corporate power and planning for idealized laws of supply and demand. The confusion is multiplied by the contradiction whereby those actually engaged in planning retain ideological loyalty to the sanctity of economic and political relationships derived from the theory of perfect competition (Battistella and Chester 1972).

The ascension of the rationalist approach coincided with a period of increased activity in the restructuring of health services. The attainment of a more rational organizational pattern of hospital and physicians' services, with fewer but larger vertically-integrated units of production caring for defined populations, was an aspiration that transcended political differences in the health politics of the 1970s. The commonly agreed upon goal was to reconstruct health services delivery from a "cottage industry" to a modern corporate structure (Battistella 1972a). Since then, the influence of this orientation has multiplied considerably and now constitutes the main parameters within which policy is conducted (Battistella and Buchanan 1987).

The language and values of the rationalist approach have broad appeal. They capture a rich cultural folklore extolling the innate superiority of market forces over those of government. Their allure encompasses persons believing in the efficacy of scientific management, whether in the planning of health services or in the running of complex corporate enterprises.

The popularity of the rationalist approach facilitated the establishment of a consensus for change forceful enough to overcome the status quo in the organization of health services. The merger and consolidation movement among non-governmental community hospitals is but one significant example. Roughly two-fifths of all hospitals and one-third of all hospital beds in the United States can now be counted as components of multihospital systems. Between 1977 and 1984 the number of community general hospitals in multi-unit arrangements rose from 24 percent to 43 percent (Eastaugh 1987). Possibly more significant, given the strong tradition of solo fee–for–service medicine in the United States, is the growth of bureaucratic-contractual modes of medical practice. The percentage of office-based private practitioners in some form of group practice, not necessarily prepaid, presently approximates 50 percent, and an equal percentage now receive at least part of their income on a time-related basis, such as salary (U.S. Senate 1984). Additionally, about one-fourth of the nation's physicians have standing financial arrangements with hospitals (U.S. Senate 1984).

The ramifications of the rationalist approach for the restructuring of health services are manifold. Rationalist logic and values are imbedded in a number of diverse developments of the 1970s, such as health planning, health maintenance organizations, professional standards review organizations (since revised and renamed professional review organizations), and the imposition of quotas on the supply of medical graduates by specialty. It is unlikely that change of such magnitude could have occurred in such a brief period of time if the policy issues had remained as highly politicized as they were during the peak influence of the normative approach.

Shortcomings of the Rationalist Approach

In retrospect, much of the optimism accompanying the introduction of rationalist methods was misguided. Far more was promised than could be delivered (Battistella and Smith 1974), and many intrinsic weakness of the rationalist approach have become evident.

First, the claims that decisions should be based on facts alone and facts speak for themselves are vacuous. They suggest that irrefutably valid data are readily obtainable and that analytic methods for the accumulation of facts are value free. Policy decisions about Medicaid reimbursement for abortions, for example, are predominantly valuative ones. The same applies to national health insurance.

Second, the assumptions contained in rationalist models inadequately penetrate the complex environment in which decisions are taken. There

is nothing indisputably objective in the assignment of interest rates for establishing the relationship between values at different points in
time or the assignment of the opportunity cost of
capital diverted from more productive alternative
expenditures. These decisions are a matter of
judgment. They involve assumptions about the
future that are speculative, and they reflect the
values of the analyst. The assignment of high interest and discount rates discriminates against
taking actions that produce long-run benefits in
preference for the short run. The bias is compounded whenever the economy is beset by high
inflation.

Third, many aspects of good medical care are
difficult to quantify. For example, how is the increased quality of life experienced after kidney
transplantation measured and compared to the
quality of life of a kidney patient surviving on
dialysis? Overall, the purpose of medical intervention has become more ambiguous. The concept of cure has no application to the vast number of health problems constituting the bulk of
health needs today, such as chronic and mental
diseases and disabilities. Given the low likelihood of achieving a cure for disorders of this
sort, the total effect of medical intervention is
more important to assess, and this too is highly
subjective. Whether people are satisfied with the
caliber of medical services they receive and
whether they view themselves to be in good or
poor health are social-psychological phenomena
which are difficult to measure and have important effects on utilization of services and treatment outcomes.

For the most part, quantification in cost-benefit forms of analysis works best when what is
being studied is accurately reflected in conventional market activities and prices. Oftentimes,
the pressures for quantification so disregard
common sense that the equating of health-pro-
gram benefits with market values induces socially corrosive consequences. For instance,
when discounted future earnings are used to
quantify the value of saving lives, investments
in white male infants, because of differences in
expected lifetime earnings, are easier to justify
than are investments in black male infants.
Women are similarly disadvantaged by this
methodology, as are the elderly.

Fourth, rationality frequently is used as a guise

for action based on the philosophical precepts of
competitive market theory in which selfishness
and greed have been elevated to the status of a
moral system. The philosophical case of rational
analysis does not accept that medical acts are an
important aspect of the human relationship of
giving and receiving, constituting the moral experience of mutual help (Campbell 1978).

Fifth, the mounting realization that many
health policy issues are highly subjective and
qualitative suggests that allegedly objective techniques may be less important in the future. One
such issue involves medical technology and ethical rights to treatment and dignified death. Another centers on entitlements to publicly supported health services. The tradeoff between economic productivity and the quality of the environment is another example of the saliency of
issues that cannot be resolved independently of
political and social values. The controversy engendered by the medicalization of abortion and
court-ordered death sentences underscores the
moral dimensions of contemporary health policy.

Generally speaking, the application of the rational approach has not succeeded in meeting its
economic and efficiency objectives because the
delivery of health care is judged not only in efficiency terms but also in terms of fairness. If anything, there is reason to believe that it may have
exacerbated governmental efforts to contain
health care expenditures. Indeed, the "rational"
models behind the government's cost-containment strategy helped create situations in which
health care providers were given "perverse" economic incentives to defeat controls. Assessing
performance with commercial accounting principles, which measures success by profit and loss
responses to economic incentives, encouraged
providers to circumnavigate cost controls by arti-
ficially inflating the number of procedures performed or by underproviding medically appropriate services, depending on the method of reimbursement. Due to the inability of the rational
models to capture the complexities of the health
field, government found itself in the bizarre position of reimbursing hospitals for the services of
financial experts whose jobs entail devising ways
to manipulate or subvert cost-cutting policies
(Battistella and Eastaugh 1980a, 1980b).

Additional unintended consequences may

arise in the future from the application of the scientific management paradigm to services that are intrinsically labor intensive and highly personalized in nature. The scientific management outlook not only contains a bias for technological expansion capable of undermining priorities for cost containment, but it has a bureaucratic proclivity at variance with the essentially human dimensions of the doctor-patient relationship.

It is shortsighted to assume that most health policy problems can be solved by subjecting the medical profession to management discipline and control, especially with respect to primary care (Battistella and Rundall 1978a, 1978b). Such an assumption understates the value to society of the doctor-patient relationship in which the bond of mutual confidence and respect is the key for minimizing disruptions in social and economic activities, many of which are associated with anxieties and symptoms for which no clinical cause can be established. Given the limitations on the life span and the aging of the population, good health increasingly is the result "of physician and patient working together, often in the face of uncertainty and fear" (Fuchs 1974) rather than simple, one-time interventions ordered by the physician.

Neoconservative Approach

Interest groups which have successfully advocated larger health spending certainly merit recognition for corresponding improvements both in medical technology and in social and territorial equity. These successes, however, have not been without their consequences. Ironically, much opposition to future spending increases originates in the contention that present-day totals are too large. Health spending is regarded variously as having reached the stage of diminishing marginal social benefit or as a hindrance to economic growth. When considered in the light of a troubled national economy, the chances of sustaining currently high rates of annual increases in health spending are problematic.

Upwardly spiraling prices for health services which increase faster than the general rate of inflation attract inquiries about waste and inefficiency that buttress fears about throwing good money after bad. Inflation, moreover, feeds skepticism about whether a positive relationship continues to exist between health status and aggregate health outlays. Indeed, it is now generally accepted that non-health services, such as housing, nutrition, lifestyle, and environmental safety, are far more important to the quality of life and that the benefits of early diagnosis and treatment have been greatly overstated (McKinlay and McKinlay 1977; Ratcliffe et al. 1984). Counter evidence, for example, a 10 percent increase in per capita medical care use is associated with a 1.5 percent decrease in mortality rates (Hadley 1982), is either lost in the mass of criticism or interpreted as confirmation of the diminishing returns from health spending (Altman and Morgan 1983).

New economic circumstances foreshadow a readjustment of the liberal agenda for health services' reform. Although not always explicit in health policy polemics, the liberal platform traditionally rested on a number of well-reasoned assumptions. Most important of all was the belief that economic growth would produce the resources to create a more just society without anyone's suffering along the way. Prosperity would be sustained, moreover, by a sufficiently high birth rate for maintaining demand and by a large enough supply of gainfully employed workers to generate the funds to pay for health and social services allocated to the aged and the disabled (Donnison 1979). The favorable economic and political conditions prevailing at the time of the introduction of Medicare and Medicaid furthermore were expected to continue, thereby lessening the chances of a financially-driven backlash against an expanding government role. The crowning goal of reform was a system of universal health insurance in which comprehensive services were provided free at the time of use on the basis of medical need. These expectations, however, have been shaken by unforeseen economic and social developments.

Paradoxically, the same economic circumstances also produced a severe testing of orthodox conservative doctrine. Despite numerous external signs of a repudiation of planning and regulation and a preference for free-market solutions, current national health policy initiatives do not signify a triumph of conservative perseverance. While scarcity has reappeared according to prophecy, the chances of health care being redefined as a private good remain too remote to contemplate. No discernible improvements have occurred in closing the gaps between the theory of self-regulating competition and the actual practice of health services delivery. If anything, the gaps have become larger and more obvious. Turn-of-the-century views of the marketplace are too discordant with contemporary exigencies for rationalization and budgetary planning. Furthermore, uncategorical castigations of governmental intervention in the health sector are profoundly indifferent to public opinion and political reality. Medicare and Medicaid are not, as contended by pro-market dogmatists, a folly perpetrated out of ignorance, irrationality, or the machinations of special interest groups, but are an expression of the genuine will of the American people. Government-sponsored health programs are wanted because, as Fuchs (1979) has put it, they meet certain wants better than the alternatives do. Arcane arguments about whether health care services meet the test of a private or public good are largely irrelevant. Health has become established in public opinion as so sufficiently meritorious that it is regarded more as a right than a privilege.

On the other hand, it is equally naive for liberals to expect that a resurgence of economic growth will appreciably expand government's share of total health spending along the lines of the British National Health Service. Since 1983 the economy has enjoyed the longest peacetime expansion in the postwar era. Yet, the government's ability to absorb costly new social programs remains severely restricted. This by itself does not, however, indicate an end to governmental responsibility for redistributive justice. Public expectations for equity are too powerful for elected officials to disregard. Political reaction against inequality is intensified by the mounting misfortunes of many Americans, as reflected in the increasingly potent coalitions of consumers and health-care providers disturbed by problems of paying both for long-term nursing-home care and home-care services for the aged, and for the extension of health insurance coverage to the uninsured and underinsured.

The invocation of absolutes from the political left or the right belies the complexities of contemporary policy. The paramount imperatives for social cohesion point to an innovative search for balance and moderation in the pursuit of interdependent goals of equity and efficiency (Fuchs 1979). Acknowledgement of the necessity for a trade-off between these two goals constitutes the basis for a new political consensus joining pragmatically minded persons from left and right of center of the health policy spectrum.

In the policy literature the term "neoconservative" is commonly used as a designation for politically influential and intellectually stimulating left-of-center individuals who agree on the need for a more eclectic and pragmatic approach to social change. This conclusion results from their reexamination of many liberal precepts behind the social and political reforms of the past several decades (Steinfels 1979).

Neoconservatives may differ on important issues such as defense spending, affirmative action, and abortion, but they remain supportive of the basic contours of the welfare state. Neoconservatives also concur that the partnership between government and the private sector should be redefined to better accommodate the changing complexities of a mature economy in which low-productivity service industries constitute the principal source of employment. The dilemma of reconciling political aspirations for equality in an era of economic limits is an overarching preoccupation.

What constitutes ground for a distinct school of thought is an outlook emphasizing the constraints on political power to effect change and the virtues of public restraint in dealing with many social problems. In addition to focusing on the difficulties of establishing and sustaining the necessary consensus for effective action in today's social and political environment, neoconservatives are alert to the lengthening administrative and technical lead times required for the solution of many problems. This perspective prompts them to conclude that far more harm than good results from the sharp and erratic short-term actions typical of many current government policies. Neoconservatives also share a deep faith in individual opportunity and achievement, rather than parity among social groups through affirmative-action quotas, as the best pathway to human progress (Steinfels 1979).

The neoconservative label continues as a code word for pragmatism when applied to the field of health policy. Since the onset of macroeconomic malaise in the early 1970's, a heightened regard for what is affordable and attainable has diminished and blurred differences in how all but extreme conservatives and liberals approach health policy issues. This convergence, is apparent, for instance, in the broad-based Congressional support for free enterprise incentives as practical instruments for overcoming the strong resistance to restructuring and managerial reforms within the health sector (Battistella and Buchanan 1987). More so than any other single word, pragmatism best conveys the dominant intellect within the health-policymaking mainstream today.

The ability of the health sector to enlarge its share of the gross national product from 4.5 percent in 1950 to over 11 percent in 1988 was in large part due to the prevalence and depth of trust in some key assumptions, which collectively constituted the prevailing conventional wisdom. Among these were the following. First, concentrated, large-scale spending for biomedical research and development will significantly improve the population's life expectancy and health levels. Second, the best place to care for patients is in the hospital, since that is where the best technology and medical services are concentrated. Third, medical specialization is both necessary and desirable. In an era of rapid proliferation of knowledge and rising public expectations for technical competence, general practice and family medicine are outmoded. Fourth, spending for health services is finite because of the eventual satiation of unmet medical needs and the benefits of preventive medicine and health education. And fifth, the role of government in health services should be confined to restoring and buttressing the capital requirements of high-technology services and the purchasing power of consumers (Battistella 1972b).

Dissatisfaction among policy makers with the unintended consequences and failures of actions taken in accordance with these assumptions contributed to many of the present uncertainties about the future of public intervention in health care delivery. Contrary to a scenario of uninterrupted progress, it became increasingly evident during the 1970s that (1) spending opportunities for health services were limitless; (2) development of high-technology medical services was reaching the stage of diminishing marginal social benefits; (3) neglect of generalist, first-contact medical services was very costly in economic and human terms; (4) modern medical diagnosis and treatment inadvertently contributed to a surprisingly large amount of illness and disability; (5) there was an oversupply of hospital beds; (6) increasing the supply of physicians was not the solution to problems of maldistribution by location and type of practice; (7) it was perilous to rely on professional self-regulation alone for the attainment of goals of economy and quality; (8) unrealistically high public confidence in the benefits of medical treatment was resulting in the medicalization of many social problems that could be better dealt with through other means; and (9) the magnitude of health spending was an impediment to economic growth.

Skepticism and disillusionment about the value of health services were fostered by a succession of highly critical publications beginning early in the 1970s, both in the United States and abroad (Carlson 1975; Cochrane 1972; Fuchs 1974; Illich 1976; Lalonde 1974; Maxwell 1974; McKeown 1976; Pocincki et al. 1973; Powles 1973; Torrey 1974; U.S. House of Representatives 1976; U.S. Department of Health, Education and Welfare 1976).

The disassociation of many prominent health liberals from the conventional wisdom is possibly best exemplified in the specially prepared 1977 edition of *Daedalus,* "Doing Better and Feeling Worse: Health in the United States," edited by Dr. John H. Knowles (Knowles 1977). The issue contained a number of far-ranging revisionist interpretations by politically and intellectually influential authors such as David E. Rogers, Donald S. Frederickson, Lewis Thomas, and Renee Fox. The contributions to the publication were linked by a concern that despite the accomplishments of the U.S. health care system, things had recently gone badly and new solutions were required.

While harboring many dissimilar views, health policy neoconservatives have a common outlook regarding some of the more important choices affecting the future of health policy. Given the recency of conversion to this outlook,however, the neoconservative movement is less established in experience than in the extrapolation of logical consequences and probabilities.[1]

---

[1]The writings of Wildavsky (1979) and Glazer (1971) provide some insights into the application of the neoconservative philosophy to health care, as they are members of the broader neoconservative establishment who have commented specifically on health policy.

For the most part, health neoconservatives remain committed to the basic goals of the welfare state and retain a preference for equity over efficiency. On the other hand, they accept the reality of resource scarcity and concede the shortcomings of orthodox liberal doctrine geared to the uncompromised growth of health services and governmental intervention. Pragmatism is a distinguishing feature.

Health neoconservatives remain open to the possibility that pricing may be acceptable, but only under carefully specified conditions. In an age of limits, what purpose is served by encumbering public financing with services that are of questionable medical value? Assuming that appropriate technology assessment capabilities exist, it is both practical and desirable from a health-promotion and cost-savings standpoint to restrict public financing to services determined to meet safety and efficacy standards (U.S. Office of Technology Assessment 1980). Surely services of unproven safety have no place in the market in a society obligated to protect the health of its citizens, although nonharmful services of questionable efficacy might be left to the market. Nor is it defensible to continue payments for medically questionable and inappropriate diagnostic and treatment services when low income groups are being deprived of essential services because of constraints on federal and state government spending. The amount of money now spent on medically valueless or questionable procedures is generally conceded to equal 25 percent or more of all outlays (Mitchell and Virts 1986; Wolfe 1988).

The shortcomings of quantitative models and techniques notwithstanding, neoconservatives generally support efforts to better establish the effectiveness and costs of health services in comparison with alternative expenditures. In the interest of informed decision making, neoconservatives require, however, that the hidden values of putatively objective methods be made explicit and that the analyses not be skewed in ways that fail to capture the highly subjective contributions of health services (Wildavsky 1979).

Pricing may also be acceptable to pragmatists looking for ways to supplement revenues for health services, provided that price does not deter early diagnosis and treatment of efficacious services. In this respect, aggressive cost recovery through the assignment of patient charges based on income and ability to pay is increasingly advocated as a method for husbanding scarce public resources targeted for truly needy persons.

The experience of the 1970s suggests that even liberals not easily associated with neoconservatism recognize and support practical uses of the market. For example, in the case of health maintenance organization policy, liberal legislators and union allies sought to accelerate the growth of prepaid group practice by turning competitive market rhetoric against forces of organized medicine which in the past had successfully used the same tactic in defense of solo fee-for-service practice. Thus confronted, organized medicine no longer was able to condemn the transfiguration of solo fee-for-service practice as socialist-inspired malice (Ehrbar 1977). Nor did liberals hesitate to support the aggressive antitrust measures used by the Federal Trade Commission (FTC) to weaken the monopoly powers of the health professions—a move dramatically counter to long-standing historical justifications for the insulation of health services from unbridled competition and for the bestowal of professional privilege (Iglehart 1978).

Neoconservatives are inclined, furthermore, to believe that the principle of universalism at the core of liberal health policy is politically untenable in a poorly performing economy, and that the interests of the disadvantaged can be protected by the substitution of the principle of selectivity. The concept of a totally publicly financed and government operated service is dismissed as economically and politically unrealistic.

Shortcomings of the Neoconservative Approach

The shortcomings of the neoconservative approach in health policy approximate those of the generic neoconservative movement itself. Proponents of this approach often are viewed as having abandoned their commitment to justice and equity for political expediency. Neoconservativism lacks a clear and simple vision of a "just" society, promulgating instead an eclectic mix of applied principles fraught with ambiguity and inconsistency. Rather than proceeding along a single line, neoconservatives prefer multipronged strategies incorporating elements of regulation and competition. In the world of realpolitik to which they are attuned, the normal rules of mathematics are suspended and the shortest distance between two points is seldom a straight line. While brilliantly inspired, it is doubtful, however, whether the blurring of ideological divisions is conducive to generating and sustaining disciplined political energy for the long-term commitments necessitated by the complexity of many contemporary policy issues.

Putting an end to ideology implies, moreover, a narrow conceptualization of efficiency incompatible with democratic aspirations. In a democracy, ideological exchange serves a valuable function by educating people and alerting them to visions of what is right and just rather than what is workable.

Another hazard is the suppression of equity to economic priorities. With the tide of politics running in a fiscally conservative direction, the pressures for containing costs and governmental outlays are very strong. Eligibility and benefit reductions in government programs are unquestionably useful for budget-balancing purposes, but unless care is taken to minimize invidious privilege the social problems they create can far outweigh any of the economic savings (Fein 1980). The trade-off between efficiency and equity raises some disturbing questions, especially with respect to restricting publicly financed services solely to persons in need. If it makes good economic sense not to give services free to persons who can afford to pay for them privately, what are the longer run political and moral consequences of a system of health services segmented by differences in employment status, income, and age? Are programs for the poor destined to provide poor services whenever competition for scarce resources occurs between social groups?

The Neo-Marxist Approach

During the heyday of the normative era, defenders of the status quo in U.S. medicine displayed a penchant for reducing proposals for health services reform to the level of Marxist-inspired subversion and conspiracy. As a tactic for arousing public suspicion and diverting legislative attention from the substantive complexities of health policy, appeals to fears of subversive foreign ideologies were highly successful. From today's perspective, however, the spirit of reform was far less radical than the rhetoric suggested.

Health reformers promulgated the social aims of medicine: community integration, social and economic role performance, and disease prevention and health promotion. Proponents of social medicine stressed that society has an obligation to protect the health of its members and that social and economic conditions have an important effect on health and disease. They also shared a belief in the value of scientific investigation and study for improving the organization and delivery of health services (Rosen 1958).

Ironically, it was not until the normative approach was in the process of being displaced by rationalism that the Marxist presence was experienced openly in the U.S. health policy scene. Whether this was due to the political exhaustion of right-wing critics or the complacency of traditional health care reformers after passage of Medicare and Medicaid in the mid-1960s is difficult to establish.

Perhaps it represented an outpouring of frustration of the part of the Vietnam War generation whose idealism was shattered by the persistence of poverty and discrimination in an affluent society. Although still outside the mainstream of health policy, the insights and positions of the Marxist perspective are the subject of curiosity among policy makers as well as scholars and students.

To what extent recent Marxist writing qualifies for the "neo" designation is difficult to say. Much of it is steeped in classical themes of social class oppression resulting from capitalists' ownership of the modes of production and their resolute pursuit of profits above all else, including environmental protection, the safety and efficacy of foods and drugs, and the health of workers. The apotheosis of the working class as uncorrupted by materialism also persists, as does belief in the remedial effects of nationalization (Elling 1977; Krause 1977; Mckinlay 1979; Sidel 1977).

The chief difference today is in the focus. Rather than proceeding within the framework of entrepreneurial capitalism, contemporary Marxist analysis deals with the effects of new concentrations of power in advanced industrial societies. Hence inquiry is directed at managerial capitalism (the power of national and multinational corporations) and science and technology. Industrialism is regarded as an ideology, independent of private or state ownership, in which health and health services are subordinated to productivity and capital accumulation goals.

From this perspective, power gravitates one-sidedly to the managers of capital (not the owners), to technocrats possessing the necessary skills and knowledge, and to bureaucracies administering and regulating economic activity. One of the consequences is that traditional class conflict is replaced by tension between those at the top responsible for running industrialized society and those at the bottom—the consumers of goods and services. Thus, social class has largely lost its importance as a category of social analysis. Due to welfare state policies, the working class in developed capitalist societies has been absorbed as part of the larger consumer mass and subject to the manipulation of a corporate elite (Waitzkin 1978).

Applied to the health sector, the conflict pits the medical bureaucracy (notably the medical profession) and the health services delivery system against consumers and patients. The result is manifested in an increase in illness attributable to physicians and health care institutions. In order to perpetuate its power, the medical profession finds it advantageous to medically addict the population (Navarro 1977a).

The neo-Marxist approach has added to the confusion in health policy for the same reason that neoconservatism has. It encompasses a polyglot body of interests ranging at the extremes from stalwart believers in the continuing relevance of Marxist doctrine to anarchistic-leaning proponents of libertarianism. Analyses pivot on subtle but important distinctions between consumption and production in the attribution of responsibility for social problems and whether identifiable interests are the actual perpetrators or agents of oppression (Navarro 1977b).

Despite its underlying utopianism and romanticism, the neo-Marxist school has made some important contributions, particularly the debunking of a number of myths prevalent in the norma-

tive period and the steering of public attention to some new realizations. First, belief in the power of morality as an engine for social justice has waned. Neo-Marxist writers have argued with some success that past reforms are not solely due to the intrinsic altruism of human nature.

They contend that change is unlikely without the manipulation of events by powerful, self-serving interests in the private sector, such as insurance companies and hospital supply and pharmaceutical corporations. Medicare and Medicaid have been reinterpreted in this light, as have the Flexner-inspired reforms of medical education (Berliner 1973; Berliner 1975; Bodenheimer 1977).

In a related vein, the self-esteem and public repute of reformers have been assailed by charges that professed humanitarian motives are but a neat (not always conscious) disguise for paternalism and elitism. Reformers who are upper class in family background and/or education are less trustworthy than others when examined in this light (Frankenberg 1977).

As viewed by Navarro (1973), the neo-Marxist emphasis on economic structure and class relations contrasts sharply with the importance given by power-elite theorists to the role of personalities in struggles for reform. Besides romanticizing the contribution of individuals, power-elite writers tend to see change in terms of conflict resolution among different groups and actors in which control of knowledge, technology, money, and the legal right to perform specified services determine the outcome (Alford 1975; Feldstein 1977; Marmor 1973).

Second, belief in the benevolence of the medical profession has diminished, and even moderate observers have become alert to the potential use of professionalism as a cover for group aggrandizement (Begun 1981; Wohl 1984). Marxist-spirited critics form part of a circle of skeptics divided in ideology but united in their distrust of the profession. Left-of-center critics are inclined to curtail professional freedom and to demythologize medicine in order to free patients from medical oppression (Ehrenreich and Ehrenreich 1974).

Bureaucratic discipline in publicly accountable organizations, together with opportunities for citizen participation in the planning, monitoring, and evaluation of services, is the preferred alternative. For the sake of individual freedom and economic efficiency, right-of-center critics recommend going still further—the weakening of restrictions on entry to medical practice, on the employment of physicians in bureaucratic organizations, and on competition among organized medical providers (Freidson 1970).

Illich (1976, 1977) has called for more radical measures: (1) the total debureaucratization of society; (2) the breaking down of professional and other monopolies; (3) the return to classical market competition in which enlightened self-interest prevails; and (4) the maximum restoration of individual self-reliance and autonomy in all matters, including self-responsibility for health. In advanced industrial society, bureaucracy and professionalism, rather than capitalist or class exploitation, are deemed the omnipresent danger to individual freedom and the exercise of free will.

A third contribution of neo-Marxism has been that belief in the monolithic structure of organized medicine has dissolved. Until the mid-1960s, the stereotype of an all-powerful, reactionary American Medical Association entered into most policy deliberations. The medical schools and teaching hospitals, in contrast, seemed to be honorable exceptions. This image was an inaccurate one that sidetracked awareness of the implications of a shift in real power to scientific and technological interests.

Neo-Marxist observers were among the first to report that the major teaching hospitals and medical centers had become the chief obstacle to making quality health services more widely available to low-income populations. Few recognized at the time that the enormous capital requirements of high-technology, superspecialty medicine were being served without proper consideration for cost-effectiveness or the availability of primary health care to underserved populations (Ehrenreich and Ehrenreich 1970).

Neo-Marxists not only were among the first to understand the powerful forces in biomedical science and technology causing medical centers to take on many of the features of private corporations, but they also pointed the way for an analysis of the implications of this trend for the provision of medically questionable procedures and the availability of first-contact services attuned to everyday health needs (Kotelchuck 1976).

Finally, belief that medicine possesses little in common with big business has declined. The corporatization of U.S. medicine and the attractiveness of investments in the health economy to major financial and industrial corporations are subjects developed by neo-Marxist analysts (Salmon 1977) and popularized by others in terms of the medical-industrial complex (Relman 1980; Starr 1982; Wohl 1984).

Shortcomings of the Neo-Marxist Approach

To be sure, conceptualization of health services as an instrument in the service of a ruling establishment is not without insight. The drawing of connections between medicine and the structural features of society opens the mind to the realization that reforms are not always conducted purely for humanitarian reasons. The manner in which analysts with a Marxist orientation examine industrialization as a process cutting across national differences in ideology allows the identification of factors more fruitful than those bound to individual personalities or highly localized circumstances. On the other hand, this approach has a number of weaknesses.

First, the presumption of selfish intent is one sided. In taking a pessimistic view of the motives of the powerful, neo-Marxism suffers the same limitation ascribed to conservative believers in the doctrine of market competition, the only difference being that the latter see selfishness as universal to human nature. For example, it is improbable, given the array of interests involved, that health programs introduced during the turbulent sixties (neighborhood health centers, community mental health centers, citizen participation in comprehensive health planning, were designed solely or principally to repress insurgency by buying off indigenous leaders with good-paying jobs, by using demonstration projects as a way to dodge action, or by indoctrinating Blacks and Hispanics to middle-class values (Higgins 1980). This goes too far in discounting the spirit of reform instrumental in the passage of legislation and the administration of new programs.

Second, neo-Marxist analyses are frustrating to follow. They tend to rely heavily on assertion instead of data. The theory often suggests a conspiratorial group design to keep and expand controls. The proclivity is to generalize on the basis of a series of policy decisions that may not be representative. For example, although it may indeed be true that some of the health programs launched during the sixties were meant to curb unrest, it is doubtful whether this motive applies to all of the many changes in health care, housing, education, and social security enacted during this period. Not all the recipients were in a frame of mind to revolt (Higgins 1980). Undoubtedly more complex reasons were involved in the cases of Medicare and Medicaid, to cite only two examples.

Finally, there is a disturbing disregard for precision in the use of concepts and categories. Neo-Marxist writing is encased in confrontational-pugnacious rhetoric that deters serious reflection and thoughtful analysis, by appealing more to prejudice than intellect. It seldom is clear just what is meant by "the ruling class," "the state," or "the system." Vagueness as to who makes policy and who has responsibility for implementation and administration complicates the task of establishing relationships with the ruling class. Similarly, many categories suggest a homogeneity that does not always hold up on close inspection (Higgins 1980).

Future Prospects for Equity in Health Services

There are many reasons to doubt that progress in equity will continue unabated. A general recognition that the once-affluent economy has entered an age of limits, coupled with mounting political disillusionment with the liberal ideology behind recent health and welfare reforms, suggests that it will be difficult to sustain past gains, let alone move ahead (Russell 1980). Indeed, the present resurgence of conservative political doctrine and the return from near obscurity of rhetoric extolling the virtues of minimalist government, can be interpreted to bode ill for the future of welfare-state policies.

The vulnerability of publicly financed health services is compounded by the disintegration of confidence in propositions about the relationship between health and medicine and by the waning status and power of the medical profession. Contrary to what was long accepted as true, health spending is now seen to inhibit economic growth, and the medical profession is denounced as an impediment to cost-effective, high quality patient care.

Worry about the future of equity in health services is understandable in the present circumstance. Economic stringency and the sheer size and importance of the health sector invite scrutiny and a search for economies (U.S. Joint Economic Committee 1980a). Progress in the pursuit of equity may have to be deferred until budget deficits decline (Oxford Analytica 1986; Amara, Morrison and Schmid 1988). What is worse, fiscal policy may require cutbacks in the scope of benefits currently provided under government programs, and sacrifices unevenly distributed by geography and social class. It is unlikely in the long run, however, that any or all of these events will culminate in the restoration of classical conservative doctrine and the return of health services to the status of a private good in which rationing is conducted by unhindered play of the competitive market (Ginzberg 1985).

The doctrine of market competition is no better equipped to withstand empirical testing today than it was in the past. If anything, its premises have been rendered more outmoded by social and economic progress. Insofar as market forces have acquired currency as instruments for overcoming entrenched resistance to overdue improvements in health services finance and delivery, it is generally understood that competition must be managed. Otherwise, treatment costs such as overlap, duplication and the exploitation of financial incentives, would be worse than the disease itself. The scope of this understanding is manifest in the hitherto politically inconceivable methods now routinely applied by government and other purchasers of health care to shrink excess capacity through prospective reimbursement and to subject clinical decision-making to systematic monitoring and evaluation through mandatory reporting and peer review (Battistella and Buchanan 1987).

The possibility that the continuing domination of presidential elections by conservative loyalists will affect a redefinition of the public-good status of health care belies the limitations on political power and omits the significance of structural factors impacting on health policy in a highly developed society. More so than in parliamentary democracies, government in the United States speaks with many voices. The independence of the permanent bureaucracy and the role of special interest groups in national political life add to the constraints imposed by the constitutional separation of powers.

Were equity for the poor the only issue, the reestablishment of health services as a private good would be politically less difficult. The economic significance of the health sector in the modern economy, both as a major employer and as an important consumer of the goods and services produced by suppliers in private industry, further hinders the prospects for radical transformation. The powerful interlocking interests which benefit from controlling nearly 12 percent of a $5 trillion economy are inclined to accept change slowly (Amara, Morrison and Schmid 1988).

The already extensive system of political alliances dependent on the maintenance of high levels of spending for health services will spread further as middle-class fears deepen about the prospects for family income security in the event of serious illness. Indeed, this was a principal motivation in the 1988 Medicare amendments which sought to provide elderly Americans protection against rarely occurring but costly out-of-pocket expenditures associated with catastrophic acute illness. This concern is also what drives senior citizens and their adult offspring to press hard for comparable protection against the cost of long-term nursing home care. People today are living longer and expect to lead higher quality lives, both which increase health-services utilization. Consequently, future demand for health services is destined to remain high.

Of greater short-run significance are the imperatives for addressing certain deficiencies in existing financial mechanisms and delivery system capabilities, of which the cost of nursing home care is but one example. The large number of uninsured Americans, totalling 37 million or 15 percent of the population, is a particularly urgent priority (Robert Wood Johnson Foundation 1987). In comparison with insured persons, the uninsured, 70 percent of whom are low-income workers and their dependents, encounter greater

difficulty in obtaining health care (Freeman et. al. 1987). Furthermore, they complicate the financial difficulties of service-oriented providers situated in economically deprived areas. A resurgence of the uncompensated care problem, virtually eliminated in the mid-1960s by generous employer-provided benefits and by the liberal provisions originally contained in Medicare and Medicaid, induces financially-driven providers to discriminate against the uninsured and penalizes those providers who persevere in rendering treatment by medical need instead of ability to pay (Punch 1984). Measures enacted by state government to save money through cutbacks in Medicaid spending, including restrictions in eligibility, reduced benefits and lower provider reimbursement, add to the financial problems experienced by hospitals and physicians caring for low-income groups.

A closely related priority is the unacceptably high rate of infant mortality, especially among racial minorities (Institute of Medicine 1988). The poor standing of the United States in comparison with what most other highly industrialized nations have accomplished is a source of national embarrassment. A more compelling reason to improve the situation arises from concerns over a looming labor shortage and the need to raise the quality of the labor force in order to compete better in international markets.

A final example of the short-term pressure for higher government spending centers on the enormous medical, economic, and social implications of the AIDS crisis (Scitovsky and Rice 1987). At the minimum, a substantial boost in outlays for the care of victims entering the terminal phase of the disease will preclude the closing of surplus hospital beds in geographic areas where the problem is heavily concentrated.

Regardless of the initial justification, once government is engaged in the financing of health services, it becomes entrapped in a series of internal contradictions. Public financing inevitably leads to issues of accessibility and costs, the solutions to which lead to attempts to get more value for money spent through better management and more productive organization of health services. As discussed earlier, these pressures already have spurred a considerable amount of rationalization in the health sector (Battistella and Buchanan 1987). It is improbable that the pressures for rationalization will soon end. There are few alternatives open to government, and some are more appealing in the abstract than in practice.

The first is to reeducate people about the limitations of scientific medicine and the need to become less dependent on physicians (Kass 1975). This alternative misses the socio-psychological point of why people seek organized health services. It glosses over the fact that people often are not emotionally and physically free to reject medicine (Pellegrino 1979). It also loses sight of the large social and economic functions of health services. In focusing too much on short-term expediency, this strategy for cost containment could be counterproductive.

In addition to the danger of improper treatment, self-responsibility begs the question of how illness should be validated to minimize disruptions in day-to-day community functioning. Chaos would ensue if people were allowed to determine on their own that they were too sick to carry out their normally assigned duties. Easily quantifiable effects, in terms of job absenteeism, lost productivity, declining quality of services, and expenditures for sick leave and disability entitlements, would only partially reveal the negative externalities.

In putting the blame for illness on the individual, self-responsibility solutions divert policy from more important social and environmental causes of bad health (Guttmacher 1979). They also tend to overstate the capabilities of behavior modification techniques for dealing with the problem. And they lead to the politically naive conclusion that society should and can withhold free treatment from those whose illness can be presumed to be the result of their own foolishness (Battistella 1978b).

A second alternative the government can follow centers on the elimination or control of environmental hazards, through regulation and economic incentives for the installation of anti-pollution devices, and occupational safety and health measures. Ironically, the costs of introducing such measures endanger both profits and jobs, with the result that interests standing to gain the most in the long run (workers and local community economies) often are the most vociferous critics of such reforms. At the macro level, the costs involved can be an obstacle to the accumulation of capital for financing investments necessary to economic growth and improving international competitiveness. Because the economic burdens are much lower when corrective measures are built into the design of new physical plants, it makes more sense to adopt an incremental approach tied to the scheduled obsolescence of buildings and production process (Battistella 1978b; Mosher 1980).

A third alternative involves the restriction of public financing to health services that meet rigorous standards for safety, efficacy, and cost efficiency. This has extraordinary appeal on humanitarian, scientific, and economic grounds. However, as described earlier, there are many methodological and ethical pitfalls in the conduct of analyses of this sort, and the findings remain too unreliable to provide unequivocal guidance to policymakers. Despite serious shortcomings, this alternative is deeply imbedded in the mindset of the generation of decision makers new to health services policy and administration (Battistella and Rundall 1978b). Therefore, its influence will expand. Indeed, the establishment of a national system of technology assessment is an idea whose time has arrived, as evidenced in the widening coalition of powerful political interests now committed to this objective (National Leadership Commission 1989). Inadequately tested technology and insufficient information about the outcomes of clinical procedures today are widely regarded as serious deterrents to cost-effective high-quality care. Along with advances in computerized information processing, this climate of opinion sanctions the use of quality of patient care controls previously dismissed as technologically unfeasible or too controversial.

More specifically, the federal government recently has made its Medicare data bank available to accelerate development of clinical guidelines for identifying and eliminating medically ineffective procedures (Garland 1988). Parallel with this, the American Medical Association, in cooperation with the Rand Corporation, is developing clinical practice parameters to guide doctors away from medically ineffective, questionable, and occasionally dangerous treatment decisions (AMA, Rand Plan Joint Effort 1988). The cumulative effect of these efforts could substantially boost equity, provided savings are earmarked for improving access among low-income groups and for elevating the range and quality of services available to populations afflicted with conditions that have remained peripheral to the priorities of modern medicine—the disabled, the mentally ill, the chronically sick, and the frail aged.

Systematic monitoring and evaluation of the efficacy and cost effectiveness of health services may also have larger beneficial social and economic consequences. Inevitably, it will illuminate examples of how public funds can be spent to better coordinate health services with economic-growth objectives. For whatever reason, U.S. policy has been indifferent to investment-in-human-capital health programs. Thus, the absence of an organized system of maternal and child health services ranks as an exception to the rule found in most developed economies. Together with the prospects for higher productivity from a qualitatively strengthened labor force, maternal and child health services produce far greater yields in lower future treatment costs than do adult disease prevention and health education investments.

As health professionals begin to apply cost-benefit logic to compete more successfully for scarce public resources, recognition of the returns from simple and inexpensive industrial medical programs will also improve. In this connection, astutely managed hospitals entering an era of steady-state budgeting will capitalize on the opportunity to develop specialized prevention and treatment programs for employers seeking ways to manage their financial liabilities for occupationally related disorders.

A fourth alternative that government is already pursuing involves managing the supply of health personnel and facilities. The combination of regulations and economic incentives currently found in the health sector is predicated, as mentioned earlier, on the belief that the usual laws of market competition do not prevail. Regardless of whether they are pursued in or outside the framework of formal health planning, government measures to control the availability of physicians and hospital beds inevitably are ultimately accountable to political demands for equity in their distribution among medically underserved populations. This, too, augurs well for equity in the years ahead (Battistella and Buchanan 1987).

A fifth alternative is market competition. Although much discussed throughout the 1980s as heralding a major shift in national health policy, the actual significance of the federal government's so-called competitive health strategy is engulfed in speculation. Believers in the superiority of orthodox competitive economic theory interpret it as a long-awaited vindication of faith. On the other hand, groups believing in the power of the state to improve the quality of life fear that the political popularity of competitive-market language among conservatives portends a disengagement of government from the health sector. The practical use to which rhetoric is employed by politicians for getting things done in a pluralistic society is conducive to hyperbole. Political pragmatists generally subscribe to the adage that in human affairs, reason is occasionally the compass but emotion is always the steam. As pointed out earlier in discussing the substantial progress made in the rationalization of health services, there are numerous practical advantages to ascribing vaunted cultural folk symbols to facilitate controversial change.

When pondered in this context, proposals for increasing the role of competition in health services take on a significance considerably removed from literal translations. Competition has become a metaphor for a major restructuring of traditional practices in the financing, organization, and delivery of personal health services. Some of the more notable aims of this effort include (1) the replacement of retrospective reimbursement with prospective payment systems; (2) the transfer of assumption of financial risks from payers (employers insurance companies and government) to providers; (3) the imposition of restrictions on consumer freedom of choice through the assignment of individuals to organized groups of providers agreeing to provide a specified range of benefits for a fixed sum; (4) the introduction of controls on the supply of practitioners by specialty, possibly including their distribution; and (5) the transformation of health services from small-scale to large-scale units of production, conducive to the application of scientific management techniques for production and quality control.[1] In practice, therefore,

---

[1] In many instances the more subtle and politically feasible aims of the "procompetition movement" actually are antithetical to the classical free market model. This further demonstrates a gap between rhetoric and reality in the movement to increase "competition" in the medical marketplace.

the competitive market strategy has numerous objectives. If introduced often in the name of cost containment, these objectives also have important positive ramifications for the availability and quality of health services.

A sixth alternative is creative financing. The Catastrophic Coverage Act of 1988 for instance, sought to enhance the financial peace of mind of 32 million elderly and disabled Americans without affecting either the budget problem or taxes for the general public, despite requiring a massive growth in new outlays estimated at nearly $31 billion over its first five years. Instead, the aged themselves were to pay for the most significant expansion of benefits under the Medicare program since its enactment in 1965. The money was to come from two sources: higher monthly premium payments for all Medicare enrollees and a special surtax applicable only to upper income elderly. For the first time ever, the elderly were asked to pay for the entire cost of an entitlement expansion package. Even more unusual was the provision compelling the well-to-do aged to subsidize the cost of services for their less fortunate cohorts, with the amount they were required to pay tied to how much they owed in federal income taxes (Iglehart 1989).

While highly appealing to members of Congress ensnared by budgetary constraints, the brief history of the Catastrophic Coverage Act suggests that the application of the surtax concept to other social programs will depend on how well it is received by key constituencies. Upon reading the fine print and comprehending the added tax on their federal income tax liability, many high-income elderly denounced the surtax. Some thought it unfair for them to assume additional charges not asked of their lower-income counterparts, whereas others complained that the additional benefits were not worth the additional premium.

Much to the surprise of many political observers who assumed that a majority of voters and members of Congress would endorse the progressive tax provision of the Catastrophic Coverage Act, the upper-income elderly subject to the surtax were successful in forcing Congress to repeal the program. However, considering the intractable nature of the dilemma confronting politicians of having to provide more with the same or lesser amount of money, there is and

will be no escape from the fiscal requirement for the self financing of any new benefits in the years ahead.

For instance, one can anticipate that Medicare will become even more self supporting in the future. Because of improvements in the economic position of the aged, due to the indexing of Social Security retirement income, better private pensions, and appreciation of real estate values, there is a general perception that they have less need of government subsidies than was the situation when Medicare was enacted over a quarter of a century ago (U.S. Congressional Record 1988).

Notwithstanding the opposition of the high income elderly, continuation of the present economic circumstances also foreshadows higher charges based on ability to pay, elimination of the $45,000 limit on earnings subject to Medicare's Part A hospital insurance tax, and possibly the treatment of Medicare benefits as taxable income. An important precedent was established in 1984 when formerly tax exempt retiree Social Security payments became taxable for upper-income recipients. In addition to reconsideration of the tax-free status of Medicare benefits, Congressional interest in altering the tax-exempt status of fringe benefits among the gainfully employed, particularly employer provided health insurance, is bound to deepen. Earmarked revenues thus acquired would do much to assure equity for the truly needy as defined by liberalized means testing. Considering the state of the federal budget deficit, there appears little chance that Medicare will be expanded to include the cost of custodial nursing home care, unless the beneficiaries of this expanded coverage pay all or most of the cost.

The combined effect of increased competition for limited public funds and greater gains in living standards accruing recently to the elderly in comparison with younger claimants to government assistance drastically constricts the role of general revenues in financing any significant expansion of Medicare benefits for the foreseeable future. Within the context of heavier reliance on self-financing mechanisms, any political controversy stirred by the extension of social insurance into the long-term care area most likely will center principally on the extent to which beneficiary charges ought to be uniform or related to ability to pay. In addition to premiums and surtaxes, other revenue sources might include estate taxes and some level of state financial participation.

Some type of public-private mix is a strong possibility. In this connection, private long-term care insurance could evolve into a useful supplement in much the same way as medigap policies now relieve pressures for higher government Medicare spending while simultaneously insulating aged premium holders from the out-of-pocket costs of deductibles and coinsurance built into the Medicare program. Although the availability of private long-term care insurance is burgeoning, the prospects are slim that it is capable of providing more than partial protection against the large-sized costs of carative-custodial services. As summarized by Rivlin and Weiner (1988), even the most favorable projections indicate that by the year 2020 private insurance marketed directly to older people will remain unaffordable to anywhere from 55 to 75 percent of the elderly. Nor is it anticipated that private insurance will be capable of covering much more than 7 to 12 percent of total nursing home expenditures. Although it is unlikely that private insurance will substantially lower public spending, it nevertheless could substantially protect the elderly against out-of-pocket expenditures necessitated by any coverage gaps and co-payment requirements in an expanded Medicare program (Rivlin and Weiner 1988).

Mandating financial responsibility for social programs to state government and the private sector is another alternative which the federal government can be expected to pursue vigorously. Several provisions of the aborted Catastrophic Coverage Act of 1988 enunciated this strategy (U.S. House of Representatives 1988). On behalf of low- income aged, the states were to be required, over a four-year period, to use Medicaid funds to pay for the out-of-pocket charges such as premiums, deductibles and coinsurance imposed on Medicare enrollees. If fully implemented this provision would have insulated about 2.5 million elderly and disabled persons with incomes at or below the federally defined poverty line from the Medicare program's cost-sharing requirements. The states also were required to extend Medicaid coverage to pregnant women and infants up to age one whose family incomes do not exceed the federally defined pov-

erty line, with the costs borne by general revenues.

Business and industry are similarly viewed as the solution to the problem of the uninsured. Massachusetts, Hawaii and several other states already require employers to provide health insurance for workers (Enthoven and Kronick 1989). Once again, with the fiscal restrictions being what they are, the federal government will be tempted to follow suit (Fuchs 1987; U.S. Senate, 1988). This approach is grounded in the realization that health insurance for all but the old, disabled and very poor is principally obtained through employer group plans. It builds on federal precedents beginning in the 1970s which require that employers with twenty-five or more workers offer an HMO option if a qualified HMO exists in their area; firms with twenty or more employees who do provide health benefits offer qualified employees and their families the option of continued coverage at group rates when faced with loss of their coverage due to specified circumstances; employers filing for bankruptcy continue health insurance coverage for retirees; and firms employing workers aged sixty-five to sixty-nine enroll them together with their spouses aged sixty-five to sixty-nine in the company's health insurance plan which then becomes the primary payer for all claims in place of Medicare (Fuchs 1987).

Concerns that the competitiveness of small firms is undermined by higher labor costs do not dissuade proponents of mandated health benefits. Presumably, increases will be passed on to consumers with impunity. Equally unsupportive are major employers already providing health insurance as a condition of employment. Inasmuch as the latter pay higher insurance premiums whenever hospitals try to offset losses from the care of the uninsured by charging insured workers more, big business objects to what it considers an unfair subsidy of firms which save on production costs by not providing fringe benefits (Jones and Feuerherd 1988). Proponents of mandated benefits also tend to disregard criticism that the ability of business and industry to compete in international trade will suffer because of higher payroll costs. Typically, only large firms are engaged in exporting and they already provide such insurance. Moreover, compared with other highly industrialized countries, American industry bears a considerably smaller burden in terms of payroll financed social programs (Fuchs 1987). Nevertheless, many employers will resist this proposal, if for no other reason than it opens the door to other Congressional proposals which look to business to fund costly new programs such as parental leave and child day care services. Given the signs of a growing Congressional determination to pursue mandated benefits, however, enlightened employers may take a different view. Instead of moving in a haphazard, benefit-by-benefit manner, a more comprehensive approach may prevail that examines what constitutes a reasonable minimum benefit package that all employers would offer.

The perverse effects attributable to piecemeal growth of government mandates stimulate practical concerns for greater consistency in establishing affordable requirements. All fifty states have enacted laws that vary considerably in the scope and cost of employer mandates. Firms offering group health insurance are required to pay for a diverse mix of services ranging from the conventional (e.g., home care, outpatient services, mental health, alcohol and drug treatment) to the highly controversial (e.g., wigs, acupuncture, in vitro fertilization). Over the past two decades nearly 700 such mandates have been enacted. Maryland, for instance, has more than thirty mandates. At least thirty-seven states require coverage for chiropractors and some insist that they be reimbursed the same as physicians. In two states insurers must reimburse for the services of naturopaths. Still others require payment for midwives, psychologists and social workers (Stipp 1988).

While the intent of preventing employers from offering skeletal health plans is sound, the unintended consequences of such mandating are highly detrimental. Among small employers not offering health insurance coverage, estimates are that one in five do so to avoid the higher premiums attributed to mandates. Possibly one-fourth of the nation's 37 million uninsured persons lack coverage because of mandates which raise premium charges by 12 percent on average (Stipp 1988).

These additional costs account, in part, for the enormous growth in self insurance among large and medium-size firms. Whereas in 1976 self insurance accounted for only 5 percent of all health insurance, today it accounts for over 40 percent. More than 70 percent of persons who work for companies with more than 500 employees are covered by self-insured programs (Jensen and Gable 1988). Under federal law, self-insured plans are exempt from most state regulations and from state taxes on health insurance premiums. This option, however, is beyond the financial reach of small-sized companies, since a few big claims would be disastrous. Only 14 percent of firms with fewer than 50 employees are self insured. Concern for the negative consequences of mandating has led a dozen or more states to require a financial impact report before approving any new mandate (Stipp 1988). Clearly, good intentions do not always produce good results. The risk to big firms is not as serious an issue since they already are providing such benefits.

The tensions described in this inquiry into the political economy of health services did not occur overnight, nor can they be attributed mainly to the policies of competing political parties. They were observable in the early 1970s, and the implications were evident in broad outline (Battistella 1972a). Indeed, it could be seen as early as then that comprehensive universal health insurance paid entirely by government was impractical (Battistella 1973). The only subsequent major changes that have occurred involve matters of degree more so than of kind and a broadening awareness within the health community that things will not improve soon regardless of the outcome of national political elections. Evidence from many other highly industrialized nations of widely differing political and economic backgrounds suggests that the causes of the reformulation of postwar health policies are structural in nature. They are the likely manifestation of a process of adjustment to the large-scale institutional changes resulting from the transition from industrialization to a service economy (Battistella 1978; deKervasdoue, Kimberly and Rodwin 1984).

The complexities of the changes now occurring in social, political, and economic institutions are a reminder that establishing the right balance in health policies between equity and efficiency will not be easy. The enormous challenge of accommodating public policy to an unfamiliar decision-making environment, in which selectivity rather than universality is becoming the rule, deserves the attention of all groups committed to the preservation of equity in an era of limits.

REFERENCES

Alford, Robert R. 1975. *Health Care Politics: Ideological and interest group barriers to reform.* Chicago: University of Chicago Press.

Altman, Drew E. and Douglas H. Morgan. 1982. The role of state and local government in health. *Health Affairs* 3:7–31.

Amara, Roy, J. Ian Morrison and Gregory Schmid. 1988. *Looking ahead at american health care.* Washington, D.C.: McGraw-Hill, Health Information Center.

AMA, Rand Plan Joint Effort on Physician Practice Parameters 1988. *Medicine and health perspectives* (October 17): 1.

Another Upset For Health Planning. 1987 *Medicine and health perspectives.* (October 5):3–4.

Arrow, Kenneth J. 1963. Uncertainty and welfare economics of medical care. *American Economic Review* 53:941–969.

Battistella, Roger M. 1972a. Rationalization of health services: political and social assumptions. *International Journal of Health Services* 2:331–348.

Battistella, Roger M. 1972b. Post-industrial Europe: Implications for health services structure. *International Journal of Health Services* 2:465–476.

Battistella, Roger M. 1973. Towards national health insurance in the USA: An examination of leading proposals. *Acta Hospitalia* 13:3–22.

Battistella, Roger M. 1978a. Health policy development in other highly industrialized nations. In *Health care policy in a changing environment,* edited by Roger M. Battistella and Thomas G. Randall, 23–51. San Francisco: McCutchan Publishing Co.

Battistella, Roger M. 1978b. Individual responsibility for disease prevention and health maintenance: Potential for productive interventions. In *Health care policy in a changing environment,* edited by Roger M. Battistella and Thomas G. Rundall, 274–293. San Francisco: McCutchan Publishing Co.

Battistella, Roger M. 1985. Receptivity of hospitals to market competition: Image and reality. *Health Care Management* 10:19–26.

Battistella, Roger M. and Theodore E. Chester. 1972. Role of management in health services in Britain and the United States. *The Lancet* 1:626–630.

Battistella, Roger M. and Steven R. Eastaugh. 1980a. Hospital cost containment: The hidden perils of regulation. *Bulletin of the New York Academy of Medicine* 56:62–82.

Battistella, Roger M. and Steven R. Eastaugh. 1980b. Hospital cost containment. In Regulating health care: The struggle for control. *Proceedings of the Academy of Political Science* 33, edited by Arthur Levin, 192–205.

Battistella, Roger M. and Thomas G. Rundall, eds. 1978a. *Health care policy in a changing environment.* San Francisco: McCutchan Publishing Co.

Battistella, Roger M. and Thomas G. Rundall, eds. 1978b. The future of primary health services in the U.S.: Issues, and options. In *Health care policy in a changing environment* 294–319. San Francisco: McCutchan Publishing Co.

Battistella, Roger M. and David B. Smith. 1974. Towards a definition of health services management: A humanist orientation. *International Journal of Health Services* 4:701–721.

Battistella, Roger M. and John R. C. Wheeler. 1978. Ideology, economics, and the future of national health insurance. In *Health care policy in a changing environment,* edited by Roger M. Battistella and Thomas G. Rundall, 373–390. San Francisco: McCutchan Publishing Co.

Battistella, Roger M. and Thomas P. Weil. 1986. Pro-competitive health policy: Benefits and perils. *Frontiers of Health Services Management* 2:3–27.

Battistella, Roger M. and Robert J. Buchanan. 1987. National health policy: Efficiency-equity syncretism. *Social Justice Review* 1:329–360.

Begun, James W. 1981. *Professionalism and the public interest: Price and quality in optometry.* Cambridge: MIT Press.

Berliner, Howard. 1973. The origins of health insurance for the aged. *International Journal of Health Services* 3:465–474.

Berliner, Howard. 1975. A larger perspective on the Flexner Report. *International Journal of Health Services* 5:573–592.

Bodenheimer, Thomas, Steven Cummings and Elizabeth Harding. 1977. Capitalizing on Illness: The Health Insurance Industry. In *Health and medical care in the U.S.: A Critical Analysis,* edited by Vicente Navarro, 69–84. Farmingdale, N.Y.: Baywood Publications.

Bowler, Jenneth M., Robert T. Kuderle and Theodore R. Marmor. 1978. The political economy of national health insurance: Policy analysis and political evaluation. In *Toward a national health policy,* edited by Kenneth M. Friedman and Stuart H. Rakoff. Lexington, MA.: Lexington Books.

Bulgaro, Patrick J. and Arthur Y. Webb. 1980. Federal-state conflicts in cost control. In Regulating health care: The struggle for control, edited by Arthur Levin, 92–110. New York: *Proceedings of the Academy of Political Science 33.*

Campbell, Alastair V. 1978. *Medicine, health, and justice: The Problem of priorities.* New York: Churchill Livingstone: 1–5.

Carlson, Rick. 1975. *The end of medicine.* New York: John Wiley & Sons.

Christensen, Sandra and Rick Kasten. 1988. Covering catastrophic expenses under Medicare. *Health Affairs* 7:65–93.

Clare, F. Lawrence, Ernell Spratley, Paul Schwab, and John K. Iglehart. 1987. Trends in health personnel. *Health Affairs* 6:90–103.

Cochrane, A. L. 1972. *Effectiveness and efficiency: Random reflections on health services.* London: Nuffield Provincial Hospitals Trust.

Cohen, Marc A., Eileen J. Tell and Stanley S. Wallack. 1986. The lifetime risks and costs of nursing home use among the elderly. *Medical Care* 24:1161–72.

Commission on Hospital Care. 1947. *Hospital care in the United States.* New York: The Commonwealth Fund.

Council on Wage and Price Stability. 1976. *The problem of rising health care costs.* Washington D.C.: Executive Office of the President.

Davis, Michael M. 1975. *Medical care for tomorrow.* New York: Harper.

Donabedian, Avedis. 1973. *Aspects of medical care administration.* Cambridge: Harvard University Press: 1–30.

Donnison, David. 1979. Social policy since Titmuss. *Journal of Social Policy* 8:145–156.

Ebenstein, William, Herman C. Pritchett, Henry A. Turner, and Dean Mann. 1970. *American democracy in world perspective.* New York: Harper and Row, 2d ed.: 510–541.

Eastaugh, Steven R. 1987. *Financing health care: Economic efficiency and equity.* Dover, Massachusetts: Auburn House.

Ehrbar, A. F. 1977. A radical prescription for medical care. *Fortune* 95:164ff.

Ehrenreich, Barbara and John Ehrenreich, eds. 1970. *The American health empire.* New York: Vintage Books.

Ehrenreich, Barbara and John Ehrenreich. 1974. Health care and social control. *Social Policy* 5:26–40.

Elling, Ray H. 1977. Industrialization and occupational health in under-developed countries. *International Journal of Health Services* 7:209–235.

Enthoven, Alain and Richard Kronick. 1989. A consumer-choice health plan for the 1990s. *The New England Journal of Medicine* 320:94–101.

Feldstein, Paul J. 1977. *Health associations and the demand for legislation: The political economy of health.* Cambridge: Ballinger Publishing Co.

Fein, Rashi. 1980. Social and economic attitudes shaping American health policy, Milbank Memorial Fund Quarterly. *Health and Society* 58:350–385.

Fein, Rashi. 1986. *Medical Care, Medical Costs: The search for a health insurance policy.* Cambridge: Harvard University Press.

Frankenberg, Ronald. 1977. Functionalism and after? Theory and developments in social science applied to the health field. In *Health and medical care in the U.S.: Critical analysis,* edited by Vincente Navarro. Farmingdale, New York: Baywood Publications.

Freeman, Howard E., Robert J. Blendon, Linda H. Aiken, Seymour Sudman, Connie F. Mullnix, and Christopher R. Corey. 1987. Americans report On their access to health care. *Health Affairs* 6:6–18.

Freidson, Elliot. 1970. *Professional Dominance: The social structure of medical care.* New York: Atherton.

Friedman, Milton. 1962. *Capitalism and freedom.* Chicago: Phoenix Books.

Fuchs, Beth C. 1987. Mandated employer provided health insurance. Issue Brief, Congressional Research Service, Order Code 1B87168. Washington, D.C.: The Library of Congress.

Fuchs, Victor. 1974. *Who shall live?* New York: Basic Books.

Fuchs, Victor. 1979. The economics of health in a post-industrial society. *The Public Interest* 56:3–20.

Garland, Susan B. 1988. Almost everybody wants to see doctor bills under the knife. *Business Week* 3085:79.

Ginzberg, Eli. 1978. Health reform: The outlook for the 1980's. *Inquiry* 15:311–326.

Ginzberg, Eli. 1985. *American medicine: The power shift.* Totowa, New Jersey: Rowman and Allanheld:81–148.

Glazer, Nathan. 1971. Paradoxes of health care. *The Public Interest* 22:62–77.

Guttamacher, Sally. 1979. Whole in body, mind and spirit: holistic health and the limits of medicine. *Hastings Center Report* 9:15–21.

Hadley, Jack. 1982. *More medical care, better health?* Washington, D.C.: Urban Institute.

Harris, Richard. 1966. *A sacred trust.* New York: New American Library.

Higgins, Joan. 1980. Social control theories of social policy. *Journal of Social Policy* 9:1–23.

Iglehart, John K. 1978. Adding a dose of competition to the health care industry. *National Journal* 10:1602–1606.

Iglehart, John K. 1989. Medicare's new benefits: Catastrophic health insurance. *The New England Journal of Medicine* 320:329–335.

Illich, Ivan. 1976. *Medical nemesis: The expropriation of health.* New York: Pantheon Books.

Illich, Ivan. 1977. *Disabling professions.* London: Boyars.

Institute of Medicine. 1988. *Prenatal care: Reaching mothers, reaching infants.* Washington D.C.: National Academy Press.

Janowitz, Morris. 1976. *Social control of the welfare state.* New York: Elsevier:41–71.

Jensen, Gail A. and Jon R. Gabel. 1988. The erosion of purchased health insurance. *Inquiry* 25:328–343.

Jonas, Steven. 1981. Population data for health and health care. In Health care delivery in the United States, edited by Steven Jonas 37–60. New York: Springer Publishing Co.

Jones, Arthur and Joseph Feuerherd. 1988. Tedicare. *Financial World* 15:8.

Journal of the American Medical Association. 1980. 243:850.

Kass, Leon R. 1975. Regarding the end of medicine and the pursuit of health. *The Public Interest* 40:11–42.

Knowles, John K. 1977. *Doing better, feeling worse: Health in the United States.* New York: W. K. Norton.

Kotelchuck, David. 1976. *Prognosis negative: Crisis in the health care system.* New York: Vintage.

Krause, Elliot, A. 1977. *Power and illness: The political sociology of health and medical care.* New York: Elsevier.

Lalonde, Marc. 1974. *A new perspective on the health of Canadians.* Ottawa: Ministry of National Health and Welfare.

Lindsay, Cotton L. 1980. *New directions in public health care.* San Francisco: Institute for Contemporary Studies.

Marmor, Theodore, R. 1973. *The politics of medicine.* Chicago: Aldine.

Maxwell, Robert J. 1974 *Health care: The growing dilemma.* New York: McKinsey.

McKeown, Thomas. 1976. *The role of medicine: Dream, mirage or nemesis?* London: Nuffield Provincial Hospitals Trust.

McKinlay, John. 1979. A case for refocusing upstream: The economy of illness. In *Patient, physicians, and illness,* edited by E. Gartly Jaco, 9–25. New York: The Free Press, 3rd edition.

McKinlay, John B. and Sonja A. McKinlay. 1977. The questionable contribution of medical measures to the decline of mortality in the United States in the 20th century. *The Milbank Memorial Fund Quarterly* 55:405–426.

Mitchell, Samuel A. and John R. Virtz. 1986. Health care cost containment: What is too much? *Health Affairs* 5:112–120.

Mosher, Lawrence. 1980. Industry takes aim at the clear air act. *National Journal* 12:1927–1930.

Myers, Robert J. 1989. A catastrophic act? it depends. Op.Ed., *The Wall Street Journal,* A-12.

National Leadership Commission on Health Care. 1989. *For The health of a nation.* Washington, D.C.: National Leadership Commission on Health Care.

Navarro, Vicente. 1976. *Medicine under capitalism.* New York: Prodist, 189–192.

Navarro, Vicente. 1977a. *Health and medical care in the U.S.: A critical analysis.* Farmingdale, N.Y.: Baywood Publications.

Navarro, Vicente, ed. 1977b. The industrialization of fetishism or the fetishism of industrialization: A critique of Ivan Illich. In *Health and medical care in the U.S.: A critical analysis* 38–58. Farmingdale, N.Y.: Baywood Publications.

Organization for Economic Co-operation and Development. 1987. *The control and management of government expenditure.* Paris: OECD.

Oxford Analytica. 1986. *American perspective.* Boston: Houghton Mifflin.

Parsons, Talcott. 1951. *The social system.* New York: The Free Press, 428–479.

Pellegrino, Edmund D. 1979. Toward a reconstruction of medical morality: The primacy of the act of profession and the fact of illness. *The Journal of Medicine and Philosophy* 4:32–56.

Pocincki, Leon S., Stuart J. Dogger and Barbara P. Schwartz. 1973. The incidence of iatrogenic illness. In *Report of the Secretary's Commission on medical malpractice,* Pub. No. (OS) 73–89. Appendix. Washington D.C. Department of Health, Education, and Welfare: 50–70.

Powles, John. 1973. On the limitations of modern medicine. *Medicine and Man* 1:1–28.

Punch, Linda. 1984. Hospitals may reduce indigent care as competition rules out cost shifting. *Modern Healthcare* 5:30–33.

Ratcliffe, John, Lawrence Wallack, Francis Fagnani, and Victor G. Rodwin. 1984. Perspectives on prevention: Health promotion vs. health protection. In *The end of an illusion: The future of health policy in western industrialized nations,* edited by Jean deKervasdoue, John R. Kimberly and Victor G. Rodwin, 56–84. Berkeley: University of California Press.

Relman, Arnold S. 1988. The new medical-industrial complex. *The New England Journal of Medicine* 303:963–970.

Rivlin, Alice M. amd Joshua M. Weiner. 1988. *Caring for the disabled elderly.* Washington, D.C.: The Brookings Institution:59–82.

Robert Wood Johnson Foundation. 1987. Access to health care in the United States: Results of a 1986 Survey. *Special report number 2.* Princeton, New Jersey: Robert Wood Johnson Foundation.

Roemer, Milton I. 1980a. The foreign experience in health service policy. In Regulating health care: The struggle for control. *Proceedings of the Academy of Political Science,* edited by Arthur Levin. 33:206–223.

Roemer, Milton I. 1980b. Optimism on attaining health care equity. *Medical Care* 18:775–781.

Rosen, George. 1958. *A history of public health.* New York: M.D. Publications, 450–495.

Rushmer, Robert F. 1980. *National priorities for health: Past, present, and projected.* New York: John Wiley & Sons:3–40.

Russell, Louise B. 1980. Medical care. In *Setting national priorities: Agenda for the 1980's,* edited by Joseph A. Pechman, 169–203. Washington D.C.: The Brookings Institute.

Salmon, J. W. 1977. Monopoly capital and its reorganization of the health sector. *Review of Radical Political Economics* 8:125–133.

Scitovsky, Anne A., and Dorothy P. Rice. 1987. Estimates of the direct and indirect costs of acquired immunodeficiency syndrome in the United States. *Public Health Reports* 102:5–17.

Schieber, George J. and Jean-Pierre Poullier. 1987. Recent trends in international health care spending. *Health Affairs* 6:105–112.

Sidel, Victor W. and Ruth Sidel. 1977. *A healthy state.* New York: Pantheon Books.

Simanis, Joseph G. and John R. Coleman. 1980. Health care expenditures in nine industrialized countries. *Social Security Bulletin* 43:3–8.

Smith, David G. 1978. Policy analysis and liberal arts. In *Teaching policy studies,* edited by William D. Coplin, 37–44. Lexington, Mass.: Lexington Books.

Starr, Paul. 1982. *The social transformation of American medicine.* New York: Basic Books.

Steinfels, Peter. 1979. *The neoconservatives: The men who are changing America's politics.* New York: Simon & Schuster.

Stipp, David. 1988. Laws on health benefits raise firms' ire. *The Wall Street Journal,* p.B6.

Thurow, Lester, C. 1980. *The zero-sum society.* New York: Basic Books: 7.

Torrey, Fuller. 1974. *The death of psychiatry.* Radnor, Penn: Chilton.

U.S. Bureau of Labor Statistics. 1988. CPI detailed report. (August)

U.S. Congress. House. Sub-Committee on Oversight and Investigations of the Committee on Interstate and Foreign Commerce. 1976. *Report of the cost and quality of health care: Unnecessary surgery.* 94th Congress, Second Session.

U.S. Congress. House. 1988. Medicare Catastrophic Coverage Act of 1988. *Report 100–661,* 100th Congress, Second Session, 255.

U.S. Congress. Office of Technology Assessment. 1976b. *Development of medical technology: Opportunities for assessment.* Washington, D.C.: USGPO.

U.S. Congress. Office of Technology Assessment. 1980. *The implications of cost effectiveness analysis of medical technologies.* Washington, D.C.: USGPO.

U.S. Congress. Senate, Special Committee on Aging. 1984. *Medicare: Paying the physician: History, issues and options.* 98th Congress, Second Session, Washington D.C.: USGPO.

U.S. Congress. Senate, Committee on Labor and Human Resources. 1988. Background information on S.1265: The Minimum Health Benefits for All Workers Act of 1988.

U.S. Congress. The Joint Economic Committee. 1980a. *Issues in federal finance: Special study on economic change.* 96th Congress, First Session, July 1979. Washington, D.C., USGPO.

U.S. Congress. The Joint Economic Committee. 1980b. The social costs of unemployment. 96th Congress, First Session, October 31, 1979. Washington, D.C., USGPO.

U.S. *Congressional Record.* 1988. Senator George Mitchell 100th Congress, Second Session, Vol. 134, No. 52, April 21.

U.S. Department of Health Education and Welfare. 1975. *Forward plan for health FY. 1977–81.* Pub. No. (OS)76–50024, Washington, D.C., DHEW.

U.S. Department of Health, Education and Welfare. 1976. Theme: Preparing for national health insurance, *Forward Plan for Health, FY 1978-82,* Pub. No. (OS)76–50046, Washington, D.C., DHEW.

U.S. Department of Health, Education and Welfare. 1980. *Health, United States: 1979.* DHEW Pub. No. (PHS) 80–1232, Washington D.C., USGPO.

U.S. Department of Health and Human Services. 1981. *Health, United States 1980.* DHHS Pub. No. (PHS) 81–1232, Washington D.C., USGPO.

U.S. Department of Health and Human Services. 1986. *Catastrophic illness expenses, report to the President.* November, 1986.

U.S. General Accounting Office. 1987. *Medicare: Catastrophic illness insurance.*

Waitzkin, Howard. 1978. A Marxist view of medical care. *Annals of Internal Medicine* 89:264–278.

Waldo, Daniel and Helen Lazenby. 1984. Demographic characteristics and health care use and expenditures by the aged in the United States. *Health Care Financing Review* 6:1–29.

Wildavsky, Aaron. 1979. *Speaking truth to power: The art and craft of policy analysis.* Boston: Little Brown and Co.

Wohl, Stanley. 1984. *The medical industrial complex.* New York: Harmony Books.

Wolfe, Sydney. 1988. *Waste not, want not. The Wall Street Journal, Special Report on Medicine and Health,* April 22:30R–31R.

Part Two

Health Policy and the Political Structure

Chapter 5

Presidential Leadership and Health Policy

William W. Lammers

The search for sources of improvement in health policies persistently turns to questions of presidential leadership. The emphasis given to President Johnson's role in the establishment of Medicare and criticisms of President Carter for being ineffective on health policy issues reflect the significant role attributed to presidential leadership in explanations of past decisions. As federal health costs and total societal allocations for health care rise in the 1990s, questions of presidential leadership are destined to increase.

In assessing health policy formation, it is important to recognize that presidents clearly do have a potential for influencing some policy steps. In responses to new issues such as AIDS or a potential flu epidemic, presidents may have a significant role in generating public attention and in promoting a specific policy response. Presidential influence in producing minor changes in existing policies or specialized new policy initiatives can also, over time, produce substantial modifications in health policy.

The persistent debate regarding presidential roles, however, revolves around presidential actions pertaining to broad changes in major policies involving access to health care and the organization and reimbursement of health care providers. Because of their broad impact, changes in these policy areas are also characterized by extensive interest group and legislative action. Debates in the 1980s over possible improvements in health care access for the medically indigent, long-term care financing assistance for the elderly, and physician reimbursement changes within Medicare illustrate the potential for extensive conflict over major health policies. Proposals for broad changes in access and reimbursement policies thus raise especially important questions about presidential leadership.[1]

---

[1]The distinction among types of policy change used in this analysis draws from Light (1988). As in that study, it is recognized that not all instances of broad changes in major policies are of an identical magnitude. Nonetheless, focusing on a sin-

In developing an understanding of both future prospects for policy change and the nature of past decisions, it is essential to consider the manner in which presidents have been contributing to changes in health policy. To do so, basic questions need to be addressed: First, what are the major ways in which presidents have been involved in the formation of health care policy? Second, what does the record of presidential involvement with basic changes in major health policy suggest regarding the nature and importance of presidential leadership? Third, given past patterns, in what ways might presidents contribute to future policy changes? To address these questions, the following discussion will first develop a framework for considering various types of presidential health policy making roles. Selected case studies of presidential action in attempted changes in major policies are then used to examine the impact of presidential involvement. Those interpretations are in turn used to consider potential future presidential leadership roles for health policy.

Presidential Policymaking Goals

The manner in which presidents may influence major changes in health policy involves actions throughout all phases of a policy formation and implementation cycle. The advantages involved in considering presidential behavior on the basis of a policy cycle approach have been extensively discussed in such works as Ripley and Franklin (1984) and Kingdon (1984). Presidential roles can be categorized as involving five basic components: issue raising; promotion of policy approaches; support building with key interests; legislative bargaining and focusing; and policy implementation. As the following review suggests, presidents have a potential for significant contributions in the shaping of major health policies on each dimension of the policy formation cycle.

Issue Raising Activities

Issue raising activities are clearly essential in the policy formation cycle. The enactment of a

new policy is generally preceded by a variety of actions which first create a widespread sense that something needs to be done, and—as action becomes imminent—that something will be done. Social conditions, in other words, do not automatically produce the attitude that there is a problem which requires solution (Kingdon 1984). Specific actions are necessary to produce a perception that a problem requiring attention does exist. In the issue raising process, presidents have multiple opportunities. Periodically, presidents have chosen to emphasize major health policy issues in their election campaigns. According to Fishel (1985), presidents have often been quite specific in campaign discussions involving not just the importance of various health policy issues, but also their endorsement of specific proposals. Those commitments have included, for example, strong emphasis on the importance of enacting a Medicare program by Presidents Kennedy and Johnson and several major campaign discussions of national health insurance by President Carter.

Once elected, presidents possess a number of potential issue raising opportunities. One important opportunity involves inclusion of health policy concerns in their major addresses. Because of the widely recognized competition for space in State of the Union addresses, an indication of concern for a health policy issue is seen as an important indication of priorities within an administration. Presidential emphasis is thus likely to increase discussion by other political leaders.

Presidents also may direct attention toward health issues by undertaking major statements. While this has been done with major messages to Congress on several occasion, health policy has not been a focus for major televised addresses. In choosing topics for their major addresses to the nation, presidents have quite strikingly never made health policy the focus for one of their occasional dramatic presentations (King and Ragsdale 1988). As they select topics for their major speeches, which tend to occur only four or five times a year, foreign policy, economic, and energy topics have predominated. Considerable attention, however, can be gained if a President prepares a major statement to be submitted to Congress. This was the vehicle used by President Nixon, for example, in his promo-

gle category of policy change facilitates a more precise analysis than could otherwise be undertaken.

tion of health maintenance organizations along with an extensive set of reform proposals in 1971. In these contexts, presidents depend upon the media and the actions of other political leaders to expand the level of interest in their focusing on health policy issues.

Presidents may also employ presidential commissions in an effort to generate interest in a policy issue. Often, one of the important roles of a commission will be to increase interest in an issue by documenting the magnitude of the problem being confronted and thus adding a sense of urgency to the commission's specific proposals. According to both Flitner (1986) and Wolanin (1975), commissions have been a more constructive tool of presidential leadership than is sometimes suggested. The skeptical view that presidents use commissions as a vehicle for reducing interest in an issue by creating a rationale for avoiding discussion of new proposals until after a commission has acted is often overstated. In recent years, however, presidents have been less inclined to use commissions as a part of their issue raising activities.

The significance of presidential roles in the issue raising process is also apparent when one considers presidential capacities for discouraging interest in a potential health policy issue. This can be achieved directly by emphasizing information which reduces the severity of a problem being discussed by others, or by employing the need for "additional study" as a basis for postponing immediate consideration. Indirectly, presidents may also contribute to the avoidance of interest in a health issue by giving major priorities to other issues. In 1977, for example, President Carter warned that the passage of his energy program constituted the "moral equivalent of war" while not giving a similar cry of alarm for his more slowly developing proposals for national health insurance (Kellerman 1984).

The presidential potential for undertaking issue raising roles, while substantial, is nonetheless likely to be shared. Presidents have the advantage of extensive media coverage when they choose to act, and multiple potential strategies for their issue raising actions. Nonetheless, the intense competition among issue areas (and the possibility of presidential disinterest in changing health policy) reduces the frequency with which the president is likely to devote major attention to health policy. In the issue raising aspects of change in health policy, one thus may find a sharing of important activity with interest groups, legislators, experts from outside governmental circles, and segments of the media.

Design of Specific Proposals

The second component of presidential policy-making activity involves the development and promotion of specific policy proposals. As health policy options grow in number and complexity, the presidential role in shaping proposals has assumed increasing importance. Actors involved with policy design issues include both the White House staff and presidential appointees within the federal bureaucracy.

Although presidents have differed in their specific organization of the White House staff and the Executive Office of the President, several key roles have emerged. On the White House Staff, a Domestic Council member or other domestic advisers will now invariably have a major health policy role. Stewart Eisenstadt for President Carter exemplifies a strong use of this role, which included a major involvement in the negotiations between President Carter and Senator Kennedy over health insurance proposals (Califano 1981). In the Reagan White House, several individuals fulfilled major roles at different times, including David Winston as a major proponent of competitive policy designs during Reagan's first term.

Because of the major budgetary implications of health policy proposals, a key role is also increasingly fulfilled by the Office of Management and Budget (OMB). Within that approximately 600 person organization, either the budget director or one of his deputies will be extensively involved with the financial aspects of new health policy proposals. The persistent expressions of concern regarding the costs of national health insurance proposals from OMB in the Carter Presidency and David Stockman's involvement with health cost considerations during the Reagan Presidency exemplify the importance of that role. Staff specialization within OMB encompasses health policy analysis as a key role—including coordination of proposals—and the development of recommendations for signing or vetoing legislation which has been passed by Congress (Wildavsky 1988).

A president may also take a significant step in the shaping of health policy proposals with the choice of top personnel in the Department of Health and Human Services (DHHS). The Secretary of DHHS and the Assistant Secretary for Planning and Evaluation frequently have extremely important policy design roles. In the Carter Administration, for example, Joseph Califano assumed a crucial role as proposals for national health insurance were developed. In helping President Carter design cost control policies as a top priority while moving more cautiously on plans for an expansion of beneficiaries, Califano clearly illustrated the importance of the Secretary's role. Similarly, the choice of Otis Bowen as Secretary of DHHS in 1985 had a major impact on the shape of Medicare catastrophic insurance proposals during President Reagan's second term. Since its initial formation as a consolidating step in 1978, the Health Care Financing Administration (HCFA) has occupied an important position in the development of proposed changes in health policy. As head of the agency responsible for administering both Medicare and Medicaid, the Director of HCFA has been called upon in recent years by both Congress and the president to develop new proposals in such basic areas as hospital reimbursement practices within Medicare.

In the appointment process, presidents often find themselves constrained by interest group actions and at least a potential for congressional resistance. Because of the absence of confirmation requirements and their less visible public roles, presidents generally have an easier time exercising their judgments without serious resistance on staff choices than in the determination of cabinet officers and their top subordinates (Pfiffner 1988). The selection of secretaries for DHHS, in particular, is likely to produce an intense interest group struggle. In 1961, for example, President Kennedy concluded that personal lobbying of at least one key Senator would be essential to insure the appointment of Wilbur Cohen to a top position within the (then named) Department of Health, Education, and Welfare (David 1985). In 1969, the selection of the Assistant Secretary for Health produced intense American Medical Association resistance and ulti-

mately a retreat by President Nixon from his initially proposed candidate. More recently, selection processes at DHHS have been complicated by the intensity of interest group efforts to focus attention on a potential appointee's position surrounding federal government policies on abortion. The intense competition among interest groups on top appointments is a clear indication of the importance which is attached to these positions as areas for either encouraging or discouraging the development of specific policy proposals.

The presidential role in shaping the policy designs which are likely to emerge from their administration may also be substantially shared. Once political appointees have been selected, there may be important contributions from higher levels within the civil service. This is particularly apt to occur when presidents ask new appointees to produce major proposals in a short period of time. As viewed by Kingdon (1984), the growing importance of technical knowledge regarding health policy options has increased the significance of top civil service roles in the development of specific alternatives. In other segments of the political system, the growth of capacities for policy analysis on the part of legislative staffs and outside experts in universities and private consulting firms has increased the potential for policy design concepts to emerge without direct presidential involvement.

Building Political Support

The third component of potential presidential policymaking activity surrounds efforts to build political support for new health policies. Potentially, this may involve election campaign activities which serve not only to popularize an issue but to create additional support for a specific policy proposal. Democratic presidents, for example, have on occasion campaigned in support of specific policies for expanding access to health care. Regarding the likely use of this role, however, such students of presidential elections as Seligman and Covington (1988) have argued that presidents are not likely to run campaigns that create strong coalitions for future action. In their view, presidents have increasingly devoted their campaigns to general themes while leaving the development of specific support for policies to their subsequent actions as president.

The promotion of support for health policy proposals while enjoying the prominence of the White House is clearly a role which presidents may choose to exercise. Since the 1960s, presidents have increased very dramatically their range of appearances before various interest groups (Hart 1987; King and Ragsdale 1988; Lammers 1982). Some of this activity, as Hart has emphasized, involves an effort to increase presidential popularity and personal support more than voter commitment to new policy initiatives. In addition, the presidential interaction with major interests may involve an important negotiating role with groups skeptical of a new policy initiative.

Several presidents have illustrated quite forcefully the manner in which the presidential role may involve direct interaction with interest groups. In a dramatic effort to increase support for his Medicare proposals in May, 1962, for example, President Kennedy arranged to address a rally of senior citizens in Madison Square Garden. Using a different format some years later, President Carter staged a lengthy question and answer session with members of the American Association of Retired Persons in an effort to build support for his approach to issues affecting the elderly. In 1983, President Reagan illustrated the importance of presidential involvement with groups questioning aspects of his health policies when he traveled to Chicago to address the annual meeting of the American Medical Association.

In their relationship to interest groups, presidents may also seek to use the "going public" approach to presidential leadership with Congress (Kernell 1986). In this strategy, presidents encourage those who are already supportive of a policy change to engage congressional action through direct communication. An early illustration of this technique was President Kennedy's effort to enlist interest groups to push Congress on Medicare.

As presidents undertake their support building roles, there may be important aspects of delegation within their Administration. If a president chooses to make a major push, cabinet members are likely to be used on the network weekend talk shows as well as the speaking circuit. There may also be significant negotiating with key interests by either a top staff member or a cabinet member who has some degree of authority in speaking for the president. A central aspect of a president's support building role may thus involve the values and political skills of the people presidents initially select and the extent to which they encourage their people to undertake significant support building roles.

Legislative Focusing and Bargaining

Relationships with Congress constitute a fourth key component of the president's role in the policy cycle. This relationship will generally include actions by both the Legislative Liaison Office within the White House Staff and extensive testimony by key administration officials to committees of Congress. When efforts to achieve broad changes in major policies are involved, there is also a real possibility for direct presidential action. These actions may include direct bargaining with legislators and efforts to keep Congress moving forward through a focusing of legislative direction (Light 1988).

In their bargaining relationships with individual congressmen, presidents may confront substantial limitations. Interpretations of legislative voting by Fisher (1981) and Ripley (1983) have emphasized the limited resources which presidents have for changing votes on the part of individual legislators who are inclined by constituency, ideological, party, or interest group commitments to take opposing positions. In efforts to gain additional support, patronage may help a president, especially early in an administration. On a few key votes in a legislative session a president may also decide to bargain with offers of favors for a legislator's district. A president taking a strong promotive as well as bargaining interest may also become involved with cross-policy-area trades. Support on a major health policy proposal, for instance, may be traded for presidential support on another policy issue of interest to a legislator. The problem for a president, however, is that there are limited opportunities for changing votes in relationship to the large number of issues on which a president is likely to confront significant resistance. It is precisely because of the problems which presidents confront with these "inside" strategies that Kernell (1986) has concluded that presidents are increasingly likely to use the support building roles with the voters as they undertake a strategy of "going public."

The potential for a significant presidential impact on Congress may also involve actions which help to keep legislation moving forward rather than becoming deadlocked among competing proposals and positions, or being abandoned as attention turns to other issues. Light (1988) has characterized these actions as involving a focusing of congressional action. In this context, presidents may not be trying to force their own specific proposal as much as seeking an accommodation among interests which will allow a major final measure to emerge. President Johnson's actions preventing "kiss of death" amendments to Medicare which would prove detrimental to successful final passage constitute a major illustration of this role (Harris 1966). At key points, a president or a top aid may also intervene at the committee stage in an effort to keep Congress moving forward on a workable final enactment of a major proposal. Despite the frequent constraints seen on the part of presidents in terms of changing the votes of individual congressmen, the emphasis on a focusing role provides an important additional perspective on the manner in which a president may fulfill a significant policy-making role.

Promotion of Policy Implementation

The final aspect of presidential health policy-making roles surrounds the crucial question of how policies will actually be implemented. Often, as stressed by Thompson (1981), implementation questions will be resolved at the level of bureaucratic and congressional committee politics with little direct presidential involvement. In the implementation of a new policy, a president's top health planners and on occasion, the president directly, may nonetheless be involved with important decisions. President Johnson, for example, met with eleven representatives of the American Medical Association directly in the oval office and delivered a spirited "pep talk" in his effort to encourage a speedy implementation of Medicare (Harris 1966). A president may encourage an administrative unit to go slow while pointing to problems, or to make a major commitment of organizational resources in the pursuit of policy goals. Frequently, the specific question surrounds the speed (or lack thereof) with which agencies such as the Health Care Financing Administration will develop newly required regulations. Rather frequently, stipulated legislative startups for new programs will confront lengthy delays before new regulations actually appear in the Federal Register. In addition, interpretations of legislation may involve a major change in the actual administration of a new policy. Although the oversight function of new programs is clearly shared with Congress, presidential action (or inaction) can also have an important impact on such major access-related programs as Medicare and Medicaid.

Conclusion

Presidents have a potential for involvement at each stage in the policy formation cycle. Potentially, those roles may be substantially shared with other participants in the policy process. If an issue has clearly been placed on the agenda by actions of legislators, interest group leaders, a previous president, or the media, a new president's primary role may involve other aspects of the policy formation cycle. Similarly, there may be substantial legislative involvement with questions of policy design and at least aspects of the support building, negotiating, and bargaining processes. To examine more closely the nature of presidential leadership during the policy formation cycle, it is thus essential to turn directly to an analysis of recent attempts at broad changes in major health policies.

Case Studies of Presidential Leadership

All recent presidents have been significantly involved with controversies surrounding major health policies. In several instances presidents have successfully contributed to policy changes, while in other situations their proposals have gone down to decisive defeat. To assess presidential health policy leadership, the following discussion reviews major cases of attempted policy change for each president who was elected since 1960. The cases being reviewed begin with the roles of Presidents Kennedy and Johnson in the establishment of Medicare and Medicaid. This is then followed by an analysis of President Nixon's role in the development of legislation promoting health maintenance organizations (HMOs) and his involvement in the issue of national health insurance. For the Carter Presidency, two unsuccessful policy initiatives are addressed. These involved the cautious promotion of national health insurance and a vigorous attempt to establish hospital cost containment regulations. Finally, for the Reagan Presidency, the controversies being considered are the establishment of prospective payment as a means of reimbursing hospitals under Medicare in 1983 and the expansion of Medicare through the enactment of the Catastrophic Health Insurance Act in 1988.

In examining the nature of presidential policymaking in each case, it is important to recognize that presidents have pursued their goals while experiencing substantially different degrees of political opportunity. These important differences in political opportunity include: (1) magnitude of electoral support; (2) levels of electoral support for a proposed policy change; (3) levels of personal popularity for the president; (4) budgetary prospects; (5) size of the president's party in Congress; and (6) their relationships and potential collaborative activities with interest groups and legislative leaders. In addition, presidential effectiveness in handling policymaking roles has been a function of personal values and differing political styles and skills. How, then, have presidents exercised leadership on major health policies?

President Kennedy

The roles of Presidents Kennedy and Johnson in the adoption of Medicare and Medicaid have been the subject of continuing interest for stu-

dents of health policy. Initial analyses by Feingold (1966), Harris (1966), Marmor (1973) and Sundquist (1968) have been supplemented by David (1985) and new interpretations of presidential leadership roles. In reviewing the nature of presidential leadership on each dimension of the policy cycle, a picture emerges in which presidential leadership was frequently significant, but in the context of key roles was also at least partly fulfilled by legislators, interest groups, and administrative officials.

Turning first to issue raising activity, President Kennedy contributed in several ways. First, he was quite familiar with the issue when he began to pursue the Democratic Party's presidential nomination, having served as one of three Senators on a Senate Subcommittee on Aging that held hearings on the original Medical Care for the Elderly proposals in 1959. During the 1960 campaign, Medicare was promoted as part of Kennedy's general commitment to a more active domestic agenda. Throughout the campaign and in his years as president, Kennedy also encouraged the efforts of the National Council of Senior Citizens. This labor-backed organization formed initially as part of "Citizens for Kennedy" in 1960, was a consistently ardent advocate of health care for the elderly (Pratt 1976).

In terms of major speeches, Kennedy took the unusual step of addressing a major rally of senior citizens in Madison Square Garden on May 20, 1962. While a success with the committed members of the audience, it proved to be a much less effective action in the quest for general public support (David 1985). In 1961, Kennedy became the first president to author a major message to Congress solely on issues of health care for the elderly (David 1985).[2] However, Kennedy was reluctant to make Medicare his number one legislative issue, and as both Marmor (1973) and David (1985) note, chose to discontinue a high level push for the program once it became clear that it faced probable defeat in the House Ways and Means Committee. In 1963, for example, he declared the adoption of a tax cut, rather than passage of Medicare, to be his top legislative prior-

---

[2]Statements regarding public speaking roles on health policy are based upon a review of all presidential public speaking on health policy matters as reported in the Public Papers of the Presidents between 1960 and 1987. For a discussion of that research, see Lammers (1982).

ity. Thus Kennedy's contribution to the high position Medicare had on the issue agenda during his administration was in a context of collaboration that found legislative leaders and groups such as the National Council of Senior Citizens also making a major contribution. The issue had been receiving substantial attention from a variety of legislative leaders and some interest groups by the time Kennedy emerged on the presidential campaign scene in 1959, and those actions continued along with Kennedy's involvement with the issue.

The design of specific proposals for health care reform found the White House primarily endorsing the basic policy design which had emerged in 1959. As emphasized by Poen (1979) and Derthick (1979), the general policy strategy which emerged for focusing on the elderly had its primary gestation with the actions of such key administrative officials as first Oscar Ewing in 1951–1952 and then Wilbur Cohen in the Department of Health, Education and Welfare (HEW). Actions by legislators and key figures in the Department of Health, Education and Welfare during the Eisenhower Administration produced a series of more specific proposals in the 1957–1960 period. For the design of a specific new proposal, however, Kennedy established a task force (headed by Wilbur Cohen) which in turn proposed a substantial expansion in the number of individuals being covered as well as specifics on the financing procedures for the program. In early February, 1961, President Kennedy submitted a comprehensive proposal to Congress which contained the basic provisions he had supported as a Senator in 1959, but was in one respect more limited. In particular, the new package of health cost assistance for the elderly was to emphasize hospital care with some inclusion of nursing home coverage, but no assistance for physician services was provided. Moreover, little change was made in the basic program as alternatives were debated in Congress. As a result, by 1963 Kennedy was increasingly concerned with the extent to which his legislation was not covering medical costs other than those involving hospitalization.

Kennedy's inability to achieve passage of his Medicare proposals ultimately centered around his difficulties with legislative bargaining and the specific resistance he encountered within the House Ways and Means Committee. Because of the early opposition of six southern Democrats, including the influential chairman, Wilbur Mills (Dem., Ark.), the opponents of Medicare on the Ways and Means committee were in a clear majority. The Kennedy Administration thus concurred with his congressional supporters not to put a formal vote against the measure on record in 1961, and no further Ways and Means hearings on Medicare were held in either 1962 or 1963. In part because he feared the loss of Ways and Means Committee support for his trade and tax proposals, Kennedy decided to avoid extensive arm twisting efforts (Marmor 1973). He similarly decided to avoid an attempt at circumventing the committee (through a discharge petition) and instead sought to keep the issue before the public with the hope of subsequent congressional response to public pressure. Additional action was being reviewed at the time of his assassination in November, 1963, however, and a quiet effort to increase the size of the pro-Medicare bloc on the Ways and Means Committee had enlarged the group of likely supporters of new legislation in 1964 (Marmor 1973).

In reviewing Kennedy's record, it is clear that he faced major limitations in his degree of political opportunity. To his potential advantage, he was a popular president and he could point to public opinion polls showing majorities in favor of a Medicare program (Marmor 1973). Conversely, however, he had been elected by a slim (50.1 percent) margin and faced a Congress in which the importance of conservative southern Democrats as both a voting bloc and in key committee chairmanships restricted his potential for developing legislative support. In addition, the American Medical Association was leading a major lobbying effort against broad-scale federal involvement with health care for the elderly.

Students of Kennedy's role have in turn produced differing lines of emphasis on the level of skill with which the pursuit of Medicare was pursued. Marmor (1973), for example, places substantial emphasis on the limitations Kennedy confronted because of the ideological composition of Congress. Harris (1966), on the other hand, emphasizes the disadvantages Kennedy faced as a result of the opposition of the AMA and its intense lobbying efforts against Medicare. Finally, revisionists such as Parmet (1983) have questioned the extent to which Kennedy was willing to make a vigorous commitment in behalf of such domestic reforms as Medicare.

Ultimately, the question of whether greater skill and commitment on the part of President Kennedy could have produced at least some expansion in health care assistance for the elderly during the 1961–63 period is difficult to resolve. From the vantagepoint of congressional studies which stress the difficulties presidents have in trying to bargain with individual legislators, there would seem to be fairly substantial justification for emphasizing the inherent difficulties President Kennedy faced during his tenure. Perhaps most centrally, however, the Kennedy experience underscores the importance of the need for both favorable political opportunity and effective leadership skills if a broad new policy step is to occur.

President Johnson

President Johnson achieved the passage of Medicare in 1965 in the context of both an unusually favorable level of political opportunity and an effective use of leadership skills on some aspects of the policy formation cycle. The dimensions of Johnson's favorable political opportunity were most substantial. He had been reelected by a landslide of over 60 percent in 1964, and enjoyed high levels of personal popularity. Within Congress he enjoyed an increase of 32 Democratic seats in the House, and a growth in likely support for a variety of his Great Society programs. In addition, Medicare enjoyed substantial general support in the general public, and the program's most vocal opponent—the American Medical Association—suffered a serious loss as many of the candidates it had backed in the 1964 election were defeated. Finally, in terms of budgetary prospects, the substantial economic growth experienced after the tax cut in 1964 made the promotion of new expenditures more plausible than in 1961.

At the same time, President Johnson fulfilled leadership roles on several aspects of the policy formation cycle. Regarding issue raising activity, the previous actions by President Kennedy, interest group leaders, and legislative proponents had served to keep medical care for the elderly quite forcefully on the nation's issue agenda prior to Johnson's sudden assumption of the presidency. While President Johnson did eagerly pursue the advocacy of Medicare in the 1964 campaign, he helped thwart the passage of a smaller legislative package before the election which would have eliminated both a good campaign issue and the potential for a more extensive effort after the election. Finally, in the legislative battle itself in 1965, Johnson stressed the issue in his State of the Union Address and made occasional references to it in his press conferences.

Regarding the policy design which ultimately emerged, Johnson found himself in the position of responding to a proposed expansion rather than initiating a major new step. The fundamental change in policy design which preceded legislative enactment occurred when Ways and Means Chairman Mills engaged in a dramatic switch in his positions. Mills proposed that the new program add physician services to the original hospital cost assistance, and also include a component (called Medicaid) to assist needy individuals of all ages. Since the proposal for assistance based upon need was being advocated by the American Medical Association in an effort to prevent the passage of Medicare for all elderly persons, their lobbyists were dismayed when that basic component was suggested as an addition to Medicare (David 1985). President Johnson quickly read a summary of the concepts and indicated his approval. In the design of a bill with broader coverage than initially proposed and also a hurriedly constructed design for assistance to some individuals solely on the basis of need, President Johnson and his top health advisers were responding to ideas initially emerging from the House Ways and Means Committee.

On two other policy design issues, President Johnson also had a significant role. Regarding reimbursement policies for Medicare, Johnson contributed to the nature of the final design when he quietly agreed to provisions which avoided governmental determination of the payment levels for physicians and hospitals in the program. Rather than attempting to fight the political battles which would surround the American Medical Association's vehement opposition to reimbursement based upon any policy other than "usual and customary reimbursement," President Johnson supported the provisions which gave physicians an opportunity for private decisions (and subsequent rapid increases) in the fees charged to both Medicare and Medicaid patients. Finally, regarding implementation aspects of the original policy design, President Johnson also supported designs which gave a rapid start to the hospital insurance program, but ultimately involved substantial delay in both Medicaid generally and in the development of regulations for the nursing homes which would be operating as a part of the new program (Vladeck 1980).

The president's most important roles were clearly those of helping to steer the measure through Congress along with some degree of support building among key interests. In an effort to prompt legislative action, President Johnson arranged to have Medicare given the symbolic position of the number one bill (House File 1 and Senate File 1) introduced into the new Congress in 1965. There were also efforts on Johnson's part to sway some legislators by making a number of helpful calls to legislators in support of the Medicare program (David 1985). Although observers such as Bowels (1987) feel that Johnson's general record on direct legislative contact is sometimes overstated, in this instance there was a selective but strategic use of presidential intervention. Most centrally, Johnson contributed to the thwarting of an attempt by Senator Long (Dem., La.) to shift the emphasis of the program toward catastrophic health insurance (i.e., for those who were in the hospital for more than sixty days) when the measure reached the Senate Finance Committee (David 1985). The importance of Johnson's role with Congress, then, could best be characterized as one of steering or focusing the process rather than directly converting large numbers of reluctant legislators.

In assessing the passage of Medicare and Medicaid, it is essential to recognize that multiple factors were involved. First, the issue was on the agenda, substantial support had been built through the course of more than a half-decade of increasing public debate, and substantial attention had been given to the development of specific proposals. Second, the election of 1964 created a presidency with substantial political opportunity—large legislative majorities and an ability to point to public support for new policy initiatives. Third, the involvement of President

Johnson with portions of the legislative focusing roles represented an aspect of presidential leadership in which this president was well suited. Formerly the majority leader of the Senate, he brought to the presidency a unique experience in promoting the passage of legislation as well as substantial energy and enthusiasm for pursuing presidential leadership in Congress. While the events of 1965 thus demonstrate the successful use of several leadership roles, the high level of political opportunity also suggests that major advantages in political opportunity as well as the impact of a politically skilled president are likely to be essential when policymakers undertake major changes in policies for access to health care.

President Nixon

The turbulent years of the Nixon Presidency occurred in the context of mixed opportunities for presidential leadership. In 1969, he entered office as a minority president, having received only 43 percent of the vote. In addition, he was the first newly elected President in over a century to face opposition party control of both houses of Congress. While his second term began with the advantage of a decisive re-election victory (60 percent of the popular vote) his personal support with the electorate fell dramatically as a result of the Watergate scandal. In terms of health policy, concern over both private and public health care costs led to proposals for both cost containment and expanded access to care (Starr 1982). In this context, the Nixon Administration chose to pursue a major effort to transform the organization and reimbursement of health care providers and engage itself with the issue of national health insurance.

The actions leading to federal support of Health Maintenance Organizations (HMOs) in 1973 represent a particularly controversial aspect of health policy development during the Nixon Presidency. The proposal for governmental encouragement of prepaid health plans which emphasized preventative health efforts found the Nixon Presidency performing unusually active issue raising and policy design roles, with the president paradoxically also engaging in interest group and legislative bargaining efforts which reduced the scope of the final legislation. As the final compromise emerged, Congress got the broad goals desired by liberally-oriented reformers, and the Nixon Administration won in the desire to provide limited funding.

The emergence of HMOs as a new approach for controlling health costs is a fascinating story of presidential health policy leadership. In the desire to find some strategy which would assist in the control of health costs, top officials in Nixon's Department of Health, Education, and Welfare turned to the ideas being advanced by Paul Ellwood, Jr., a physician and head of a Minneapolis based policy study group (Brown 1983). There was an initial receptiveness based upon a sense of urgency in the face of the President's promise of new strategies for cost control, combined with a desire to do something different. Nixon was initially enthusiastic about the concept of federal HMO encouragement, and included that approach as a centerpiece in his major health policy statement submitted to Congress in early 1971. To an unusually high degree, President Nixon and his top health advisers were thus responsible for choosing a particular policy approach as the preferred strategy for fighting the rapid increases in health care costs in the private sector. Quite strikingly, as they took that step they were promoting a strategy which initially had the support of only a third of the public (Brown 1983). Although the concept of prepaid health plans had been in existence for several decades, it is doubtful that HMOs would have emerged as a major focus for changes in health care organization without the strong actions of President Nixon.

The unusual aspect of HMO politics during the Nixon Presidency surrounded his subsequent retreat from a support building role. The stage for Nixon's shift was set as the Democratic majorities in Congress (and in particular Senator Edward Kennedy) became increasingly interested in using HMOs to advance a variety of related policy objectives, while the American Medical Association expressed increasing alarm over the prospect of federal support for a significant shift away from independent physician and fee for service forms of organization (Falkson 1980). By 1973, as a modified bill was passed, legislative bargaining occurred in which the Nixon Administration

expressed substantial concern regarding the size of the future HMO effort. Thus the Nixon Administration's role was significant in somewhat contradictory ways—in raising an issue and promoting interest in a new policy approach, but also in working to restrict the scope of the new initiatives when Congress began to promote a major expansion. In the implementation phase, the Nixon Administration was left with a difficult law to administer, and through the 1970s the level of HMO development fell substantially below the original optimistic projections.

On policies which might expand access to health care, the inability of federal policymakers to reach an agreement on new policy steps during the Nixon Presidency provides a second important direct indication of the importance of—and difficulties surrounding—presidential leadership. The Nixon Years were characterized by extensive interest in expanded access to health care, but a disagreement among interest groups, the White House and Congress on policy techniques and an inability of key policymakers to negotiate their differences in preferred policy approaches. Beginning in 1970, Walter Reuther and the United Auto Workers helped to form a labor-supported coalition for fundamental change in health policy with the establishment of the Committee of One Hundred for National Health Insurance. The labor proposal, which also had the endorsement of such liberal legislators as Senator Kennedy, called for federal funding, comprehensive coverage, and use of the federal government (rather than private insurance companies) in the administration of the new plan. For proponents, this step represented the logical extension of Medicare and its coverage of the elderly population.

The Nixon plan included a continuation of private policies, with the government providing insurance for those not covered by private plans. Administration of the plan was to be carried out by existing insurance companies, and the government's financial contribution was to be 75 percent of an individual's medical costs up to an annual maximum of $1,500.00. Interestingly, Casper Weinberger, as Secretary of Health, Education and Welfare, was a particularly strong proponent of this plan. As a broad third alternative, the debate within Congress included the catastrophic insurance approach which had been advocated for almost a decade by Senator Long. In the catastrophic approach, individuals were to be assisted with medical costs when they reached variously defined maximum levels in a given year.

The scope of differences among policy designs clearly made negotiation difficult. In addition, the widely shared assumption that the Congress being elected in 1974 would be more liberal than the previously constituted Congress appears to have contributed to an interest in "holding out" on the part of those endorsing approaches which had been initially promoted by labor in 1970. As a potential advantage for negotiations, however, that same perception motivated an increased interest in passing some bill on the part of the private health insurance companies and those generally opposed to a broader commitment to national health insurance.

Although the negotiation of a compromise in 1973–74 would have been difficult, some action may have been possible. John Kingdon (1984) concluded from his study of issue agendas that there was some opportunity for significant action on national health insurance in the early 1970s. Similarly, Paul Starr (1982) views the early 1970s as a period in which a conservative accommodation to the liberal policy agenda in a number of areas was making significant action possible.

President Nixon nonetheless did not undertake an extensive effort to promote legislative bargaining or to facilitate negotiation among key parties in either his first term or in 1973. In reviewing Nixon's relationships with Congress, Bowles (1987), concluded that he was reluctant to get directly involved, and preferred written notes rather than direct personal contact. More generally, Nixon was a foreign policy oriented president who usually expressed little interest in maneuvering on domestic legislation. While one can not prove that a more skilled and personally committed president could have achieved a major public financing measure in the early 1970s, President Nixon's weakness in internal legislative relationships stood in marked contrast to President Johnson's direct involvement in both encouraging a basic negotiated compromise and then working to insure that the compromise was not derailed by competing interests.

On health policy, just as in so many other areas, the Nixon Presidency was an unusual period in American politics. On the specific development of HMOs, the Nixon Presidency showed the importance of presidential action in developing new policy approaches. Regarding national health insurance, a president who was concerned about his slide in the polls could propose a fairly substantial change. Yet conversely, his continuing Watergate-based problems, coupled with limited efforts at presidential leadership, reduced chances for significant new action on access to health care.

President Ford

In his brief interlude in office, President Ford quite dramatically displayed the problems which can confront a president who is weak on virtually all of the components of political opportunity. The absence of the legitimation which comes by winning an election was an initial handicap, and Ford's popularity fell by some 17 percentage points in the wake of his pardon of Richard Nixon. After the congressional elections in 1974, the size of the Republican delegation fell to only 144 House seats and 37 Senate seats, and the President was confronted by late 1974 with the necessity of trying to reduce the dual impact of a recession and inflation. To make matters even worse, there was a rapid increase in Medicare and Medicaid costs in the 1975–1976 period, thus intensifying budgetary concerns (Starr 1982). In the wake of these constraints, President Ford withdrew references to national health insurance in his State of the Union Address in 1976. Although Ford never really sought national health insurance, it is also true that he confronted a situation in which chances for major expansion in access to health care had clearly declined.

President Carter

The Carter Years also produced a clear lack of success in presidential efforts to achieve broad changes in major health policies. As in the Nixon-Ford period, a substantial number of adjustments in health policy did occur. On the two related and highly visible issues of hospital cost control and expanded access through the adoption of one of the competing proposals for national health insurance, however, the Carter Administration was unable to achieve congressional action.

Carter's lack of success occurred in the context of political opportunities which were clearly mixed. He had been elected by a two million vote majority and was fairly popular in his first months in office. He also enjoyed partisan majorities in both houses of Congress, with the Democrats holding 292 House seats and 61 Senate seats. Relationships with Congress nonetheless faced potential problems from the outset. Committee chairmen were in several instances quite skeptical of the new president, Senator Kennedy stood as a potential future rival, and the Democratic majorities cloaked major differences over the appropriate next directions for the Democratic Party. Furthermore, support for policy changes within the electorate was more uncertain in the face of rising inflation and growing concern over the nation's poor economic performance (Starr 1982). On access to health care, although a slim majority of the public favored some help for those without any health insurance, there was also a 62 percent majority in favor of keeping the existing system (Braverman 1978).

The fight for hospital cost control legislation represented a major attempt at decisive presidential leadership and yet resulted in a resounding defeat. In the evolution of this controversy, President Carter, the HEW Secretary, Joseph Califano, and the president's legislative liaison staff all attempted significant leadership roles. The net result, however, was that Congress rejected hospital cost control plans in both 1978 and 1979. These defeats included an original proposal which provided a cap on hospital costs in relationship to the consumer price index and a 1979 proposal which excluded nonprofessional wages from a more flexible cap (in an effort to win union support) and provisions designed to protect areas experiencing rapid population growth. Ultimately, rather than restrictions on the annual rate of increases in reimbursement the hospitals could obtain, the only new development was a hospital industry pledge to constrain the annual rate of increase which had been running at approximately 15 percent.

President Carter and his administration clearly sought a major role throughout each aspect of the policy cycle. In part with the encouragement of Secretary Califano, Carter began promoting cost control in his frequent talk shows and local appearances throughout the country in the spring of 1977. Press conference references were also fairly extensive, and he frequently included hospital cost control in his major speeches, including the 1978 State of the Union Address. The design of both cost control measures was undertaken at the Department of Health and Human Services (formerly HEW), and included the efforts to design a more acceptable second proposal in late 1978.

In the support building and legislative bargaining activities, President Carter was also personally involved. In speeches to special groups, talk show sessions, and in references within his major speeches, President Carter constantly emphasized the importance of hospital cost control. His efforts behind the second proposal in 1979 were especially extensive (Jones 1987; Califano 1981). As he confronted a key committee vote, Carter used the telephone in a quest for legislative support. On several occasions, individual meetings were also held at the White House with key individual legislators. The nature of political divisions and actions by the hospital lobby, however, ultimately proved to be too much for the President to overcome. Analyses of legislative voting by Mueller (1986) and Feldstein and Melnick (1984) point to Carter's inability to modify resistance based upon a combination of ideological skepticism about additional regulation, advantages in being supportive of the hospital association's political action committees, and concern for the impact of the legislation on more rapidly growing areas.

In an extensive review of Carter's relationships with Congress, Jones (1987) emphasizes the underlying difficulty of the task the President faced on this issue. Hospital cost control was viewed by several of those he interviewed as an issue around which opposition was easily formed because of concerns in the industry and within geographic areas which felt a relatively greater need for an expansion in hospital facilities. Yet at the same time, the potential beneficiaries constituted a more diffuse and less readily mobilized group of supporters. For Jones, the underlying power relationships within the policy arena made this a difficult issue for a president regardless of his level of skill in dealing with Congress.

Turning to national health insurance, President Carter clearly had difficulty determining the direction and leadership role he wanted to undertake. During the presidential campaign in 1976, he endorsed national health insurance quite specifically in the context of a determined effort to gain the support of such major union groups as the United Auto Workers (UAW) (Fishel 1985; Califano 1981). In an effort to placate union concerns that he was moving too slowly, in 1977 he also delivered a major address to the UAW supporting the concept of national health insurance and included references to health insurance in a variety of public appearances. The overall thrust of Carter's issue raising role, however, was to tie cost control with additional access as a related issue rather than seeking to build support for a rapid, broad-based expansion in national health insurance.

On the specific question of policy design, President Carter had considerable difficulty controlling developments. With the encouragement of both Secretary Califano and his budgetary cost conscious economic advisers, Carter sought to get cost control measures in place first and to take a relatively cautious role in expanding direct federal financing to additional groups. This orientation did not satisfy either Senator Kennedy or major segments of the labor coalition which supported broad-based plans for federal health insurance. In the midst of this controversy, the development of a specific policy proposal became increasingly difficult during 1978, and ultimately the Carter Administration introduced a catastrophic insurance bill which was considered to be quite unsatisfactory by such supporters of national health insurance as Senator Kennedy and the labor-based coalition for national health insurance. Carter's proposal did not get beyond the committee stage during his tenure, and the impetus for national health insurance eroded substantially by 1979–1980.

The Carter Presidency thus again underscores the extent to which multiple conditions are necessary for presidents to have success in providing a significant role surrounding changes in major aspects of health policy. President Carter is often judged to have been a relatively poor utilizer of the degree of political opportunity which he had

with Congress. In this evaluation, emphasis is often focused on Carter's tendency not to focus on a few key legislative items and his lack of enjoyment of the legislative bargaining role (Kellerman 1984). Nonetheless, the difficulties apparent in Carter's seeking to gain agreement on the scope of new policy designs for national health proposals would seem to underscore the extent to which not only presidential skill, but also a fortunate convergence of political opportunity and multiple contributing roles within Congress and the interest group structures are necessary to achieve a significant modification in policies relating to either access to health care or reimbursement policies.

President Reagan

The Reagan Years constitute an extremely important period in any assessment of presidential health policy leadership. Overall health policy developments in the 1980s produced a substantial degree of change. In 1981 and 1982, the Reagan Administration was partly successful in gaining congressional support for its proposed extensive cuts in a variety of programs. Fairly significant changes were made in Medicare and Medicaid, with the Administration emphasizing greater out of pocket payments for the elderly and Congress focusing on tighter control on the reimbursement of providers. The most dramatic new steps, however, were the 1983 changes in the method of paying hospitals and the establishment of an expanded catastrophic health benefit under Medicare in 1988.

The successes of the Reagan Presidency in promoting changes in health policy occurred in the context of a fairly high degree of political opportunity. President Reagan was elected quite decisively in 1980 and overwhelmingly in 1984. Although his popularity fell sharply during the recession in 1982, he enjoyed greater long-term personal popularity than any president since Johnson's popularity began to decline in 1965. In dealing with Congress, Reagan faced Democratic control in the House, but a Senate which was in Republican hands between 1981 and 1986. In terms of the Congresses which Reagan confronted, there was initially a period of reluctance to thwart a popular president with at least the potential for influencing legislative races. This was then followed by the emergence after the 1986 elections of a Congress which was increasingly assertive on a variety of domestic policy issues.

Budgetary issues also contributed to the nature of political opportunities for major policy change. The rapid increases in governmental costs for health care provided an important incentive for federal policymakers to address reimbursement issues that affected the cost to government for each specific service being rendered. Conversely, however, the growth of the budgetary deficit provided a reduced opportunity for measures which added directly to the federal deficit. In this context, Reagan exercised quite different roles in the areas of hospital reimbursement and catastrophic insurance.

The change in hospital reimbursement within Medicare in 1983 was a somewhat surprising development because it represented both a significant policy shift without extensive direct presidential leadership and a change which one might have expected to be not only strongly opposed by the health provider lobbies but also a Republican President as well. Yet the federal government did move from reimbursing hospitals under Medicare on the basis of usual and customary fees to a system of prospective payment based upon some 467 different diagnostic related groups. Rather strikingly, an Administration which had entered office promoting major shifts toward greater competition as a vehicle for controlling health costs became a major advocate of a policy approach which had been receiving encouragement from the Health Care Financing Administration during the Carter Presidency, and which involved a substantial expansion in the governmental price setting role. How could this change occur?

The successful promotion of Medicare's prospective payment for hospitals by the Reagan Administration occurred in the context of a complex set of events. Within top White House circles, there was an inability to agree upon proposals such as a voucher system which would directly foster competition among health care providers.[3] At the same time, health policy lead-

ers within Congress continued to express concern regarding the substantial annual inflation in health service costs and pressed the Health Care Financing Administration for new proposals. From the standpoint of the hospitals, (and most forcefully the for-profit hospitals) concern regarding the possibility of more far reaching future changes created an interest in achieving the best possible compromise as of 1983.

Quite strikingly, there is little indication of a significant personal role for President Reagan on most aspects of the movement to prospective payment. There were no presidential addresses on hospital cost containment or significant references to it in any of his major speeches. The primary thrust of Reagan's issue raising activity dealt with problems of fraud and abuse in the Medicaid program and a major tour in the spring of 1982 touting a proposed "swap" of Medicaid and income support programs between the federal government and the states. Similarly, in a major address to the House of Delegates of the American Medical Association in 1983, Reagan made no reference to the changes in hospital reimbursement policies.

In terms of the effort to develop alternatives, the Reagan White House was clearly unable to develop a pro competition proposal on hospital rates which would satisfy various key constituencies. Initially, Health and Human Services Secretary Richard Schweiker indicated at the beginning of 1982 that a pro competition strategy would be forthcoming from the Administration, but found himself supporting the prospective payment system by the end of the year. The policy debate resulted in an approach that had been encouraged by the Health Care Financing Administration through an experiment in New Jersey in the late 1970s, and encouraged by Congress in requests for an administration study. The prospective payment system received the endorsement of the Reagan White House.

The development of support for prospective payment as the preferred policy approach to hospital cost control involved agency officials and legislators as well as representatives of the

---

³This conclusion is drawn in part from the weekly summaries of

health policy which are contained in McGraw-Hill's *Washington Report on Medicine and Health.* Subsequent interpretations in the Reagan cases draw substantially from a review of that publication since 1981, plus the *Congressional Quarterly Weekly Report* for periods of legislative involvement.

Reagan White House. Representatives of the Health Care Financing Administration, in the wake of their required report, testified before Congress in support of the proposal. In legislative hearings, major interest groups indicated their positions, with the for-profit hospitals in particular seeking to shape prospective payment schemes in a manner which was most compatible with their interests. In part, all of the provider based groups were anxious to insure that any scheme would apply only to governmental programs and not payment by private insurance companies. The more widespread "all payers" system to regulate private as well as public payments to hospitals, which had been established in a few states by 1983, constituted a common point of opposition among the health care providers. In an additional step designed to placate fears from the hospital industry, the legislation as proposed by the Administration also avoided confronting the difficult question of the manner in which capital costs would be reimbursed under Medicare, thus leaving a system in place which most hospitals preferred.

In the promotion of President Reagan's legislative program in Congress, his legislative liaison team effort helped to create a sense in early 1983 that this proposal was on a "fast track" and that those who wanted some action taken in an effort to curb increases in hospital reimbursement should not ask too many questions (Demkovich 1983). Some supporters felt that the proposal would not accomplish much because of the potential for "creative" adjustment on the part of hospitals through the use of a multiple admission strategy, but nonetheless took the position that it was the best piece of legislation that could gain passage at that time. In the quest for support, the primary thrust by administration lobbyists was that the proposed legislation was a compromise step which could be taken quickly.

In the movement toward rapid congressional approval, there is little indication of intense lobbying of specific legislators. Strategically, the positioning of the prospective payment plan within the extensively negotiated and far reaching proposal for modifying Social Security clearly facilitated a limited legislative debate (Light 1985). The most important vote on prospective payment came in the House of Representatives, and the measure passed by a convincing 282–148 margin. In the Senate, only token opposition emerged as the measure was passed with only eight dissenting votes.

The Reagan Administration thus provided an important, but shared, role in the establishment of the prospective payment system. On issue raising activity and on legislative bargaining, there seems to have been a limited role. Congress was clearly ready to do something about the costs of services within Medicare. At the same time, the Administration did seize upon a policy design which had the potential for fairly broad support among both legislators and affected interests. In developing a proposal which would have at least cautious support among major hospital lobby groups, the Administration clearly provided access for the American Hospital Association. At the same time, the Administration was willing to confront the continued opposition of the American Medical Association—and its fears that steps taken for hospitals would be subsequently used as a precedent for changes in the manner in which physicians were reimbursed under Medicare. Finally, it should also be emphasized that in the wake of its legislative victory the Reagan Administration successfully resisted efforts by the hospital industry to achieve delays in implementing the new program. Thus in 1983, a reform characterized by Demkovich (1983) as "The most significant change in Medicare in seventeen years" began to alter the manner in which hospitals were reimbursed for the care provided within Medicare.

The establishment of catastrophic health care benefits within Medicare in 1988 represented a second major health policy change during the Reagan Presidency. In providing for major increases in hospital coverage, the new legislation was often characterized as the most substantial increase in access to health care since the establishment of Medicare in 1965. Along with expanded access, however, the program also contained a major new financing approach. Rather than being funded through increases in the Medicare tax paid by employees, the new program was designed to have the elderly themselves provide the additional funds through a combination of increased Medicare payments and a special tax on elderly persons with substantial incomes. Once again, significant roles were undertaken by administrative and legislative leaders, some interest group representatives, as well as by President Reagan.

In contrast to the President's virtual public silence on the hospital reimbursement issue, interest in catastrophic insurance was encouraged by Reagan's public role. Beginning in 1983, catastrophic insurance received a brief but recurrent inclusion in each State of the Union Address. In the issue raising role, Reagan's level of emphasis on catastrophic health insurance never approached the frequency of emphasis which occurred on such policy questions as responses to drug abuse. Nonetheless, with his periodic references to catastrophic health care costs, Reagan helped to create a political environment which was conducive to some form of legislative action.

President Reagan, whether intentionally or not, also contributed to the pursuit of a new catastrophic insurance program with his nomination of Otis Bowen, an Indiana physician and former governor, as Secretary of Health and Human Services in late 1985. At his confirmation hearings, Bowen very forcefully emphasized the importance he attached to the development of improved protection against the costs of catastrophic illnesses.

By the time Secretary Bowen actually reported his plan to the Reagan Administration in late 1986, there was also considerable interest in the issue within Congress. That interest could be traced to three factors. First, the Democratic gains in Congress (including the successful return to majority party status in the Senate) increased a sense of assertiveness on domestic policy. Second, the obvious weakening of the Reagan Presidency following the revelations surrounding the Iran-contra scandal also contributed to a sense of assertiveness within Congress. Third, discussion of the catastrophic insurance proposal was generating an increasing expectation that some action would be taken. Thus as the Reagan White House debated the merits of Bowen's proposal, Republican as well as Democratic members of the House Energy and Commerce Committee were sending word to the president that they were about ready to act whether the White House submitted the Bowen proposal or not. Reagan's subsequent endorsement of the Bowen proposal and submission to Congress was an important step in its signalling of presidential support, but it did not represent the seizing of an

initiative which would otherwise have remained dormant in Congress as of early 1987.

In the development of the design for catastrophic insurance which finally emerged, significant roles were performed within both the Reagan Administration and in Congress. The final bill was considerably broader than had originally been proposed by Secretary Bowen and, in turn, President Reagan. Not only was a prescription drug benefit added along with limited new provisions for home care, but also the states were required to expand coverage for the elderly poor under Medicaid, and the payment formulas were substantially modified. Besides emerging as a more comprehensive program, the final bill also represented a compromise of significant differences between the original House and Senate versions.

Once the initial proposal began to evolve in Congress, the Administration also contributed to the program design in one very important respect. The position taken by Secretary Bowen against the inclusion of a long term care benefit, along with the continuing discussion of the threat of a presidential veto, served to reduce potential support for an attack on long-term care costs in the context of the proposed catastrophic insurance measure.

President Reagan did take some important steps in maintaining support for a catastrophic insurance package. Along with his initial indication of support in his health message to Congress, he also used his radio address on Feb 14, 1988 to express his concern for the development of a catastrophic insurance package. President Reagan's support was a significant step in the movement toward a catastrophic insurance proposal, since his support made resistance on the part of the program's conservative opponents considerably more difficult.

The role of legislative leaders in shaping the final legislation was also very substantial. At points, interest group opposition was quite intense, as groups such as the Pharmaceutical Manufacturers Association fought against aspects of the prescription drug benefit which they felt would encourage future policies to move away from the use of brand-name (toward generic) medications. There were also substantial pressures for a larger bill, with lobbyists for the elderly and legislators such as Senator Kennedy and Congressman Henry Waxman (Dem., Calif.) promoting measures which would begin to address the question of financial assistance for long term care. The actions of the Reagan Administration in supporting a limited bill thus both increased the likelihood that some legislation would emerge and also decreased the likelihood that a bill would emerge which addressed the more substantial health care access issue for the elderly—the financing of long-term care.

The Reagan Presidency thus produced additional indications of the ways in which a president might contribute in the development of access and reimbursement reforms. In the enactment of prospective payment reform within Medicare in 1983, the Reagan Administration performed an important role in the negotiations with affected provider interests and in designing a proposal which would have a good chance of rapid passage. In the establishment of the Catastrophic Health Insurance Act of 1988, there was some initial issue raising activity and an important advocacy role by Otis Bowen. At the same time, policymaking roles in both instances were substantially shared. Congress had also been seeking some cost control design in 1981–1982, and on the expansion of Medicare in 1988, legislative initiatives and bargaining among interest groups made important contributions in the developments that allowed a final bill to emerge.

Ultimately, perhaps the most important lesson from the two successful reform efforts in the Reagan Presidency surrounded the extent to which political opportunity for a president was being shaped by the budgetary aspects of his proposals. Increasing concern with health care costs created a climate in which legislators were anxious to address approaches that would help reduce payment rates for the federal government. In turn, the passage of the catastrophic coverage demonstrated the importance of a financing mechanism which avoided direct competition for scarce revenue through the use of fees and an additional tax to be paid by the elderly.

Lesson and Implications

Presidential actions surrounding major health policy changes suggest important conclusions regarding both past performances and future leadership prospects. On the basis of past performances and the total cost and demographic change factors which are now shaping health policy concerns, presidents should be expected to fulfill definite roles if there is to be successful achievement of major changes in health policy. Presidential leadership will be an essential, but not sufficient, force for major change.

The first lesson from the case studies is that successful presidential leadership in achieving significant changes in major health policies can occur only when a convergence of political opportunity and political skill and commitment occurs. In the instances in which presidents were unsuccessful with their initiatives, aspects of political opportunity were lacking. The presidents who were unsuccessful in these cases (Kennedy, Nixon on national health insurance, and Carter) all confronted major limitations surrounding at least one of the following factors: lack of a working majority in Congress, lack of electoral support for their presidency, lack of personal popularity, and intense interest group opposition. A president who lacks political skill and commitment may further decrease chances for major policy change, but it is unlikely that a president who lacks strong political opportunities will be successful even if he possesses substantial political skill and a desire to pursue major new initiatives.

The second lesson from the case studies is that actions leading to major policy change are characterized by a substantial sharing of roles, but with major instances of change occurring with presidents undertaking actions in at least some aspects of the policy formation cycle.

Turning first to issue raising roles, presidents have made differing contributions. Presidents Kennedy and Johnson acted as part of a major focus on health policy problems of the elderly which began among interest groups and legislative advocates. President Nixon very clearly contributed to an interest in HMOs as both a general cost control issue and a specific choice of a policy design. On national health insurance proposals, Nixon undertook little specific action, in the context of a period in which a large number of proposals were already on the congressional agenda.

Presidents Carter and Reagan had different experiences with the issue raising process. Carter gave some attention to national health insurance but quite quickly acted to try to slow the movement for at least the more sweeping proposals. Conversely, on hospital cost containment, he did make major and unsuccessful national appeals. For Reagan, changes in medicare reimbursement were not addressed as a public issue, but the actions involving catastrophic insurance did involve initial presidential encouragement. A major issue raising effort, in sum, has been sufficient to insure neither new legislation nor a requirement for ultimate success.

Questions of policy design have seen important actions taken in several contexts by our recent presidents and their top health policy specialists. Here again, however, the role has often been shared at key points with members of Congress. Medicare, in particular, underwent major expansion in the Ways and Means Committee. Nixon's development of proposals for HMOs was very distinctly the product of his Department of Health, Education and Welfare, but was also modified by Congress. Carter's proposals for cost control and Reagan's design of a new method of Medicare reimbursement for hospitals involved major administration proposals, but followed initial legislative and administrative interest.

On the access proposals of Nixon and Carter, their ultimately unsuccessful ideas constituted one set of proposals among a large group of access proposals being considered. Reagan's design of an access proposal in the form of expanding Medicare to include catastrophic coverage also underwent significant modification—but with basic policy dimensions having been outlined by Secretary Bowen.

In balance, it appears that presidents do not have to dominate the policy design process in order for a successful proposal to emerge. Because of the growth in legislative staff and the emergence of significant consultative activity on aspects of health policy, there is a substantial potential for aspects of policy design to be worked out in the context of modifications in presidential proposals. Efforts at major change are likely to be substantially reduced, however, if the process of movement toward a final policy design does not involve a significant presidential role involving interest group interactions and a focusing of the legislative process to avoid tendencies toward stalemate.

In the area of political support building, presidents have not spent extensive amounts of time working with potentially supportive constituencies surrounding potential beneficiaries of expanded access. Speeches such as President Kennedy's address to senior citizen groups in Madison Square Garden are very rare. The actions by presidential aides, more than the presidents themselves, have been important in support building roles. Presidents themselves may also have important roles, however, in the specific negotiations with groups skeptical about initial proposals.

The relationship with Congress also involves a major presidential role. The case studies have not produced instances in which presidents have successfully changed large numbers of votes among Congressmen who were disposed by constituency, ideology, or party orientations to take a different position. Johnson's success in 1965, for example, is not significantly attributed to his efforts to change the votes of rank and file members of Congress. Although operating from a much weaker position in 1978–79, Carter's inability to achieve his hospital cost control legislation nicely illustrates the difficulties involved in trying to change the position of significant numbers of legislators.

The presidential relationship with Congress takes on major importance, however, in other respects. Presidents have often had important roles in insuring that some form of legislation would move forward. A steering of the legislative process was important for Johnson in 1964–65 and in Reagan's hurrying of the legislative response on Medicare's prospective payment scheme. Often an important role has involved helping to prevent "kiss of death" amendments in which opponents will amend a bill in an effort to increase chances for ultimate defeat of the entire package. Because health policy involves so many competing choices among specific techniques, the significance of the steering role is thereby increased.

As presidents relate to Congress, a key question is whether presidents will seek to promote either the higher or lower levels of a change likely to be supported by a legislative majority. On Medicare, President Johnson enthusiastically backed those who sought to provide a broader program in 1965. In other instances, such as the passage of the Catastrophic Health Insurance Act of 1988, the choice of technique and magnitude of effort involved an attempt to restrict congressional expansion of the initial proposal. On hospital reimbursement, the Reagan Administration was not willing to endorse an "all payers" system, and thus acted to reduce pressures for a more encompassing form of hospital rate regulation. Similarly, Nixon on HMO legislation ultimately ended up supporting more limited financing of the new initiative than was being advocated by many members of Congress.

The case studies have also suggested that presidents can have important roles in the context of the implementation phase of the policy cycle. Legislative enactments in 1965, 1973, and 1983 produced a necessity for implementation decisions. Quite persistently, the health care providers who have opposed aspects of legislation in Congress have sought a subsequent modification through presidential decisions in implementing new policy steps. Generally, those debates have involved issues of speed in startup actions and the specific interpretation of reimbursement practices being established with the new legislation.

Given past experiences, what might be expected in the future? In the coming years, as in the recent past, there is a potential for substantial sharing of issue raising roles and at least some of the efforts at interest–group support building. The president's role in helping to focus agreement on specific policy design choices seem likely to assume greater importance. This is likely to occur because of the tremendous range of choices possible in the design of health policy options. Given that range of choices, presidential leadership can be extremely important in avoiding deadlocks which occur as supporters of competing approaches each becomes firmly wedded to the favored approach.

The presidential role in negotiating with key interests also seems likely to take on increasing importance. The tremendous economic stakes that such interests as physicians, hospitals, and insurance companies have in both access and reimbursement decisions, plus the magnitude of their political resources, are likely to make future interactions between presidents and such groups as the American Medical Association, the American Hospital Association, and the Hospital Insurance Association of American extremely important in the possible development of major changes in health policy.

Ultimately, instances of significant presidential health policy leaderships roles in achieving broad changes in health policy are likely to occur infrequently. In terms of political opportunity, instances of divided government appear to be the predominant pattern in Washington, and presidents appear to have increasing problems in maintaining personal support. Budgetary considerations, in turn, are likely to offer opportunities for reimbursement policy changes but also operate as a constraint on access policies which involve additional expenditures. On a personal level, presidents may also lack the necessary skills and the requisite commitment to health policy issues.

For those interested in health policy change, four conclusions are thus warranted. First, potentials for sequential adjustments involving less fundamental change deserve careful consideration. While incremental adjustments are less dramatic, a series of changes can produce substantial amounts of change over a several year period. Medicaid, for example, has been substantially altered since its creation without one dominant occurrence in which a fundamental change was enacted. Second, the nature of collaborative roles in which the magnitude of a president's contribution is somewhat reduced deserves to be explored. Strong advocates of additional public support for access to health care within Congress, for example, may find that pushing a more reluctant president can lead to bargaining roles in which presidents are somewhat reactive to proposals for an expansion of initial presidential initiatives. Third, precisely because opportunities for changes in health policy through strong acts of presidential leadership tend to occur infrequently, it is essential for those who are interested in major changes to work toward the creation of those opportunities for presidential leadership. Fourth, when those opportunities do occur, their uniqueness should be fully recognized. The infrequency of instances in which presidents seem likely to be able to provide leadership resulting in major changes in health policy underscores the importance of actions which maximize those opportunities when they do occur.

REFERENCES

Bowles, Nigel. 1987. *The White House and Capital Hill: The politics of presidential persuasion.* New York: Oxford University Press.

Braverman, Jordan. 1978. *Crisis in health care.* Washington, D.C.: Acropolis Books, LTD.

Brown, Lawrence D. 1983. *Politics and health care organization: HMOs as federal policy.* Washington, D.C.: Brookings Institution.

Califano, Joseph A., Jr. 1981. *Governing America.* New York: Simon and Schuster.

Congressional Quarterly Almanac. 1978. Hospital cost control. Washington, D.C.: Congressional Quarterly.

Congressional Quarterly Weekly Report (Select issues). Washington, D.C.: Congressional Quarterly.

David, Sheri I. 1985. *With dignity: The search for medicare and medicaid.* Westport, CT.: Greenwood Press.

Demkovich, Linda. 1983. Who says Congress can't move fast? Just ask hospitals about Medicare. *National Journal.* (April 2): 704–707.

Falkson, Joseph L. 1980. *HMOs and the politics of health system reform.* Chicago: American Hospital Association and Robert J. Brady, Co.

Feingold, Eugene. 1966. *Medicare: Policy and politics.* San Francisco: Chandler Publishing Co.

Feldstein, Paul J. and Glenn Melnick. 1984. Congressional voting behavior on hospital legislation: An explorational study. *Journal of Health Politics, Policy and Law.* 8:686–700.

Fishel, Jeff. 1985. *Presidents and promises.* Washington, D.C.: CQ Press.

Fisher, Louis. 1981. *The politics of shared power: Congress and the executive.* Washington, D.C.: Congressional Quarterly Press.

Flitner, David Jr. 1986. *The Politics of presidential commissions.* Dobbs Ferry, N.Y.: Transitional Publishers, Inc.

Harris, Richard. 1966. *A sacred trust.* New York: New American Library.

Hart, Roderick P. 1987. *The sound of leadership: presidential communication in the modern age.* Chicago: University of Chicago Press.

Johnson, Haynes. 1980. *In the absence of power.* New York: Viking Press.

Kellerman, Barabara. 1984 *The political presidency.* New York: VikingPress.

Jones, Charles. 1988. *The trusteeship presidency: Jimmy Carter and the U.S. Congress.* Baton Rouge, LA.: Louisiana State University Press.

Kernell, Samuel. 1986. *Going public: New strategies of presidential leadership.* Washington, D.C.: CQ Press.

King, Gary and Lyn Ragsdale. 1988. *The elusive executive: Discovering statistical patterns in the presidency.* Washington, D.C.: CQ Press.

Kingdon, John W. 1984. *Agendas, alternatives, and public policies.* Boston: Little, Brown.

Lammers, William W. 1982. Presidential attention-focusing activities. In *The president and the public,* edited by Doris Graber, 145–171. Philadelphia: Institute for the Human Issues.

Light, Paul. 1985. *Artful work: The politics of social security reform.* New York: Random House.

Light, Paul C. 1988. "The focusing skill and presidential influence in Congress." In *Congressional politics,* edited by Christopher Deering, 239–261. Chicago, IL.: The Dorsey Press.

Lefkowitz, Bonnie. 1983. *Health planning: Lessons for the future.* Rockville, MD.: Aspen Systems Corporation.

McGraw-Hill (weekly). Washington report on medicine and health. Washington, D.C.: McGraw-Hill, Inc.

Marmor, Theodore R. 1973. *The politics of Medicare.* New York: Aldine Publishing Co.

Mueller, Keith J. 1986. An analysis of congressional health policy voting in the 1970s. *Journal of Health, Politics, Policy and Law.* 11:117–135.

Parmet, Herbert S. 1983. *J.F.K., the presidency of John F. Kennedy.* New York: Dial Press.

Pfiffner, James P. 1988. *The strategic presidency: Hitting the ground running.* Chicago: The Dorsey Press.

Poen, Monte M. 1979. *Harry S. Truman versus the medical lobby: The genesis of Medicare.* Columbia, MO.: University of Missouri Press.

Pratt, Henry J. 1976. *The gray lobby.* Chicago: University of Chicago Press.

Public papers of the presidents (Annual). Washington, D.C.: Government Printing Office.

Ripley, Randall. 1983. *Congress: Process and policy.* New York: Norton.

Ripley, Randall. 1984. *Congress, the bureaucracy, and public policy.* Homewood, IL.: Dorsey Press.

Seligman, Lester G. and Cary R. Covington. 1989. *The coalitional presidency.* Chicago: The Dorsey Press.

Starr, Paul. 1982. *The social transformation of American medicine.* New York: Basic Books.

Sundquist, James L. 1968. *Politics and policy: The Eisenhower, Kennedy and Johnson years.* Washington, D.C.: The Brookings Institute.

Thompson, Frank J. 1981. *Health policy and the bureaucracy: Politics and implementation.* Cambridge: The MIT Press.

Vladeck, Bruce C. 1980. *Tender unloving care.* New York: Basic Books.

Wildavsky, Aaron. 1988. *The new politics of the budgetary process.* Glencoe, IL.: Scott, Foresman/Little Brown.

Wolanin, Thomas F. 1975. *Presidential advisory commissions: Truman to Nixon.* Madison: University of Wisconsin Press.

Chapter 6

Congress and Health Policy:

The Legacy of Reform and Retrenchment

David Falcone

Lynn C. Hartwig

Congressional health policy encompasses legislative decisions directly affecting principle actors and institutions in their roles in the health field. Several identifiable legislative structures which deal with bills that directly affect the organization, delivery, and financing of health services can be identified. It is our contention that there is little to distinguish the politics of health legislation other than (a) this structural differentiation in Congress, whereby responsibilities are assigned for health issues, and (b) the particular "concentration of interest" that characterizes pressure group demands in the health policy arena (Falcone 1980–1981, 1983).

The legislative process with regard to health issues is not immune to the factors that have affected all policy areas over the past twenty years. In her book, *Stability and Change in Congress*, Barbara Hinckley (1983) asks "what is the effect, if any, of congressional variations on environmental policy, or education, or any other policy area?"

Hinckley is not the only observer of legislative behavior who has asked this type of question. A highly controversial body of literature has challenged the traditional political science view that places significance on procedural reform (Dye 1980). The studies making up this literature—referred to, among other labels, as "determinants analyses"—have at least forced people to consider, in qualitative as well as quantitative terms, whether the variations in structure and process that have been the foci of reform efforts, such as the professionalization and institutionalization of state legislatures, have been merely coincidental with, rather than causes of, policy change.

In this chapter, after discussing what we mean by health policy, we will delineate the major reforms in congressional procedure of the 1970s, assess their impact on legislative decision making in health and examine the question of whether these changes have made any significant difference in health policy.

Procedurally, we note that the influence of the

general budget policy process has grown in importance relative to the specific health policy process. We hypothesize that disjointed incrementalism (which we will use interchangeably with decrementalism) remains an appropriate description of the *health* policy process even if more rationalistic "models" better fit the budgetary process.

Substantively, the general conclusion reached is that it is nearly impossible to ascribe policy developments, or the lack of them, in the health field to variations in the structure and process of congressional decision making. This is not to say that the reforms were insignificant, only that changes in both policy and procedure may also spring, among other sources, from economic and, perhaps consequently, ideological variables, from the substance and style of the Presidency, and from "rational" evaluations of the efficacy, efficiency, and effectiveness of past policies.

Health Policy

Several types of policy directly affect or seek to affect health. Those that come readily to mind are primarily legislative, but they also include judicial and executive decisions. Specific subjects include the rates of production, geographic and specialty distribution of health personnel, health care financing, assurance of the quality of health personnel, institutions and services, occupational safety and environmental protection, and attempts to limit consumption of destructive substances such as alcohol, tobacco and synthetic carcinogens. In some instances, the indirect effects on health of housing, income maintenance, or other welfare policies may be even more consequential than the direct effects of policies that patently deal with health (Falcone 1983; Feldstein 1988). Nevertheless, it is useful to limit the conception of health policy to the conventional notion of public decisions that seek primarily to affect health or principal actors, both professional and institutional, in their roles in the health arena. Using this restriction allows statements to be made such as the one posited above that some other policies may ultimately have a more telling impact on health than more strictly

health policies, or that there is a need for integrating different policy areas (health and welfare are perhaps those most frequently cited).

Health Legislation, Nixon to Reagan: Surge and Decline

This section reviews legislative developments in the health arena through four time periods (see table 6–1) in an attempt to depict the forward thrust in policy activity, particularly from 1965 through 1975, followed by a diminution of government intervention from the late 1970s through the late 1980s. The 1970s were a period of major congressional reform, and a research question examined here is the influence of this reform on congressional decision making in explaining this policy shift.

Before 1960, health care policy in the United States focused on improving the quality of care through activities of the health professions and state governments. After the Flexner Report in 1910, for example, a number of medical schools in this country were closed as the educational process for physicians was standardized and the basis for scientific and specialty medicine was created in the basic science departments of educational institutions. At the same time, states passed licensing laws restricting entry into practice to graduates of accredited schools (Stevens 1971).

Federal public health activities were limited to hospitals for special populations to communicable disease control, and to some maternal and child health programs. These functions were overshadowed after World War II by the passage of Hill-Burton legislation and the buildup in the 1950s and early 1960s of the research programs of the National Institutes of Health (NIH). The first major federal social policy thrust on the other hand, the Social Security Act (SSA) of 1935, purposefully omitted health proposals from its content. Framers of the act feared medical profession opposition would subvert the entire program. While some of the above policies, such as the reduction in medical school openings, negatively affected access, others, such as Hill-Burton, increased access and improved the quality of the facilities in small communities.

Development of Medical Policy in the United States Over Four Time Periods: 1900–1988

Time period	1900–1960	1961–1972	1973–1980	1981–1988
Goal	Quality	Access	Cost effectiveness	Decrementalism
Objectives	Upgrade medical education Strengthen scientific basis of medicine Strengthen specialty training and practice Upgrade medical practice	Increase number of physicians and other health professionals Improve geographic distribution Improve ability to pay Improve specialty distribution	Control capital expansion Reduce use of expensive technology Control number of providers Reduce use of institutions	Decentralization/Devolution Control federal budget
Policies	Pass state licensing laws Close medical schools Standardize medical education through accreditation Fund biomedical research Fund hospital construction Hill-Burton	Expand medical schools Build new schools *CHP NHSC Medicare AHEC Rural health initiatives EPSDT Primary care programs including family medicine	PSRO HSA HMO Prevention/promotion programs Center for health technology Primary care programs as cost control mechanism	Block grants Medicine prospective payment for hospital care Medicare Cuts Catastrophic health insurance

TABLE 6–1

*CHP Comprehensive health planning; NHSC, National Health Services Corps; AHEC, Area Health Education Center; EPSDT, Early and Periodic Screening, Diagnosis and Treatment; PSRO, professional standards review organizations; HSA, Health Services Administration; HMO, Health Maintenance Organization.

In 1960 a new emphasis upon access as a goal, and the shift to greater federal involvement in policy decisions generally, resulted in a fifteen-year period of legislation designed to reduce financial, geographical, organizational, and other barriers to care. The decision makers placed their faith in input and process policies, assuming that the outcome would be beneficial; that is, if resources were provided them, people would get the health care they needed and improved health status would result. Within a very short period, federal health policies laid the foundation for increases in facilities, personnel, and money. Amendments to the Hill-Burton legislation, PL 87-395, PL 88-442, and PL 91-296, provided support for outpatient facilities, nursing homes, and the modernization of hospital and health care facilities in urban areas.

In 1963 health manpower legislation, PL 88-129, authorized support to medical schools for the first time. Later, legislation encouraged existing schools to expand enrollment, funded new schools, supported programs to train new health practitioners and primary care physicians, and created Area Health Education Center (AHEC) programs. Federal policies were directed at preventing an impending physician shortage that was predicted in numerous studies in the 1940s, 1950s, and early 1960s (Sorkin 1977).

The legislative debates over the Hill-Burton legislation, health manpower, and research funding were mild compared to the debates that raged over national health insurance. Several factors limited controversy. For one thing, it was difficult to argue with the need for physicians, hospitals, or research. In addition, the policies were perceived as essentially distributive in nature, benefiting the professional and academic interest group constituencies without directly depriving anyone else of support.

Far more controversial was legislation that finally passed creating national health insurance for those over sixty-five and for the poor. Marmor (1973) charts Medicare's progress from impossible in the 1950s to enactment in 1965 and notes that the House Ways and Means Committee had a central role, first in preventing passage and then, after the 1964 election made the legislation virtually inevitable, in greatly expanding the Johnson administration's proposals.

While policymakers from 1961 to 1964 focused public attention on the battles between the American Medical Association (AMA) and AFL-CIO, the most crucial negotiations took place between then Assistant Secretary of Health, Education and Welfare Wilbur Cohen and Ways and Means Chairman Wilbur Mills (Dem., Ark.) According to Marmor's analysis, Mills had the political sensitivity, power, and technical expertise to block legislation before 1964 and then to steer his own version of Medicare through the Ways and Means Committee and the House. Many of the legislative reforms in the 1970s were aimed directly at breaking Mills' power on Ways and Means, and it is doubtful whether by 1980 any member of Congress could exercise the control Mills did through "Persuasion, entreaty, authoritative expertise and control of the agenda" (Marmor 1973).

Other key elements of President Johnson's health policy were Regional Medical Programs (RMP) designed to help move the latest medical knowledge into communities through a cooperative arrangement between academic institutions and community physicians, and Comprehensive Health Planning (CHP). As with many federal programs, CHP began as a permissive program and later became mandatory.

Health legislative activity continued under the Nixon administration, and in 1970 eleven major acts of legislation were passed, including such new areas as occupational health and safety, alcohol abuse, and the National Health Service Corps. In 1971 the President's declared war on cancer resulted in substantially increased support for comprehensive programs targeting this disease.

The major features of legislation passed between 1961 and 1971 were improved access through increased numbers of physicians and other health professionals, construction of facilities, and payment for care. Policy makers before 1972 showed little concern for either actual or future cost as legislation was passed creating program upon program. At the end of this period, health policy, as other policy areas, changed in three ways: (1) the magnitude of government spending at all levels in health rose both in absolute terms from $6.6 billion in 1960 to $104.2 billion in 1980 and as a percent of total health expenditures from 24.7 percent to 42.2 percent (Gibson and Waldo 1982); (2) policy and decision making shifted to the federal level; and (3) the goals of the policy process became implicitly more redistributive and explicitly aimed at improving access to health care.

By 1972 the costs of these programs had become visible, whereas their effectiveness measured in terms of improved health status had not. The prospect of some form of national health insurance seemed imminent, and the consequent effect on inflation was viewed with alarm by federal policymakers (Russell 1977). A significant change in the rhetoric of the health policy debate was evident in Congress by 1972 during consideration of professional standards review organization (PSRO) legislation and discussion of the National Health Planning and Resources Development Act (PL 93–641). Cost containment was the prevailing justification for peer review. Policymakers believed that if unnecessary hospitalization and surgery could be averted, Medicare and Medicaid cost could be reduced. The containment of costs was also the justification for a stronger health planning law. As time for the legislative authority of Hill-Burton, Regional Medical Programs, and Comprehensive Health Planning began to run out, Congress recognized that government programs had proliferated in an uncoordinated fashion and that inflation in the health system was significantly greater than general inflation. For those in health policy circles desiring to expand health insurance in the United States, regulation was one method of centralizing control of the system. On January 4, 1975, a few days after the National Health Planning and Resources Development Act was signed into law, a staff member of the Subcommittee on Health of the Senate Labor and Public Welfare Committee told an audience of health planners that "you are providing the foundation of an effective, efficient national health insurance program" (Biles 1975).

Ironically, the same year that PL 93–641 was passed, the health manpower legislation was allowed to expire. For two years Congress was unable to pass renewal authorization. While the new health planning system was given authority to determine the need for health professionals, it had no control over the training or distribution of physicians. After ten years of federal funding of health professionals' education, Congress realized that, while the medical schools had responded to federal policy by increasing the output of physicians, nearly doubling the number of student spaces by 1974, the increased numbers had not altered geographical and specialty maldistributions. Suggested solutions that would be

less costly were to direct physicians into primary care, use nonphysician health personnel, and increase the number of areas receiving members of the National Health Service Corps. Differences between proposals supported by Senator Edward Kennedy (Dem., Mass.) and Congressman Paul Rogers (Dem., Fla.) prevented final congressional action (LeRoy and Lee 1977). Rogers' philosophy ultimately was reflected in the Health Professions Assistance Act of 1976. Medical students were not required to enter primary care specialties or practice in underserved areas, but medical schools were required to have 50 percent of their graduates entering primary care residencies by 1980; more coercive policies might have been considered if this goal were not met. The critical concept was primary care, and Congress chose the least controversial but also least meaningful definition—graduates entering internal medicine, family medicine, pediatrics, and obstetrics-gynecology.

Cost containment was also used as justification for the Health Maintenance Organization legislation passed during the Nixon presidency, although with an entirely different rationale than PSROs and HSAs. The purpose of federal support of HMOs was to instill competition in the health care system and to encourage effective preventive medical care. Senator Kennedy's attempt to turn the administration bill into a much stronger initiative to reform the health system resulted in a bill that contained proposals (such as open enrollment) making it difficult for federal HMOs to compete. AMA pressure resulted in a bill that provided limited funds for feasibility studies and development grants (Price 1975). Subsequent revisions of the act created a more economically realistic set of criteria for HMO development, but far fewer applicants than had been expected qualified for federal status.

Between 1970 and 1975, Congress created a host of new programs. The prevailing ideology still expected government to provide solutions to the problems identified in the health system. But instead of the open-ended financing of the 1960s, such programs needed to be justified in terms of cost effectiveness. New program costs had to be offset by saving to the system. This belief, and the presence of two subcommittee chairmen (Rogers and Kennedy) intent on establishing reputations in the health arena, made the period a particularly productive one.

As health care costs continued to escalate at rates above general inflation during the Carter presidency, the Democrats were divided over how to proceed. Senator Kennedy argued that costs could be controlled only by centralizing the insurance system. The President and more fiscally conservative senators and representatives feared that until a mechanism was in place to control at least hospital costs, expansion of the insurance system could strain the federal budget to the breaking point. National health insurance took a back seat to proposals to control fraud and abuse in the system and change hospital reimbursement to a formula reflecting historical costs and growth in the GNP. Carter was successful in the former, but not in the latter, effort. The Hospital Cost Containment Act failed to pass in the 95th and 96th Congresses largely due to lobbying efforts on the part of the hospital industry and initial success of its "Voluntary Effort" cost-containment program. In addition, the difference between general inflation and that in the hospital sector briefly decreased, thereby temporarily quelling the desire for reform.

With the election of Ronald Reagan, the terms of the health policy debate were significantly altered. After twenty years of government expansion, Reagan promised to balance the budget and to reduce the size and scope of federal activity. Congressional policy making was caught between a popular president and growing concern in both the public and private sectors over the federal deficit. Initially, Reagan's proposals spared Medicare, but when Congress showed a willingness to include this program in serious budget cuts, the Administration "soon came around" (Iglehart 1985). The President's initial budget proposed replacing the categorical grant structure with two block grants for health and preventive services. Responsibility for allocating resources among the programs would be shifted to the states. The amount of funds transferred to the states for the programs would be reduced by 25 percent on the argument that states would have lower administrative costs and duplication of effort could be reduced. For other programs such as the health planning system, PSROs, HMO support, health professions support and the National Health Service Corps, Reagan proposed

defunding entirely. For Medicaid, he proposed a cap on the federal contribution. Within a year of taking office, he proposed a swap calling for, among other things, federalizing Medicaid and turning the food stamp program over to the states.

Congress was forced to respond to Reagan's agenda, and while substantial changes were made in the block grant proposal (four block grants were created with restrictions on funding and ten programs were left out of the block grants), many of the other Reagan proposals were incorporated in the Omnibus Reconciliation Budget Act of 1981. Federal contributions for Medicaid were reduced by 3 percent in fiscal 1982, 4 percent in fiscal 1983 and 4.5 percent in fiscal 1984, and the out-of-pocket costs borne by beneficiaries increased by 25 percent. Congressman Henry Waxman (Dem., Calif.), chairman of the House Energy and Commerce Subcommittee on Health and the Environment, was more successful than any other legislator in countering the Administration's proposals, and the continued authorization of many health programs was the result of his efforts, efforts that were often in vain when the programs went unfunded (Iglehart 1983).

By 1985 the health planning system had been dismantled and funding for HMOs and the new scholarships for the National Health Service Corps had ceased, but the competitive, deregulated health system Reagan envisioned never materialized. No coherent competitive strategy ever emerged from the Reagan Administration. What became obvious during the budget debates of 1981 and 1982 was that Reagan's focus would be on controlling the cost of federal programs, particularly Medicare and Medicaid, not attempting to restructure the private sector, as Carter's hospital cost containment legislation had sought. Congress preferred to reduce spending for all programs rather than discontinue them. And by the end of Reagan's first term, spending cuts were beginning to be restored, including a major expansion of the Medicaid program to include poor women and children in households not previously eligible, a proposal originating in Waxman's subcommittee.

Since discretionary health spending (i.e., all programs other than Medicare and Medicaid) accounted for only 14 percent of the total federal health outlays and Medicare alone accounted for 60 percent (Davis 1981), it was obvious that Medicare and Medicaid costs had to be contained to effect significant budget reductions. During the period 1980 through 1987, Congress enacted more than thirty laws that affected the Medicare and Medicaid programs. An analysis by the General Accounting Office (GAO 1988) of the five laws[1] having the most telling effects on program and beneficiary costs concluded that had prior cost growth trends continued, actual inflation-adjusted Medicare costs would have been about $17.3 billion more than they actually were.

Congressional health policy making in the Reagan years was characterized by changes in both process and content. Decision making shifted from the authorizing and appropriating processes, to the budget reconciliation process. Health subcommittees came to play a much smaller role than they had previously. Traditional interest groups found they were much less able to follow policy proposals as they emerged in consolidated budget acts, let alone influence the process (Lawton 1981).

The policy process within Congress in the 1980s was conditioned by two environmental factors—the election of Reagan and the budget deficit. By 1981 even the most committed government interventonist had to bow before the reality of the costs of social programs put in place in the 1960s and 1970s. Policy making became a zero-sum game. Explicit redistribution was necessary between government policy arenas (e.g., defense and domestic policy) and among groups and classes of citizens (e.g., young and old). As Price (1985) has observed, Congress is better at distributing benefits than redistributing them, generating ideas and representing particular interests, rather than enacting policies which are integrative, and broadly representative of a national interest. Congress in the 1980s found itself in a dilemma of having to enact policies it was least equipped structurally and least comfortable politically to address. It reacted by (1) avoiding making decisions until the last possible

moment, which resulted in government run by continuing resolution for days to months after the start of fiscal years, and (2) making policy through the budget reconciliation process, largely invisible to outsiders, and for which accountability largely disappeared. We now turn to a more rounded assessment of the relationship between the congressional process and policy.

Health Policy and the Legislative Process

Fifteen years ago we would have described the U.S. Congress by noting that it was distinctive among Western democratic legislative assemblies with respect to the power it has retained vis-a-vis the executive, despite the fact that the complexities of policy formation have increasingly placed the responsibility for policy initiation, priority determination, and formulation with the executive branch of government.[2] Whereas most legislatures have had as their principle function the refinement of executive proposals, Congress has remained comparatively capable both of generating policy and of posing the threat of thwarting executive initiatives so that, at least, the calculus of anticipated legislative reaction has been a significant factor in influencing the shape of major policies.

This may still be an accurate distinction, but it is certainly not as definite as before. The reasons why Congress has joined in the often bemoaned decline of legislatures (Loewenberg 1971) are complex and interrelated: the executive's near monopoly on information needed to make decisions; the fact that perhaps more than ever in twentieth-century legislative history senators and representatives need not adhere to party guidelines in their campaign rhetoric or voting behavior, thus creating a power vacuum in Congress that is exploitable by a vigorous president; the tendency toward plebiscitary democracy that is furthered although, as the Ford and Carter administrations' experiences attest, certainly not determined, by the president's preemptory access to the mass media; and the reliance on vari-

---

[1]They are the Omnibus Budget Reconciliation Act of 1981, the Tax Equity and Fiscal Responsibility Act of 1982, the Deficit Reduction Act of 1984, the Consolidated Omnibus Budget Reconciliation Act of 1985, and the Omnibus Budget Reconciliation Act of 1986.

[2]We borrow this "staging" of the policy process from Van Loon and Whittington (1987).

ants of neo-Keynesian economics (albeit perhaps implicity) and the resultant blending of fiscal, monetary, and social programs in such a way that a single source ultimately must interdigitate the ingredients of the overall policy mix. In any event, it is clear that a death knell for Congress would be premature, even if the policy initiation capability of this institution has been compromised. This is as true of health legislation as it is other arenas of congressional concern.

Key Structures in the Health Policy Legislative Process

Congressional decision making is so fluid and complex (e.g., each session of the House and Senate establishes its own procedures although some are emminently predictable), that it is an oversimplification to single out the components of the legislative process responsible for health policy. Nevertheless, it is fairly clear that certain standing committees are central: most notably Ways and Means and Commerce in the House, Finance and Labor and Human Resources in the Senate. Their respective turfs are not so readily indentifiable since committees are regularly engaged in jurisdictional disputes and because some proponents of legislation use the machine gun approach in advancing their causes; that is, they target several committees in the hope that one will be a hit.

Given norms of subspecialization partly owing to the complexity of modern legislation, particularly health legislation, subcommittees are key working units in the congressional process. There traditionally (at least during the period covered by this review of major changes in health policy) has been a Senate Subcommittee on Health within the Committee on Labor and Human Resources (formerly the Committee on Labor and Public Welfare). With the changeover in party control of the Senate in 1981, however, the new chairman of the full committee, Senator Orrin Hatch (Rep., Utah) formerly the ranking minority member of the subcommittee, retained his full measure of discretion over health issues by dissolving the subcommittee, thus leaving health affairs to the full committee. This arrangement

remained in place when the Democrats returned to power in 1986.

In addition, there periodically are select committees (i.e., those struck with responsibility for issues of emerging importance), such as the Senate Special and House Select Committee on Aging, that consider health issues. Moreover, all legislation must undergo the scrutiny of the House Rules Committee and the Senate and House Budget Committees. Finally, the Appropriations Committees of both houses are divided into subcommittees with functional responsibilities, one of which is health. Their support is crucial, since many authorizations are beefed up, watered down, or even (although this usually is a breach of collegiality), actually inaugurated at this stage (Redman 1974). Every prospective grantsman, for example, has keenly felt the meaning of the phrase "authorized but not appropriated." Authorizations usually cover a period of several years, whereas appropriations are voted on yearly.

Other committees occasionally assume prominence in dealing with health issues when their central concerns intersect with this policy area. For example, the Banking and Currency Committees were especially important during the early to mid 1970s because of the impact of the Economic Stabilization Program (wage and price controls), over which they had jurisdiction, on health care institutions.

The potential confusion in the legislative process surrounding the health arena mirrors the difficulty in labeling health policies: most not only seek to affect quality of care, access, and financing but also, explicitly or implicitly, call for regulation and redistribution of resources. For example, consideration of National Health Insurance (NHI) schemes could require decisions about revenue (House Ways and Means Committee and the Senate Finance Committee), health services delivery (Interstate and Foreign Commerce Committee in the House and the Labor and Human Resources Committee in the Senate), federal-state relations (Judiciary in each house), and the organization of government to administer the plan (Government Operations in the House and Senate).

The effects of fragmentation of responsibilities in the congressional process traditionally have been mitigated to varying degrees by an agile and vigorous leadership, norms of reciprocity and specialization, as well as presidential direction. The 1970s reforms, however, may have undercut the informal structures and processes that "greased the skids" of this very frictional mechanism. The irony in this turn of events is that the intention of the reformers was to smooth the way for "liberal" legislation.

Congressional Reforms of the 1970s

Between 1970 and 1975 Congress, particularly the House of Representatives, passed a series of primarily procedural reforms (Congressional Quarterly 1976). The major reforms are outlined in table 6–2 according to how they affected congressional structures, processes, and resources.

From 1911 until the late 1960s a pattern of legislative decision making evolved around powerful committee chairmen who rose to their positions by virtue of their ability to be reelected. Many of these posts, especially the critical positions on Rules and Ways and Means, were held by conservative southern Democrats who were adept at delaying or defeating liberal legislation.

The 1964 election dramatically changed the context of policymaking and the characteristics of Congress. The reforms of the 1970s date to this election. From the Johnson landslide of 1964 to that of the Congressional Democrats in 1974, the composition of Congress reflected the proportional increase in the number of young voters, and the growing demand of minorities and women for influence and power. Murphy (1974) has characterized the whole movement as a "new politics" involving three major effects on Congress. The first was a significant decline in the power of the conservative coalition. Southern Democrats in both houses of Congress were being challenged by Republicans in general elections; primary competition was greater; and the constituency in the suburbs, traditionally Republican strongholds, became less conservative. The second and related change was that the composition of the House became more diverse. Black membership increased from five in 1960 to sixteen in 1974. Although their numbers did not increase, women began to play a more important role. Finally, public interest lobbying forces,

such as that of Ralph Nader and the Sierra Club, emerged as a counterbalance to the traditional interest groups.

Reforms were so numerous during the 1970s and affected so many areas of congressional activity that the particular problems to which they were directed are difficult to discern (Jones 1977). The problems appear, however, to fall into the following five categories:

1. An unequal and ineffective relationship with the executive
2. The concentration of power in senior committee chairmen
3. Too many barriers in congressional procedure, which allowed a minority of legislators to block programs
4. The inability of junior members, particularly freshmen, to play an active role in the legislative process
5. A weak party structure and inability to effect party platform commitments

The reform movement began with the formation of the Democratic Study Group, an unofficial alliance of liberals concerned about social policy legislation. In 1968 they pushed to revive the Democratic caucus, and in 1973 they were instrumental in creating the Democratic Steering and Policy Committee. Through procedural reforms, power and authority were transferred to these structures and away from the House Ways and Means and Rules Committees, which were viewed as major stumbling blocks for liberal legislation.

Initially, the reforms worked to the benefit of the liberals who proposed them. The rejuvenated caucus and Steering and Policy Committee provided a forum for discussion. The majority of the Democrats were relatively liberal and therefore could control votes taken within the party caucus. The freshman and junior members had been guaranteed seats on major committees and subcommittees hitherto impossible to achieve and, at the height of the reformists' power, three senior committee chairmen (all conservative Southern Democrats) were removed from their posts. The visibility of the legislative process was

1970–1988 Major Congressional Reforms and Their Impact on Congressional Structures, Processes, and Resources

Congressional Reform	Structure	Process	Resource
Legislative Reorganization Act of 1970		Written committee rules Teller votes on House floor recorded Role call votes in closed committee made public	
Caucus Rule Changes 1971	Committee on Committees no longer needs to consider seniority in choosing chairman	Ten Democrats can request separate vote on chairman Can hold only one sub-committee chairmanship	
Caucus Rule Change 1973	Steering and Policy Committee created	Caucus must meet regularly even without quorum Open committee meetings Secret vote for chairman can be requested Each Democrat guaranteed one major assignment Majority of caucus can force right to amend on floor	
Subcommittee Bill of Rights 1973	Established subcommittee jurisdictions Set party ratios	Subcommittee chairmen to be elected by full committee caucus Committee chairman must send bill to subcommittee within 2 weeks Guaranteed each member major subcommittee	Provided subcommittee budgets
Hansen Reforms No. 988, October 1974	Required all committees to exercise oversight responsibility through special committee or assign to standing committee	House Democrats required to meet to organize in December	

Congressional Reform	Structure	Process	Resource
Caucus rule changes December 1974	Committee assignments to be made by Steering and Policy Committee All committees with over 20 members must have at least four subcommittees Expanded Ways and Means from 25 to 37 members Speaker to nominate Rules Committee members	Secret vote for chairman required Chairman of Appropriations Subcommittees to be elected	
Congressional Budget and Impoundment Act of 1974	Created budget committees	Required budget figures be set then reconciled by end of year Conference Committee opened	Created Congressional Budget Office Increased staff of overall subcommittee and minority component
Caucus rule changes 1975			
Implementation of Reconciliation 1980		Enforced 1974 Budget Act	
Balanced Budget and Emergency Deficit Control Act of 1985 (Gramm-Rudman-Hollings)		Tied expenditure and revenue decisions to deficit reduction targets	

TABLE 6–2 (continued)

Source: Congressional Quarterly, Inside Congress, Washington: Congressional Quarterly, 1976, updated by authors.

enhanced when teller votes were recorded, committee sessions were opened to the public, and the budget acts required explicit priority setting in the appropriations process. With this increased visibility, coalition building and compromises became more difficult to negotiate. Members found their interest group constituencies paying closer attention to their voting record and uninterested in the necessity to sometimes "make deals."

The intended outcomes of the reforms were to strengthen the party leadership, remove barriers in the legislative process, and democratize (i.e., give more power to more members) the decision making structure. Observers of the reforms (Reiselback 1977; Ornstein and Rhode 1977; Oleszek 1977) maintain that the cumulative effect was to decentralize power so severely that committee chairmen could no longer manage their committees. The sharing of authority and expertise (e.g., staff) with subcommittee chairmen led to the characterization of the 1970s as an era of "subcommittee government" (Davidson 1977).

The effect of the reforms on the health subcommittees proved less crucial than in other areas. Rogers and Kennedy, though very different in style, were able to get their bills skillfully to conference. Rogers' subcommittee was known as one of the most productive in the House. During the Ninety-second Congress more than one-third (twenty) of the total bills reported by the Commerce Committee were in the area of health, and all cleared the House (Price 1978).

Health care issues, especially research, personnel training, and hospital building remained popular. The lower level of AMA opposition and the emergence of interest groups representing numerous other health constituencies meant considerable demand for legislation viewed as distributive or self-regulatory (Feldstein 1977).

By the late 1970s, when legislation was increasingly viewed as redistributive, the presence of all these groups, their ability to focus almost exclusively on a small number of subcommittee members, and the addition, at least in the House Subcommittee, of more conservative members, prevented Chairman Rogers from mobilizing a moderate, centrist consensus. It appears that the reforms have weakened party and, thereby, congressional leadership. Interest groups that had

exploited the hierarchy in the 1960s now proceeded to take advantage of the lack of leadership in the mid- to late-1970s by obstructing those policies they viewed as undesirable.

The Impact of the Budget Containment Movement of the 1980s

The policy impact of major procedural reforms of the 1970s has been partially obscured by the effects of the budget containment movement of the 1980s. The reforms did produce results (Sinclair 1985; Hinckley 1983; Dodd and Openheimer 1985): The committee chairs still do not wield the power they once did; the process of their selection remains more open; subcommittees have assumed more ability to initiate, refine and obstruct. However, assessing the impact of these changes on the politics of congressional decision making and on the shape and pace of policy in general, and health policy in particular, is confounded somewhat by the recognition in the late 1970s and early 1980s that fiscal responsibility would have to guide congressional behavior more visibly than ever before. Policies previously regarded as distributive are now seen as patently redistributive (Ellwood 1985; Schick 1983).

Much attention has been focussed on the Gramm-Rudman-Hollings legislation as an enforcer of fiscal responsibility. In fact, the budget reconciliation movement began with the Congressional Budget and Impoundment Control Act of 1974, which created the House and Senate Budget Committees and contained provisions that made members go on record for higher spending, or taxes, or deficits, if Congress could not live within its own budget guidelines.

Describing the subsequent transfer of power from the appropriations to the budget committees, John Ellwood (1985, 328–29) notes:

> During the first stage of the development of the new procedures (1975 through 1979), both budget committees and especially the House Budget Committee, acted as brokers for the claimants within each chamber. Their budget resolutions frequently reflected a balance among the wants of the various committees, the party leaders, and the president. In this role the committees were traffic cops of a bottom-up (that is, from the sub-

committees and committees) budgetary process. Over time, however, the budget committees became budget guardians because they alone were in a position to add up the effects of the incremental requests and actions of the other committees. The appropriations committees had abandoned their role as guardians of the purse and had become claimants for federal money. The budget committees were able to build their power to the extent that they could work their will on the budget process.

The budget consciousness movement is manifest in the titles of the major bills affecting health policy in the 1980s: the Omnibus Reconciliation Act of 1981; the Tax Equity and Fiscal Responsibility Act of 1982; the Deficit Reduction Act of 1984; the Consolidated Omnibus reconciliation Act of 1985; and the Omnibus Reconciliation Act of 1986. The shift of power and responsibility from authorization and appropriations committees by centralizing costs as well as benefits, made partisan and ideological cleavages more pronounced, relative to clientele and interest group bargaining. It thereby gave the congressional leadership more power relative to committee and subcommittee chairmen.

This development is related to a centralizing tendency in the bureaucracy, with budget requests aggregated at the Office of Management and Budget and interagency allocations then made on a top-down basis. Ellwood (1985) contends that this dynamic has lessened the validity of disjointed incrementalism and made more descriptive a "rational" synoptic model which envisions economic reasoning exerting increasing influence on policy.

His observation is apt if one examines *general* trends in U.S. policy, which have been the result of compromises struck between supporters of presidential and congressional leadership budget proposals. The former have tended to be geared to deficit reduction targets which reflect a commitment to maintenance (at least) of defense expenditure levels and downscaling of domestic programs, a related ideological (or economic) commitment to reduction in the tax burden on those regarded as most prone to produce and consume in accordance with Supply–side economics. "Alternative budgets" proposed by congressional leaders, on the other hand, have taken a decidedly different tack; they propose transfers

from defense to domestic programs. But within the *health* policy arena, disjointed incrementalism is perhaps more evident than ever in the two largest health programs: Medicare and Medicaid. (Hinckley and Hill 1988).

By and large, Medicare and Medicaid have been regarded as "uncontrollable" categories of expenditure, although their growth in fact has been marked by a decrease in the rate of acceleration of government spending. This "negative growth" has occurred largely through almost arbitrary marginal program cuts: physician per visit reimbursement levels have been frozen and they have been forced to bill at a rate in effect when services were rendered rather than in the next year; the nursing care differential was eliminated from hospital reimbursement; indirect medical education allowances have been reduced; hospitals now are prospectively reimbursed; Medicare enrollees' deductibles and Part B premiums have been raised to the extent that, as a proportion of their incomes, out-of-pocket health expenditures by the elderly now are higher than before Medicare.

This "decrementalism" thus has been disjointed: within reduced expenditure outlay ceilings and revenue enhancement targets, hospitals, physicians, and program enrollees have borne, to varying extents at different times, the marginal brunt of efforts to keep federal budgets under control. The federal budget cuts, either in coverage under entitlements or net expenditures on entitlements, have occurred in seemingly uncoordinated fashion; they have been guided by expectations about where there was the most fat or where they would be least politically painful to impose rather than by systematic cost-benefit analysis.

This micro-view seemingly contrasts with Ellwood's (1985) more macroscopic view in which OMB–aggregated budgets, tempered by presidential preferences, are pitted against Congressional Budget Office shaped budgets pushed by congressional leaders. These views, however are reconcilable. Within major health programs, the chess pieces in this titanic game are still maneuvered under the gaze of special interests who have high stakes in the size and location of the expenditure decrements.

Further, Ellwood focuses his attention on manifestly redistributive policy. Increasingly, as demonstrated by the DRG system brought in under Prospective Payment, NHI initiatives which would rely on mandated employer benefits, and proposals to remove or qualify the tax exemptions of not-for-profit hospitals, redistribution is being effected (albeit perhaps implicitly and haphazardly) via regulation. Regulative policy eludes many of the generalizations Ellwood (1985) makes about overall revenue and expenditure policies. The relationship between the congressional process and regulative policy within the context of the new shape of legislative-executive interaction clearly needs new research in light of old typologies.

Whatever the comparative utility of frameworks for viewing the legislative process, and whether that utility varies by policy scope, function, or area, we must confront the question posed by Hinckley. What difference does the congressional process make on policy; what impacts on policy, not just process, are attributable to congressional reforms of the early 1970s and the heightened budget consciousness of the late 1970s and 1980s?

Framework for Assessing the Impact of Congressional Reform

At the outset of this discussion it should be pointed out that it is assumed that the procedural reforms in the 1970s represented a significant alteration in the power structure of Congress, and the reconciliation process did heighten Congress' sense of fiscal responsibility. If this seems to be a banal proposition, consider another view: that the reforms and reconciliation process amounted to what Alford (1976) in another context referred to as "dynamics without change." The reforms could have been merely cosmetic, simply exchanging subcommittees for full committees as the principal fiefdoms in the feudal domain of congressional decision making; reconciliation could simply have replaced appropriations committees with budget committees. (In this view, what we have regarded as a set of independent variables affecting policy change really amounts to a constant and, for this reason alone, cannot be expected to have explanatory power.) Of course, this would not be the first time that

legislative decision making structures have led to an elaboration of other ones to fulfill the function performed by the originals. Recall the effects of the Legislative Reorganization Act of 1946, whereby the number of committees was sharply reduced only to result in a proliferation of subcommittees. Congressional history can serve as a mine for testimonials to the observation that *plus ca change, le plus c'est la meme chose* (The more things change, the more they stay the same).

However, even eschewing such procedural nihilism, as most observers of congressional behavior have done, and assuming that the legislative changes noted were more than chimerical, there are still difficulties in attributing health policy trends to the legislative developments of the 1970s and 80s. Other potential causes of policy retrenchment have to be considered.

Economic Circumstances

Perhaps the most obvious of the coincidental and interrelated causal factors that compete with legislative reform is the economic downturn that began in the 1970s. This trend illuminates the fact that many health policies are reallocative and that they, therefore, rest on the presumption that there will be resources to allocate. Theories of public finance (Bird 1971; Dye 1980) that view government expenditures as led by "luxury" categories such as health and welfare and that posit the existence of a ratchet effect that underlies an irreversible incrementalism have to be reconsidered. In short, the law of expanding state activity, which envisions almost inexorable "progress," should be called into question for reasons quite apart from changes in congressional behavior patterns. The dynamics of that law (and its variants) also could be used to explain decrementalism.

As for the deficit problem that has most preoccupied Congress and the executive as it has become more and more visible, we are sensitive to the fact that there are strongly conflicting views on whether it really should be such a major concern (e.g., GAO 1988; Morris 1989; Freidman 1988). Nevertheless, unless one assumes very persuasive and pervasive disingenuity on the part of the leadership of both parties, the deficit has been *perceived* as critical and perception *is* reality in viewing constraints on government expenditure programs.

Experience of Government Health Programs

Another factor coinciding with congressional change as an explanation of policy change has been the experience of government programs. By way of illustration, Medicare and Medicaid have been far more expensive than predicted and have been accompanied by numerous regulations not unanticipated by watchful observers. Mechanic (1981) has observed that the hesitant and, therefore, perhaps awkward approach to government-sponsored health insurance programs has disaffected both the right and left sides of the ideological spectrum. Medicaid, in particular, has not resulted in easily available and accessible services for those citizens it targets; moreover, it has been costly both in terms of outright public expenditures and the administrative superstructure it has promoted. Consequently, on pragmatic grounds alone, the efficacy and effectiveness of further government ventures into the financing and regulation of health services delivery could be questioned.

There is also a less cynical interpretation of the impact that experience with government health programs has had; that is, such programs have actually achieved a measure of success and, therefore, have quieted demands for policy change. Most obviously, Medicare has helped make a wide (if not totally comprehensive) range of services accessible to the heaviest users of health care. Medicaid covers the designated poor, although in a less than ideally humanitarian fashion. And what perhaps most escapes public attention is that government tax expenditures in effect subsidize the private health insurance industry. This has had more than a trivial effect on the numbers of people covered and is somewhat analogous to the more explicit government subsidization of sickness funds in the Federal Republic of Germany and Sweden, for example. The fact that the income tax exemption accorded employer paid health insurance premiums is a form of government expenditure, in terms of foregone revenues to the Treasury (Surrey and McDaniel 1985), did not go unnoticed by the Reagan administration and Republican Senate, which considered the termination of such indirect government support as a means of curtailing government expenditures by putting potential consumers at greater risk and, at the same time, generating revenues. Nor have health care tax expenditures escaped the attention of the House Ways and Means Subcommittee (Falcone and Warren 1988). In this policy posture, the government is perhaps further mending the patchwork quilt of programs that has forestalled a more comprehensive health policy.

Another impact of government programs has been the increasing trend toward oligopsony (or bilateral oligopoly) that they have furthered. As Marmor et al. (1976) and others have pointed out, concentrated interests result in decision makers becoming more cost-conscious purchasers of health services. This historical observation is corroborated by cross-national comparison: those nations in which a single unit of government (whether national as in Great Britain or provincial as in Canada) is a large subsidizer of health services tend to exhibit more concern about medical care cost inflation than nations in which financial responsibility is divided among levels of government (e.g., the nation and communes in Sweden, the federal government and landers in the Federal Republic of Germany) or among governments and other sources of funds (e.g., France with parallel public and private financing).

The United States still falls in the mixed, pluralistic source of funding classification, but, over time, expenditures have become increasingly centralized. Medicare has had a more profound effect than Medicaid in this regard (Marmor et al. 1976), but the sheer amounts of money required to underwrite the Medicaid program have also piqued the fiscal sensitivity of federal, state, and county governments. Obviously, the experience with the government programs factor overlaps the economic constraints factor as they compete with congressional change for explanatory power regarding policy change.

Ideological Orientation

In addition to the cynicism and cost consciousness engendered by government health programs and the resource limitations faced by recent Congresses, there has perhaps also been an ideological shift to the right. This has not been a distinctively U.S. phenomenon, as it seems that in every nation the basic role of the state is being questioned. Whether this reemphasis on major ideological issues is a separable phenomenon from the shrinking of available resources is problematic. Furthermore, it is tempting to read more fundamental shifts in attitudes into electoral results than is warranted, especially in view of the unusually low turnout (51 percent) in the 1980 presidential election which, more than any, was signalled as a harbinger of change. Also, the electoral success of Democratic legislators since then should mitigate the temptation to view the "Reagan Revolution" as the result of an ideological groundswell on the part of the public, even the attentive public.[4] On the other hand, taking the *intensity* as well as the direction of opinion into consideration, one could view growth in conservatism as a major development in U.S. political behavior. Members of the attentive public, whose opinions are most important in policy formulation, have challenged the traditional idea that government should assume responsibility for potentially private matters, at least in the economic realm. In light of this attitudinal movement in favor of reprivatization (or, at least, a climate of opinion not conducive to intensified government activity), the retrenchment is as understandable, if not explainable, by conventional, civics-text notions about the responsiveness of legislators to their constituents' preferences, as it is on the basis of economic, pragmatic or procedural considerations.

Again, however, the impact of ideology on policy is questionable. First, it is nearly impossible to separate the rhetoric that underlies policy change from that which merely is convenient to justify it. Second, whatever the causal mechanism involved, the media seem to have adjudged that there has been an ideological shift, and that may amount to a self-fulfilling prophesy in that the assessment is as important as the phenomenon being analyzed. Third, ideological constraint, even among the elite (i.e., political leaders) is limited. Support for process reform is rarely divorced from substantial policy implications (e.g., those who favor limitations on debate typically oppose the positions of those who likely will be using the filibuster or other tactics to obstruct legislation). Finally, to summarize the effects of ideology, this classification is simply too convenient. Political language is often couched in ideological terms, and *post factum* analyses of political events tempt people to exchange ideas in the coin of the realm. Historians and journalists perhaps are especially prone to succumb to this fallacy, but other social scientists are not immune to such entrapment.

Presidential Character

Another variable that is analytically troublesome from the standpoint of isolating its effects from other influences on policy that have been mentioned is the role assumed by the president. If one were trying to explain policy primarily on the basis of the types of behavior that constitute what Barber (1972) calls "presidential character," Lyndon Johnson's legislative dexterity could be considered a major factor behind the policy innovations of the mid-1960s; Nixon's Machiavellian pragmatism could be cited as an important influence supporting the drive for NHI during the late 1960s and early 1970s; and the Watergate scandal could be partially credited for the demise of this same policy movement. The weaknesses of the Ford and Carter administrations, for perhaps different reasons, would be adduced to explain the subsequent lack of dynamism in any policy area, and, of course, there has been the "Reagan Revolution" orchestrated by the "Great Communicator" and (not pejoratively) some of his near utopian counsellors. But, of course, all these could be questioned in an analytical perspective that included the other effects on policy previously mentioned. For example, except in the most heroic view possible, one cannot discount the impact of economic factors, over which the president clearly has less than total control, on his policy initiation capacity. In addition, some reforms, notably the Anti-Impoundment Act, were specifically designed to undercut the executive's unilateral discretion. Thus, the decline of

---

[4]There is some evidence from a *New York Times*/CBS News poll of January 1986 that Reagan's popularity did not reflect support for his view of the proper scale of federal policy. See R.W. Apple. Poll on Reagan: High popularity still continuing. *New York Times*, 30 January 1986, cited in Brown (1988).

presidential prerogatives on policy during the Nixon, Ford and Carter administrations were not caused solely by weaknesses in these presidents alone. Nor did Reagan's leadership capability (at least with respect to securing the confidence of the public) enable him to leave behind a healthy treasury.

Conclusion

Legislative events over the past twenty years undoubtedly have affected health policy, but their explanatory power is difficult to determine in a systematic research design. It could be argued that health policy, not unlike welfare, education, or other social policies, is now undergoing the retrenchment required by the economic constraints now facing U.S. decision makers as well as leaders of other Western nations. This retrenchment may be linked primarily to legislative reform, government experience with health programs, presidential leadership, a shift in ideological perspective, or, more likely, a combination of these interacting factors. What is important to remember is that health policy is swept in the overall direction of government activity and that, for whatever reason or collection of reasons cited above, it may be that traditional theories of public finance will have to be reformulated to take into account the possibility of a diminution of productivity, and, thus, by the logic of the theories themselves, a reduction in the scope of government activity. As changes in legislative structure and procedure occur, one has to be on guard against the temptation to weigh them too heavily in assessing their significance in the determination of health and other social policies. This cautionary note is particularly applicable to the evaluation of the demonstrated incapability of Congress to mount a successful counterinitiative to the Reagan administration's budgetary and related social policy proposals. It seems that the weakening of the leadership structure in the 1970s and the deficit induced reconciliation process have been partially accountable for this turn of events, but the other variables considered in this discourse also seem to have come into play.

While noting that in examining health policy trends, public finance theories have to be refor-

mulated, we also have suggested that different descriptive models, disjointed incrementalism and a "synoptic" framework, might be more appropriate, respectively, in viewing the health policy and overall policy process. Finally, we think it at least a feasible hypothesis that while distributive politics and policies have given way to redistributive politics and policies, perhaps regulative policy will be used more and more to effect preferred redistributions.

REFERENCES

Alford, Robert. 1976. *Health politics: Dynamics without change.* Chicago: University of Chicago Press.

Barber, James D. 1972. *Presidential character.* Englewood Cliffs, N.J.: Prentice-Hall.

Biles, Bryan. 1975. Regional orientation session health resources planning. Unedited transcript of remarks. Atlanta, Georgia, January 13–14.

Bird, Richard. 1970. *The growth of government spending in Canada.* Toronto: Canadian Tax Foundation.

Blumstein, James F. 1977. Inflation and quality: The case of PSRO's In *Health: A victim or cause of inflation,* edited by Michael Subkoff, 245–295. New York: Prodist.

Brown, Larry. 1986. Introduction to a decade of transition. *Journal of Health Politics, Policy and Law* 11:569–584.

Brown, Michael K. 1988. The segmented welfare system: Distributive conflict and retrenchment in the United States, 1968–1984. In *Remaking the welfare state: Retrenchment and social policy in American and Europe,* edited by M.K. Brown, 182–205. Philadelphia: Temple University Press.

Congressional Budget Office. 1981. *The impact of PSRO's on health care costs: Update of CEO's 1979 evaluation.* Washington, D.C.: U.S. Library of Congress.

Congressional Quarterly. 1976. *Inside congress.* Washington: Congressional Quarterly Press.

Cooper, Theodore. 1976. Federal health policy. *Journal of Health Politics, Policy and Law* 1:9–12.

Davidson, Roger. 1977. Breaking up those cozy triangles: An impossible dream?" In *Legislative reform and public policy,* edited by Susan Welch and John G. Peters' 30–53. New York: Praeger Publishers.

Davis, Karen. 1987. Reagan administration health policy. *Journal of Public Health Policy* 2:312–331.

Davis, Karen and Cathy Schoen. 1978. *Health and the war on poverty: A ten year appraisal.* Washington, D.C.: The Brookings Institution.

Dood, Lawrence C. and Bruce I. Oppenheimer, 1985. The house in transition. In *Congress reconsidered,*

3rd ed, edited by L.C. Dodd and B. Oppeheimer, 380–411. Washington, DC: Congressional Quarterly Press.

Dye, Thomas. 1980. *Understanding public policy.* Englewood Cliffs, N.J.: Prentice-Hall, 4th edition.

Ellwood, John W. 1985. The great exception: the congressional budget process in an age of decentralization. In *Congress reconsidered,* 3rd ed., edited by L.C. Dodd and B.I. Oppenheimer, 345–362. Washington, DC: Congressional Quarterly Press.

Etzioni, Amatai. 1967. Mixed scanning: A 'third' approach to decision-making. *Public Administration Review* 27:385–42.

Falcone, David. 1983. Health policy analysis and health policy. In *Encyclopedia of policy sciences,* edited by Stuart Nagel, 753–775. N.Y.: Marcel Dekker.

Falcone, David and Warren David. 1988. The shadow price of pluralism: the use of tax expenditures to subsidize hospital care in the United States. *Journal of Health Politics, Policy and Law* 13:735–751.

Feldstein, Paul. 1977. *Health associations and the demand for legislation.* Cambridge: Ballinger Publishing Co.

Feldstein, Paul 1988. *Health economics,* 3rd ed. N.Y.: John Wiley & Sons.

Friedman, Milton. 1988. Straight talk about deficits. *Wall Street Journal,* December 14.

Gibson, Robert M. and Daniel R. Waldo. 1981. National health expenditures. *Health Care Financing Review* 4:1–35.

Department of Health, Education and Welfare. 1978. *Health 1976–77.* Washington, D.C.: United States Government Printing Office.

Hinckley, Barbara. 1983. *Stability and change in Congress,* 3rd ed. N.Y.: Harper and Row.

Katherine Hinckley and Bette Hill. 1988. Biting the bullet? Post-1980 congressional process and Medicare/Medicaid decisions. Paper presented at the 1988 Annual Meeting of the American Political Science Association, Washington, D.C., September 2–4.

Iglehart, John K. 1988. The administration's assault on domestic spending and the threat to health care programs. *New England Journal of Medicine* 312:525–528.

Iglehart, John K. 1988. The administration responds to cost spiral. *New England Journal of Medicine* 305:1359–1364.

Iglehart, John K. 1983. The Reagan record on health policy. *New England Journal of Medicine* 308:232–236.

Jones, Charles. 1977. How reform changes Congress. In *Legislative reform and public policy,* edited by Susan Welch and John Peters, 11–29. New York: Praeger Publishers.

Lawton, Stephen. 1981. Budget reconciliation. *New England Journal of Medicine,* 305:1297–1300.

Leroy, Lauren and Philip Lee. 1977. *Deliberations and compromise.* Cambridge: Ballinger Publishing Co.

Loewenberg, Gerhard. 1971. *Modern parliaments: Change or decline.* New York: Aldine Publishing Co.

Marmor, Theodore. 1973. *The politics of Medicare.* New York: Aldine Publishing Co.

Marmor, Theodore, Donald Wittmann, and Thomas Heagy. 1976. The Politics of Medical Inflation. *Journal of health politics, policy and law* 4:69–84.

Mechanic, David. 1981. Some dilemmas in health policy. *Milbank Memorial Fund Quarterly/Health and Society* 59:1–15.

Morris, Charles R. 1989. Deficit figuring doesn't add up. *New York Times Magazine* February 12.

Murphy, Thomas P. 1974. *The new politics Congress.* Lexington, Mass.: Lexington Books.

Oleszek, Walter, J. 1977. A perspective on congressional reform. In *Legislative reform and public policy,* edited by Susan Welch and John Peters, 3–10. New York: Praeger Publishing Co.

Ornstein, Norman and David W. Rohde. 1977. Revolt from within: Congressional change, legislative policy, and the House Commerce Committee." In *Legislative reform and public policy,* edited by Susan Welch and John Peters, 247–256. New York: Praeger Publishing Co.

Price, David. 1975. *The commerce committees.* New York: Grossman.

Price, David, E. 1978. Policymaking in congressional committees: The Impact of 'Environmental' Factors. *American Political Science Review* 72:548–574.

Price, David. 1985. Congressional committees in the policy process. In *Congress reconsidered,* 3rd Edition, edited by Lawrence Dodd and Bruce Oppenheimer, 290–311. Washington, DC: Congressional Quarterly Press.

Redman, Eric. 1974. *The dance of legislation.* New York: Simon & Schuster.

Rieselback, Leroy N. 1977. *Congressional reform in the 70s.* Morristown, N.J.: General Learning Press.

Russell, Louise. 1977. Inflation and the federal role in health. In *Health: A victim or cause of inflation,* edited by Michael Zubkoff, 225–244. New York: Prodist.

Sinclair, Barbara. 1985. Agenda, policy and alignment change. In *Congress reconsidered,* 3rd ed., edited by Lawrence Dodd and Bruce Oppenheimer, 300–314. Washington, D.C.: Congressional Quarterly Press.

Sorkin, Alan L. 1977. *Health manpower.* Lexington, Mass.: D.C. Heath.

Stevens, Rosemary. 1971. *American medicine and the public interest.* New Haven: Yale University Press.

Surrey, Stanley and Paul McDaniel. 1985. *Tax expenditure.* Cambridge, MA: Harvard.

United States General Accounting Office. 1988. *The budget deficit.* Washington, D.C.: Government Printing Office.

United States General Accounting Office. 1988. *Medicare and Medicaid: Updated effects of recent legislation on program and beneficiary costs.* Washington D.C.: Government Printing Office.

U.S. Senate. Committee on the Budget. 1988. The congressional budget process: An explanation. 100th Congress, 2nd Session, *Proceedings,* 100–89.

Van Loon, Richard J. and Michael Whittington. 1987. *The Canadian political system.* Toronto: McGraw-Hill.

Wilson, Florence and Duncan Neuhauser. 1976. *Health services in the United States,* Cambridge: Ballinger Publishing Co.

Chapter 7

The Role of Law in Health Policy

Tom Christoffel

Governments operate by enacting and implementing laws. These laws provide the mechanism and the framework for health politics and policies. The unique balancing of authority between federal and state governments and among legislative, executive, and judicial branches of government established two centuries ago under the United States Constitution forms the rules of the game within which health policy and politics are carried out in this country. The rules can help or hinder the attainment of any particular policy goal.

By means of the laws they enact and enforce, the various levels and branches of government touch virtually all aspects of health and medical care, everything from immunization policies to toxic waste cleanup, from decisions to terminate life-support to intervention in cases of child abuse, from the requiring of airbags in automobiles to the operation of health departments. It is not too much to say that to understand health politics and policy in the United States, it is necessary to have some understanding of law and the legal system in the United States, especially the role of the judiciary in overseeing the legal system.

The Health "System"

In the United States, government came late to assuring direct responsibility for the public health and health care needs of its citizens. Thomas Jefferson once observed that, "Without health there is no happiness. And attention to health, then, should take the place of every other object." (Foley 1967) Yet for the first half of the nation's history, this view did not translate into governmental concern with the health of its citizens. The concept of "medical police," that is, government protecting the public's health, developed in Europe in the 1700s, but it was not until the late 1800s that such a concept began to take hold in the United States. On the state level, the

135

first state board of health created to conduct broad health programs (other than quarantine) was not established until 1855, and the first state school health law was not enacted until 1906. On the national level, a federal port quarantine authority was not established until 1878. The federal role in health was so limited that in an 1886 decision, the U.S. Supreme Court went out of its way to criticize the lack of federal health-related actions.[1] It was only with the enactment of such legislation as the Pure Food and Drug Act of 1906 and the Venereal Disease Act of 1918 that a clear role in health policy began to emerge for the national government.

Once started, however, governmental involvement in matters affecting the public's health and access to medical care increased steadily. Yet given the importance of health—to all citizens and to the life of the nation as a whole—it is striking that the United States does not have a more comprehensive, better coordinated set of health policies. Unlike virtually all other industrialized nations, the U.S. lacks a coordinated national system of health insurance coverage. Health planning in the United States never really amounted to much and, in recent years, has given way to reliance on something called "market forces." The U.S. health care system is best characterized as a fragmented, uncoordinated, incomplete hodgepodge of health services and public health protections. There are many reasons for this state of affairs, not the least of which are the peculiarities that result from a sharing of political and legal authority between federal and state governments (Christoffel 1982, Ch. 2, 4, 5). For example, medical care is provided or paid for by a patchwork of federal, state, and local programs, each with its own eligibility and coverage guidelines. In addition, each governmental level is itself uncoordinated. As Rand Rosenblatt (1978, 243) has noted:

> For the past thirty years, federal health care policy has been characterized by frustration and contradiction. On the one hand, Congress has repeatedly enacted laws to secure consumer access to quality health care at a reasonable cost and has appropriated billions of dollars to

achieve these ends. On the other hand, federal statutes and, more frequently, administrative practice have failed to establish effective regulatory control over the providers of health care (doctors and hospitals) who largely determine the use, quality, and price of the publicly funded services, or even over the federal and state officials who administer the programs.

Similarly, fragmentation has characterized efforts to reduce motor-vehicle injuries, a significant cause of death in the U.S. The National Highway Traffic Safety Administration, for example, enforces vehicle standards while the Federal Highway Administration focuses on the roads designed for the vehicles to travel upon. The states, on the other hand, license vehicles and drivers, build roads, and enforce traffic laws. In addition, local governments also build, maintain, and police streets and highways.

This fragmented state of affairs did not result from happenstance, nor is it without its supporters. Both Madisonian and contemporary interest-group liberalism are based on a fragmented, pluralistic model in which the absence of a coordinated system serves as a defense against centralized control and tryanny. And many people champion the concept of a "laboratory of the states," that is, the fact that states can experiment with differing approaches to social problems and benefit from each other's mistakes and successes. But regardless of whether a fragmented governmental structure is good or bad, it does resist easy comprehension. The study of health policy in the United States must therefore require as a prerequisite some knowledge of law and the legal system. Such an understanding, however, is not easily come by. Not even legal academics can agree on what law is all about.

The Function of Law in Society

At the beginning of this century, law in the U.S. was viewed in terms of classical jurisprudence (Monahan and Walker 1986, 479), or: ——————

> the belief that a single, correct legal solution could be reached in every case by the application of logic to a set of natural, self-evident principles. Classical jurisprudence understood the process of deciding cases to be purely rational and

---

[1] *Morgan's Louisiana and Texas R.R. and Steamship Company v. Louisiana State Board of Health.* 118 U.S. 455 (1886), as quoted in Kagan.

exclusively deductive and thus produced a formal and mechanical approach to decision making.

This view was supplanted during the early decades of the 20th Century with a less rigid view that considered law as a kind of pragmatic, commonsense set of commands, colored by political and public policy considerations and rooted in the traditions, customs, and history of society. Sociology, economics, and experience replaced logic (Mensch 1982, 18–39). Legal scholars such as Roscoe Pound, who defined the function of law quite simply as "social control through the systematic application of the force of politically organized society," along with Justices Oliver Wendell Holmes and Benjamin Cardozo, argued that rules of law were not "final truths" but instead "working hypotheses, continually retested in those great laboratories of law, the courts" (Pine 1988, 659–660)" Still, law continued to be viewed as an ultimately fair, impartial, and positive social force, a relatively objective distillation of society's values.

There is little disagreement today over law being *the* systematic social control mechanism. But there is considerable debate over the nature of that mechanism. Does law represent an overall societal consensus or does it represent particular interests within the society? Is law an objective and impartial force existing outside of, or above, the political arena, or are law and politics parts of the same whole? How does one determine whether a particular law is "good" or "bad"? These questions cannot be adequately addressed in this short essay, but the several competing modern perspectives can be outlined.

Over the past two decades, three major new intellectual movements have developed within the nation's law schools. The first is the law and economics movement, which evaluates and explains legal rules and institutions from an economic perspective, using market competition and efficiency as the standards to determine which laws are socially appropriate. Richard Posner, a leading advocate of this approach, notes (1975, 854–856) that:

> The basis of an economic approach to law is the assumption that the people involved with the legal system act as rational maximizers of their satisfactions. . . . (C)riminals, contracting parties, automobile drivers, prosecutors, and others subject to legal constraints or involved in legal proceedings act in their relation to the legal system as intelligent (not omniscient) maximizers of their satisfactions. . . . (T)he legal system itself— its doctrines, procedures, and institutions—has been strongly influenced by a concern (more often implicit than explicit) with promoting economic efficiency.

Law and economics advocates view their approach as a way of understanding and improving a legal system that is—or can be made to be— neutral and objective.

A second intellectual perspective on law, that of the law and society movement, uses sociological concepts and theories to define the law in terms of law as it is actually implemented, not simply law as it is written down in statutes, regulations, or even judicial opinions. The law and society approach is therefore concerned with empirical studies of the actual operation and impact of laws. From this perspective, law is seen as political, rather than objective and rational (Taylor 1982, 173–174):

> While the power of law as an institution pervades society, the institution is in turn influenced by various political and economic interests within society. . . . As the social scientific evidence documents, not only may interests external to the law influence its institutional nature, but they may also establish alternative and partly independent legal systems.

The critical legal studies movement, the most controversial of the three intellectual perspectives on law, also views the law as being neither an objective nor a necessarily rational set of rules. But critical legal study adherents go on to interpret law as a form of politics and policy that serves the interests of particular political and economic interests, providing a set of rules and values compatible with those interests. According to this third perspective, law is neither rational, just, impartial, nor natural; it reproduces rather than resolves social contradictions. In the words of one proponent of this view (Kennedy 1985):

> the existing rules in force, the law as we have chosen to make it through our various law-making institutions, is profoundly implicated in distributional, social injustice in our society. The

system by which the rich and powerful, white and male, stay rich and powerful, generation after generation, has a very strong legal component. . . . The rules we have chosen as rules of the game reproduce social injustice generation after generation. And the . . . presentation of the rules of the game as the consequence, to some extent, of a neutral, legal, analytic process, makes things that are rotten and unjust look natural, inevitable, logical and inherently fair. So that if you are a loser, it's your own fault.

What do these three views of the law say regarding health policy? The law and economics school would say that much of health care regulation fails the cost-benefit test and that the marketplace can provide health services much more efficiently than can government. The law and society school, while not advocating a market alternative, would note that much health-related legislation has failed, that is, licensure protects the provider more than the consumer; despite Medicare, the elderly pay more out-of-pocket for their medical care than they did in 1965, and prevention programs pale as compared to current knowledge of what should and could be done. Finally, the critical legal studies school would suggest that, contrary to the portrayal of Washington health politics as a game in which the provider groups are simply more adept and better financed than other players, health policy is actually developed within a system of laws so slanted that the advocates of public health and improved access to health care services cannot succeed no matter how adept and energetic they may be.

The Legal System

What then is law, and what role does it play in health policy? The answer depends on where you sit. For health policy advocates, law can be considered rules of the game—to be used or overcome. This means that better understanding of law and the legal system can lead to more effective use of the policy development process and the policy implementation apparatus. As one commentator notes (Clune 1983, 123):

> Because law is politics, enormous room for creativity, adaptation, and negotiation exists. Political law can be liberating; autonomous law (if it really existed other than as an ideology) would be confining.

But a legal mystique—what one observer has called a "veil of dignified mystery"—often deters nonlawyers from attempting to deal with legal principles and concepts in the same way they would with other political issues. The law is seen as arcane and mysterious, understandable only by those who have dedicated their professional careers to the task. Because of this perspective, little effort is made to become informed in this area. This lapse is similar to that made by most people without training in the health professions, who know amazingly little about how their bodies work or about disease processes, and are ready to place their fate unquestioningly in the hands of "experts."

Certainly law is far from being the mystery the nonlawyer believes it to be. "On the contrary," wrote one well-known iconoclastic law professor, "law deals almost exclusively with the ordinary facts and occurrences of everyday business and government and living. . . . Lawyers would always like to believe that the principles they say they work with are something more than a complicated way of talking about simple, tangible, non-legal matters; but they are not" (Rodell 1939, 4 and 6).

Actually, there is no single U.S. legal system, but rather the differing systems of the fifty states, the U.S., territories, plus the federal legal system. Each of these systems has evolved in its own way, each with its own constitution, its own legislation, and its own judicial decisions. The result is a complex and voluminous set of laws. These laws are best understood if viewed in terms of a system that divides the powers of government into three separate branches—legislative, executive, and judicial—with a constitution establishing the framework. Each of the three branches creates law in varying form, so that on both the state and federal levels, four different "types" of law can be distinguished. Based on the origin or authority for each, these are constitutional-based law, legislatively-based law, administratively-based law (or regulations), and judicially-based, or common, law.

Constitutional law

The U.S. Constitution provides the basic legal authority for the nation. It defines the powers, limits, and functions of the federal government.

By ratifiying the Constitution the states gave up certain governmental powers to a federal government of higher authority. The U.S. Constitution is broad vague, and general in wording and therefore open to interpretation as to application and meaning. State constitutions, which provide the same type of legal definitional authority for the states and their subdivisions, tend to be more specifically worded.

Statutory law

The enactments of Congress and the state legislatures (statutes) and of municipal bodies (ordinances) represent governmental policy choices, translating public needs and demands into programs and restrictions. These enactments govern a wide variety of human endeavors by declaring, commanding, prohibiting, establishing, and funding. They must be consistent with the U.S. Constitution (and in the case of state and local enactments, with the individual state constitutions).

Regulatory law

Statutes may represent policy choices, but legislative bodies lack the time, expertise, or flexibility to make their enactments operable. Detailed rules and regulations translate broadly-worded statutes into operating standards. Regulations are developed by executive-branch and independent administrative agencies to carry out broad legislative mandates. Regulations have the full force of law. They must, however, be derived from and be consistent with this legislative authority.

Common law

When a court is called upon to resolve a legal dispute in an area in which no statutory law applies, the court will be guided by what other courts—or the same court—have previously decided in similar disputes. These *precedents* become a type of law in themselves. The principle is that a past decision, specifically the rationale for its outcome, must be respected by a court when it next confronts the same question. Thus common law consists of legal precedent as found in the decisions of the most authoritative courts. In addition, it includes the loose collection of legal custom, tradition, and precedent as developed by the federal and state courts. This "judge-made" law controls the many areas of human activity for which the legislative branch has not established statutory policies.

These four areas of law—constitutional, statutory, regulatory, and common law—exist on both the federal and state levels. A critical issue today, just as it was 200 years ago, is how the federal and state legal systems interact. In theory, the federal government can legislate only in those areas in which the Constitution has explicitly granted it authority to act. Since health is not mentioned in the Constitution, federal authority to legislate and regulate on health matters would seem to be non-existent. Yet this is obviously not how things stand, as evidenced by Medicare, the National Institutes of Health, the Occupational Safety and Health Administration, Food and Drug Administration, and a myriad of other health-related federal programs, laws, and bureaucracies.

The explanation is quite simple. Two of the greatest sources of federal authority are the power to spend and the power to regulate interstate commerce, powers conferred upon the federal government in the U.S. Constitution. Article I, Section 8, Clause 1 of that document provides that "The Congress shall have power to lay and collect taxes, duties, imposts, and excises, to pay the debts and provide for the common defence and general welfare of the United States. . . ." And so many federal health-related programs, such as Medicare, are spending programs which carry with them a multitude of requirements that must be met (by patients, providers, and or states) in order to qualify for funding: who pays the piper calls the tune. Article I, Section 8, Clause 3 of the Constitution gives Congress the power "To regulate commerce with foreign Nations, and among the several States. . . ." And so many other federal health-related programs, such as the Occupational Safety and Health Act, are based on this Congressional authority to regulate interstate commerce, a power that has been broadly interpreted by the U.S. Supreme Court.

Whenever Congress has legislated in a particular area, its control over that area has legal authority superior to that of any state or local claim.

Where the maintenance of a uniform system of interstate commerce is involved, such federal "pre-emption" is even more readily established. Thus, for example, the federal government has assumed authority over nuclear power, including issues relating to public health and safety, and thereby pre-empted state authority to regulate nuclear-power-plant safety.[2,3] And while protection of public health and safety has traditionally been a state governmental function, Congress has claimed—and the courts have upheld—superior authority to establish rules by which hazardous substances may be transported through populated areas.[4]

Regardless of the level of government involved, the past several decades have witnessed an increasingly important role for administrative (regulatory) agencies, particularly as regards health issues. Yet it should be noted that on the national level less than $2 billion (or 0.2 percent of the federal budget) is spent annually to fund the combined regulatory efforts of the Environmental Protection Agency, the Occupational Safety and Health Administration, the Food and Drug Administration, the National Highway Traffic Safety Administration, the Consumer Product Safety Commission, and the food safety programs of the Department of Agriculture (Bollier and Claybrook 1986, 210).

In theory, administrative agencies merely implement policies established by the legislative branch. For example, Congress enacts a Food, Drug and Cosmetic Act and the Food and Drug Administration applies that Act to the broad range of foods, drugs, cosmetics, and medical devices that come under its statutory jurisdiction. But the fact is that administrative agencies play a significant policy role. In part this is due to the fact that even in establishing overall policy by enacting statutes, legislative bodies cannot avoid leaving much room for interpretation—that is, policy choices—when the statute is implemented. In addition, legislative bodies often purposely avoid making policy choices by handing an issue over to the administrative agency or, more cynically, make what appears to be a popular policy choice by enacting a statute without providing the relevant agency with the necessary resources, clear legislative language, or specific guidelines to effectively implement the policy.

The Role of the Courts

Constitutional, statutory, regulatory, and common law form the basic building blocks for the legal system, but the system is not self-enforcing. When the abstractions of the law must be applied to a specific fact situation, interpretation is called for, and interpretation is what judges do best. As Rodell noted many years ago (1939, 22–23):

> practically every lawyer thinks and talks of The Law as a sort of omnipotent, omniscient presence hovering around like God over the affairs of men. . . . The strange thing is, however, that lawyers . . . are never able to agree about the presence or its interpretation, when it comes down to applying The Law to a simple, specific factual problem. If the lawyers agreed, there would never be a law case, for every law case results of course from a legal dispute as to what The Law is. If the lawyers agreed, we would not have appellate courts reversing the judgments of trial courts and super-appellate courts reversing the judgments of appellate courts, and super-super-appellate courts—or supreme courts—reversing the judgments of super-appellate courts.

It is in the leeway afforded them in interpreting the law that judges bring their political perspectives to bear on it. As Justice Holmes once noted, "The true grounds of decisions are consideration of policy and of social advantage, and it is vain to suppose that solutions can be attained merely by logic and the general propositions of law which nobody disputes."[5] Or, as another distinguished jurist put it (Craven 1972, 977):

> I believe that there are only two kinds of judges at all levels of courts: those who are admittedly (maybe not to the public) result-oriented, and those who are also result-oriented but either do

---

[2]*Vermont Yankee Nuclear Power Corp. v. Natural Resources Defense Council, Inc.* 435 U.S. 519 (1978).

[3]*Pacific Gas & Electric Co. v. State Energy Resources Conservation and Development Commission.* 461 U.S. 190 (1983)

[4]*City of New York v. United States Department of Transportation.* 715 F.2d 732 (1983).

[5]*Dissenting in Vegelahn v. Gunter.* 167 Mass. 92 (1896) at pp. 105–106.

not know it or decline for various purposes to admit it.

An interesting insight into the political nature of judicial interpretation was brought out in an unsuccessful effort during the Reagan Administration to elevate a U.S. Court of Appeals Judge, Robert H. Bork, to the U.S. Supreme Court. Bork sought to portray himself as a non-ideological and flexible jurist or, if he had to be categorized, as a "strict constructionist" interested in limiting the role of the judiciary. Yet, an analysis of Judge Bork's vote in all cases in which he wrote the opinion or in which he disagreed with fellow judges while on the Court of Appeals disclosed that the only consistent predictor of how he would vote was the identity of the parties involved. One reviewer noted (Claybrook 1987, 23) that:

> in cases where the government is a party, Judge Bork exercised judicial restraint and voted against consumers, environmental groups, workers, and individuals almost 100 percent of the time. In that same category of cases [i.e., where government was a party], he was a judicial activist and voted for business 100 percent of the time.

The greatest power exercised by the judiciary in interpreting the Law is the power to declare federal and state laws—laws enacted by Congress or state legislatures and signed by the President or Governor—unconstitutional and therefore null and void. But there are other ways in which courts exercise their authority to interpret what the law is. They interpret the meaning of statutes, which often contain language that is broad and vague. They determine how statutory law shall be applied to specific fact situations. And the courts exercise these same powers of nullification, interpretation, and application over regulatory laws and regulatory agencies.

Regulatory law and regulatory agencies are of particular importance in the health policy area, and it is important to understand the basic principles involved. It has been well established that Congress can make broad delegations of authority to administrative agencies. It is also quite clear that the regulations promulgated by these agencies have the full force of law. But at the same time, there are controls on the agencies. First, Congress can restrict or remove regulatory

authority previously given and/or mandate specific regulatory actions. Second, Congress can provide procedural rules and safeguards, as it has by enacting an Administrative Procedures Act.[6] And third, administrative agency actions are subject to judicial review, with the potential for invalidation of agency regulations or agency enforcement actions.

The federal Administrative Procedures Act establishes basic procedural safeguards and general and specific judicial review authority over the regulatory agencies of the federal government. The Act specifies the procedures agencies must follow when engaged in rule making and adjudication. A major thrust of the Act is to protect public input into the process of rule making. Administrative agency activity must be consistent with the rest of the legal system: that is, the Constitution, relevant statues, and common law. Judicial review of agency activity is therefore important in overseeing and assuring this consistency. Standards for judicial review are outlined in the Act. Such review is not aimed at determining whether the administrative agency acted wisely, but at whether the agency has (1) exceeded its constitutional or statutory authority, (2) properly interpreted the applicable law, (3) conducted a fair proceeding, (4) avoided arbitrary, capricious, and unreasonable action, and (5) reached a decision supported by substantial evidence on the record. It should be readily apparent that these criteria are openended and vague enough to allow courts considerable latitude in overseeing agency actions.

The U.S. Supreme Court has held that, although the standards courts are to follow in reviewing agency decisions are technically narrow ones, they should include a searching and careful inquiry to determine "whether the decision was based on consideration of the relevant factors and whether there has been a clear error of judgment."[7] The courts have also made it easier to initiate judicial challenges and Congress has also joined in broadening "standing" to initiate such challenges.

Congress has also augmented the Administrative Procedure Act with a Freedom of Informa-

---

[6]5 U.S.C. Sec. 551 et seq.

[7]*Citizens to Preserve Overton Park, Inc. v. Volpe.* 401 U.S. 402 (1971).

tion Act[8] (allowing public access to agency files and information), a Federal Advisory Committee Act[9] (regulating the operations of committees advising Federal agencies), and a Government in the Sunshine Act[10] (requiring that decisionmaking meetings of collegial administrative agencies be open to the public).

Since administrative agencies exercise considerable discretion, their policy decisions are therefore subjected to considerable challenge. According to former Environmental Protection Agency Administrator William Ruckelshaus, over 80 percent of that Agency's regulations were challenged in court, with the result that close to 30 percent were significantly changed (1984, 134).

Most judicial review involves requests by affected parties to alter an agency decision that fails to meet the relevant legal requirements. Courts are less likely to intervene when an agency has acted, but acted in an ineffective, inadequate, or limited manner. Judicial intervention may also be sought for an order to require an agency decision where one has been avoided, but this is generally quite difficult to accomplish unless the agency has completely failed to act in a situation where action has been specifically mandated by the legislative body (e.g., failure to collect taxes). Administrative agencies generally have some degree of discretion in determining when and when not to initiate particular actions, and the courts are loathe to second-guess agency expertise and compel action in such instances. This would be especially the case when agency action would require the expenditure of significant amounts of tax funds. Cases in which courts have ordered such expenditures, for example, to improve prison conditions, are relatively rare primarily because courts are limited in their ability to enforce their orders in the face of executive and legislative branch recalcitrance. See, for example, *Wyatt v. Stickney*,[11] a case involving court mandated minimal requirements for a state mental health system.

---

[8] 5 U.S.C. Sec. 552.

[9] 5 U.S.C. App. I.

[10] 5 U.S.C. Sec. 552b.

[11] 325 F. Supp 781 (M.D.Ala. 1971), 334 F.Supp. 1341 (M.D.Ala. 1971), 344 F.Supp. 373 (M.D.Ala. 1972), *aff'd sub nom Wyatt v. Aderholt,* 503 F.2d 1305 (5th Cir. 1974).

Science and Law

The possibility of judicial review makes the courts major players in governmental policymaking. This policy involvement cannot and should not be ignored, although it raises discomforting questions for those lawyers and legal scholars who adhere to the less critical views of how law operates. Tushnet has made the important observation that "for lawyers . . . there has to be a difference between judges and legislators; otherwise the distinction between law and politics collapses" (1986, 506).

Judicial disclaimers notwithstanding, the fact is that judges play a significant political role in the United States. And since the health area is so heavily influenced by law and regulation, the courts are major factors in health politics and policy. In fact, the interaction of health and the law has provided some of the most interesting, perplexing, and important legal challenges and judical decisions of the past two decades.

Health law is a subcategory of law, with its historical roots most firmly in the areas of forensic medicine and public health law. Recent developments in this field have been so rapid and dramatic as to be without precedent. Lawyers have become so involved in practically all aspects of health and health care that they could almost be considered a new category of health professional. It has become routine for lawyers—and courts—to be involved in health-related matters ranging from termination of treatment to implementation of quality assurance programs. Among the many areas of law encompassed under the health law rubric that have undergone significant change in recent years are antitrust, refusal of treatment, mental health law, and genetics and the law. Other health-policy-related areas of legal change and controversy are reproductive rights, access to care, mandated review of the quality and cost of health care, nursing home regulation, and the various legal issues surrounding the AIDS crisis (including data confidentiality, compulsory testing, new drug approval, and discrimination).

It is impossible to provide even a cursory review of the changing health law landscape in a single essay. But some examples of legal developments can be given for each of the four major types of law (Constitutional, statutory, regulatory, and common law), thus providing some suggestion of how change has taken place.

Constitutional

The U.S. Supreme Court did not specifically recognize a Constitutional right to privacy until 1965, in the case of *Griswold v. Connecticut*.[12] This decision, invalidating a Connecticut law that made it illegal for anyone to use or prescribe contraceptives, established the principle that certain areas of intimate human activity were Constitutionally protected from state and federal restriction and control. This principle was extended in subsequent federal and state court decisions to prevent governmental intrusion into individual decisions regarding abortion,[13] termination of treatment,[14] and other "personal intimacies of the home, the family, marriage, motherhood, procreation, and child rearing" (*Paris Adult Theatre I v. Slaton*[15]). While these privacy decisions have definitely not been without controversy and criticism, there can be no denying that they have significantly altered the legal relationship between government and the individual.

Statutory

A variety of federal statutes enacted during the 1960's and 1970's have had significant impacts on health policy and politics. Medicare,[16] Medicaid,[17] and attendant cost control systems (e.g., Diagnostic Related Groups) have had a far reaching, albeit inadequate, impact on the way in which health care services are organized and delivered in the United States. Environmental protection laws, such as the Clean Air Act[18] and

Clean Water Act[19], expanded the right of individuals to sue governmental agencies to stop or compel action. And the establishment of federal agencies to oversee occupational safety and health (Occupational Safety and Health Act),[20] motor vehicle safety (National Traffic and Motor Vehicle Safety Act[21] and Highway Safety Act[22]) and product safety (Consumer Product Safety Act[23]) shifted the political debate over these issues into federal administrative forums.

Regulatory

The creation of new federal agencies, such as the Consumer Product Safety Commission, sharply altered the regulatory landscape for health and safety related issues. There were several other developments during the past two decades that also contributed to a new regulatory picture. Congressional enactment of the Freedom of Information Act as an amendment to the Administrative Procedures Act made it much easier for people outside of government to find out what government is or is not doing. This has altered the politics of advocacy on health and other issues.

A series of court decisions applying antitrust laws to the health professions have also served to alter the health policy and politics equation, opening the door to advertising by physicians and other health professionals, weakening the professional control of physicians, and changing health insurance practices (Busey et al. 1988).

Finally, increased judicial emphasis on procedural fairness, especially in the administration of governmental entitlement programs, has made the courts active players in the health policy area.[24,25]

Common law

It might seem that malpractice should top the list of common law developments of particular

---

[12]381 U.S. 479 (1965).

[13]*Roe v. Wade* 410 U.S. 113 (1973).

[14]>*In the Matter of Karen Quinlan*. 70 N.J. 10, 355 A.2d 647 (1976).

[15]*Paris Adult Theatre I v. Slaton*. 413 U.S. 49 (1973).

[16]42 U.S.C. Sec. 1395 et seq.

[17]42 U.S.C. Sec. 1396 et seq.

[18]42 U.S.C. Sec. 1857 et seq.

[19]33 U.S.C. Sec. 1251 et seq.

[20]29 U.S.C. Sec. 651 et seq.

[21]15 U.S.C. Sec. 1381 et seq.

[22]23 U.S.C. Sec. 402 et seq.

[23]15 U.S.C. 2051–2081.

[24]*Goldberg v. Kelly*. 397 U.S. 254 (1970).

[25]*Mathews v. Eldridge*. 424 U.S. 319 (1976).

significance during the past two decades. But this prominence may be more apparent than real. The basic law of medical malpractice has changed little in recent years except to the extent that many state legislatures have by statute limited the patient's ability to sue successfully for harm caused by negligent health professionals. This has been done in the name of malpractice "crises," although it is unclear to what extent, if any, patients are suing more often or for larger awards (Saks 1986).

A more substantive change can be seen in a related area of common law: product liability. State courts have evolved a theory of strict liability for unreasonable product hazard, a theory in which negligent manufacture is not a prerequisite. This legal theory has been pressed with particular force in those areas where government regulation has not adequately protected consumers. The potential high cost to manufacturers and retailers from successful product liability lawsuits can provide a strong incentive to eliminate hazards to the public (Teret 1981; Teret 1986; Teret and Jacobs 1989). A study by the Rand Corporation concluded that:

> Of all the various external social pressures, product liability has the greatest influence on product design decisions (Eads and Reuter 1984, 289).

The many changes that have occurred—and are occurring—at the interface of health and the law reflect several important forces at work. One is technological; dramatic advances in medical science and technology have created or exacerbated areas of legal and ethical uncertainty (Office of Technology Assessment 1988; Annas 1988). This would include advances in cardiopulmonary life support, in genetic screening and testing, in life expectancy itself, and in the resulting higher cost of high-tech medical care. Another factor affecting health law has been the general expansion of civil rights and liberties in the society, leading to a heightened concern over matters of patient autonomy and consent, confidentiality of information, and equal access to high-quality health care. Finally, the fact that the health care system has been rapidly transformed from a cottage industry into a "medical-industrial complex" has simultaneously depersonalized the system while increasing monetary incentives.

The fact that the health policy process is so

interwoven with law, and that the law is continually in flux, means that health policy debates and bureaucratic controversies have increasingly been moved into the courts for resolution. As Federal Appellate Judge David Bazelon has noted (1981, 210):

> Scientific questions touching life and health are increasingly dealt with through government regulation. That change prompted me to observe in 1971 that we "stand on the threshold of a new era" in the collaboration between administrative agencies and reviewing courts.

This raises an interesting technical problem: judges rarely have science backgrounds, but they nevertheless have to deal with many difficult scientific issues. Did the U.S. Environmental Protection Agency go beyond the scientific evidence in promulgating a standard limiting the lead content of gasoline to 0.5 grams/gallon? Can it be said that lead in automobile emissions "will endanger public health"?[26] Is it possible to establish some factual connection between the radioactivity dispersed after atmospheric testing of nuclear weapons and the cancers and leukemia suffered by nearby residents?[27] Can terminally ill patients be denied access to drugs that have not been approved by the Food and Drug Administration?[28] Is AIDS a handicap within the meaning of the Rehabilitation Act of 1973?[29] (Parmet 1987, 61–72.) What constitutes the "withholding of medically indicated treatment from a disabled infant with a life-threatening condition"?[30] (Lantos 1987, 444–447.) Questions like these often have no clear-cut answer. As the appellate court in *Ethyl v. EPA* noted:

> Even scientific "facts" are not certain, but only theories with high probabilities of validity. Scientists typically speak not of certainty, but of probability . . . (R)egulators seek to prevent harm that often cannot be labeled "certain" until after it occurs. . . . Questions involving the environ-

---

[26]*Ethyl Corp v. EPA.* 541 F.2d 1 (D.C. Cir. 1976) (*en banc*), *cert. denied*, 426 U.S. 941 (1976).

[27]*Allen v. United States.* 588 F. Suppl. 247 (D. Utah 1984), *rev'd on other grounds*, 816 F.2d 1417 (10th Cir. 1987).

[28]*United States v. Rutherford.* 442 U.S. 544 (1979).

[29]*School Board of Nassau County v. Arline.* 107 S. Ct. 1123 (1987).

[30]*Bowen v. American Hospital Association.* 106 S. Ct. 2101 (1986).

ment are particularly prone to uncertainty. Technological man has altered his world in ways never before experienced or anticipated. The health effects of such alterations are often unknown, sometimes unknowable. While a concerned Congress has passed legislation providing for protection of the public health against gross environmental modifications, the regulators entrusted with the enforcement of such laws have not thereby been endowed with prescience that removes all doubt from their decision-making. Rather, speculation, conflicts in evidence, and theoretical extrapolation typify their every action. How else can they act, given a mandate to protect the public health but only a slight or nonexistent data base upon which to draw?

Just as Congress and the regulatory agencies it has created have had to grapple with such difficult problems, so too the courts have been drawn into these policy debates and been forced to address the problems.

How do the courts conduct their review of administrative actions? And how well do they conduct it? Judge Bazelon described (1981, 211) a minimal standard of review when he noted that:

> In reviewing regulatory decisions, the court does not reweigh the agency's evidence and reasons. Just as common law courts might leave fact and value questions to the jury, a reviewing court leaves factual conclusions and policy choices to the agency. Courts lack the technical competence to resolve scientific controversies; they lack the popular mandate and accountability to make the critical value choices that this kind of regulation requires. The court's role is rather to monitor the agency's decision-making process—to stand outside both the expert and political debate and to assure that all the issues are thoroughly ventilated.

But despite Judge Bazelon's disclaimers, the courts have indeed been forced to resolve controversies involving complicated questions of science and technology. Many of Judge Bazelon's fellow judges are more candid in admitting to their involvement in weighing technical issues and making factual and policy judgments. Appellate courts have entered the technical arena by relying on the lower court and agency records before them, as well as on appellate briefs and on the type of short-lived expertise that comes from reviewing such materials. From time to

time suggestions have been put forward to establish special "science courts" or to provide judges with "science clerks" in the same manner in which they now make use of law clerks. But these suggestions have never garnered significant support (Bazelon 1977; Leventhal 1974; Markey 1977; Whitney 1973; Talbot 1978).

Conclusion

Policy and law could both be said to be aspects of human interaction that are resistent to clear definition yet clearly of great significance. A common theme in public policy literature is that "policy" is a slippery term which resists definition. As Fred Frohock puts it, "defining policy in a neat phrase is probably as difficult and fruitless as looking for a single-phrase definition of politics" (1979, p. 8). Others, such as Thomas Dye (1984), content themselves with defining public policy as "whatever government chooses to do or not do." Similarly, legal academics are currently involved in intense debate over the true nature of law. Although there is general agreement among legal scholars that law is a mechanism of social control and conflict resolution, the agreement stops there.

How does one attempt to understand the interaction of these two slippery areas of activity? The most sensible viewpoint is probably the pragmatic one: law and policy are part and parcel of politics. Law affects politics by defining the rules of the game. Law, in turn, is affected by political—that is, policy—decisions. To understand something about politics and policy one must understand something about law and the legal system—and vice versa.

For the health policy advocate, one of the main things this interrelationship suggests is that policy, politics, and law should not be compartmentalized. Only by looking at the big picture is it possible to understand and operate within the health policy system. In particular, by better understanding the role of law in health politics and policy, it becomes possible to use the system and the rules of the game in the way most effective to attaining a particular policy agenda. Conversely, however, specific advances most readily can be made by focusing narrowly on specific actions, that is, by careful forum shopping. If Congress seems to be the most sympathetic and promising forum, seek statutory change. If an administrative agency seems to be the most sympathetic and promising forum, seek a regulatory response. And when neither of these forums works effectively, consider using common law approaches to achieve what statutory and regulatory law would normally do better. For example, while a regulatory approach to safety and health protection would generally be the most effective, regulation is not always politically feasible. In such cases, private litigation may serve a critical role.

It is easy to see why Thomas Jefferson suggested that attention to health "should take the place of every other object." What is harder to understand is why it has taken this nation so long to focus that attention. But focus it has, so that in the last third of the 20th Century health has become a leading political and public policy concern. By almost any benchmark, health care ranks as one of the largest industries in the U.S. The Department of Health and Human Services oversees the largest budget of all of the Federal agencies. A day does not go by without at least one health-policy-related issue receiving major attention in the national media.

It is striking that it took so long for the importance of health policy to receive formal academic recognition. For example, the Book Review Editor of the *New England Journal of Medicine* notes that in 1960 only 3.4 percent of the books received for review by the *Journal* were health policy related. By the 1970s and 1980s this percentage had risen to, and plateaued at, around 10 percent (Moore 1985). Despite this publication increase, the Editor notes that the quality of health policy literature has tended to be low. "Many of the books seem pedestrian, unimaginative, not blessed with any new vision, new techniques, or new insights. . . . As compared with the current dynamic literature in such areas as molecular biology and genetics, microvascular surgery, neonatology, cardiology, or microbiology, this literature would have to be considered disappointing." (Moore, 1985, 1167)

And yet health status is a function of public policy. A community can have the level of health it is willing to pay for, in terms of funds appropriated and legal restrictions and regulations adopted. If this principle were better understood, health policy and politics could be developed in a more rational and effective way.

REFERENCES

Annas, George J. 1988. *Judging medicine.* Clifton, N.J.: The Humana Press.

Bazelon, David L. 1977. Coping with technology through the legal process. *Cornell Law Review* 62:817–832.

Bazelon, David L. 1981. Science and uncertainty. *Harvard Environmental Law Review* 5:209–215.

Bollier, David and Joan Claybrook. 1986. *Freedom from harm: The civilizing influence of health, safety and environmental regulation.* Washington, D.C.: Public Citizen & Democracy Project.

Busey, Roxanne C., Philip A. Proger, and Donald R. Schmidt. 1988. *The antitrust health care handbook.* Chicago: American Bar Association.

Christoffel, Tom. 1982. *Health and the law: A handbook for health professionals.* New York: The Free Press, Chapters 2, 4, and 5.

Claybrook, Joan. 1987. Judging Judge Bork on his record. *Public Citizen* 7(6):23.

Clune, William H. III. 1983. A political model of implementation and implications of the model for public policy, research and the changing role of lawyers. *Iowa Law Review,* 69:47–125.

Craven, J. Braxton, Jr. 1972. Paean to pragmatism. *North Carolina Law Review* 50:977.

Dye, Thomas. 1984. *Understanding public policy,* Fifth Edition, Englewood Cliffs, N.J.: Prentice-Hall.

Eads, George and Peter Reuter. 1984. Designing safer products: Corporate responses to product liability law and regulation. *Journal of Products Liability* 7:263–294.

Foley, J.P., ed. 1967. *Jeffersonian cyclopedia: A comprehensive collection of the views of Thomas Jefferson,* Vol. I. New York: Russell and Russell, as quoted in *Health care delivery in the United States,* Second Edition, edited by Steven Jonas, 21. 1981. New York: Springer Publishing Company.

Frohock, Fred. 1979. *Public policy: Scope and logic.* Englewood Cliffs, N.J.: Prentice-Hall: 8.

Kagan, Morris. 1977. Federal public health: Reflections of a changing Constitution. In *Legacies in law and medicine,* edited by C. Burns, 216–217. New York: Science History Publications.

Kennedy, Duncan. 1985. Remarks at *A discussion on critical legal studies at the Harvard Law School.* New York City, May 13, 1985, Occasional Paper No. 1 of the Harvard Society for Law & Public Policy.

Lantos, John. 1987. Baby Doe five years later. *New England Journal of Medicine* 317:444–447.

Leventhal, Harold O. 1974. Environmental decision making and the role of the courts. *University of Pennsylvania Law Review* 122:509–555.

Mensch, Elizabeth. 1982. The history of mainstream legal thought. In *The politics of law,* edited by David Kairys, 18–39. New York: Pantheon Books.

Monahan, John and Laurens Walker. 1986. Social authority: Obtaining, evaluating, and establishing social science in law. *University of Pennsylvania Law Review* 134:477–517.

Markey, Howard. 1977. A forum for technocracy? A report on the science court proposal. *Judicature* 60:364–371.

Moore, Francis D. 1985. The Health Policy Book Literature. *New England Journal of Medicine* 313:1165–1167.

U.S. Congress, Office of Technology Assessment. 1988. *Biology, medicine, and the Bill of Rights— Special report,* OTA-CIT-371. Washington, D.C.: USGPO.

Parmet, Wendy E. 1987. AIDS and the limits of discrimination law. *Law, Medicine and Health Care* 15:61–72.

Pine, Rachael N. 1988. Speculation and reality: The role of facts in judicial protection of fundamental rights. *University of Pennsylvania Law Review* 136:655–727.

Posner, Richard A. 1975. The economic approach to law. *Texas Law Review* 53:757–778, as reprinted, 1979. In *Readings in jurisprudence and legal philosophy,* edited by Philip Suchman, 854–856. Boston: Little, Brown and Company.

Rodell, Fred. 1939. *Woe unto you, lawyers!.* Republished, 1980, New York: Berkley Books.

Rosenblatt, Rand E. 1978. Health care reform and administrative law: A structural approach. *Yale Law Journal* 88:243–336.

Ruckelshaus, William. 1985. Environmental negotiation: A new way of winning. Address to the Conservation Foundations's Second National Conference on Environmental Dispute Resolution, October 1, 1984. As quoted in Lawrence Susskind and Gerard McMahon. 1985. The theory and practice of negotiated rulemaking. *Yale Journal on Regulation* 3:133–165.

Saks, Michael J. 1986. In search of the 'lawsuit crisis'. *Law, Medicine and Health Care* 14:77–82.

Talbot, Richard E. 1978. Science court: A possible way to obtain scientific certainty for decisions based on scientific fact? *Environmental Law* 8:827–850.

Taylor, George H. 1982. Deconstructing the law. *Yale Law & Policy Review* 1:158–185.

Teret, Stephen P. 1981. Injury control and product liability. *Journal of Public Health Policy* 2:49–57.

Teret, Stephen P. 1986. Litigating for the public's health. *American Journal of Public Health* 76:1027–1029.

Teret, Stephen P. and Michael Jacobs. 1989. Prevention and torts: The role of litigation in injury control. *Law, Medicine and Health Care* 17:17–22.

Tushnet, Mark. 1986. Critical legal studies: An introduction to its origins and underpinnings. *Journal of Legal Education* 36:505–517.

Whitney, Scott C. 1973. The case for creating a special environmental court system. *William and Mary Law Review* 33:41–56.

Chapter 8

The Enduring Challenge of Health Policy Implementation

Frank J. Thompson

The experience of social programs in the United States over the last quarter century has relentlessly reaffirmed a major message: the politics played out after a bill becomes law is as important as that in evidence before passage. Early studies of implementation often chose painful examples to drive this point home. For example, Pressman and Wildavsky (1979) and Bardach (1977) chronicled tales of good policy intentions gone sour through underperformance, delay, soaring costs and other factors. They reinforced the dominant theme of the 1970s that "the great American weakness . . . lies in implementation" (Heclo and Wildlavsky 1974, 12). Subsequent studies did not so uniformly support this gloomy picture. Toward the end of the 1970s, for example, various analysts took to specifying conditions that contributed to implementation success (Rodgers and Bullock 1976; Sabatier and Mazmanian 1979).

The emergence of the study of implementation has to some extent found expression in the study of health policy. Two major types of studies stand out. One type focuses on the experience of particular programs such as the complex bargaining that transpired between medical providers and the federal bureaucracy after the birth of Medicare (Feder 1977). In a similar vein, another analysis plumbs the troubles encountered in implementing Medicaid's Early and Periodic Screening, Diagnosis and Treatment program (EPSDT). This program, which emphasized medical outreach in order to reduce death and disease among infants and children, met with repeated delays and other woes, initially reaching a small percentage of those targeted for assistance. On the brighter side, however, there is evidence that state EPSDT programs improved their performance over time (Goggin 1987). Still other work has attempted to penetrate the dynamics of implementation through a comparative analysis of the evolution of a number of health programs (Thompson 1981).

Aside from these efforts to assess implementation processes, another stream of analysis looks more to the future, attempting to anticipate the implementation problems that various health reforms might face (Marmor 1980). In 1980, for example, the Urban Institute released a 721-page volume that explored many of the issues that would surface in implementing a national health insurance program (Feder et al. 1980). Such matters as physician reimbursement, hospital payment, patient cost sharing, and utilization review received judicious scrutiny in this tome.

Although existing works on health policy implementation have fostered understanding, further inquiry is important. Much remains to be done in order to enhance the capacity to describe, explain, and predict implementation processes, outputs and outcomes. In a related vein, analysts must grapple with the normative issues of implementation and must sharpen their capacity to advise policymakers and others on suitable implementation strategies.

This essay lays a partial foundation for the subsequent exploration of health policy implementation by focusing on certain critical factors and dynamics that characterize these processes in the United States. In this regard, it initially considers some key ingredients of implementation processes. It then examines several forces that leave their mark on implementation. These include (a) the policy mandate (or founding statute) which serves both as a source of program hypotheses and of the particular tools, instruments or technologies that implementors use; (b) the capacity of administrative agencies with particular attention paid to the implications of a political culture that casts the federal bureaucracy in a negative light, and to the erosion of the federal service during the 1980s; (c) the implementation challenges embedded in administration by proxy; that is, the reliance on other governments or private parties to deliver public programs; and (d) the forces that influence the presence or absence of program fixers in the agency's environment.

Implementation Ingredients

Health policy implementation is a deceptively simple phrase. Its meaning seems obvious until matters of formal definition arise; then consensus vanishes. Some, for example, might adopt the common sense notion that health policy implementation involves the carrying out of some formally stated policy. Reasonable as this may seem, other students of the subject would object. Sensitive to the way in which implementation can transform original program goals, some analysts emphasize that implementation is less the carrying out of policy than the evolution of policy (e.g., Farrar et al. 1980). The complexities of implementation will no doubt fuel debate concerning appropriate definitions and metaphors well into the future (Lester et al. 1987). For present purposes, this essay considers health policy implementation to be the program processes that occur in response to a health policy mandate. These processes lead to some output (e.g., the delivery of care to a patient in a Veterans Administration Medical Center) and outcome (e.g., the veteran's health improves). Implementation processes feature strategic, routine, and fortuitous aspects (in the sense of chance rather than good fortune).

Bardach (1977, 57–58) captures the strategic aspect of implementation when he defines it as "the playing out of a number of loosely interrelated games whereby . . . elements are withheld from or delivered to the program assembly process on particular terms." Hence, the implementation of health programs finds various participants (e.g., medical providers, consumer groups, program administrators, unions, key congressional subcommittees) with diverse perceptions and goals mobilizing power resources, forming coalitions, and consciously plotting gambits. Each participant hopes to prevail in the implementation games of special concern to them. Bargaining and compromise often occur. The program assembled as a result of strategic maneuvering in countless games may, of course, differ so greatly from the one envisioned by the founding statute as to undercut any notion of implementation as the "carrying out" of a health policy.

The bureaucratic processes that promulgate health program rules often serve as one important focal point for strategic interaction. Major administrative regulations and guidelines are not simply imposed. Rather civil servants draft them with the intention of giving various interest groups a chance to respond. When the bureaucracy publishes a "Notice of Proposed Rulemaking" in the *Federal Register* the reaction can at times be particularly intense as a case involving the National Health Planning and Resources Development Act (PL 93–641) illustrates. In response to this law, federal administrators in 1977 issued tentative guidelines aimed at reducing excess hospital beds and underused facilities. Among other things, the guidelines suggested that rural hospitals deliver at least 500 babies annually if they were to maintain a maternity ward and delivery room. The guidelines also implied that, regardless of location, inability by a hospital to achieve an average of 80 percent occupancy of its beds would be interpreted as a sign of excess capacity.

The guidelines elicited a massive protest, especially from rural areas. All told federal civil servants received 55,000 written communications on the guidelines, nearly all of which were negative. Some congressional offices received as many as 10,000 communications. Following this gusher of complaints, the House of Representatives unanimously adopted a resolution demanding that the final guidelines reflect the needs of rural areas to a greater degree (Zwick 1978). The Department of Health, Education and Welfare (DHEW) subsequently eased the standards somewhat. Final guidelines took pains to mention that Health Systems Agencies (HSA) could, after careful analysis, depart from federal standards in reviewing grant proposals and construction requests. In seven of eleven issue areas, federal civil servants modified standards to take into account the concerns of those in rural areas. For example, the new guidelines made no explicit reference to the number of deliveries an obstetrical unit in a rural hospital should achieve. Instead, the guidelines focused only on hospitals providing care for "complicated obstetrical problems" (Thompson 1981).

Strategic considerations also shape decisions concerning whether to promulgate any rules at all. The specification of rules need not proceed in some neat, linear fashion once Congress gives civil servants a statute to implement. Consider, for example, the Hill-Burton program that Congress launched in 1946 to spur the construction of hospital facilities. The statute called for equal protection of racial minorities and required hos-

pitals receiving grants to provide some free service to the medically indigent. It was not until October 1978, however, that DHEW promulgated rules governing "free service" that possessed any teeth at all. During the program's first thirty years, DHEW administrators avoided the conflict with the hospital industry that enforcement of this provision would create. The decision to issue relatively stringent regulations came only after considerable court action and related agitation by representatives of the poor during the 1970s.

In addition to the strategic considerations, standard operating procedures and other informal decision rules are major ingredients of implementation processes. These procedures and rules greatly simplify choices for administrators, allowing them to make some decisions almost unthinkingly. Certainly, officials make many choices without the strategic consciousness suggested by the game metaphor. For example, Medicare administrators follow certain routines in determining whether someone is eligible to receive benefits from that program. Standard operating procedures facilitate the reliable performance of tasks by ordinary people. An inability to develop these procedures almost invariably undermines prospects for program success (Kelman 1984).

Ultimately, the strategic and routine combine with chance events to create an implementation mosaic. Conveying the importance of the fortuitous has presented difficulties for social scientists who by training tend to emphasize regular or predictable patterns of interaction. Work by Cohen et al. (1972), Kingdom (1984) and others, however, represents an intriguing effort to deal with implementation's random qualities. Implementation viewed as a process of organized anarchy could in part be portrayed as the product of four streams: problems, solutions, participants, and choice opportunities. Although none of the streams is completely independent of the others, the model holds that implementation decisions often derive from a somewhat fortuitous confluence of the four. For instance, the purchase of new computers and utilization review software (a solution) by the VA plus the hiring of a new medical director could give those concerned (participants) with the excessive prescription of certain drugs and services (the problem) a chance (choice opportunity) to correct the excess.

The strategic, the routine, and the fortuitous thus comprise key ingredients of the implementation of health policy. But what factors shape the particular implementation patterns that emerge and their consequences? Rather than present a laundry list of variables, this chapter will focus on several particularly important ones.

Health Statutes as Pivotal Hypotheses

Observers have often equated implementation difficulties with the "bureaucracy problem." There is undoubtedly something to those definitions of the bureaucracy that refer to it as an organization that cannot learn from its mistakes (Crozier 1964). The errors of health administrators often push a program toward certain policy pitfalls. But the difficulties faced in implementing health policy stem only in part from a bureaucratic propensity to err. The founding statute and subsequent legislative amendments also do much to rig the implementation game.

A health policy embedded in a statute is in essence a hypothesis. it specifies that if a, b, c, and so on, are done at time one, then x, y, z, and so on, will result at time two. As hypotheses, policies vary enormously in their precision and plausibility. Precision is a function of the degree to which a policy defines terms, quantifies objectives, specifies timetables for obtaining them, indicates priorities among objectives, and prescribes the administrative structure and procedures to be used in implementing the program (Sabatier and Mazmanian 1979). With these dimensions in mind, policies can be arranged on a continuum from precise to less precise.

Ultimately, the health policy hypothesis achieves some level of plausibility. At times, a formal policy lacks plausibility in that it calls for arrangements that seem destined to foster ineffectiveness, waste, or some other program failure. At other times, the causal notions built into the policy hypothesis ostensibly make sense. For example, the assumption embedded in the Comprehensive Health Manpower Training Act (PL 92–257) that medical schools would increase their enrollments if the federal government used capitation grants to reward them financially for doing so seemed reasonable at the time Congress passed the law in 1971. And, in fact, the law subsequently fueled increases in medical school enrollments.

In considering the implications of the statute for implementation processes, an important caveat deserves mention. A health policy may at times perform certain symbolic functions and engender significant sociopolitical outcomes regardless of whether or not officials vigorously move to implement it. The passage of laws that the bureaucracy does not or cannot implement energetically may at least reinforce commitment to important values in the health arena. In some cases, it buys time for government to pick the moment or to develop the means for delivering on these value commitments.

In considering statutory hypotheses, some analysts have emphasized the importance of precision. This viewpoint has been termed a top-down perspective—one that sees clear specification of goals and means as critical and tends to judge implementation in terms of the degree to which administrators comply with the law (Palumbo 1987, 93). Precise policy mandates possess considerable appeal in a democratic society. They seem consistent with the rule of law and the thwarting of unaccountable bureaucratic power (Lowi 1969). Aside from keeping elected officials in the driver's seat, several observers have emphasized the role of precision in fostering the efficiency and effectiveness of program implementation (e.g., Sabatier and Mazmanian 1979; Montjoy and O'Toole 1979). Observers credit precise mandates with giving an agency a major weapon to turn against those who oppose its mission. Specific statutes also win praise for reducing prospects that an agency's officials will dissipate energy by skirmishing with one another over how to interpret the law. In addition, such mandates allegedly expedite program evaluation and, thereby, the detection and correction of errors. While no one sees precise statutes as a panacea, a substantial bias towards precision exists in much of the writing on implementation as well as in the conventional wisdom of society.

The alleged virtues of precise health statutes cannot be slighted. Indeed, one intriguing analysis (Foltz 1975) of the difficulties faced in implementing the EPSDT program implies that ambiguous policy had much to do with the problems encountered. Other research (Thompson 1981) indicates that the vague goals of the National Health Planning and Resources Development Act of 1974 contributed to some of the problems officials faced in implementing this program.

But other evidence from the health arena indicates that precision is no elixir. In its original form, for example, the Health Maintenance Organization Act of 1973 was a precise policy for the near impossible. The law (Falkson 1980) which provided various grants, loans, and loan guarantees to spur the development of health maintenance organizations (HMOs), was highly detailed. But some of the specific requirements built into the law seriously threatened its plausibility. Among other things, the statute required subsidized HMOs to provide a very rich mix of services and periodically provide open enrollment. These provisos raised serious questions as to whether these HMOs would be able to compete with other plans. The case of the HMO legislation illustrates how political processes in Congress can at times thwart the application of reasonable theories. It is evident that processes of bargaining, compromise, and coalition formation give birth to ambiguous law. What needs to be stressed is that the same processes directed toward statutory precision can lead to a splicing of incongruous, albeit specific, provisions into a single law.

If precise laws at times undermine effectiveness, vague laws can on occasion spawn creative adaptation, that is, change that helps a program escape policy pitfalls. In 1970, for example, Congress passed an ambiguous, four-page statute that authorized placement of Public Health Service (PHS) physicians in shortage areas as part of what was subsequently called the National Health Service Corps (NHSC). Given this foggy mandate, the program underwent considerable change during the 1970s. At first, agency officials stressed the objective of retaining NHSC physicians in private practice within shortage areas after their departure from the Corps—an effort that met with little success. By the end of the decade, however, agency officials had turned their backs on that concern. Instead, they stressed the placement of such physicians in federally supported organizations that provided care to the poor (e.g., community health centers). They emphasized reenlistment in the NHSC after

a physician's term of duty had expired rather than placement in the private sector. It is at least arguable that this shift permitted the program to achieve a higher level of effectiveness. Retention rates rose along with physician productivity (Thompson 1981). The Reagan Administration subsequently gutted the program, but its utility for illustrating creative program evolution remains.

The experience of the NHSC supports the arguments of implementation theorists who cling to a bottom-up or backward-mapping perspective (e.g., Elmore 1979, 1987). Among other things, this perspective emphasizes the importance of focusing on the street-level phase of implementation where the delivery of income, service or goods occurs (e.g., the provision of care to a patient). It questions the wisdom of clear policy mandates and plays down the virtues of hierarchical control. Instead, it values administrative discretion especially "at the point where the problem is most immediate" (Elmore 1979, 605). Certain "choice" theorists provide further support for this perspective. In this regard, March (1978, 595, 603) has argued that when decision makers have confused and contradictory preferences, "precision misrepresents them." In this view, decision making involves guesses not only about the future consequence of various alternatives but about preferences for these consequences. At times, people learn what they want by doing it. Recognition of this phenomenon has driven students of choice to the conclusion that vague tastes or goals may at times be intelligent rather than stupid.

Debates about administrative discretion and the importance of statutory precision cannot be settled without understanding context. Under what circumstances will less precise statutes more readily foster positive program results? Several conditions, among others, suggest themselves (Thompson 1984).

First, statutory ambiguity more readily fosters creative evolution when Congress cannot turn to a good underlying theory in drafting legislation and problems seem so pressing that something must be done (throwing money at the problem may be the only hope). For example, Congress is probably incapable of drafting a plausible statute that specifies in great detail how best to allocate research funds to reduce the cancer mortality rate.

Second, specific health statutes seem less fruitful when rapidly changing social and economic factors promise to threaten the validity of any precisely worded hypothesis. For example, knowledge of which substances qualify as carcinogens in the workplace and the precise effects of some level of exposure to them remains in a constant state of flux. Therefore, an occupational safety and health law that precisely established maximum exposure levels for some finite set of toxic substances would be destined for rapid obsolesence.

Third, creative program evolution in the face of an ambiguous mandate occurs more readily when a tempered consensus exists within the implementing agency as to its fundamental mission and this mission is not completely at odds with the *general* thrust of the statute. In the case of the National Health Service Corps, for example, top officials responsible for the program shared a strong commitment to delivering care to the disadvantaged through certain kinds of group medical practices. Without internal accord of this kind, vague legislation tends to generate internal tensions. Dysfunctional delay often surfaces as civil servants fight with one another over the proper definition of program goals.

The wrong kind of consensus can, of course, dramatically impair implementation. Hence, tempered commitment looms large in importance. Such commitment exists within an implementing agency when its key personnel strike a reasonable balance between skepticism (or hostility) and dogma (or zealotry). Skepticism or hostility can breed sabotage or lethargic program implementation. The concept of tempered commitment also recognizes that too much commitment (dogma, zealotry) can hurt a program if implementors are "true believers" who fail to acknowledge evidence of program shortcomings, tenaciously clinging to certain strategies and techniques no matter how dysfunctional. If officials are to facilitate the creative adaptation of a program, they need to remain open to information that certain initiatives do not work and of the potential need to formulate alternative policy hypotheses.

Fourth, foggy health statues more readily foster creative evolution if the bureaucracy faces an environment relatively free of interest groups intensely opposed to the program's effective or ef-

ficient administration. Where such resistance exists, program officials tend to need well-crafted, precise grants of statutory authority or persistent backing from oversight actors. If, for example, Congress wants Medicare officials to stand up to hospitals and physicians on issues involving their payment, it probably needs to strengthen the position of the bureaucracy with clear grants of authority.

Finally, precise legislation becomes less appealing when doubt exists about the efficacy of overhead actors, especially Congress.[1] Efficacy increases to the degree that these actors possess the capacity and incentive to formulate theoretically sound and coherent policies as well as to engage in error correction (Thompson 1984, 10). Efficacious overhead actors effectively exploit the knowledge base available in society to guide policy development. Any attempt to calibrate the efficacy of overhead institutions faces thorny empirical and normative questions. Nonetheless, informed speculation is possible.

Some students of Congress have argued that certain dynamics make it increasingly difficult for that body to draft coherent legislation. One thesis holds that, as many in Congress came to view the office as a stepping stone rather than a capstone to their careers, the incentive for showmanship and quick recognition broadened and "the formerly widespread pride in legislative craftsmanship . . . steadily declined" (Ornstein 1981, 369). More fundamentally, the fragmentation of power within Congress may well; have vitiated congressional efficacy in drafting laws. This fragmentation springs from a quest by members of Congress for personal clout that in turn tends to scatter power to subcommittees. Fragmentation has resulted in a situation in which many subcommittees can claim jurisdiction over a single health bill. As access points for interest groups multiply,the coalition formation process becomes less predictable and legislation increasingly seeks to satisfy a multitude of particular interests. The statutory sum of the particular interests often fails to equal a coherent whole (Davidson 1981; Sinclair 1981). If arguments such as these are correct, it could well mean that efforts to draft precise legislation run high risks of spawning implausible policy hypotheses.

---

[1]Overhead actors also include the President and the courts.

No doubt other conditions also boost the correlation between statutory ambiguity and creative program evolution. The central point should be clear, however. Students of health policy implementation must pay careful attention to statutes and other written mandates governing programs (e.g., administrative regulations, court opinions). These mandates set major rules of the game, powerfully influence behavior, and define standards of accountability. An analysis of statutes also provides major clues as to whether any subsequent program failures stem from faulty program design or from inadequate implementation. In this sense, advocates of a top-down perspective on implementation are quite correct. But those who espouse a backward mapping perspective are equally sagacious in their skepticism about the inherent desirability of statutory precision. Precision hardly qualifies as an unmitigated blessing. The optimal level of clarity varies depending on certain contingencies related to the implementing agency and its environment.

The Elusive Link to Policy Type

In their quest to develop better empirical theory, students of implementation have attempted to conceptualize policy typologies that would allow them to predict certain implementation challenges. One approach, for instance, emphasizes that the use of certain *tools* presents predictable problems (Salamon 1989). These tools include direct government delivery of a service, good, or income (e.g., care at the Veterans Administration Medical Center), regulation (e.g., the occupational safety and health program), tax policy (e.g., the deduction of medical expenses above some amount from taxable income), loans and loan guarantees (e.g., to encourage the development of HMOs), insurance (e.g., Medicare), and more. Others attempt to forge their typologies around the concept of *policy instruments*— that is, "an authoritative choice of means to accomplish a purpose" (Elmore 1987, 175). Still others prefer to base their analysis on such general policy categories as distributive, redistributive, competitive regulatory and protective regulatory (Ripley and Franklin 1982). So far, however, no firm consensus exists as to the theo-

retical supremacy of any one typology. Since health policies come in many forms, the development of such a typology could facilitate understanding of their implementation.

Without attempting a synoptic classification, one can illustrate the implementation issues posed by different kinds of policies by focusing on two prevalent types of technologies—regulatory and allocative.[2] Most policies comprise a mix of these two types of activities although a policy often emphasizes one or the other of the technologies. Technology here does not refer to hardware, but instead, to the repertoire of practices and means through which public agencies seek to accomplish certain ends.

Regulatory Technology[3]

A regulatory technology calls on the public agency to prescribe and control behavior for a designated group in its task environment. For instance, the Occupational Safety and Health Administration (OSHA) seeks to protect workers from hazards to their health in the workplace. Like other regulatory programs, it features the promulgation of rules or standards (e.g., specifying acceptable levels of exposure to toxic substances), the monitoring of groups to determine compliance with standards and the imposition of penalties for failure to comply. Each component of regulatory technology poses perplexing implementation problems.

In the cases of rule promulgation, questions involving priorities are often central. For instance, the health standards of OSHA cover only a small number of the known carcinogens. If agency officials wish to promulgate new stan-

---

[2]It would be useful to develop subtypes of these two general kinds of technologies. For instance, the degree to which a policy overlays a regulatory or allocative technology with an induced technology makes a difference. Induced technologies require a government agency to coax private firms, private nonprofit grantees, or other governmental entities to undertake critical implementation tasks. Some of the challenges of an induced technology receive consideration in the section of this chapter dealing with administration by proxy (Levine et al. 1989).

[3]Much of the discussion of regulatory and allocative technologies draws extensively on Levine, Peters and Thompson (In Press).

dards, which carcinogens should receive attention first? Should it be those that affect the most workers? Those that have the severest effect on the workers exposed to them? Those housed in industries with less political power to make trouble for the agency? Those where affected firms can comply with the new standard at less economic cost? Those that have caught the attention of the media? The answers are far from obvious. Similar conundrums can confront implementors when they weigh the desirability and feasibility of spending agency resources on getting rid of obsolete rules already on the books (Thompson 1982).

The deployment of investigatory resources in order to achieve the efficient and effective enforcement of existing standards also presents major implementation challenges. Difficult strategic questions abound. For instance, which kinds of violations of standards should receive more attention? Which groups or sectors in society should be targeted for greater surveillance? The risks of misspent effort are substantial. For instance, complex dynamics have pushed OSHA to assign a higher priority to "safety" rather than "health" regulation. Safety hazards are those that tend to produce immediate injuries such as a broken leg or electrocution; health threats are those that engender occupational illness (e.g., cancer)—often after many years of exposure to a toxic substance. OSHA's bias toward safety exists even though most knowledgeable observers believe that health, rather than safety enforcement, should receive priority (Thompson and Scicchitano 1987).

The targeting of scarce enforcement resources also intersects with issues of responsiveness. Implementing agents have a strong incentive to dispatch inspectors to investigate citizen complaints about health hazards. Great responsiveness to citizen complaints, can, however, lead to the distortion of an agency's enforcement priorities whereby compliance officers spend more time investigating trivial rather than major infractions of the rules. Following criticism for its slow handling of complaints of severely ill workers in the late 1970s, for instance, OSHA executives placed a higher priority on following up complaints. Eventually, however, this practice produced a situation in some regions where responses to complaints consumed nearly all of the inspection staff's time. The agency soon came under criticism for allowing complaints to impede efforts to target workplaces with the most serious hazards.

The implementation of a regulatory technology also involves important choices concerning the response to infractions. In general terms, agencies may pursue a legalistic or consultative approach. Under the former, top managers urge inspectors to cite all infractions, however minor, and to seek stiff penalties. Under the latter, executives encourage inspectors to use their judgment. Compliance officers have more discretion to size up the situation and to refrain from issuing citations and proposing penalties if they believe that hazards can be abated more effectively in other ways. The legalistic version allows managers to defend themselves against charges of playing favorites or caving in to industry. However, this strategy tends to engender considerable hostility as the agency comes to be perceived as picayune and unreasonable. A consultative approach can militate against an image of unreasonableness. The risk is that enforcement officers may go beyond the proper bounds of discretion. Inspectors may do favors for employers when they should not. The approach can easily breed suspicion of corruption or excessive leniency.

Allocative Technology

Health policies featuring allocative technologies also tend to produce predictable challenges. An allocative technology involves the overt delivery of income, services, or goods to groups of individuals who (usually) apply for them. While those who manage regulatory technologies often meet resistance from their basic target group, those who oversee allocative technologies often face the problem of being so popular as to be swamped with demands for program benefits. In this regard problems frequently revolve around targeting and the management of supply.

Implementors Can Miss the Target

Federal laws generally deem certain categories of individuals or entities eligible to apply for and receive program benefits. These eligibility decisions may stem from entitlement policies such as Medicaid where once an individual meets certain standards, the state must supply a range of health care benefits to him or her. In other cases, groups compete with one another (e.g., communities applying for Hill-Burton hospital funds, scientists competing for grant support from the National Institutes of Health). Here eligibility for benefits implies not only meeting certain basic criteria but convincing program officials of the merits of one's case relative to the competition.

In the case of entitlement programs, eligibility errors often present a targeting problem. How can one ensure that only those eligible for program benefits actually receive them? In the case of Medicaid the answer to this question remains far from obvious. Intake workers in social service agencies must frequently interpret complex eligibility regulations. To compound problems, low pay for intake workers often heightens turnover among them and reduces expertise. Nor can one take for granted that valid information about a Medicaid applicant will flow to the intake worker in timely fashion. For example, an applicant's income and wealth often pose an important variable in an eligibility decision. The intake worker may not, however, be able to obtain accurate information about these factors. How can one be sure that an applicant who claims he has no bank account is telling the truth?

Where implementing agencies make funding decisions in a more competitive context, they confront the obvious problem of investing resources in the most deserving case—of targeting resources where they will do the most "good." In the case of programs that distribute resources on a geographic basis, pork barrel dynamics often surface. In an effort to serve their constituents, members of Congress seek to spread program benefits into many congressional districts. This can lead to a dispersion of scarce resources from critical targets. In essence, a substantial sum of money gets transferred from the neediest areas in order to maintain the coalition that provides continued funding and authorization for the program (Bardach 1977). For instance, the placement of Veterans Administration facilities has as much to do with placating key senators and representatives as with maximizing the access of veterans to care.

Supply: Access and Quality

Becoming eligible for program benefits does not guarantee receipt of these benefits. Access may be quite limited. In the case of Medicaid, for instance, many physicians refuse to treat those who are eligible. Or an eligible individual may live in a remote area far from medical facilities. Demanding forms, long queues, busy phone lines, limited business hours, deductibles and copayments may also curtail access to medical providers. Alternatively, program beneficiaries may at times suffer from too much access to services. If Veterans Administration hospitals have large numbers of beds, many veterans may remain in the hospital well beyond a medically justifiable point. Excessive hospital stays not only waste resources; they expose patients to certain diseases that they might otherwise avoid. Hence, too much access may spawn "flat-of-the-curve medicine" whereby greater medical inputs yield no appreciable improvement in health (Enthoven 1978).

Quality also looms as a basic challenge in the implementation of allocative technologies. For instance, where the health care agency delivers a service, does it provide the right amount and blend of different types? Where products are allocated (new VA facilities) do they meet societally defined standards of acceptability? Judgments about quality are typically quite complex. Considerable debate persists about what "quality medical care" means and how it can be monitored and measured.

As this discussion suggests, different technologies pose particular challenges for implementors. Advancement in implementation theory depends upon progress in coming to grips more specifically with the link between the types of technologies embedded in policies and subsequent implementation challenges.

Federal Agencies: Crisis of Capacity?

The statute and policy type comprise, of course, only part of the equation. The commitment and capacity of public agencies formally charged with implementing a program greatly affect its destiny. In general, program prospects improve when key personnel sustain tempered commitment (that which strikes a balance between dogma and skepticism) toward a program. The presence of an agency culture that facilitates such commitment also helps.

In turn, capacity depends on the presence of the following factors, among others:

adequate resources in the form of money, personnel, information, status (or prestige), authority, and physical facilities and equipment; the presence of skilled personnel looms particularly large in importance.

skilled management sensitive to the technical core of the agency and to the art of administrative politics;

a set of standard operating procedures conducive to the accomplishment of program objectives.

The Problem of Bureaucratic Status

While recognizing the significance of personnel and a host of other factors related to administrative capacity, this section focuses on an agency resource that has received less attention in the implementation literature—agency status, or prestige. Status ranks among the most important resources an implementing agency can possess. Its general reputation for competent and humane action influences its access to other resources and can greatly facilitate or impede implementation. At least to a degree, what the public thinks makes it so.

The political culture of the United States casts the federal government and its bureaucracy in a negative light. Waldo (1980, 17) has gone so far as to suggest that "the ineffectiveness and inefficiency" of the public sector is a belief "so widely and firmly held that one . . . can regard it as a unifying theme of our creed. . . ." Survey after survey bears testimony to this conclusion. For instance, one study found a substantial majority of respondents convinced that the federal government hires too many people and that these personnel do not have to work as hard as those employed in the private sector (Gallup Opinion Index 1977). Another reported that over three quarters of respondents believed that people in

government waste a lot of their tax money (Public Opinion 1987, 27).

Some view the low status of the federal bureaucracy as a plus, as a vehicle for curtailing bureaucratic arrogance and for keeping civil servants on their toes. But the disadvantage of a sullied reputation can outweigh the benefits. Specifically, it can contribute to a climate for implementation weakness and failure by engendering defensiveness, dependence, and defeatism.

First, the relatively low status of federal managers may exacerbate the tendency for policy implementation to become a defensive and nonexperimental exercise where officials spend much time maneuvering to avoid scrutiny, blame and responsibility (Bardach 1977, 37). Avoiding scandal, fraud, and embarrassment rather than performing tends to become the salient administrative concern. Such an orientation corrodes the bureaucracy's willingness to experiment with potentially useful but risky initiatives. It may, for example, help account for the initial reluctance of Medicare officials to embrace HMOs and other modes of prospective payment more fully. It may also help explain why OSHA administrators have tended to adopt a rigidly legalistic approach to compliance even in the face of evidence that a more flexible posture might better serve safety and health objectives.

Second, the political culture heightens the dependence of federal executives on overhead actors or groups in their environment. Lacking status, it becomes all the more important for public agencies to cultivate support. A successful quest for such support need not, however, bode well for program accomplishments. At times constituencies that back a program push it away from one trap into the grips of another. Thus, the presence of a supportive milieu should prompt the following question: At what price has the support been purchased? The support that health care providers gave Medicare for example, partly derived from the program's tolerance of the medical sector's inefficiencies. Given the bureaucracy's limited status as well as the considerable power of the medical lobby, such tolerance may well have been necessary to ensure the effectiveness of the program during its early years. But the United States today would probably be better served by the emergence of a more conflictive milieu around the program—one that would feature major governmental forays to encourage greater sensitivity to cost in the delivery of care. Although those responsible for administering Medicare have taken some steps to constrain payments to providers, they have hardly been zealous in this regard.

The limited status of the bureaucracy fuels the desire of civil servants to avoid conflicts with health care providers over issues of cost effectiveness. With public understanding of issues of medical payment minimal and the bureaucracy viewed as nearly incapable of doing anything right, top administrators negotiate or bargain from weakness. If open conflict erupts, the risk runs high that the public will side with the providers of care rather than with the civil servants. One by-product of this more general circumstance is a regulate and retreat syndrome. Aware of the highly developed entrepreneurial skills of health care providers, yet not indifferent to the goal of more cost-effective implementation, bureaucrats in the health arena often attempt to gain control over the situation by issuing countless pages of regulations. Health care providers see many of these regulations as excessive and niggling; they often manage to apply sufficient pressure to persuade federal civil servants to back off from initial provisions. Given these and related dynamics, regulations constantly seem to be in a state of flux, thereby complicating the administration of the program and conveying inconsistency (Glaser 1978; Price 1978). This syndrome reinforces the image of an ineffectual federal bureaucracy.

Third, the negative strain in the political culture can induce *defeatism* among federal executives (Levine et al In Press). Defeatism refers to a kind of inferiority complex whereby an executive takes too limited a view of what can be accomplished. Defensiveness and defeatism are closely related. However, while defensive managers may nonetheless be entrepreneurial and strive to accomplish ambitious goals, defeatism implies resignation to subpar performance. The executives tend to give up too easily out of a conviction that forces "out there" will prevent them from doing what needs to be done. In a certain sense, the executives, themselves, come to accept the cultural stereotype.

Defensiveness, dependence and defeatism heighten the risk of a self-fulfilling prophecy with respect to program implementation. At worst, they can reinforce the theme pervasive in the broader political culture. Portrayed as ineffectual, federal managers risk becoming so. In all probability, most executives resist such tendencies. Many of them in fact set high standards of creativity and effectiveness in managing health programs. Several factors help buffer them from the self-fulfilling impact of a negative political culture. The subcultures surrounding particular agencies serve as one such buffer. While the public may rail against government bureaucracy in general, they often respect the importance and competence of certain agencies in particular (e.g., the National Institutes of Health). Moreover, a skilled executive can help create a favorable image for his or her agency (Ferman and Levin 1987). Executives may effectively cultivate a reputation for enlightenment and competence with the media by obtaining visible program results, by careful presentation of self and agency to the media, or in other ways. Nonetheless, the blame-the-bureaucrat strain in the political culture makes implementation more trying.

The Reagan Legacy

Much of the rhetoric of the Reagan Administration reinforced negative views of federal administrative agencies. This rhetoric along with other developments in all probability precipitated an erosion in federal administrative capacity during the 1980s (Levine et al.). In particular, concern mounted that the federal government was losing the struggle to attract and retain top quality executives. The top echelons of the career services (the Senior Executive Service, or SES) seemed particularly threatened. For instance, high resignation rates among the SES fueled concern that a "brain drain" had occurred. The full meaning of any brain drain becomes more apparent when one realizes that as of the late 1980s, about one-third of the SES members were scientists and engineers; one-fifth were other professionals such as attorneys, economists, accountants and medical officers (U.S. President's Commission on Compensation 1988).

Pay, politicization, cutbacks and red tape sparked recruitment and retention problems in the skilled professional and executive positions of the federal service. By the end of the 1980s, a broad consensus existed about the inadequacies of federal pay. President Reagan's Commission on the Compensation of Career Federal Executives (1988, 4, 30) reported in 1988 that "the Federal Government is at a substantial disadvantage in competing for the best of our nation's executive talent." More specifically, it concluded that from 1979 to 1987 real SES pay had slightly declined. Politicization also exacerbated problems. Reagan ideologues often manifested profound distrust of the career civil service. In many agencies, political executives went out of their way to limit the role of career civil servants. Declining morale and diminished agency performance often resulted. An environment of retrenchment also contributed to difficulties in recruitment and retention. Facing cuts in personnel and other resources, top executives and professionals had even more incentive to look for greener occupational pastures. Finally, the restrictive, control-oriented nature of many management systems within the federal government probably persuaded some that they could not realize their professional potential in federal agencies.

Federal health bureaucracies have not, of course, escaped these enervating forces. For example, stagnant federal pay scales have heightened prospects that the National Institutes of Health will not be able to retain their most able scientists. At a time when the Centers for Disease Control faced growing responsibilities in the battle against AIDS, it suffered cutbacks in personnel (Panem 1988).

Hence, the risk of a self-fulfilling prophecy loomed large as the 1990s dawned. Fueled in substantial measure by negative stereotypes about federal bureaucracies, events threatened to undermine the ability of these agencies to achieve high levels of efficiency and effectiveness. This development could in turn fuel negative cultural sentiments. However, a growing sense of the potential magnitude of the capacity problem had become more evident among policymakers of all ideological stripes by the end of the 1980s. For instance, neither presidential candidate in 1988 engaged in much bureaucrat bashing. Moreover, the creation of a National Commission on the Public Service with funding from such private organizations as the Ford

Foundation and the Rockefeller Foundation could conceivably help arrest decline. Chaired by Paul Volcker, the widely respected former Chairman of the Federal Reserve Board, the Commission dedicated itself to strengthening the career services of government (National Commission on the Public Service 1989). Efforts such as this could ultimately reduce the risk of self-fulfilling prophecy.

Administration By Proxy

The relatively low status of the federal bureaucracy as well as the fear of centralized political authority embedded in the nation's cultural heritage have fueled use of administration by proxy. To a marked degree, the federal government depends on private entities in an effort to accomplish its purposes in the health arena. It also turns much implementation of federal policy over to state and local governments. Each practice adds new dimensions to the challenges of implementation.

Privatization: All that Glitters Is Not Gold

A major administrative legacy of the Reagan Administration was the sparking of more explicit consideration of privatization as an implementation strategy. Definitions of privatization vary. In part the concept implies load shedding whereby government withdraws completely from a program. More to the point here, it denotes practices where government pays money or otherwise ensures that private parties provide certain goods and services. Such arrangements have, of course, long prevailed in the health care arena. Insurance companies and private medical providers have from the start played pivotal roles in the Medicare and Medicaid programs. Even efforts to regulate medical providers, such as the 1974 health planning law or the statute establishing Professional Review Organizations (to conduct utilization and quality review), have allowed private entities to act as implementing agents.

The privatization models in the health arena have tended to come in two major flavors: direct and consumer-driven. Direct arrangements more explicitly and exclusively involve government officials in the role of purchaser. In the purest case, government contracts with a provider (e.g., a Health Systems Agency) to perform a particular service (e.g., conduct planning and certain regulatory activities in a given geographical area). Consumer-driven models rely more on the presumed beneficiaries of government programs to pick the provider. For instance, older citizens eligible for Medicare have substantial latitude to choose their physicians and hospitals. The federal government then pays the provider or reimburses the Medicare recipient for the service rendered. To be sure, the federal government may attempt to exert quality and cost control by certifying only some providers for reimbursement (e.g., hospitals X and Y but not Z). But program beneficiaries continue to have considerable freedom to select among various providers.

Proponents of privatization believe that it facilitates efficiency and effectiveness. A market model lies at the heart of this justification. The idealized scenario runs as follows. Private agents compete vigorously with one another to become the supplier of some governmental good or service. This competition stimulates a drive for efficiency. Providers seek to impress purchasers with the amount and quality of the output they deliver relative to its cost. Government officials or clients (in the consumer-driven model) have access to this information and readily understand it. They choose the most efficient alternative. If providers fail to deliver the promised service or product at a reasonable cost, purchasers move on to another provider. Hence, government programs presumably come to enjoy the efficiency and effectiveness that competition can produce.

Attractive as this model appears, its dynamics repeatedly break down in operation. Nowhere has this been more common than in the health arena. Space does not permit a comprehensive discussion of the problems of privatized implementation in the health arena. Suffice it to note that competition among insurance companies and medical providers is often limited. Moreover, the competition that occurs does not necessarily lead to a quest for efficiency. Providers can often generate additional demand for their service by providing more intensive treatment. Troubled patients with few handy scorecards to judge quality and with costs substantially covered by Medi-

care or other third party payors often fail to search extensively for the most efficient and effective medical care. Aside from these general difficulties, government problems in calibrating inducements for private proxies deserve note.

Inducement schedules for medical providers have repeatedly posed problems. For instance, payment practices prevalent in Medicare's history gave physicians and hospitals minimal incentive to seek out the most efficient treatment for different kinds of clients. Hospitals tended to get paid more if they allowed their costs to rise. Under the customary, prevailing and reasonable charge formula used to pay physicians, doctors who wanted to receive higher payments in the future possessed ample incentives to boost their fees in a given year. In the case of hospitals, the shift in 1983 to a payment strategy based on Diagnosis Related Groups curtailed some of the tendency to provide excess service. But it also threatened efficiency by heightening the risk that patients would be discharged "quicker and sicker."

Dealings with insurance companies also illustrate some of the problems of private contracting. Are health insurance companies the masters or servants of government? Under Medicare, these companies have possessed vast discretion and have been far from easy for the federal bureaucracy to harness. Early claims by insurance companies that their close relationships with physicians would allow them to establish effective payment and utilization review practices tended to be long on promise and short on delivery. Federal frustration with the performance of these companies grew to a point that in 1973 DHEW established the Perkins committee to examine Medicare's contracts with the insurance industry. Among other things, the committee urged DHEW to develop a more systematic means for measuring carrier performance, spell out methods for rewarding good performance, define ways of terminating those carriers doing poorly, and improve cost reporting and accounting. Subsequently, DHEW inched toward implementing these recommendations (U.S. House committee on Appropriations 1977).

But problems persisted. Consider, for example, the insurance companies that pay hospitals for serving Medicare patients. Despite soaring program costs, these intermediaries often revealed little commitment to evaluating hospital cost claims critically. This stemmed, first, from an inability of the federal bureaucracy to write specific instructions governing reimbursement under the complicated cost-based payment system required by law. Second, it arose from the performance standards applied to these companies. Federal Medicare officials put pressure on the intermediaries to process claims quickly and to hold down administrative costs per claim processed. To spend time examining claims for excess charges could lead to delays in processing and a reputation for being a "bad intermediary." Third, the statutory provision giving hospitals the right to nominate the intermediaries that reimburse them impeded careful evaluation of hospitals' claims. An intermediary who tried to get tough with a hospital faced the prospect of being "fired" and seeing the hospital shift to an intermediary with a reputation for being a softer touch. Finally, the private business interests of the intermediaries militated against an aggressive posture toward hospitals. As one DHEW official noted, these companies were "in business outside of Medicare. . . . They have their private business to pursue and one does not gain in business by making enemies. One does make enemies when he begins to tighten the purse strings of the person who he's trying to work with" (U.S. House Committee on Ways and Means 1979).

The private concerns of companies also militated against efficient administration of the program in another respect. Insurance companies have often attempted to make the government pay a disproportionate share of their overhead costs. By so doing, they have enhanced their competitive position in private markets. Problems such as these have led Feder and Holahan (1980) to conclude that "as long as administrative agents are active in a private market, conflicts of interest remain likely."

Keeping the contractors accountable may be a particular problem in the United States. Sharkansky (1979) suggests that the United States proves less successful in controlling the margins of the state than either Israel or Australia. He points to the entrepreneurial culture of the United States as one source of the problem (as opposed, for instance, to the culture of compliance that is more manifest in Australia). But he also ascribes the accountability problem to the antigovern-

ment sentiments that permeate U.S. political culture. This hostility makes it difficult for government ever to seem "right" in dealing with private sector institutions. Leaders of insurance companies sense this weakness and are not above exploiting it.

Antigovernment sentiments also serve as cultural blinders with respect to more direct efforts by public agencies to deliver care. Some evidence (Thompson and Campbell 1981) suggests that Washington's prime long-term venture into "socialized medicine," the VA medical network, yields results at least as good as, if not better than, programs that rely on private sector providers. Another study argues that the ability to respond rapidly to epidemics like AIDS requires a large cadre of civil-servant scientists rather than massive reliance on extramural grants to scientists in universities (Panem 1988). Hence, analysts need to keep an open mind about the possible advantages of more direct governmental administration of various health programs. The use of private contractors and grantees at times makes considerable sense from an implementation perspective. But no automatic assumptions about the superiority of this strategy seem warranted.

State Implementing Agents: Boon or Barrier?

Fear of centralized political power has also spawned interest in using state and local governments as agents of implementation. Students of implementation have at times portrayed such involvement as problematic—as representing another veto point or decision site at which Washington's policies can flounder. Others, however, see this approach as fostering an innovative and responsive administration that can facilitate the achievement of desirable program ends. In considering these alternatives, issues of state commitment and capacity loom large.[4]

---

[4]Local governments are also important implementing agents in the health arena and deserve analysis in their own right. For present purposes, however, let it suffice to note that many of the observations about state capacity and commitment also apply to local jurisdictions.

State Commitment

Commitment refers to whether actors in the dominant coalition within states seek to implement federal programs efficiently and effectively. If state officials generally share federal objectives, they can often help the federal government achieve a level of effectiveness beyond that otherwise achievable. But where state officials lack sympathy for federal programs, they can easily impede the attainment of policy goals.

When state officials possess little interest in implementing a federal policy, Washington usually confronts major difficulties in forcing them to do so. A neat hierarchical model does not apply to federal-state relations in the health arena. Rather a kind of bargaining or negotiation at arms length often characterizes these relationships. The central government and the states make bids and counterbids with each trying to get something of what they want (Ingram 1977). This process as well as other modes of federal-state interaction may yield less than impressive outcomes. Even after federal administrators made concessions to the states with respect to the EPSDT program, for example, many state officials continued to view the program with little enthusiasm. Medicaid posed a number of problems for the states—soaring costs, lack of effective claims systems, abuse by medical providers, and more. In the face of these problems, EPSDT essentially asked the states to drum up additional business. Not surprisingly, many of the states failed to place a high priority on launching vigorous out-reach programs for poor children.

The example of EPSDT also points to the reluctance of the central government to penalize the states for noncompliance. The penalties available to federal officials are usually blunt; they often threaten to harm program clients more than the officials responsible for lethargic implementation. In the case of EPSDT, the federal government could withhold one percent of the federal share of payments to the Aid to Families with Dependent Children (AFDC) program. Imposition of this penalty would in essence victimize the poor for the failures of state officials. The limited prestige of the federal bureaucracy and the fear of conflict that this generates also reduces the appeal of penalties. The DHEW administrators knew that withholding money from states with poor EPSDT records would provoke opposition from state officials and certain members of Congress; HEW might well lack the resources to prevail in this conflict, and a defeat could further undermine its prestige.

The EPSDT episode should not be read as a sign that the states invariably lack commitment to federal policies that seek to meet the medical needs of the poor. When Congress approved the Medicaid program in 1965, the federal bureaucracy was almost overrun by states eager to obtain federal dollars. Even when the costs of Medicaid became more obvious to state officials, many of them moved to cover more services under the program and did not constrain eligibility for care (Thompson 1986).

As a general rule, however, the limits to state commitment more readily surface in the case of health policies that involve taxation of the more affluent to serve the poor (redistributive). Analysts note that advocates for the poor tend to be weaker in the states than in Washington (Brown 1984). In a related vein some have stressed the role of *migration theory* in sapping commitment to redistributive programs. This theory holds that competition among states for economic resources spawns a bid-down effect. Decisions by jurisdictions to provide the most generous benefits permitted under federal programs for the disadvantaged could drive up state taxes (since federal programs usually require some kind of matching allocation by the state). At some threshold higher taxes for redistributive ends tend to discourage firms and affluent individuals from remaining in or moving to the state thereby eroding its revenue capacity. Simultaneously, generous redistributive programs may entice needy people to move to the state thereby draining public resources still further. On a local level, victims of AIDS have flocked to San Francisco, a jurisdiction which has committed itself to more humane and generous treatment for those with the disease (Panem 1988). The exact empirical dynamics of the migration model and its explanatory power relative to other political and administrative models waits to be determined. However, migration theory has enough plausibility and empirical support to be taken very seriously at least as a partial explanation for the limits to state commitment (Peterson and Rom 1988).[5]

---

[5] The evidence suggests that certain political characteristics of states also affect commitment to redistributive programs (Peterson and Rom 1988).

It deserves note, however, that a common professionalism among state and local administrators may partially check the tendency for redistributive programs to encounter more resistance (Peterson et al. 1986). Health professionals at the federal and state levels often share a common commitment to ensuring greater access to medical care for the deprived. Where they can buffer themselves sufficiently from countervailing political forces in a state, the level of state commitment to redistributive health programs may well be higher. Still, the weight of migration theory seems likely to impose severe limits on generosity.

State Capacity

In the past, skepticism dominated assessments of state capacity to implement federal programs. Their legislatures lacked professional staffs; their top elected officials (especially governors) lacked authority over many line agencies; relatively low pay and patronage characterized personnel administration; their election processes inhibited minority voting.

According to recent analysis, these days are gone. One extensive survey of state capacity points to a "profound restructuring of the state governmental landscape" in the 1960s and 1970s. The report finds state governments to be "more representative, more responsive, more activist, and more professional in their operations than they ever have been" (U.S. Advisory Commission on Intergovernmental Relations 1985, 365). Others express less sanguine views about the implications of state government reform (Murphy 1981). On balance, however, it appears highly probable that most states have bolstered their administrative capacity. Agencies responsible for implementing health policy have benefited from this trend. Moreover, any gap between the administrative capacity of the states and that of the federal government has probably diminished since the mid-1970s. As noted earlier, the 1980s ushered in forces that eroded the capacity of Washington's bureaucracies.

To the extent that states have suffered blows to their capacity in the last decade, the tendency of electorates to restrict state discretion to tax and spend stands out. In the period from 1976 through 1981, 19 states, including larger ones

such as California and Michigan, enacted such restrictions. As with commitment, states vary greatly in capacity. Nor can one safely assume that states are converging along this dimension. For instance, some evidence suggests a growing disparity among the states in their revenue capacity (Thompson 1986, 664–665).

As the 1990s commenced, however, the chief concern about the states as implementing agents of federal policy centered less on capacity than commitment, especially in the case of redistributive health programs. However, worries about commitment diminish to the degree that professionals with common backgrounds hold positions in state and federal agencies, and Washington absorbs a greater percentage of the costs of redistributive programs. In particular, Washington's willingness to pay more of the price tag reduces the bite of migration theory. The theory becomes less applicable because state commitment to program generosity does not require it to raise taxes or siphon off funds from programs aimed at the middle class. Hence, a national health insurance plan which assigned an important implementing role to the states could achieve high levels of efficiency, effectiveness, and responsiveness if the federal government would foot all or a major share of the bill.

In Quest of the Fixer

Implementation problems generated by the statute (program design, the policy hypothesis), the limited status of federal agencies, other capacity problems,and the difficulties of administration by proxy hardly need be insurmountable if the task environment of the implementing agency contains forces conducive to program repair. In this regard, few concepts have a more revered place in discussions of implementation than that of the fixer. A fixer is some actor or coalition that carefully monitors a program, accurately diagnoses where it has gone astray, and intervenes to correct a problem (Bardach 1977, 274). A fixer can help compensate for errors that seem destined to afflict a founding statute. Wildavsky (1979) has even cautioned against the stultifying impact of trying too hard to avoid mistakes in the forging of original policies. Better to expect errors and pick up after oneself.[6]

But fixers are often in short supply, especially within the ranks of oversight institutions. Uncertainty and the more general problems of learning compose part of the problem. It is not always clear what ails a program or how to fix it. Moreover, learning from past experience is far from automatic. In reacting to the past, decision makers frequently "develop myths, fictions, legends, folklore and illusions" (March and Olsen 1976, 59).

One can, however, easily exaggerate uncertainty and learning disabilities as major factors crippling the efforts of fixers. Members of Congress probably never had so much access to analytically derived information as they did during the 1970s and 1980s. The General Accounting Office, the Congressional Budget Office, the Office of Technology Assessment and others turned out countless studies. The problem was not so much error detection as motivating elected officials to undertake error correction. In this regard, interest group activity and the media often inhibited efforts to deal with problems.

Interest Groups and the Media

The forces that appear to debilitate a program are almost always of direct benefit to some group. These groups frequently develop powerful incentives to perpetuate program "weakness." Hospitals and physicians, for example, hardly view Medicare's payment practices as flawed just because they fail to provide them with much incentive to control costs. Reforms aimed at making consumers and medical providers more aware of cost factors in the health arena (be they market reforms or those calling for more centralized control by the federal government) can expect to encounter considerable resistance. The barriers to repair may well become even larger. Relman (1980, 963–970) has warned of the rise of a "new medical industrial complex" consisting

of "a large and growing network of private corporations engaged in the business of supplying health care services to patients for a profit." In his view the rise of this complex will "probably hinder rather than facilitate rational debate on national health-care policy."

In addition to interest groups, the media compose another outside force that can inhibit error correction. As a rule, implementation problems do not make for interesting news stories. When the media do cover implementation, they tend to examine cases of egregious abuse rather than the more systemic problems that often possess far more relevance for program performance. Media people, for example frequently pay considerable attention to scandals such as outright fraud by medical providers or clients, while giving short shrift to the seemingly dry, technical, but more important issues concerning payment formulas and the day-to-day incentives they establish for medical providers. One cannot count on the media, then, to focus attention on the most critical problems calling for repair.

The AIDS epidemic illustrates how media coverage can fuel alarm and make implementation more difficult. By early 1983, the U.S. Public Health Service (PHS) faced mounting evidence that AIDS could be transmitted by heterosexual sex and by direct contact with blood or blood products containing the AIDS virus. In response, PHS scientists conducted several studies including epidemiologic research in Zaire, an African country where AIDS afflicted women about as frequently as men. In the spring, of 1985, a scientist from the Centers for Disease Control touched upon the preliminary results of the Zairian study in a lecture at the University of California, Berkeley. The study showed that African household members who lived with an AIDS victim were three times more likely to develop AIDS than those who did not live with the victim. The study posited that the Zairian finding could emanate from such factors as ritualistic blood letting or scarification, different sexual practices, and poor sanitation. Drawing on additional evidence from the United States, the study did *not* isolate casual contact with AIDS victims as a source of the epidemic. News reports of the lecture, however, conveyed the impression that casual contact spread AIDS (Panem 1988, 125–127). Public acceptance of this view has at times exacerbated problems

---

[6]As employed here, the concept of fixing focuses on all kinds of repair, from changes in the policy mandate to changes within the confines of existing law. Of course, "fixing" is ineluctably intertwined with normative judgments. One person's fix can be another person's breakdown.

of providing services for AIDS patients (e.g., community hostility which makes it impossible for children with the disease to attend school, and difficulties in recruiting employees to care for AIDS victims).

Oversight and Fixing

Interest group pressures, media propensities, and other forces frequently provide little incentive for members of Congress to become fixers. Members of Congress frequently sense that voters will judge them less in terms of how well the system works than in terms of how well they can explain individual acts. Rather than engage in fixing programs, legislators often divest their attention to casework or the blame-the-bureaucracy gambit. Members of Congress have grown increasingly interested in cultivating voters through a potpourri of constituent services and frequently intercede on behalf of citizens who must deal with the bureaucracy. Casework yields much political profit for a member of Congress. It creates far fewer enemies than does taking stands on issues that affect programs as a whole. It often does little, however, to strengthen their performance as program fixers (Fiorina 1977). Aside from this tendency, Congress often plays the blame-the-bureaucracy game. The low status of agencies tempts members of Congress to increase their political popularity by blaming or ridiculing the bureaucracy rather than by helping it diagnose and correct errors. They often prefer the accusatory finger to the helping hand. Members of Congress have, for example, berated federal Medicaid officials for lax administration while simultaneously refusing to provide the staff or funds that might help officials monitor and control developments.

The behavioral propensities of Congress illustrate the importance of drawing a firm distinction between greater oversight and fixing. Until now, the issue with respect to Congress has been framed too much in terms of control. When and how does Congress exert leverage over the bureaucracy? Can it hold federal agencies accountable? These and other questions are important since they go to the heart of critical issues of democratic theory. But a Congress that zealously

monitors a program can at times hurt more than it helps. Members of Congress may, for instance, lean on regulators to go easy on medical providers in their districts. Or they may seek information in ways potentially detrimental to the functioning of programs. In the early 1980s, for instance, Ted Weiss, a representative from New York, convened congressional hearings on the AIDS problem and focused in part on the performance of the Centers for Disease Control (CDC). In conducting this oversight, Weiss insisted that his committee should have the right of access to all personnel and files at the agency. Responding to professional ethics and realizing that cooperation from the gay community in researching AIDS would be greatly impaired if subjects perceived that oversight committees had access to their files, CDC resisted. Subsequently, the agency and the oversight committee compromised. Committee investigators would have access to the files but only with all subject or patient identifiers removed (Panem 1988, 31–35). In these and other ways, congressional intervention does not necessarily serve the interests of efficiency, effectiveness and accountability.

It would, of course, be a gross distortion to portray the media, interest groups such as medical providers, and Congress as inevitable obstacles to fixing. Elected officials often rise to the challenge as do top government executives and the courts. The media and interest groups at times generate the pressures needed for program repair.

Moreover, the mammoth federal budget deficit, the relentlessly rising demand for health care stemming in part from increases in those over 75, and health care price boosts that persistently outpace the general inflation rate may well galvanize efficiency-minded fixers. For instance, abandonment of Medicare's cost-based reimbursement system for hospitals in favor of more prospectively determined payment based on DRGs has, for all its limits, generated a better set of problems for health policymakers to tackle in the future.

While cost pressures heighten the quest for program repairs that emphasize more health bang for the buck, these pressures also bring risk. Attempts at repair could spawn cost savings but at disproportionately reduced benefits to program beneficiaries (thereby fostering neither efficiency nor effectiveness). Financial stringency also means that fixes costing appreciable amounts of money (e.g., certain proposals to expand government health insurance) face a very stiff head wind.

Conclusion

Numerous pitfalls can sidetrack implementation. A faulty statute, public agencies lacking in capacity or commitment, the convolutions of attempting to get private entities to do government's work, and the absence of fixers can all impede programs. In considering these possibilities, however, one should not cross the line into administrative hypochondria. By most reasonable standards, many health programs get implemented, and they work.

But what are the pertinent standards? How can success and failure be judged? Multiple evaluative criteria suggest themselves, including accountability, efficiency, and effectiveness. Do implementing agents operate within the bounds set by law when they administer a health program (compliance, accountability)? Given some level of program accomplishments, do implementing agents hold down waste and score well in getting substantial returns for each dollar spent (efficiency)? Does the program do well on pertinent measures of accomplishment such as increasing access to medical care, enhancing the quality of care, constraining medical costs and, ultimately, improving the health of the populace (effectiveness)? Beyond these specific questions does the program seem to engender benign political and economic consequences (eg., bolster the legitimacy of government by allowing it to appear as a competent and humane problem solver)? Does it reinforce efforts to build the long term capacity of implementing agents? Does it fundamentally affect the allocation of authority and power within a given health arena (Elmore 1987, 176–177)? These questions, among others, point to important evaluative dimensions.

It would require a Panglossian temperament to expect a health program to perform well on all major dimensions. Short of such a troublefree existence, however, a program can still score impressive achievements. In this regard, consider-

able evidence suggests that initiatives such as Medicare, Medicaid, the Veterans Administration medical program, and the National Health Service Corps have registered significant accomplishments (Thompson 1981). Hence, the tale of implementation in the health arena is not one of woe.

The study of health policy implementation needs to be kept on the analytic front burner. Although the Reagan Administration gutted several health programs (e.g., health planning), the major regulatory and allocative programs of the federal government persist. Medicare expenditures have risen apace and consumed an increasing share of domestic policy spending. The costs of Medicaid and the Veterans Administration programs have also shot upward. Despite the Reagan Administration's pronounced sympathy for deregulation, regulatory strategies continue to attract much attention as a vehicle for constraining medical costs (Brown 1988, 45) and fighting health hazards in the environment. New challenges such as AIDS and the thirty-seven million Americans who lack health insurance await. While budget deficits make major initiatives extremely difficult, policymakers at least do not have to buck public antipathy toward a greater investment in health. As the 1980s closed, a majority of the public expressed a preference for more government spending on health; most favored providing adequate medical care to all who could not afford it even if such a step meant new taxes (*Public Opinion* 1989).[7]

Hence, the need to generate more powerful implementation theory remains stronger than ever. The stakes are high. If policies bolster the efficiency of health programs and of the medical sector more generally, painful choices about the rationing of care become less necessary. In seeking to forge better understanding of implementation both in terms of basic theory (science) and advice to policymakers (engineering, craft) (Elmore 1987), the concepts, approaches and propositions native to more general discussions of policy implementation can cast light on the health policy sphere. Also, the experience with

---

[7]The question of how much more tax the majority would be willing to pay, however, remains open, as shown by the negative response of many of the nation's elderly to the surtax requirement that ultimately killed the Catastrophic Health Insurance Act.

government programs in the health arena can sharpen and refine broader discussions of implementation. Given the complexities of implementation, this exercise will not yield a rigorous theory analogous to those found in some of the natural sciences. But it can enhance the ability to describe, explain, and predict; it can bolster efforts to assist policymakers (e.g., Lester et al. 1987).

Whatever the specific initiative pursued in studying implementation in the health area, analysts must consider more than the internal dynamics of administrative agencies, per se. Obviously, these dynamics are important to study. They probably rank among the more malleable components of implementation. But astute analysis requires a broader perspective. Thus, implementation analysis needs to address the problems of Congress as a formulator of policies and of how these policies often rig the implementation game. It needs to assess how certain qualities of political institutions, such as the weakness of political parties, affect Congress. Nor can widespread beliefs about public agencies prevalent in the political culture be ignored, given the danger they will become self-fulfilling prophencies. The role of interest groups, the media, and oversight institutions in encouraging or undermining the fixing of programs also commands consideration. The implementation of health programs does not simply revolve around the "bureaucracy problem." Instead it remains deeply intertwined with the general "health" of the political order. In sum, potent explanations or accurate predictions will not spring from a context-free theory of implementation. Further specification of the external contingencies that shape implementation looms as critical.

REFERENCES

Bardach, Eugene. 1977. *The implementation game.* Cambridge: MIT Press

Brown, Lawrence. 1984. The politics of devolution in Nixon's new federalism. In *The changing politics of federal grants,* by Lawrence D. Brown, James W. Fossett, and Kenneth T. Palmer, 54–107. Washington: Brookings

Brown, Lawrence. 1988. *Health policy in the United States: Issues and options.* New York: Ford Foundation.

Cohen, Michael D., James G. March and Johan P. Olsen. 1972. A garbage can model of organizational choice. *Administrative Science Quarterly.* 17:1–25.

Crozier, Michel. 1964. *The bureaucratic phenomenon.* Chicago: University of Chicago Press, 1964.

Davidson, Roger H. 1981. Subcommittee government: New channels for policy making. In *The new Congress,* edited by Thomas E. Mann and Norman J. Ornstein, 99–133. Washington: American Enterprise Institute.

Elmore, Richard F. 1979–80. Backward mapping: Implementation research and policy decisions. *Political Science Quarterly.* 94:601–616.

Elmore, Richard F. 1987. Instruments and strategy in public policy. *Policy Studies Review.* 7:174–186.

Enthoven, Alain C. 1978. Shattuck lecture—Cutting cost without cutting the quality of care. *New England Journal of Medicine.* 29:1229–1238.

Falkson, Joseph L. 1980. *HMO's and the politics of health system reform.* Chicago: American Hospital Association.

Farrar, Eleanor, John E. DeSanctis and David K. Cohen. 1980. The lawn party: The evolution of federal programs in local settings. *Phi Delta Kappan.* November: 161–171.

Feder, Judith M. 1977. *Medicare: The politics of federal hospital insurance.* Lexington, Mass: D.C. Health.

Feder Judith and John Holahan. 1980. Administrative Choices. In *National health insurance: Conflicting goals and policy choices,* edited by Judith Feder. John Holahan, and Theodore Marmor, 21–71. Washington: Urban Institute.

Feder, Judith, John Holahan and Theodore Marmor, eds. 1980. *National health insurance: Conflicting goals and policy choices.* Washington, D.C.: Urban Institute.

Federal Register. 1978. 43:13010–13020.

Ferman, Barbara and Martin Levin. 1987. Dilemmas of innovation and accountability: Entrepreneurs and chief executives. *Policy Studies Review.* 7:187–199.

Fiorina, Morris P. 1977. *Congress—Keystone of the Washington establishment.* New Haven: Yale University Press.

Foltz, Anne-Marie. 1975. The development of ambiguous federal policy: Early and periodic screening, diagnosis and treatment (EPSDT). *Milbank Memorial Fund Quarterly Health and Society.* 53:35–64.

The Gallup Opinion Index 146. September 1977:20–24.

Glaser, William A. 1978. *Health insurance bargaining.* New York: Gardner Press.

Goggin, Malcolm L. 1987. *Policy design and the politics of implementation.* Knoxville: University of Tennessee Press.

Heclo, Hugh and Aaron Wildavsky. 1974. *The private*

government of public money. Berkeley: University of California Press.

Ingram, Helen. 1977. Policy implementation through bargaining: The case of federal grants-in-aid. *Public Policy.* 25:499–526.

Kelman, Steven. 1984. Using implementation research to solve implementation problems: The case of energy emergency assistance. *Journal of Policy Analysis and Management.* 4:75–91.

Kingdon, John W. 1984. *Agendas, alternative and public policies.* Boston: Little, Brown.

Lester, James P., Ann O'M. Bowman, Malcolm L. Goggin, Laurence J. O'Toole, Jr. 1987. Public policy implementation: Evolution of the field and agenda for future research. *Policy Studies Review.* 7:200–216.

Levine, Charles, B. Guy Peters, and Frank J. Thompson. In Press. *Public administration: Challenges, choices, consequences.* Glenview, Ill: Scott Foresman.

Lowi, Theodore. 1969. *The end of liberalism.* New York: W.W. Norton.

March, James G. 1978. Bounded rationality. Ambiguity and the engineering of choice. *The Bell Journal of Economics.* 9:587–608.

March, James G. and Johan P. Olsen. 1976. *Ambiguity and Choice in Organizations.* Bergen: Universitetsforlaget.

Marmor, Theodore R. 1980. *National health insurance: Implementation forecast and policy choice.* New Haven: Unpublished paper.

Montjoy, Robert S. and Laurence J. O'Toole, Jr. Toward a theory of policy implementation: An organizational perspective. *Public Administration Review.* 39:465–476.

Murphy, Jerome T. 1981. The paradox of state government reform. *The Public Interest.* 64:124–139.

National Commission on the Public Service. 1989. *Leadership for America: Rebuilding the public service. The Report.* Washington.

Ornstein, Norman J. 1981. The House and the senate in a new congress. In *The new Congress,* edited by Thomas E. Mann and Normal J. Ornstein, 363–383. Washington: American Enterprise Institute.

Palumbo, Dennis J. 1987. Introduction. *Policy Studies Review.* 7:91–102.

Panem, Sandra. 1988. *The AIDS bureaucracy.* Cambridge: Harvard University Press.

Peterson, Paul E., Barry G. Rabe, and Kenneth K. Wong. 1986. *When federalism works.* Washington: Brookings

Peterson, Paul E. and Mark Rom. 1988. Federalism, welfare policy, and residential choices. Washington: Unpublished Paper.

Pressman, Jeffrey and Aaron Wildavsky. 1979. *Im-*

plementation, Berkeley: University of California Press.

Price, Don K. 1978. Planning and administrative perspectives on adequate personal health. *Milbank Memorial Fund Quarterly, Health and Society.* 56:22–50.

Public Opinion. 1987. The role of government: An issue for 1988. 90 (March/April):21–33.

Public Opinion. 1989. What Americans are saying about taxes. 11 (March/April):21–26.

Relman, Arnold C. 1980. The new medical industrial complex. *New England Journal of Medicine.* 303:963–970.

Ripley, Randall B. and Grace A. Franklin. 1982. *Bureaucracy and policy implementation.* Homewood, Ill: Dorsey Press.

Rodgers, Jr., Harrell R. and Charles S. Bullock III. 1976. *Coercion to compliance.* Lexington Mass: D.C. Heath.

Sabatier, Paul and Daniel Mazmanian. 1979. The conditions of effective implementation: A guide to accomplishing policy objectives." *Policy Analysis.* 5:481–504.

Salamon, Lester M., Ed. 1989. *Beyond privatization: The tools of government action.* Washington: Urban Institute Press.

Sharkansky, Ira. 1979. *Wither the state?* Chatham, N.J.: Chatham Publishing.

Sinclair, Barbara. 1981. Coping with uncertainty: Building coalitions in the House and the Senate. In *The new Congress,* edited by Thomas E. Mann and Norman J. Ornstein 178–287. Washington: American Enterprise Institute.

Thompson, Frank J., Chapter V with Leonard Robins and Chapter VI with Richard Campbell. 1981. *Health policy and the bureaucracy: Politics and implementation.* Cambridge: MIT Press.

Thompson, Frank J. and Richard W. Campbell. 1981. Implementation and service error: VA health care and the commercial market option. *Journal of Health Politics, Policy and Law.* 6:419–443.

Thompson, Frank J. 1982. Deregulation by the bureaucracy: OSHA and the augean quest for error correction. *Public Administration Review.* 42:202–212.

Thompson, Frank J. 1984. Policy implementation and overhead control. In *Public policy implementation,* edited by George C. Edwards, III, 3–26. Greenwich, Conn.: JAI Press.

Thompson, Frank J. 1986. New Federalism and health care policy: States and the old questions. *Journal of Health Politics, Policy and Law.* 11:647–670.

Thompson, Frank J. and Michael Scicchitano. 1987. State implementation and federal enforcement priorities: Safety versus health in OSHA and the states. *Administration and Society* 19:95–124.

U.S. Advisory Commission on Intergovernmental Relations. 1985. *The question of state government capability* Washington: USGPO.

U.S. House Committee on Appropriations. 1977. *Department of Labor and Health, Education, and Welfare Appropriations for 1978: Part 6.* Washington D.C.: USGPO.

U.S. House Committee on Ways and Means. 1979. *Intermediary performance regarding fraud and abuse.* Washington, D.C.: USGPO.

U.S. President's Commission on compensation of Career Federal Executives. 1988. *The report of the President's Commission on Compensation of Career Federal Executives.* Washington.

Waldo Dwight. 1980. *The enterprise of public administration,* Novato, Calif. Chandler and Sharp.

Wildavsky, Aaron. 1979. *Speaking truth to power.* Boston: Little, Brown.

Zwick, Daniel I. 1978. Initial development of guidelines for health planning. *Public Health Reports.* 93:407–420.

Chapter 9

An Overview of State Roles in Health Care Policy

Debra J. Lipson

States have had primary responsibility for the development of health care policy and the administration of health care programs for most of this country's history. But the advent of Medicare and Medicaid as the major public financing mechanisms for health care, along with their power to mold and influence the health care industry, cast a huge shadow over the previous dominance of state governments in health care financing and delivery. For most of the 1960s and 1970s, state governments were often viewed with distrust by those concerned with health care policy at the federal level. Those who held this attitude did not regard states as having as much commitment to the provision of health and social services to the poor as the federal government (Thompson 1986).

When he took office in 1980, however, President Ronald Reagan ushered in a new era—one characterized by the return to states of greater control and discretion over the financing, delivery and regulation of health care. In his first State of the Union address in January, 1982, the President promised cuts in taxes, cuts in federal spending and a reduction in burdensome federal regulatory requirements by giving more decision-making authority to state and local governments (Congressional Quarterly 1982). He even went so far as to propose a trade: the federal government would take over all responsibility for the Medicaid program if the states would assume complete responsibility for the Aid to Families with Dependent Children (AFDC) cash welfare program and the food stamp program in addition to other programs whose administration and funding were formerly shared by both levels of government.

Representatives of state government viewed this swap with great suspicion, fearing it was merely a ploy to reduce federal support and dump the financing burden for welfare on state governments (Demkovich 1982). Their opposition led Congress to reject Reagan's grand scheme to reorganize federal and state responsibilities. Nonetheless, during the 1980s, state governments did accept the implied challenge and began to assume greater involvement in health and social welfare policymaking. This chapter reviews evidence on how states redefined their roles during the 1980s and created new models of government innovation in the financing, delivery, and regulation of health care. It discusses five primary roles or areas of responsibility that the states assume—as payers, direct providers of services, regulators of the health care industry, implementers of federal health programs and funding mechanisms, and as innovators.

For each of these roles, this chapter will (1) describe the major trends in state activities during the 1980s (2), provide examples of how state governments defined their role vis a vis federal and local governments or in relation to the private sector, and (3) explain the variation among states in the way they carry out these various roles.

Political Context for State Involvement in Health Policymaking in the 80s

What was Reagan's motivation for returning more power to state governments? Did he truly believe that state governments were more appropriate agents for making domestic—particularly health and welfare—policy? Democrats suspected that this rhetoric was just a cover for his desire to substantially reduce government involvement in health and welfare issues. They, like many policymakers at the federal level, mistrusted state and local governments in social welfare policy. For example, participants in a January, 1980, conference on state and local government involvement in health care agreed that despite some instances where states had become more generous, such developments could quickly erode and were not uniform across the states. Participants also expressed the commonly held view that state governments were subject to more political patronage and inefficient government than the federal government (Jain 1981).

Such thinking had contributed to a host of social and health programs created at the national level during the 1960s and 1970s. In 1965, state

and local governments spent about the same amount as the federal government ($5.2 billion) on health and medical care, but by 1980, the federal government was spending twice as much as state and local governments and two and a half times more in 1985 (U.S. Department of Health and Human Services 1987).

Republican supporters of the President, on the other hand, believed that state governments were more appropriate decision-makers, closer as they are to the people affected by laws and regulations. However, they would not be as sorry as the Democrats if the result of handing over more discretion to the states was less governmental action and intervention in the health and social arena.

In the end, Congress agreed to let Reagan experiment with some transfer of control to the states. The compromise also involved Congress cutting some of the funds for the programs that Reagan proposed, though overall they appropriated more money than the Administration had requested. It fell to the largely Democratic dominated state legislatures and Democratic Governors in nearly two thirds of the states to figure out how best to respond. Their options were further constrained by reductions in state budgets that accompanied the economic recession of the early 1980s. In order to raise money to support programs previously funded with federal dollars, personal income taxes or sales taxes were raised in more than half the states between 1983 and 1986 and state tax collections rose by 33 percent (Rapoport 1982).

In the process of raising taxes and cutting back budgets there was far less divisiveness along ideological or party lines among state and local public officials than might be expected. This was especially true for social and economic programs that would likely save money in the long run. For example, Democrats and Republicans, liberals and conservatives, agreed in the majority of states to allocate increased funds for expanded prenatal care programs based on data showing that costs associated with low birthweight babies could be reduced (Herbers 1987).

David Osborne, a political and economics writer, also contends that Republican and Democratic Governors moved closer in their thinking over the past ten years, transcending the traditional patterns that separated Republicans into tax cutters and Democrats into tax raisers. In his book, *Laboratories of Democracy,* in which he reviewed the efforts of six governors to reform their states' economies while raising the level of education and welfare, he concluded that ". . . the developments in America's state capitols offer the glimmering of a new synthesis . . . [one which] defines the solution as new roles for and new relationships between our national institutions—public sector and private, labor and management, education and business. The fundamental goal is no longer to create—or to eliminate—government programs; it is to use government to change the nature of the marketplace. To boil it down to a slogan . . . the synthesis is government as partner." (Osborne 1988, 326–327)

State policymakers in today's environment prefer non-bureaucratic solutions. "Health care provides a good example: many traditional liberals have favored some kind of national health care system. When new paradigm governors look to expand health coverage, however, they are more inclined to turn to health maintenance organizations, so as to inject decentralization and competition, rather than new government bureaucracies into the system." (Osborne 1988, pp 327–28)

The rest of this chapter provides examples of the experimentation, progress and change in health care policy initiated by state governments during the 1980s as they strove to find a balance between public and private responsibilities for the public's health. It shows how state governments were able to lower the rate of growth in health care expenditures in Medicaid programs and, as a result, were able to extend its reach to cover new groups of uninsured women and children. It demonstrates how different states decided on the proper mix between regulation and competition in the health care marketplace. It presents examples of states acting to bring together all the pieces—financing, delivery, regulation and implementation—to create health care models that preceded (or may inaugurate) national programs. Finally, it provides important caveats about the limits of state governments in achieving major health policy reforms and the ongoing need for partnerships between states, the federal government, and the private sector to meet the formidable challenges of the next decade.

States as Payers of Health Care Services

States bear a large responsibility for financing health services for the poor. They fulfill this responsibility primarily through the Medicaid program, which is jointly financed by the federal and state governments. In most states, the Medicaid program accounts for more than 60 percent of all state health expenditures. Nationwide, approximately 23.2 million individuals were eligible for Medicaid in 1987. Other state-related health expenditures support general acute and mental hospitals, medical education, maternal and child health initiatives and a host of other public health programs. States also have an important role, along with city and county governments, in financing health care for the medically indigent and uninsured not covered by Medicaid.

Trends in Medicaid Spending and Eligibility

A total of $45.2 billion was spent under Medicaid by both the federal and state governments during federal fiscal year 1986, nearly double that in 1980 (Sawyer 1983; Lipson 1988a). Each state's "matching rate" or the percentage of the program's costs reimbursed by the federal government depends on a state's per capita income. The federal matching rate varies from 80 percent in a state with the lowest per capita income (Mississippi), to 50 percent which is the minimum, and most common, matching rate. This results in about 45 percent of the Medicaid program's costs paid for by the states and 55 percent by the federal government.

In return for federal support, each state is required to operate its own Medicaid program within relatively broad federal guidelines. These guidelines specify the required or allowed coverage groups and health care benefits. Within these federal parameters, states can choose to adopt a generous or restrictive program, depending on such factors as the state's economic capacity to finance Medicaid services, the influence of consumer and provider groups on state policymakers, competing priorities with other state programs, and federal financial incentives or sanctions.

This flexibility results in great variation in the Medicaid program from state to state. For example, in 1984 per recipient expenditures ranged from $737 in West Virginia to $3,069 in New York. Though the variable federal matching rate was intended to reallocate resources from the wealthier to the poorer states, this does not appear to have occurred. States with greater proportions of poor citizens actually spent less on Medicaid per person in poverty than states with lower percentages of poor people (Holahan and Cohen 1986).

Some attribute these differences to the tendency by some states, particularly in the South, to spend very little on the poor, regardless of how much money the federal government offers to help them serve this group (Sundquist 1969). But in fact federal matching rates have been found to be less important in determining state spending than their *ability* to pay. Thus, federal subsidies to poorer states appear to be insufficient as an inducement to allocate state funds on Medicaid at the same level as wealthier states (Holahan and Cohen 1986).

The problem for the poorer states—and even in some wealthier ones—is that the Medicaid program has eaten into state budgets more and more. Medicaid spending has comprised an increasing percentage of state expenditures, rising from 4 percent in 1971 to 7.7 percent in 1981 and 11.5 percent in 1988 (Farrell 1988). Throughout the 1970s, states experienced a three-fold increase in Medicaid budgets, and the rise in state Medicaid spending was more than twice the increase in state budgets overall (Clarke 1981).

One might expect that Medicaid expenditures in each state would be related to the relative size of the population in need in each state. But studies have not found a clear relationship between the proportion of poor people in a state and the percentage of the poor covered by the state's Medicaid program. Instead, differences in Medicaid coverage of the poor appear to reflect the variations among states in the income standards used to determine Medicaid eligibility (which are subject to state control) and the state's coverage of certain optional eligibility groups under the program (Holahan and Cohen 1986).

Eligibility for Medicaid varies widely among the states. When Medicaid was established by

Congress in 1965, it was intended to provide health coverage for those who qualified for public assistance as well as others who might become poor as a result of high medical expenses. According to federal law, the categories of people that *must* be covered by each state's Medicaid program include low-income women and children who are eligible for welfare (the federal-state Aid to Families with Dependent Children or AFDC program), and low-income aged, blind or disabled persons eligible for welfare in the form of cash payments by the federal Supplemental Security Income program (SSI). Thus, for the most part, Medicaid eligibility is linked to eligibility for welfare.

However, states differ greatly in setting the maximum income level required to qualify for the AFDC program, which affects the percentage of the poor population eligible for Medicaid. State Medicaid eligibility thresholds as of January, 1989 for the AFDC program ranged from $1,416 in annual income for a family of three in Alabama to $8,316 in Utah. In addition, because federal guidelines permit coverage of numerous other population groups at a state's option, certain categories of the poor, for example, families in which both parents are unemployed, are covered in some states but not others.

Less variation between state eligibility standards occurs in coverage of the aged and disabled, including those who are developmentally disabled or mentally retarded. States are required to cover aged and disabled persons whose income exceeds the SSI income requirements but who can "spend-down" to the state's medically needy standard.

Over time, the spend-down process and the high costs of caring for the aged and disabled has resulted in an increasing proportion of state Medicaid budgets being spent on this group. The latter grew from 62 percent of the total in 1975 to 74 percent of the total by 1985. and occurred at the same time that the overall percentage of elderly and disabled individuals in the program remained the same, or about 30 percent. Poor children and families continue to comprise the remaining 70 percent of Medicaid recipients (Burwell and Rymer 1987).

Medicaid Coverage of the Poor Population

Although it is generally assumed that the Medicaid program provides health insurance protection for the nation's poor, in recent years Medicaid has actually covered fewer and fewer of those individuals and families with incomes below the federal poverty level. The percentage of all poor people covered under Medicaid dropped from a high of 65 percent in 1976 to approximately 40 percent in the mid 1980s.

There are two major reasons for this trend—one related to states' inaction and the other to Federal action—both resulting in lower health care coverage for poor families. First, during the 1970s and the early 1980s, state AFDC standard of need levels (income and resources)—to which Medicaid eligibility is largely tied—remained largely unchanged in most states. Only a few states increased AFDC standard of need levels to keep pace with increases in the cost of living. Thus, as the federal poverty level increased over time, more people with incomes below the poverty level found themselves making too much money to qualify for Medicaid, but unable to afford health insurance. In addition, states themselves reduced eligibility for the Medicaid program during the early 1980s in response to state budgets strained by unemployment and the economic recession.

The federal government also exacerbated the growing rate of uninsured families. Changes in federal welfare law enacted in the Omnibus Budget Reconciliation Act (OBRA) of 1981 placed a limit on gross income (before deductions for child care and other expenses) that a family could have and still be eligible for AFDC. It also limited the amount of income which could be disregarded by states. These changes led to a decrease of almost two million people from the AFDC program (and therefore from the Medicaid program as well), or about 8.5 percent of the total caseload, mostly from the ranks of poor working people (Cromwell et al. 1984).

These gaps in Medicaid coverage have worsened the problem of medical indigence. From 1980 to 1987, the number of people without any health insurance increased by 25 percent with an estimated 37 million Americans lacking any health insurance. Most of these individuals are members of working families and between one-fourth and one-third are estimated to live in households with incomes below the poverty level. Clearly, the Medicaid program no longer fulfills the promise of providing health care protection to the neediest of citizens.

Around 1984, this situation gained greater recognition at the federal level. To a large extent, the resolution of the problem was framed and advocated by those states who were least able to finance Medicaid coverage expansions. Richard W. Riley, former Governor of South Carolina was successful in convincing his colleagues in both the Southern Governors' and the National Governors' Associations that the federal government should allow states to provide Medicaid coverage to a particularly vulnerable group of the poor—pregnant women and children—without having to make them eligible for welfare. Provision of prenatal care was critical, he said, in order to reduce terrible infant mortality rates and avoid the costs associated with hospitalization of prematurely born infants (Southern Regional Task Force on Infant Mortality 1985, pp 24–25).

One of the reasons Riley was successful in obtaining the support of the other governors was that states were beginning to implement a variety of cost containment measures, including prospective hospital reimbursement methods and experiments with the enrollment of Medicaid recipients into HMOs and other types of managed care arrangements. These strategies helped to reduce the double-digit increases in Medicaid spending that characterized the late 1970s and permitted some degree of freedom to expand eligibility.

The efforts of the governors' associations, in conjunction with other key groups, especially the Children's Defense Fund, were successful in gaining passage of a steady stream of federal legislation that incrementally expanded Medicaid coverage for *targeted* groups of people—first pregnant women and young children, and later elderly and disabled individuals, living below the poverty level. In the Deficit Reduction Act (DEFRA) of 1984 and the Consolidated Omnibus Budget Reconciliation Act of 1985 (COBRA), Congress mandated state Medicaid coverage of two previously optional eligibility groups: all pregnant women meeting the state's AFDC income and resource requirements, regardless of marital status, including married women in families with an unemployed head of household, and all financially eligible children up to age five.

An even more significant action was taken in 1986. In that year, Congress enacted the Sixth Omnibus Budget Reconciliation Act of 1986—

known as SOBRA or OBRA-86—which permitted states to provide Medicaid coverage to all pregnant women and children up to age five in households with incomes *above* the state's AFDC standard of need but below the federal poverty level. This development was significant because it broke the long-standing connection between eligibility for cash assistance (AFDC or SSI) and Medicaid. It also removed the requirement that pregnant women with incomes greater than the state AFDC level incur medical expenses above a certain percentage of their income to qualify. It simply required that total family income be under the federal poverty level.

Another important expansion of the Medicaid program was allowed by the 1986 budget reconciliation legislation. States were permitted to cover the aged and disabled who make less than the federal poverty level but still have incomes above the SSI eligibility threshold. To take advantage of this option, the state first had to extend coverage to an additional group of pregnant women and children.

Over the next two years, forty-two states and the District of Columbia picked up the option to expand eligibility to poor pregnant women and infants up to a year old—demonstrating the popularity of an approach that improved health coverage without adding people to the welfare rolls (Lipson 1988a). Even as the few remaining states were trying to figure out how to finance such an expansion, Congress struck again. Provisions contained in the Medicare Catastrophic Coverage Act of 1988, signed into law in July, 1988, mandated that state Medicaid programs cover all pregnant women and infants, up to age 1, living below the poverty level, regardless of their categorical eligibility, by July, 1990. Even more significant, the act required all state Medicaid programs to pay for the Medicare premiums, deductibles and copayments for elderly and disabled Medicare beneficiaries who make less than 100 percent of the federal poverty level.

While it is still too early to judge the effectiveness of reforms that remove financial barriers to care on improvements in infant mortality rates or other measures of health status, there is little doubt that this incremental expansion strategy— actively promoted and eagerly implemented by most state officials—will result in coverage of more of the poverty population under the Medicaid program.

Trends in Public Health Spending

As mentioned earlier, Medicaid is not the only program through which states pay for health care. The Public Health Foundation, which tracks spending by state health departments, found that total state health agency expenditures (excluding Medicaid) rose from $2.5 billion in 1976 to $6.8 billion in 1985. Personal health program expenditures on services provided outside of institutional settings showed the largest increase over this period. Federal grant and contract funds contributed 56 percent of total spending while state funds contributed 38 percent and fees and other sources made up the remaining six percent. Local health departments spent another $1.6 billion in 1985 (Public Health Foundation 1987).

State health agencies spend these dollars on a variety of public health programs, including services related to maternal and child health, communicable disease control, public health nursing, mental health, alcohol and drug abuse treatment and prevention, environmental health, health personnel and facilities, and state-operated institutions. Interestingly, most of the federal funds (64 percent) given to states for health programs come from the U.S. Department of Agriculture's Special Supplemental Food Program for Women, Infants and Children (WIC). If funding for the WIC program were excluded, state health expenditures from federal funds decreased by 9 percent from 1976 to 1985. For personal health programs, other than maternal and child health, federal funding represents less than 30 percent of total state health agency expenditures.

Since maternal and child health programs constitute about 46 percent of state health budgets, it is important to examine what types of services are delivered to mothers and children. Over half ($1.5 billion) is spent for the WIC Supplemental Food program. General maternal and child health services and family planning services comprise most of the rest. According to a 1986 survey by the Children's Defense Fund, nearly every state offered prenatal care programs for poor women ineligible for public or private maternity coverage. However due to insufficient funding, only a small proportion of low-income pregnant women who did not qualify for Medicaid were served by these programs. Less than half the states provided funding for maternity inpatient services and only two states reported the availability of any pediatric inpatient programs (Rosenbaum et al. 1988).

Since that survey was conducted, it is likely that even fewer states pay for prenatal and pediatric services to non-Medicaid eligible poor women out of state maternal and child health funds. This is because, in many states, those dollars have been reallocated to help finance the new Medicaid eligibility expansions for pregnant women and children under age five.

State Responsibility for the Medically Indigent and Uninsured

One of the more critical gap-filling functions performed by state and local health departments is financial support for general medical care provided to people who are medically indigent and do not have any health insurance. While many of these individuals are served by the public health programs just described, there are other so-called state indigent care programs—also funded and administered jointly by the state and local government. In 1985, all but ten of the fifty states had medically indigent care programs in operation on a statewide basis.[1] (Desonia and King 1985)

Estimates vary widely regarding the total state and county expenditures for health care services provided under all state indigent care programs ranging, from $2.5 billion (Desonia and King 1985, xii) to over $15 billion dollars annually (Butler, 1988 39). The numbers of individuals served by these programs is almost impossible to ascertain, given the lack of reporting systems in some states or the poor quality of the data in others. There is little doubt, however, that these state and county expenditures help to keep open the doors of some public and private health care institutions to serve the poor.

State indigent care programs can be divided into two categories: (1) general assistance-medical programs and other statewide general indigent care programs; (2) other programs that target specific services or specific population groups.

General assistance-medical programs are in place in twenty-two states, where the indigent care program is associated with a state or county general assistance program. General assistance programs (also called general relief, home relief and poor relief in some states) are state or local programs of continuing or emergency income assistance. These programs serve as the ultimate safety net for people such as single males or intact families who have little or no income and are ineligible for federally supported welfare programs such as AFDC or SSI. In nineteen of the twenty-two states, a recipient of cash payments from the general assistance program is automatically eligible for services under the medical component. Eighteen of the states with general assistance-medical programs cover essentially the same health care services as those provided under the Medicaid program. (The remaining four states—Massachusetts Michigan, Vermont, and Virginia—cover only non-hospital services.) However, states sometimes place greater restrictions on health services under their general assistance-medical programs than they do under Medicaid.

Another 25 states have indigent care programs in addition to or instead of general assistance-medical programs. These programs are characterized chiefly by their diversity. In this category are programs that provide medical services to the indigent statewide, for example, California's Medically Indigent Adult Program, as well as programs such as one in Texas that requires county governments to spend a certain amount of their locally raised taxes on health care expenses for indigent residents. It also includes state programs that channel appropriations to a state university hospital to provide care to the indigent (e.g., Iowa and Colorado). Nine states provide pharmaceutical assistance programs for their residents, which are paid for largely out of state revenues. Six of the nine restrict participation to those aged sixty-five and over whose income is below a certain level. Two other states, Illinois and New Jersey, allow both the elderly and the physically disabled to participate.

[1]These ten included: Delaware, Georgia, Idaho, Kentucky, Nebraska, New Hampshire, North Carolina, North Dakota, Tennessee, and West Virginia. Note, however, that in most of these states there were non-uniform county-based programs in operation that may have covered some or all of the state's population.

Some states operate other small programs which reach very limited target populations. These include state operated, disease-specific programs such as those targeting sickle cell anemia, cancer, and blindness. For example, Tennessee has a state-administered program that provides blood supplies and treatment to hemophiliacs unable to afford necessary care; it also operates a program to assist persons suffering from chronic renal diseases.

For many years, states have also dealt with the problem of the medically indigent by paying providers—primarily hospitals—for the cost of delivering care to the uninsured. However, throughout the 1980s, it became increasingly apparent to policymakers that reimbursing hospitals for uncompensated care costs would not address access to primary care or other outpatient care that might prevent inappropriate use of hospitals by the uninsured. And no matter how much states gave to hospitals, the growing numbers of uninsured people continued to overwhelm the budgets of many small or public hospitals.

State policymakers, tired of trying to fill a seemingly unending well of uncompensated care costs out of state general revenue funds, started to search for a more broad-based financing strategy in order to pay for care of the uninsured. Between 1982 and 1986, in over forty states, task forces and legislative study commissions were set up to gather data on the make-up of the uninsured population in their own state, analyze various options and recommend legislation or new program initiatives. Over and over, they found that approximately three of every four persons without health insurance are in poor and near-poor families in which one or both parents are working, but are not offered or cannot afford health insurance through their workplace. This led state legislators to develop strategies that target these individuals for expanded insurance options.

In their search for financing options that would not stretch state budgets more than necessary, they turned to strategies that would increase the role of the private sector.[2] However, when the proposal was debated in states such as Wiscon-

sin, Minnesota and Washington, it was strongly resisted by the business community. Instead, these states and a few others embarked on approaches that involve state subsidies to low and moderate-income families so that they can afford to purchase health insurance coverage. These programs typically contained the following features:

participation restricted to individuals whose incomes do not exceed some threshold of poverty—usually between 150 percent to 200 percent of the federal poverty guidelines—and who do not have access to an employer-sponsored group insurance plan

premiums and copayments structured according to a sliding fee scale that takes into account family income

coverage arranged through managed care systems, such as HMOs, physician case management organizations, or other entities that have built-in cost containment incentives

The Massachusetts Experiment

One state that initially was able to overcome objections by the business community to taxes or other incentives for employers to cover health insurance premiums for their full-time employees was Massachusetts. The decision to impose a tax at all was a marked departure from other states' attempts to mandate employer-based health insurance. For many years, state officials wanted to require businesses to provide insurance to their employees. However, federal law (the Employee Retirement Income Security Act or ERISA) prohibits states from doing this. Only Hawaii was able to mandate that employers cover certain workers' health insurance premiums because Congress granted the state a special exemption from the federal ERISA law. But Congress has not shown much inclination to provide any other states with this authority.

To avoid the "ERISA problem," states examined a variety of voluntary options to induce businesses to provide coverage for their employees. Various strategies were proposed for different groups of employed uninsured. One approach involved taxing employers that did not provide

[2]This same thinking gave rise to proposals like that offered at the federal level by Senator Edward Kennedy (Dem., Massachusetts)—designed to mandate or encourage who did not provide coverage to their workers to start offering that coverage.

health insurance coverage; however, raising the cost of doing business is politically difficult for states when they are concerned about losing employers to lower-cost states.

The circumstances that led to passage of an employer-based health insurance expansion for the uninsured were somewhat unique to Massachusetts. One factor was the state's existing method of paying for hospital bad debt and charity care, which was done by adding surcharges to hospital bills paid by insuring businesses. This system made explicit the subsidy that large businesses provided to firms that did not cover health insurance costs for their workers. In such a situation, the absence of some firms from the health care financing scheme becomes more noticeable. The magnitude of that subsidy became even larger when the federal government withdrew Medicare participation in the state's financing of hospital bad debt and charity care. This action prompted an increase of 4 percent in hospital surcharges. The business community realized that its financial obligation was not going to diminish, much less be phased out, unless another source of financing could be found.

Other factors that facilitated passage of the Massachusetts plan were the state's budget surplus at the time the proposal was introduced and its low unemployment rate—one of the lowest among the states, and about half the national average. This healthy economic climate made possible the financial commitment to cover those left out of employer-based plans, such as unemployed people and part-time workers making too much to qualify for Medicaid. In addition, the state's relatively generous Medicaid program left a manageable group of poor people to add to the state's financial responsibility. Other states with larger proportions of poor uninsured would have to pay much more.

Most important, the political timing was right. Massachusetts voters had already stated their preferences in a November, 1986, referendum on the question of health care, favoring by a two to one margin a comprehensive, national health program for all citizens. The support of Democratic Governor Michael Dukakis, who plunged into the issue to demonstrate his leadership and initiative as a presidential candidate, was also a key factor.

Under such auspicious circumstances, the Massachusetts Health Security Act was enacted in April, 1988. The law as enacted required that by 1992, all employers with six or more employees were to pay a tax of 12 percent on the first $14,000 of wages paid to all eligible employees (or $1,680 per year). To qualify, workers had to be employed at least thirty hours a week for more than ninety days (or twenty hours a week if a head of household or an employee of six months of more). New businesses and firms with under six employees were exempt. Employers would be able to deduct from the 12 percent tax only those amounts that represent their average expenses per employee for providing health coverage for their workers. Thus, only those firms that chose not to provide insurance at all, or provide health coverage at a cost of less than $1,680 per employee, would pay the tax.

Small employers (with five or fewer workers) were to be offered special assistance to encourage them to provide health insurance. This help would include initiatives to broker health insurance for small businesses. In 1989, the state would set up a small business health insurance pool for businesses with six or fewer full-time employees. In 1990, it would offer tax incentives to firms of fifty or fewer workers to get them to offer coverage. The state would also establish a hardship trust fund to assist firms whose liability for the medical security contribution exceeds 5 percent of gross revenue. New employers, regardless of size, were to be eligible for tax rates that were less than the 12 percent tax rate during the first two years they were in business.

Thus, Massachusetts became the first state to enact a law guaranteeing all residents health insurance coverage by either an employer or state plan. Since then, however, several bills have been introduced to repeal or drastically change the law in light of a serious downturn in the state's economy and dire budget problems. It may be that states cannot support such a lofty plan without the help of the federal government to protect them from the ups and downs of economic cycles.

Nonetheless, the "Massachusetts Miracle" inspired more than a dozen states the following year to propose payroll tax penalties of varying proportions on employers that do not provide basic health care coverage to full-time workers. It remains to be seen whether any of these states will ultimately enact legislation that involves such a strong "incentive" as tax penalties. For the most part, states remain doubtful of their financial ability to emulate the Massachusetts model. They also wonder if the federal government will step in soon with a national health program that requires employers in all states to offer health benefits to full-time workers (Lipson 1988b).

But as they wait and wonder, they are supporting other voluntary approaches to help make health insurance more affordable to employers, particularly small firms that have had trouble gaining access to the private health insurance market. For example, Oregon authorized tax credits for small businesses providing health care benefits for the first time. Many states enabled the formation of multiple employer trusts (METs) which allow small businesses to form new large groups to reduce the cost of health insurance. State governments, such as West Virginia, also explored the possibility of bringing the uninsured into existing groups by allowing small businesses to join a public employees health insurance group. Finally, states such as Michigan, Massachusetts, New Jersey, Wisconsin and Pennsylvania began to develop programs that subsidized health insurance premiums for former welfare recipients who found work in firms that did not offer health insurance.[3]

In summary, the states' role as major payers of health care services is characterized by significant variations (and limitations) in state capabilities to subsidize health care for their citizens. Such variation leads to glaring inequities in the availability of services for people in the same economic circumstances or with the same disease or health condition, but who live in different states. While almost every state tries to assure access to emergency care, only those states with better economies and tax bases are generally willing and able to provide access to basic health care for most or all of their poor citizens. And virtually every state perceives limits on its ability to provide complete medical benefits to every resident because of political and economic realities that restrict their willingness to impose taxes to support such services.

States as Direct Providers of Health Care

States have long been involved in the direct provision of health care, though their role has been much overshadowed by local governments, which have been more likely to own and operate general public hospitals. Earlier in this century, states and localities operated tuberculosis hospitals and nursing homes. These have since been phased out or turned over to local governments. States, however, continue to operate mental institutions, which by fiscal year 1985 consumed on average 64 percent of all state mental health agency expenditures (ranging from a high of 92 percent to a low of 29 percent) or about $5.3 billion across all states (Lutterman and Mazade 1987). State governments provide $9 of every $10 spent by all government entities on care for the chronically mentally ill.

States are also involved in the direct provision of services—less so in providing personal health services than assistance and support services to local health agencies in areas such as public health nursing, communicable disease control, and environmental health, including air and water pollution control, regulation of hazardous waste disposal, and food and milk control.

Trends in Direct Provision of Institutional Care for the Mentally Ill

One of the most striking changes in health care over the last thirty years has taken place in the treatment of the mentally ill. Between 1950 and 1980, the number of people in state mental institutions dropped from 560,000 to less than 140,000 (Goldman 1981), due to a number of factors including the introduction of antipsychotic and antidepressant medications, exposes in the media and by public commissions about deplorable conditions in mental institutions, and most important, the growth of the community mental health movement.

The trend towards a community-based model

---

[3]One year of continued Medicaid coverage for former AFDC recipients who obtain work will be required in all states as of July, 1990 by virtue of a provision contained in the Family Support Act of 1988, Public Law 100–485.

of care was largely spurred by the federal government during the 1960s. But, there was one unfortunate feature of the federal grant program set up in 1963 . "There was no clear mandate . . . for the community mental health centers to coordinate their efforts with state mental hospitals or to care for chronic patients. In fact, federal policymakers intentionally created a program granting federal resources to local agencies, bypassing state mental health authorities. As a result, mental health centers primarily served new populations in need of acute services and failed to meet the needs of acute and chronic patients discharged in increasing numbers from public hospitals. Homelessness and indigency were predictable outcomes for many" (Goldman and Morrissey 1985). Deinstitutionalization also led to an increase in admissions to private psychiatric inpatient hospitals and to transfers to nursing homes.

While efforts were made to redress some of these problems, notably through the development of community support programs and systems, fiscal constraints brought on by the recession in the early 1980s and the Reagan administration budget cuts, threatened or severely compromised the care of the chronically mentally ill in the community. Furthermore, entrenched interest groups made it difficult for states to quickly shift funds from institutions to community-based programs. By 1984, the National Association of State Mental Health Program Directors reported that state and county operated, inpatient mental health hospitals still consumed over 67 percent of all public mental health funds (Goodrick 1984).

In some states, however, the development of community-based systems of care for the mentally ill has been forceful and innovative in terms of financing strategies. A report issued by the Urban Institute highlighted several states that used astute approaches in reforming their state mental health systems. Florida, for example, tackled the problem of its outmoded budget system for the state's mental institutions. It began to arrange for the provision of services through management contracts with private firms enabling the state's mental hospitals to operate more independently and more efficiently than other Florida state hospitals (Cohen et al. 1988).

The report also described how Maryland tried to make sure that elderly mentally ill individuals could be legally and properly placed in nursing homes where, under certain circumstances, their costs could be shared with the federal government. The state placed them in nursing homes throughout the state to make sure that individual nursing homes would not be disqualified from participation in Medicaid by violating federal rules which require that nursing homes keep the proportion of mentally ill patients under 50 percent. It also took advantage of the states' Medicaid nursing home reimbursement system which pays more for higher-cost patients needing more care. Finally, it paid a "patient transition management fee" to homes accepting these types of patients.

Wisconsin has probably been more successful than any other state in shifting funds from hospital to community programs—so much so that it has one of the lowest inpatient hospitalization rates in the country among the mentally ill. Wisconsin achieved this over a period of almost fifteen years, primarily by shifting program and financial responsibility for hospital and community-based services to county governments. County mental health boards provide or contract for a full range of inpatient and outpatient services, which builds in incentives to keep hospitalization rates low in order to finance services to more people in the community. By 1984, Wisconsin became the first state to require that all of its counties establish Community Support Programs. The state's FY 83 budget for mental health services, $96.4 million, was split evenly between inpatient and community services and in Dane County (Madison), only 15 percent of the county budget is spent on inpatient care (Daniels 1987).

As these examples indicate, states that were faced with the pressing need to use existing resources more efficiently have gradually discovered ways to deliver care to the chronically mentally ill more appropriately.

Residual Providers of Care

Although the trend is away from direct provision of care, there are instances of care being delivered when local governments need help or the private sector is unwilling to provide certain services. Some states, such as Connecticut, do not have county health departments. In other cases, state governments have stepped in to make sure that physicians and other health personnel are available in rural areas through programs such as state health service corps or the provision of incentives such as scholarships and loans for health professionals who agree to practice in rural or other underserved areas. A few states also reduced postgraduate training requirements needed for licensing in order to encourage students to practice in an underserved region (Ziegler 1987).

Throughout the 1980s, physicians and other health professionals located in rural areas or practicing in certain specialties became more reluctant to serve patients—particularly poor pregnant women—because of the rising cost of malpractice premiums. Most states dealt with this issue through traditional tort reform approaches (e.g., caps on economic or non-economic damages, binding arbitration provisions, etc.) and increased regulation of insurance rates or practices. But several states devised other ways that had a more immediate effect on keeping doctors from leaving the practice of obstetrics.

Missouri, for example, passed a law permitting the state to assume liability for doctors practicing under an agreement with a publicly owned hospital. A pilot program in North Carolina was established to subsidize the cost of malpractice premiums for family physicians and obstetricians who agreed to provide prenatal and obstetrical services in underserved counties and to all women, regardless of ability to pay. Both Virginia and Florida enacted "no fault" liability coverage for birth-related neurologically injured babies. A special fund was established in each state to compensate the families of infants born with these injuries and remove these cases from the court system. Since the law's enactment in Virginia, one insurer removed its moratorium on coverage for obstetricians, and a new carrier began offering coverage for the first time.

Another critical public health service that is provided in most states by state and local governmental units is emergency medical services. Though meagerly funded in comparison to other state health programs, EMS is funded with state general revenues in forty-eight states, and about a dozen states supplement those funds with fines from moving traffic violations.

In general though, states are getting out of the business of providing direct services to individuals, transferring responsibility to city and county governments or to the private sector when possible. States may never be able to completely withdraw from their role as operators of state mental hospitals, but they do recognize that the patients discharged from those hospitals must receive community-based care, funded to a large extent by the state. Similarly, states have accepted responsibility to provide care to special populations or assure access to specialized services not provided by anyone else.

States as Regulators of the Health Industry

States are vested with broad legal authority to regulate almost every facet of the health care system. They license and regulate health care facilities and health professionals, restrict the content, marketing and price of health insurance (including professional liability or malpractice insurance), set and enforce environmental quality standards, and enact a variety of controls on health care costs. However, along with the federal government, states have decided that regulation is not the only approach to health care. The 1980s saw a remarkable amount of experimentation with deregulation and promotion of competition in health care.

Trends in State Regulatory Activities: Certificate-of-Need

One traditional area of state health regulation has been control over the construction of new health facilities, the addition of new services, and the purchase of new equipment. By 1974, almost half the states had enacted certificate-of-need (CON) programs. But the federal government significantly expanded its involvement in this arena with the passage of the National Health Planning and Resources Development Act, signed into law in early 1975. It set up an elaborate regulatory system that, for the, most part, bypassed state governments by setting up over 200 health systems agencies (HSAs) at the local level. The HSAs had to review and make recommendations to the state on whether to approve certificates-of-need (CONs) for new hospital and health facility construction. States were mandated to establish state health planning and development agencies, but the local HSAs were funded by (and therefore accountable to) the federal government.

As with other regulatory programs, the health planning system was targeted for elimination by the Reagan Administration. Minimum dollar thresholds that triggered reviews by HSAs and state planning agencies were lifted and states were provided with greater discretion over the types of projects, procedures, and the criteria to be considered in the review of applications. By the end of 1983, most state CON activities were concentrated on bringing the thresholds for projects subject to CON review into conformity with federal requirements. A few states adopted at least one threshold level that was higher than the minimum federal requirement, thus potentially placing their programs out of compliance with federal law. In 1983, two states, New Mexico and Idaho effectively repealed their CON statutes by refusing to reauthorize them. The CON laws in several other states contained sunset provisions that provided for an automatic repeal at a specified time, for example, Arizona, and Kansas in 1984 and Texas in 1985.

The trend toward deregulation of health planning at the state level, tacitly allowed if not specifically authorized by the federal government, continued throughout the decade. As of December 31, 1986, nine states had no certificate of need program, although Congress did not take formal action to end the National Health Planning and Resources Development act until the end of 1986. Another three states terminated their CON programs the following year (Thomas 1986).

The trend was not universal, however. Efforts to repeal CON programs failed in several states, and, in at least eighteen the CON thresholds fell below (i.e. were more stringent than) federal standards. Furthermore, even states that deregulated the CON process still required some state review of newly constructed facilities, particularly nursing homes.

Minnesota experimented with efforts that ap-peared very pro-competition at times and very pro-regulation at others. For example, the state repealed its CON program in 1984, in line with the state's preference for trying market forces to improve the efficiency of health care services and reduce health care costs (Minnesota Department of Health 1985). However, in recognition of its position as having one of the highest rates of nursing home beds per capita of any state, the state slapped an indefinite moratorium on nursing home construction. It later extended a hospital capacity expansion moratorium into the next decade.

The state's actions may not be as contradictory as they seem. The health care regulatory changes in Minnesota over the last decade demonstrate the state's strong interest in promoting marketplace solutions with an equally strong willingness to step in when necessary to protect consumers. In another example, Minnesota has been one of the leading states in fostering the development and growth of new health care plans—HMOs, PPOs, and other hybrid managed care plans. Yet, the state has also made concerted efforts to regulate these plans to make sure that consumers understand their health plan coverage and receive the benefits that are in fact covered. In addition, Minnesota became the first state (Nebraska is the only other) to equalize nursing home rates between Medicaid and private paying patients. In essence, the state did not want nursing homes competing by discriminating in their admissions based on the source of payment.

Trends in State Regulatory Activity: Hospital Rate Controls

Both the states and the federal government have tried regulatory and free-market approaches to gain control over the escalating rate of hospital costs. Hospital charges were growing at double digit rates each year in the late 1970s but efforts to cap hospital rate increases by the Carter Administration and Congress failed under an onslaught of hospital lobbying. This, in spite of studies showing that in six states where hospital rate controls were in place, hospital costs were held down 14 percent below the national average (Biles et al. 1980).

When Reagan assumed office in 1981, nine states had mandatory hospital rate setting programs and another eight asked hospitals to comply with voluntary budget reviews (Esposito 1982). Among these states was New Jersey, which since 1976 had been involved in an experiment funded by the federal Health Care Financing Administration to develop a hospital prospective rate-setting system, based on a patient's diagnosis. The case-mix system, using a set of diagnostic related groups (DRGs) was adopted in 1980, and was used to set rates to be paid by all payers, including Medicare, Medicaid and all commercial and non-profit insurance plans in the state.

Prospective payment for hospitals became a major agenda of the Department of Health and Human Services under Reagan. The plan they developed and subsequently helped to enact in federal law was based on the DRG methodology developed for and tested by the state of New Jersey. It is, in fact, somewhat ironic that the most significant increase in federal government regulation of hospital reimbursement occurred under the Reagan presidency.

With at least sixteen states using DRG-based reimbursement methodologies for their state Medicaid hospital payments as of 1988, the combination of controls achieved through Medicare and Medicaid makes hospital rate regulation a reality for those hospitals largely dependent on these two financing sources, even if private insurers' rates are not limited by the state. Total hospital rate regulation, that is control over the rates that *every* public and private payer in the state can make to hospitals, remains in two states by the end of 1988 (New Jersey, and Maryland). Another two control all payers but Medicare (New York and Massachusetts) and a number of other states employ some form of hospital rate regulation affecting non-governmental payers (e.g., Connecticut, Maine, Washington).

This situation followed a period of great swings back and forth by individual states in establishing and then eliminating hospital rate regulatory systems. For example, in 1983 Wisconsin replaced a voluntary hospital rate review program with a mandatory rate-setting program after poor cost containment results of the voluntary program. A three member commission was vested with powers to review hospital budgets, disallow

expenses and revenue, and set maximum rates. The state legislature also authorized a number of pro-competitive policies, such as lifting all but minimal regulatory controls over HMOs and PPOs and requiring HMO enrollment of Medicaid recipients and of state employees. One of the political advantages to proposing a "mixed bag" of regulatory and market-oriented solutions was that powerful interest groups, such as the state hospital association, had less political influence than usual since their attention was dispersed in so many directions. Two years later, just as the program was getting started, the legislative coalition that initially supported it fell apart, and the legislature decided to let their state's hospital rate-setting commission sunset in 1987.

Another state that seemed one of the most unlikely to swing the other way—that is, from free-market promotion back to hospital rate controls—was Nevada. There, the state allowed hospitals free reign for the most part. This policy was called into question by a gubernatorial health care cost containment commission which discovered the state's health care costs to be among the highest in the nation. As a result, the Division of Health Resources and Cost Review was established to collect and analyze cost data in order to give purchasers (primarily the state and private businesses) the information they needed to infuse more competition into the market.

When the state's Democratic Governor Richard Bryan saw the data produced by this agency, he learned that one of the primary reasons for Nevada's high health care costs was $54.7 million in pre-tax profits made by a few Las Vegas investor-owned hospitals, which he called "excessive and obscene" (Merrill 1987; Holoweiko 1988). Furthermore, the medically indigent were not able to obtain access to many hospitals in the state, while hospitals that served the poor were losing money. In response, he called upon the Nevada legislature to withstand pressure from industry lobbyists in order to reduce hospital billed charges for fiscal year 87–88, maintain a freeze through fiscal year 88–89, and permit growth in rates of no more than 4 percent above the consumer price index after that. The 1987 law also required all hospitals in the state to provide a minimum level of charity care (0.6 percent of net revenues) before it could send bills to county governments for care provided to indigent patients.

In summary, the CON and hospital rate regulation issues demonstrate that there was no clear resolution during the 1980s of the competition vs. regulation contest. While some states favored deregulation, others actually increased regulation, and some blended a mixture of the two. States demonstrated a greater willingness to let the market forces work, but if they did not—that is, if consumers or the state itself suffered in the process—the state would step in. Shirley Wester, former executive director of the American Health Planning Association predicted on the eve of the demise of the health planning program at the federal level, " It is certainly our expectation that as the negative consequences to the health care system of the competitive free-for-all become more apparent, states will increasingly move to plan for and regulate health care financing and delivery systems" (Thomas 1986)

States as Administrators of Federal Funds and Programs

Another role that states assume is that of intermediary between the federal government and local governments, but it has often been charged that states take too much time to distribute money allocated by the federal government and too much money for administrative purposes. Do the charges have merit or are they made by self-interested groups that wanted but were denied federal funds by state governments?

In terms of basic state administrative capacity, it appears that states have improved markedly over the past ten to twenty years. A 1980 study that examined this issue concluded that "states have actually strengthened both their structures and functions and their finances to the point where they are quite capable of assuming full partnership in the federal system. Indeed, by almost every measure, states have improved their ability to govern, provide services, and meet the current and anticipated future needs of their constituents" (U.S. Advisory Committee on Intergovernmental Relations 1980). Another report on the subject five years later found state governments to be " more representative, more respon-

sive, more activist and more professional in their operations that they ever have been" (U.S. Advisory Committee on Intergovernmental Relations 1985).

The judgments contained in these two reports were based on such things as the growing number of staff in state legislatures, organizational restructuring of executive branches, improved fiscal management practices, and related factors. However, other analysts questioned the conclusions of the reports, arguing that there is not necessarily a direct relationship between such factors as large legislative staffs and enhanced effectiveness in governing (Thompson 1986). Still, if one compares state with federal performance, the gaps in commitment, capacity, and progressivity between state governments and Washington seems to have diminished.

One of the severest tests of the states' ability to carry out their role as allocators of federal funds came early on in the 1980s. In one of the clearest examples of the Reagan administration's "New Federalism," DHHS was mandated to consolidate funding for over twenty categorical grant programs into four block grants: (1) maternal and child health (MCH), (2) alcohol, drug abuse and mental health (ADAMH), (3) preventive health, and (4) primary care. Concern was expressed that less popular or controversial programs, though still important for the public's health, would disappear if they were no longer required.

In fact a survey (O'Kane 1984) that examined the first few years of the block grant process found less than half the states maintained the same proportion of funding for *each* service under the MCH and ADAMH block grants as that made under the previous programs. In the process, some individual programs suffered the consequences. For example, funds for sudden infant death syndrome programs were abolished in Ohio, Alabama and Tennessee, and lead-based paint poisoning prevention programs were eliminated in Missouri and Tennessee. In addition, the preventive health block grant brought about major shifts of program categories in most states. Programs that lost ground included rodent control, emergency medical services and home health. However, the survey found that while the majority of states chose to reallocate resources to some degree, there were no major shifts in funding when all states were examined in aggregate.

Furthermore, over half of the thirty-one states responding to the question reported making a greater state funding commitment than was required for the Maternal and Child Health Block Grant (states were required to match $3 for every $4 provided by the federal government), indicating a commitment to these services. The Preventive Health and the Alcohol, Drug Abuse and Mental Health block grants required no state match, but 90 percent of the states responding to the survey reported making state appropriations. The survey concluded, "Given the difficult fiscal circumstances in many states, this indicates a real commitment to the continuing existence and effectiveness of these programs" (O'Kane 1984, 6).

States as Innovators

States have taken initiative in many arenas that demonstrated their ability to combine all of their roles—as payers, providers, regulators and federal policy implementers—to fashion entirely new delivery systems or respond to new and emerging health issues. In some of these arenas, long-term care and AIDS for example, the federal government showed great reluctance to plan effectively for adequate health care delivery and financing systems, which required the states to create their own solutions.

One of the most interesting examples has been Arizona which was the last state to enter into an agreement with the federal government to administer a Medicaid program. Before 1981, the state took virtually no responsibility for care of the poor, leaving it to local government to provide services and subsidize care in private facilities. But as county governments began to sink under the burden of this responsibility (up to 25 percent of county tax revenues went to health care), they asked the state to help them by securing federal financing. The situation reached crisis proportions in 1980 when a ballot initiative was passed limiting county tax increases.

In response, the state legislature fashioned a solution initially proposed by then-Governor, Bruce Babbitt, who suggested that the state contract with health maintenance organizations (HMOs) to provide care to the poor. Such an ap-

proach would take advantage of HMOs ability to contain costs, while leaving government with limited liability for costs that exceeded the capitated fee for each enrollee. Contractors would be selected on the basis of a competitive bidding process and paid in advance of care, assuming the risk for delivery of all required services within a set amount. In order to operate such a program, the state needed a waiver of a number of federal Medicaid rules from the federal government. Once the waiver was negotiated with the federal government, the program which became known as the Arizona Health Care Cost Containment System (AHCCCS), began in October 1982.

The innovative route, however, is often a rocky one. It was particularly so in this case because of a number of political and administrative mistakes that were made. Osborne reviewed some of these in his book, *Laboratories of Democracy*. First, legislators mandated that AHCCCS begin operations less than a year after the act was signed, "in time to campaign as saviors of the poor during the 1982 elections" (Osborne 1988, 130). The state also chose a firm that had no experience in health care to administer the complex system and, according to Osborne, "operated more like a defense contractor than a health provider," which was not surprising in that the firm, McAuto Systems Group, was a subsidiary of McDonnell-Douglas (Osborne 1988, 131). The result was a program that cost over $20 million more than originally allocated by the state and showed a consistent pattern of denial of critical health services to the poor.

Babbitt stepped in to clean up the mess by appointing a medical director who was a strict disciplinarian. State personnel were brought in to write and monitor contracts with providers, a stringent financial accounting system was instituted, and the program's operations were generally redesigned. Osborne concluded that "Arizona has shown HMO systems for Medicaid make sense, but it has also demonstrated the pitfalls other states should avoid" (Osborne 1988). Based on Arizona's experience and that of several other states that experimented with HMO models of care for the poor, about 30 states became involved in similar managed care initiatives by the end of the decade—a trend that shows little sign of abating.

One unusual feature of the Arizona Medicaid

demonstration program was its exclusion of long-term care coverage. This was enormously significant, given that nearly half of most other states' Medicaid budgets are spent on long-term care services for the elderly and disabled. In 1987, Arizona committed itself to incorporating these services into AHCCCS, using the same principles of prepayment and capitated reimbursement, seeking to recreate on a statewide level the encouraging results of an innovative model for financing and delivery of long-term care services—the social health maintenance organization (SHMO).

Arizona is but one example among a number of states (rather than the federal government) that are leading the way on almost every aspect of long-term care financing and delivery reforms. Their efforts in this arena arise from their role in administering all the major public financing programs for long-term care of the elderly—Medicaid, the Older Americans Act, Social Services Block Grants and autonomous state supported programs. Even though the vast majority of funds (over 90 percent) are still spent on institutional long-term care in nursing homes (Lipson and Donohoe 1988), current state debates over how to reform the long-term care system focus on how to expand the availability of home and community care services rather than the details of nursing home reimbursement (Justice 1988).

State initiatives in long-term care system reform include reorganization of state responsibilities so that one agency has fiscal control over expenditures for institutional and community-based services (e.g., Oregon, Texas, Washington). They also include the development of an infrastructure capable of funneling all clients needing long-term care to local agencies that can perform comprehensive assessments, refer to all appropriate services and provide case management so that all services and funding sources are coordinated in the most efficient manner. States are also experimenting with varying degrees of reliance on federal funds, state revenues, and increasingly, on the promotion of private insurance or private financing mechanisms. These are areas where the federal government has virtually no experience, suggesting that as the aging of the population occurs and the demand for long-term care grows, states will play a central role in managing the new long-term care system that must emerge.

States have also acted as innovators by filling a gap left by the federal government in responding to one of the major public health crises of our age—AIDS. In the fiscal years 1984 to 1988, states allocated more than $240 million in general revenues for programs that attempt to stem the transmission of the virus or provide services to persons with AIDS (Rowe and Ryan 1988). Nearly 80 percent of the states formed an AIDS task force, commission or other advisory group to review state policies and recommend changes to the Governor or the legislature—long before the federal government organized such a commission.

Virtually every state government, and especially those hit hardest by the epidemic (New York, California, New Jersey, Florida and Texas), have had to contend with a myriad of issues, that the federal government largely avoided during the first several years of the epidemic (Shilts 1987). They had to decide how to establish screening programs and whether to allow or require tests for the AIDS virus among various groups of the population; how to establish surveillance of HIV infection that protected the public's health while maintaining individuals' right to privacy; how to protect individual rights to confidentiality while at the same time protecting the public health; what legal actions would be necessary to reduce discrimination against persons with AIDS or HIV infection; what types of financing options could be used to pay for services needed by AIDS patients; how to provide comprehensive, coordinated medical care and support services to AIDS patients; what types of public education programs were needed; and how much to support research on the causes and treatment of AIDS.[4]

There are numerous examples of states taking the initiative to address the AIDS epidemic, with the majority of them doing so in ways that helped to reduce the panic and fear associated with AIDS. For example, in almost every state legislature where it was proposed, mandatory pre-marital testing for the human immunodeficiency virus (HIV) was defeated. Moreover, many states

---

[4]For a full discussion on state approaches to these issues, see *AIDS: A Public Health Challenge, State Issues, Policies and Programs,* by Mona Rowe and Caitlin Ryan, Intergovernmental Health Policy Project, George Washington University, October 1987.

took explicit action to extend anti-discrimination protections to people with AIDS or HIV infection. And nearly every state established public health education programs aimed at health professionals, persons displaying high risk behaviors, the general public, or all three groups.

State Roles in Health Care in the 1990s

Towards the end of 1988, commentators in the media began to assess the Reagan legacy. One journalist's review (Hamilton 1988) of the states' assumption of new roles during the previous eight years concluded, "At its best, a renewed federalism—in which the states play a more active policy-making role than the national government—can produce innovative solutions to vexing problems, allowing states to test these remedies on a small scale, discarding what doesn't work and building on what does."

As the Reagan Administration showed so clearly, the ability of the states to be creative and innovative depends on the federal government's willingness to let them take on this responsibility. After nearly a decade of experience with a shift in the locus of control to the states, however, it is important to ask whether the variation that inevitably results from a lack of federal standards leads to an unacceptable degree of inequity between citizens of different states. As the Bush administration takes charge in Washington, the debate becomes louder between those who believe state variations are confusing and unfair and those who believe state flexibility is essential for the development of creative or tailor-made solutions to local problems.

As with so many other political questions, a good part of the answer ultimately revolves around money. Some state government representatives argue that they would be happy to let the federal government take over any number of health programs, as long as states would not have to be financially obligated to help pay for them. They say this in recognition of the limits of their state budgets to accommodate all the needs they see and hear about from their constituents. But if the federal government expects states to help pay the bills, they argue, then state

flexibility is essential due to variations in state economies and tax policies.

A compromise might be to guarantee federal financing for a minimally acceptable level of health care, allowing states to provide additional services as they are able to afford. But as almost twenty five years of experience with the Medicaid program has shown, varying financial contributions by the federal government must be structured differently to help states with weaker economies finance national programs. The methodologies used to equalize states' economic capacity to finance a *minimum* package of basic health services—decided upon at the federal level—must be improved if Medicaid or any other national health program is to cover a broader number of people living in poverty.[5]

Such a proposal, however, runs into a very difficult ethical issue. If the federal government, for example, decides that organ transplants are not part of a minimum basic benefit package but some states decide to cover them anyway, state flexibility will still result in some obvious inequities. This situation was recently played out in the state of Oregon. In 1987, the state legislature decided it only had enough money in the state budget to pay for expanded eligibility for pregnant women under the Medicaid program and not enough to cover heart, liver, pancreas and bone marrow transplants. The decision was made on the basis of convincing proof that prenatal care can save money in the long-run by preventing costly complications or disabilities among children.

Within the current system, state flexibility to make this type of judgment allows the rest of the country to observe and consider the determinants and consequences of such decisions. State decisions like the one in Oregon do not necessarily mean that some state governments are miserly or uncaring. They do, however, provide important examples of how different political bodies grapple with issues on which there is no national consensus. And in that sense, we can view such discussions as helping to lay the

---

[5]Holahan and Cohen propose a detailed methodology using a capitation approach that incorporates adjustments for the number of poor people in each state and state-specific health care prices and involves high national subsidies for minimum uniform eligibility levels and a standard benefit package (Holahan and Cohen 1986, 107–113).

groundwork for policy debates at the federal level on the issue of which "high-technology" health care services can be covered under government programs.

On a more fundamental level, states are likely to continue to play a critical role in health policy-making, if for no other reason than that the federal government would like the states to maintain their existing financial contributions to health services and long-term care. As long as the states' portion of the health care expenditures remains as high as it is, they will continue to retain substantial power in any national debate on health care issues. States' experience in health care financing also suggests that they can effectively wield power in the private sector to achieve cost containment, especially if they act in conjunction with the federal government.

Regardless of how much of the bill they pay, states are not likely to give up any of their other roles—as residual providers of care to groups left out of private sector health care delivery, as regulators of health insurance and environmental standards, as monitors of the use of federal funds by local entities, and especially as innovators. And more so now than ever before, states will be relied upon by the federal government to be full partners in the administration of health programs and the regulation of the health care industry. The election of George Bush to the While House portends continued importance of states in the federalism of the early 1990s, which is consistent with the previous administration's emphasis on greater state responsibility for health and welfare decisions.

More and more policymakers and observers seem to agree that states have finally proven their ability to manage complex programs, successfully maneuver their way in and out of regulatory relationships with the private sector, and develop innovative strategies to deal with health care problems more quickly than the federal government and in ways that respond to the unique set of political and economic factors and conditions in each state.

REFERENCES

Biles, Brian, Carl Schramm, and J. Graham Atkinson. 1980. Hospital cost inflation under state rate setting. *New England Journal of Medicine* 303:664–667.

Burwell, Brian and Marilyn Rymer. 1987. Trends in Medicaid eligibility: 1975 to 1985. *Health Affairs* 6:30–35.

Butler, Patricia. 1988. *Too poor to be sick: Access to medical care for the uninsured.* Washington, D.C.: American Public Health Association.

Clarke, Gary. 1981. The role of the states in the delivery of health services. In Role of state and local governments in relation to personal health services. *American Journal of Public Health,* edited by Sager C. Jain, 59–70, 71: Supplement No. 1.

Cohen, Joel, Korbin Liu and John Holahan. 1988. Financing long-term care for the chronically mentally ill. Washington D.C.: Urban Institute.

Congressional Quarterly. 1982, *Weekly report.* (January 30) 40:178.

Cromwell, Jerry, Rachel Schurman, et al. 1984. The evolution of state Medicaid program changes. Final report prepared for the U.S. Department of Health and Human Services, Assistant Secretary for Planning and Evaluation.

Daniels, La Vonne. 1987. Retooling in the 80s—Transferring dollars from hospital to community programs. *State Health Reports,* No. 30. Washington D.C.: Intergovernmental Health Policy Project, George Washington University.

Demkovich, Linda E. 1982. Medicaid for welfare: A controversial swap. *National Journal* 14:362–368.

Desonia, Randolph and Kathleen M. King. 1985. *State programs of assistance for the medically indigent.* Washington D.C.: Intergovernmental Health Policy Project, George Washington University.

Esposito, Alfonso, Michael Hupfer, Cynthia Mason and Diane Rogler. 1982. Abstracts of state legislated hospital cost containment programs. *Health Care Financing Review* 4(2):129–158.

Farrell, Karen. 1988. *State expenditure report.* Washington D.C.: National Association of State Budget Officers.

Goldman, Howard. 1981. Defining and counting the chronically mentally ill. *Hospital and Community psychiatry* 31:21–27.

Goldman, Howard and Joseph Morrissey. 1985. The alchemy of mental health policy: Homelessness and the fourth cycle of reform. *American Journal of Public Health* 75:727–731.

Goodrick, David. 1984. Survival of public inpatient mental health systems: Strategies for constructive change. *State Health Reports* Number 11, Washington D.C.: Intergovernmental Health Policy Project, George Washington University.

Hamilton, Martha. 1988. States assuming new powers as federal policy role ebbs. *Washington Post,* August 30.

Herbers, John. 1987. The new federalism: Unplanned, innovative and here to stay. *Governing* 1:28–37.

Holahan, John and Joel Cohen. 1986. *Medicaid: The trade-off between cost containment and access to care.* Washington D.C.: Urban Institute Press.

Holoweiko, Mark. 1988. What happens when the profit motive runs wild. *Medical Economics* (July 18):150–168.

Jain, Sagar C. 1981. Introduction and summary to role of state and local governments in relation to personal health services. *American Journal of Public Health* 71: Supplement No. 1.

Justice, Diane. 1988. *State long term care reform: Development of community care systems in six states.* Washington D.C.: National Governors' Association.

Lipson, Debra J. 1988a. *Major changes in state medicaid and indigent care programs.* Washington D.C.: Intergovernmental Health Policy Project, George Washington University.

Lipson, Debra J. 1988b. Massachusetts legislation: A model for other states or a costly mistake? *Business and Health* 5(10):48–49.

Lipson, Debra J. and Elizabeth Donohoe. 1988. *State financing of long-term care services for the elderly.* Washington D.C.: Intergovernmental Health Policy Project, George Washington University.

Lutterman, Theodore, Noel Mazade, Cecil Wurster and Robert Glover. 1987. Trends in revenues and expenditures of state mental health agencies: Fiscal years 1981, 1983 and 1985. *State Health Reports* No. 34, Washington D.C.: Intergovernmental Health Policy Project, George Washington University.

Merrill, Teri. 1987. Regulation v. competition: Three states choose. *Hospitals* 61(13):34–35.

Minnesota Department of Health. 1985. *Minnesota health care markets: Cost containment and other public policy goals.* St. Paul, MN.

O'Kane, Margaret. 1984. State implementation of health block grants. *focus on . . .* No. 5. Washington, D.C.: Intergovernmental Health Policy Project, George Washington University.

Osborne, David E. 1988. *Laboratories of democracy: A new breed of governor creates models for national growth.* Boston, MA.: Harvard Business School Press.

Public Health Foundation. 1987. *Public health agencies 1987: Expenditures and sources of funds.* Publication No. 103, Washington, D.C.

Rapoport, Daniel. 1982. The states: A new priority. *National Journal* 14:73.

Rosenbaum, Sara, Dana Hughes, and Kay Johnson. 1988. Maternal and child health services for medically indigent children and pregnant women. *Medical Care* 26

Rowe, Mona and Caitlin Ryan. 1987. *AIDS: A public health challenge, state issues, policies and programs.* Washington, D.C.: Intergovernmental Health Policy Project, George Washington University.

Rowe, Mona and Caitlin Ryan. 1988. Comparing state-only expenditures for AIDS. *American Journal of Public Health* 78:424–431.

Sawyer, Darwin, Martin Ruther, Aileen Pagan-Berlucchi, and Donald N. Muse. 1983. *The Medicare and Medicaid data book, 1983.* U.S. Department of Health and Human Services, Health Care Financing Administration. Baltimore, MD.

Shilts, Randy. 1987. *And the band played on: Politics, people and the AIDS epidemic.* New York: St. Martins Press.

Southern Regional Task Force on Infant Mortality. 1985. *Final report for the children of tomorrow.* Washington, D.C.: Southern Governors' Association.

Sundquist, James. 1969. *Making federalism work.* Washington, D.C.: The Brookings Institution.

Thomas, Constance. 1986. CON changes taper off. *State Health Notes* No. 67. Washington, D.C.: Intergovernmental Health Policy Project, George Washington University.

Thompson, Frank J. 1986. New federalism and health care policy: States and the Old Questions. *Journal of Health Politics, Policy and Law* 11:647–669.

U.S. Advisory Commission on Intergovernmental Relations. 1980. ACIR and the intergovernmental system: A 20-Year Report. *Intergovernmental Perspective* 6:20.

U.S. Advisory Commission on Intergovernmental Relations. 1985. *The question of state government capability.* Washington, D.C.

U.S. Department of Health and Human Services, Health Care Financing Administration, Office of the Actuary, 1987, National health expenditures, 1986–2000. *Health Care Financing Review* 8(4):1–36.

Ziegler, Andrew. 1987. States address shortage, distribution of health professionals. *State Health Notes,* No. 75, Washington, D.C.: Intergovernmental Health Policy Project, George Washington University.

Chapter 10

The Politics of Federalism and Inter-governmental Relations in Health

Richard C. Elling
Leonard S. Robins[1]

A Brief Modern History of Federalism and Intergovernmental Relations

Interpretations and explanations of the constitutional and behavioral relationships between the nation and the states vary in accordance with broad trends in the American polity.

Post-World War II

In the 1950s and early 1960s, the major works on federalism and intergovernmental relations of Grodzins (1966) and Elazar (1984) led students of federalism to a new understanding of American intergovernmental relations by persuasively arguing that the nation and the states had always been primarily *partners* rather than competitors in the performance of governmental functions. They emphasized and favorably noted the fact that when an important problem arose that called for governmental action, both the states and the national government typically attempted to respond with appropriate action. Although strongly in favor of a major state role in United States federalism, they generally downplayed efforts at determining which level of government does what best (Grodzins 1966; Elazar 1984).

Given their perspective on intergovernmental relations, it is not surprising that they did not consider grant-in-aid programs to be a usurpation of state power by the national government. Rather, they argued that grants-in-aid typically did not substitute national power or programs for those of the states, but actually increased both state and national power. For example, when states lacked the resources to deal with a problem, the national government made those resources available by a grant-in-aid program (with both governments sharing responsibility), and

[1]The authors would like to thank Charles Backstrom and William Hathaway for their comments on an earlier draft of this chapter.

this increased rather than decreased state power. This example is not hypothetical. Grodzins (1966) and Elazar (1984) concluded that vigorous national action typically had come not when the states refused to act, but rather when they were unable to act by themselves (Grodzins 1966; Elazar 1972).

Further support for this analysis is provided by surveys of attitudes of state officials toward grants-in-aid. These surveys elicited strong support for both existing grants-in-aid and the related concept of joint national and state control over programs (Wright 1982).

The Great Society

During the Great Society years of President Lyndon Johnson, however, grant programs multiplied and proliferated in a remarkable, crazy-quilt pattern and contained conditions that were typically qualitatively different from those previously attached to grants-in-aid—different in ways that tended to increase the degree of national control relative to that of the states.

The most important change was that during this period project grants rather than formula grants became the dominant form of grant-in-aid, and the characteristics of formula grants and project grants have a major impact in determining the relative degree of national and state control over grant programs. One pair of observers wrote:

> Formula grants are grants whose funds are divided among all eligible recipients on the basis of some announced criterion that is applied proportionately across the board and without any discretion in the hands of the grant-giving officials. . . . Formula grants are distributed to all eligible jurisdictions as a matter of "right." The discretion, if there is any, lies in the hands of the recipient governments that decide how much matching money they want to use to obtain a particular federal grant. Federal influence under formula grants lies in the administrative requirements that accompany the grant, rather than in the substance of the grant (Reagan and Sanzone 1981, 58).

States are almost always the recipients of formula grants from the national government.

Project grants are considerably different from formula grants. "Project grants are made to meet specific problems and are not spread among all potential recipients according to any fixed proportions" (Reagan and Sanzone 1981, 59). Project grants thus typically operate in a manner that enhances national influence in grant programs, for the national government both creates the criteria for projects and makes the actual selection among the applications for support of projects. Project grants, moreover, frequently go to localities, special-purpose governments (e.g., school districts), or even private recipients. Although the states frequently have an important administrative role in grant programs that do not designate them as the recipients (Elazar 1984), their influence and control over these grants is less than over those grants that designate them as the recipients. In short, the new emphasis on project grants resulted in a major increase in the influence of the national government in grant-in-aid programs.

Describing these and other trends in grants-in-aid more quantitatively and systematically, one scholar contended that the following are particularly noteworthy:

1. *The Dollar Amount.* Aid to state and local governments increased from $7 billion in fiscal year 1960 to $83 billion in fiscal year 1980. During the same period federal aid went from 14.7 to 23.6 percent of state-local expenditures.

2. *Instruments.* The means by which financial assistance was transmitted expanded to include a variety of federal-state, federal-local, and federal-private transactions under formula and project categorical grants, block grants, general revenue sharing, procurement contracts, and cooperative agreements.

3. *Participants.* The extent of state and local government involvement expanded to the point where virtually all general-purpose local units and many special purpose units received assistance, thus multiplying the number of people affected by intergovernmental actions.

4. *Strings.* The conditions attached to federal programs became more extensive, expensive, and intrusive. In addition to traditional

requirements (e.g., financial reporting and audits), the federal government increasingly used federal assistance programs as vehicles for achieving national social policy goals, such as affirmative action, environmental quality, historical site preservation, and citizen participation. By the late 1970s, nearly 60 of these requirements applied to all or most programs, regardless of purpose.

5. *Bypassing.* Federal financial assistance increasingly involved transmitting money directly to local governments, neighborhood groups, private agencies, and community action agencies (Stenberg, 1980:29–31).

During this period, the number of federal grants increased from less than 100 in the 1950s to nearly 500 by the late 1970s. Nearly 100 of these grants directly or indirectly involved health and medical care. In a major survey of intergovernmental relations, the Advisory Commission on Intergovernmental Relations (ACIR) concluded that the federal government's assumption of progressively greater responsibility for dealing with domestic problems through use of grants-in-aid stood out as the dominant feature of intergovernmental relations in the decades 1959–1979 (Stenberg 1980).

The Reagan Years

In reaction to these trends, students of intergovernmental relations became increasingly critical of what they felt was an excess of national government influence in the grants-in-aid system (Elazar 1984). Additionally, they argued that grants-in-aid had grown so numerous and confusing that they had become part of the problem rather than the solution. Even some of those who approved of grants-in-aid heavily influenced by the national government, recognized that uncoordinated proliferation of narrowly targeted grant programs had made the coordinated solving of problems more difficult (Sundquist 1969). In the long run, the goal is solving problems, not delivering tightly packaged service components.

The Ronald Reagan Presidency, partly in response to these criticisms, changed the intergovernmental relations system in two fundamental ways. First, national funding for grants-in-aid

programs was significantly reduced (after adjusting for inflation). Indeed, funds for grants-in-aid programs were more sharply cut than for any other major component of national government spending (Conlan 1988). Second, national control and administrative supervision of grants-in-aid was decreased, best symbolized by the conversion of categorical into block grants.

As one final point, it is important to note that attitudes on intergovernmental relations are strongly shaped by "whose ox is being gored." For reasons that need not be analyzed here, labor and minority groups have, by and large, historically been stronger at the national than at the state level of government (Riker 1964). Consequently, they have tended to be opposed to proposals for weakening the national government's influence in grant programs. The political right, in contrast, has usually been stronger at the state and local governmental levels, and most conservatives tend to be strong advocates of proposals that would weaken national control over grant programs. Therefore, who is in political control is probably more important in shaping intergovernmental relations than intellectual philosophizing about the intergovernmental system.

A Theoretical Analysis of Federalism and Intergovernmental Relations

It was noted earlier that modern students of federalism and intergovernmental relations tend to think of the national and state governments as partners rather than rivals. Nonetheless, it is still appropriate to ask whether in theory there are certain functions which should be primarily—not exclusively—the responsibility of the national government or primarily that of the states? The answer most students of federalism and intergovernmental relations would give is yes.

The Allocation of Functions

Drawing on the economics concept of "externalities," the argument is made that states and localities are freer to spend what they think is the correct amount on education, law enforcement, and transportation services than on aiding the poor through welfare and personal medical services. The reason is that states and especially localities often fear that businesses and upper-income residents will move rather than pay for services through higher taxes, thus removing themselves from the consequences of collective decision making. Though the threat is often a bluff, it is true that the upper-income citizen receives no clear gain from higher welfare expenditures to balance the pain of higher taxes and might even consider them dysfunctional if they are believed to attract more potential welfare applicants to the state or locality.

Conversely, increased spending on education results in a benefit to all citizens as well as higher taxes, and hence higher taxes might be tacitly accepted or even advocated for this function. There is little, if any, reason in this context for business and upper-income residents to escape the consequences of collective decision making. Thus, most economists and students of federalism and intergovernmental relations argue that the national government should assume primary responsibility for welfare and personal medical services programs, with responsibility for education, transportation, and law enforcement left largely to the states (Peterson 1981; Peterson, Rabe, and Wong 1986).

Types of Federal Involvement

A second important theoretical issue concerns the range of ways in which the national government can involve itself programmatically vis-a-vis the states. There are, on a continuum from greater to lesser control, five modes of national programmatic involvement: nationally-run programs, project categorical grants, formula categorical grants, block grants, and revenue sharing. Of course, there also may be no national programmatic involvement. These modes are outlined in table 10–1, with selected health programs listed under the appropriate categories.

Nationally-run Programs

While it might seem surprising that nationally-run programs such as Medicare are included in a chapter that focuses on the relative degree of

national influence on various types of intergovernmental health programs, this is nonetheless essential. Many liberals prefer that governmental programs typically be run this way, favoring, for example, the organizational structure of Medicare over that of Medicaid. Without including this category, the clear and incorrect impression is left that a central position in the degree of national control over programs is somewhere between categorical grants and revenue sharing. Within the context of grant-in-aid programs, however, national influence is greatest in categorical grants-in-aid.

Categorical Grants

Categorical grants are typically those for specifically and narrowly defined purposes; they usually give very little discretion to the recipient government as to how it uses the grant. They are vehicles for identifying problems, setting priorities, and focusing resources on a national basis. They not only carry restrictions on the use of money, but usually also have planning, accounting, reporting, and personnel requirements (Reagan and Sanzone 1981). A categorical grant is the kind of program most people think of, in terms of both strengths and weaknesses, when they think of national grant programs. Empirical research on the operation of grant programs, however, indicates that who actually is in control is much less clear-cut than this definition implies (Ingram 1977; Radin 1972; Thompson 1981; Williams 1980). But a significant degree of national control is almost always intended in categorical programs.

Block Grants

Block grants differ from those that are categorical in the following four ways:

1. federal aid is authorized for a wide range of activities within a broadly defined functional area
2. recipients have substantial discretion in identifying problems, allocating resources, and designing programs
3. administrative, fiscal, reporting, planning, and other federal requirements are kept to

Modes of National Involvement in Programs

Nationally-Run Programs	Project Categorical Grants	Formula Categorical Grants	Block Grants	Revenue Sharing	No National Involvement
Medicare	Community Health Centers	Medicaid	Public Health Block Grant 314(d) (1966–1981)	(1972–1986)	(National Health Insurance)
Food and Drug Administration	Black Lung Clinics	State Comprehensive Mental Health Services Planning	Preventive Health Services		
	Migrant Health Centers		Maternal and Child Health		
	Health Care for the Homeless		Alcohol, Drug Abuse and Mental Health		
(Others)	(Others)	(Others)			

TABLE 10–1

the minimum amount necessary to ensure that national goals are being accomplished

4. federal aid is distributed according to a statutory formula, which has the effect of narrowing federal administrators' discretion and providing a sense of fiscal certainty to recipients (Stenberg and Walker 1977).

In short, block grants are designed to be both theoretically and operationally the opposite of categorical grants.

Revenue Sharing

Revenue sharing is, essentially, money given to the states and localities to assist them in the performance of *their* functions. It is only indirectly relevant to the question of which level of government should perform any given function. For a variety of economic, historical, political, and state constitutional reasons, states and localities have typically relied on property and sales taxes for the bulk of their revenues—regressive taxes that hit the poor very hard. The national government, in contrast, has primarily relied on the more progressive personal and corporate income taxes. A strong case can be made, therefore, that the clearest effect of revenue sharing is to substitute income taxes for sales and property taxes, that is, progressive for regressive taxes.

No National Involvement

The national government may, of course, decide not to become involved in a functional area, that is, to have no national program. This category may also seem unusual in a classification of types of national involvement, but, as the reverse of nationally-run programs, it is equally important to emphasize that the real programmatic option is often the choice between a categorical grant or no national involvement.

Interpretation

Block grants have always had difficulty in getting enacted and obtaining adequate funding. The reason is that they are not politically attractive to Congress. Students of congressional spending behavior stress that members of Congress look with favor on concrete programs that seem to meet visible needs directly and are supported by strong clientele groups, on programs over which they can exercise a considerable degree of control, and on programs that offer an opportunity for them to take personal credit for successes (Niskanen 1971). Categorical programs meet these criteria. They deal with problems such as heart disease and cancer, and by preserving a clear measure of national control, they allow members of Congress to have some influence over them and claim some of the credit for the good they accomplish. In contrast, block grants are frequently amorphous programs over which members of Congress have little control and whose "good works" are seen as coming from state and local governments.

The history of the 314(d) public health block grant in the Partnership for Health Act of 1966 provides strong evidence of the difficulty of securing adequate funding for block grants. Although not a large program ($54 million at its inception in fiscal year 1967), it was distinctive for being the first block grant enacted in modern times. Those pushing for its enactment also pledged to seek a major increase in its funding. In fact, however, funds for it were steadily cut (Robins 1974), and by 1981, when it was folded into the Preventive Health and Health Services block grant, its funding had shrunk to $9 million (Peterson, Bovbjerg, et al. 1986).

The most dramatic evidence for this proposition, however, is that the only "big ticket item" that was totally eliminated (as contrasted to merely cut) during the Reagan years was revenue sharing. Despite the fact that revenue sharing was the program that most closely fit Reagan's ideological approach to federalism, when something had to be done to cut the deficit, it was quickly seized on for elimination. The Congress, liberals and conservatives alike, acquiesced without major resistance and some liberals were even positively delighted. The only objectors were governors, state legislators, mayors, and other local officials (Conlan 1988).

Fluctuations in Degree of Control

Typically there is a long-term tendency toward the "creeping recategorization" of block grants over time. This can happen in one of two ways,

First new conditions may be attached to the block grant. An example outside of health is the Community Development Block Grant, in which targeting of funds to poor neighborhoods increased during President Jimmy Carter's Administration (Kettle 1980). Second, the block grant may be kept very small and may parallel categorical programs established to accomplish objectives that logically should have been assigned to the block grant. This was true in the case of the 314 (d) public health block grant, for Congress subsequently enacted new programs such as family planning and expanded several ongoing programs such as venereal disease control that should logically have been included in the overall public health block grant.

It is important to emphasize, however, that a similar, albeit reverse, process frequently occurs with categorical programs, that is, over time, state and local recipients frequently increase their authority as they become more knowledgeable about regulations and how they can be manipulated to serve their ends. Thus, it is essential to understand that the grants-in-aid system is not a static one and that federal, state, and local officials are constantly maneuvering within it to serve their own interests.

Finally, there are obvious institutional biases in considering the appropriate degree of control. State and local officials—whether ideologically of the left or right—feel impelled to argue that their levels of government should have more discretion in grant programs. National administrators, on the other hand, typically have an opposite point of view.

The Reagan Health Block Grants

In 1981, the Reagan Administration proposed a sweeping consolidation of twenty-six health programs into two health block grants. Congress resisted somewhat, but basically acquiesced by combining eight programs into the Maternal and Child Health block grant (MCH), eight programs into the Preventive Health and Health Services block grant (PHHS), and five programs into the Alcohol, Drug Addiction, and Mental Health block grant (ADAMH). Table 10–2 shows which

programs were absorbed into each of the health block grants.

The trends in federal appropriations for the health block grants are shown in table 10–3, with the figures for FY81 being the cumulative totals for the original programs combined into each block grant. Understanding what happened to the programs combined into health block grants requires first noting that although there were sharp reductions in funding for the new block grants (compare FY81 to FY82 funding), other health programs that continued in categorical form were cut as sharply, if not more than those that were folded into new the block grants (compare FY81 and FY82 funding for the ADAMH block grant and funding for other ADAMAHA programs in table 10–5). It equally requires extending the analysis beyond changes in the federal funding for these programs.

Trends in Total Spending for Block Grant Health Programs

Most of the programs funded with ADAMH, MCH, or PHHS dollars were funded from a variety of sources before the block grants were created. These included other federal grant programs, state funds, local government funds, fees for services, co-payments, and third party reimbursements from insurance companies. Hence, depending upon changes in support from these various sources, a given percentage reduction in federal block grant funding may or may not have been precisely mirrored in lower overall levels of financial support for specific programs.

Table 10–4 shows that in some states these programs received increased funding even as block grant funding was initially decreasing. While these increases were often not enough—especially if inflation is considered—to compensate for the decline in federal funding support, they were often very helpful in preventing sharp cutbacks in particular programs.

Various nonblock grant funding sources were more generous in some states than others. States also exhibited varying patterns of preference for certain programmatic areas over others. In Colorado, MCH-related programs fared least well and PHHS-related programs fared best. In Washing-

Categorical Programs Combined Into Each Health Block Grant*

PRESENT BLOCK GRANTS:	Maternal and Child Health Block Grant	Preventive Health and Health Services Block Grant	Alcohol, Drug Abuse, and Mental Health Grant
OLD CATEGORICAL PROGRAMS:	Maternal and Child Health Grants	314(d) Health Block Grant	Community Mental Health Centers
	Crippled Children's Services	Emergency Medical Services	Alcoholism Project Grants
	SSI-Disabled Children	Hypertension	Alcoholism Formula Grants
	Lead-Based Paint Poisoning Prevention	Urban Rodent Control	Drug Abuse Project Grants
	Genetic Diseases	Fluoridation	Drug Abuse Formula Grants
	Adolescent Pregnancy Prevention	Home Health	
	Hemophilia	Health Education and Risk Reduction	
	Sudden Infant Death Syndrome	Rape Crisis and Prevention Centers	

TABLE 10–2

*SOURCE: Adapted from THE REAGAN BLOCK GRANTS: WHAT HAVE WE LEARNED? by Petersen, Bovbjerg et al. Copyright 1986 by Urban Institute Press, Washington, D.C.

Federal Funding for Health Block Grants, FY81–88**
(in $ Millions)

Fiscal Year

Block Grant	1981*	1982	1983	1984	1985	1986	1987	1988
Maternal and Child Health (MCH)	455	374	478	399	478	457	497	527
Preventive Health and Health Services (PHHS)	93	82	86	88	89	88	90	86
Alcohol, Drug Abuse, and Mental Health	585	428	468	462	490	469	672	692

TABLE 10–3

**SOURCE*: Budget of the United States Government, _Appendices, 1984–1990._

*FY81 is the spending for the predecessor programs now in each block grant.

Changes in Total Financial Support From All Sources for Health Block Grant Programs in Selected States, FY81–83***

	Block Grant		
State	ADAMH %	MCH %	PHHS %
Colorado	4	– 11	16
Florida	4	18	4
Iowa	15	– 6	6
Kentucky	– 8	12	4
Massachusetts	14	4	– 16
Michigan	20	6	– 11
Mississippi	9	27	6
Pennsylvania	3	– 7	– 5
Texas	24	32	19
Vermont	12	32	– 17
Washington	14	12	– 6

TABLE 10–4

***SOURCE: U.S. GAO, States Have Made Few Changes in Implementing the Alcohol, Drug Abuse and Mental Health Services Grant (1984); Maternal and Child Health Block Grant Program Changes Emerging Under State Administration (1984); States Used Added Flexibility Offered by the Preventive Health and Health Services Block Grant (1984).

ton State, however, just the opposite was true. In Mississippi, Texas and Vermont total funding increases for maternal and child health-related programs exceeded those for the other two areas. But in Iowa, MCH-related programs fared least well.

Seeking to account for these interstate and interprogram differences in support requires that we turn our attention to the other sources of funds from which states and localities could draw to support particular programs.

The State Response to Block Grant Changes

Block grant champions generally argued that the states could be "trusted" to put up their own resources to support particular programs even as categorical constraints were eliminated. In addition, they believed that the greater flexibility inherent in block grants would permit states to support programs at comparable levels with fewer dollars (Williamson 1981). Opponents argued that states were likely to be unable to replace cuts of the magnitude proposed in conjunction with the transition from categorical to block grants. Many opponents also suspected that block grant advocates really didn't believe that states would step into the breach, and even hoped that they would not, with the result that overall public spending for particular domestic programs would decline (Peterson, Bovbjerg, et al. 1986).

Certainly the fact that the block grant transition coincided with the onset of the worst economic downturn of the postwar period was hardly conducive to state or local replacement of federal cuts. From a state and local perspective, the block grant cuts, and other federal aid reductions, came at the worst of all possible times. In addition, a "strategic" reluctance to replace the federal cuts was displayed by some state and local officials opposed to Reagan Administration priorities. Too readily taking up the slack created by the cuts could be used by the Administration as proof that further cuts could be undertaken.

More positively, many of the block grants, and certainly the health block grants, provided funds for programs in which states or localities had longstanding involvement. This made it likely that various state and local government officials, service providers, clients, and interest groups would strive to have their state or local government take at least some of the sting out of the federal cuts.

Early studies of the transition from categorical to block grants concluded that state replacement of federal dollar cuts was neither substantial nor consistent across programs or states (Nathan, Doolittle, and Associates 1983). Later analyses, however, uncovered evidence of more substantial state and local funding replacement. An eighteen-state Urban Institute study (Peterson 1984), for example, found that full replacement of cuts in ADAMH funding as compared to its categorical predecessors grants had occurred in twelve states. Full replacement of the cuts in the MCH and PHHS block grants occurred in eight and nine states respectively. Partial replacement occurred in several other states for each of these program areas. On the other hand, full replacement of lost federal dollars *adjusted for inflation* occurred in just five states in ADAMH and PHHS, and in only four states in the MCH block grant. Still, state and local replacement of cuts in the health block grants was greater than for many of the nonhealth block grants (Peterson 1984).

In general, it appears that the states at least partially filled the void created by reductions in federal support. The fears of some that the states would simply ratify the federal cuts were, at least in part, overexaggerated.

Changes within the Block Grants

Assessing the impact of the Reagan health block grants also requires an examination of changes in program priorities that occurred *within* individual block grants. Those who consider block grants to be a vehicle that permits states to establish their own funding priorities between types of health programs should be pleased if such changes occurred. From the point of view of those concerned about specific public health problems, however, the virtue of a categorical grant is that it assures a certain amount of funding for programs to address that problem while the folding of that program into a larger block grant introduces uncertainty. The facts are clear: priorities between categoricals folded into one or another of the three health block grants did shift, although this was more true for some block grants than others. Assessing the desirability of these shifts is difficult, but it is apparent that states did indeed exercise their newfound discretion.

In the case of the MCH block grant, one pattern dominated. Categorical programs with a history of state support tended to do better than those that were viewed as "theirs," that is, those more purely federal in origin or emphasis. Those programs whose benefits were spread across a state, and were focused on population groups that citizens viewed as especially needy also fared better in the new budget competition. Conversely those that "were concentrated in a few geographical areas and with an emphasis on population groups that are not viewed as especially needy were the losers" (Peterson, Bovbjerg, et al. 1986, 110).

The biggest MCH "winner" was Crippled Children's Services. Not only was this a function in which states had been significantly involved for a long period of time, but crippled children "proved to have wide public support," as became clear in public hearings and in expressions of local (county) priorities for MCH spending (Peterson, Bovbjerg, et al. 1986, 110).

The advent of the MCH block grant also prompted at least some states to add services. Among these was Michigan, where state officials reported that the MCH block grant provided a portion of the additional funding needed to address the state's higher than average infant mortality problem by permitting the expansion of funding for maternal and infant care programs from only nine to all local health departments (Elling 1988).

The fate of the Lead-Based Paint Poisoning prevention program contrasts sharply with that for Crippled Children's Services. Among the eight programs folded together to create the MCH block grant, this program ranked in size somewhere in the middle with a federal appropriation of $12 million in 1980. But it was "widely viewed as a big-city program that had formerly been administered by the federal government" (Peterson, Bovbjerg, et al. 1986, 110). In addition, victims of lead poisoning are more difficult to identify than are crippled children. As a result,

funding for the Lead-Based Paint Poisoning prevention program declined in most states after the creation of the MCH block grant, with several states eliminating the program entirely.

The smallest of the prior programs folded into the new MCH block—Sudden Infant Death Syndrome—also fared badly when budgets were cut, since it was another example of programs "with narrow target groups that were highly concentrated in big-city hospitals" (Pererson, Bovbjerg, et al. 1986, 110–111).

A similar underlying dynamic accounts for both the continuity and change in priorities for those programs folded into the Preventive Health and Health Services block grant. On the one hand, the U.S. General Accounting Office concluded that relative continuity in program shares reflected "a continued need for services, a desire to minimize the disruption of ongoing services and the states' basic satisfaction with most existing services because of their role in fashioning the prior programs" (U.S. GAO 1984, 22). On the other hand, nearly every state adjusted the PHHS program mix to some extent, and programmatic losers tended to be narrowly targeted programs in which past state involvement was limited. Thus, the Urban Rodent Control program lost funds in every one of the states that had such a program. Like the Lead-Based Paint Poisoning prevention program under the MCH block grant, Rodent Control was "perceived as a large-city program" (Peterson, Bovbjerg, et al. 1986, 116). State support for Emergency Medical Services, Home Health and Health Education programs were also more often than not targeted for cuts (U.S. GAO 1984).

Winners in the competition among the prior categoricals folded into the PHHS block grant included Health Incentive grants previously funded under the 314 (d) block grant as well as Hypertension and Fluoridation programs (U.S. GAO 1985).

Programmatic priorities changed least in the case of the Alcohol, Drug Abuse, and Mental Health block grant largely because Congress, in approving this block grant, placed many more restrictions on states' use of these funds than was true for either of the other two health block grants. States were required to divide total ADAMH spending between substance abuse and mental health in proportion to each area's historical share of funds received. States were also required to spend a minimum share of the block grant on substance abuse and to allocate minimum shares of these funds to both alcoholism and drug abuse efforts. They were required to allocate block grant funds to those Community Mental Health centers (CMHC) that received operating funds in FY81, although funding levels could be changed. All other CMHCs could receive funding at a state's option.

The most significant effect of this block grant was that it served to bring those service providers who had previously received categorical funding directly from the federal government into the state system for the first time. This meant that these grantees had to "better serve *state* priorities (emphasis added)" or their funding allocations would be cut. The latter occurred with considerable frequency (Peterson, Bovbjerg, et al. 1986, 129).

One final point should be made about how states chose to exercise their enhanced power to reshape program priorities. A common pattern was for states to distribute block grant dollars more *widely*. To be sure, public health needs in the states are such that almost any area of a state can put additional funds to good use. But the result of this spreading of health block grant dollars has often been adverse to the interests of large urban areas and the poor and minorities who constitute a substantial proportion of those areas' populations. Several examples from Michigan illustrate this. State officials worked with the Michigan Health Officers association to develop a formula to distribute at least 10 percent of MCH and PHHS block grant dollars for FY83 to local health departments on a per capita basis in order to address "priority health problems." The state also decided to channel MCH block grant funds for infant health care to all thirty-nine local health departments in the state, none of which had received past categorical funding for this purpose. The resulting reduction in Wayne County's (Detroit) funding share forced it to close three of thirteen health centers (Elling 1988). This reallocation certainly did not make it easier for the City of Detroit to address its very high infant mortality rate.

Local Government Responses to Health Block Grant Cuts

Health block grant funding reductions were also replaced in some cases by an infusion of funds from local governments. The extent to which this occurred depended upon several factors. One was the extent to which particular program areas had previously received funds from local governments. Another was the extent to which states cushioned various cuts by increasing their own spending rather than passing the cuts on to local units of government and service providers. Third was economic—the ability of local governments to replace cuts.

Local governments, by and large, have less ability to replace cuts than the states. This is because local economies are less diverse than state economies. This makes them more vulnerable to economic downturns. Additionally, local decisions to increase spending or taxes so as to be able to replace cuts are much more likely to place a local jurisdiction at a competitive disadvantage as far as costs to businesses or homeowners are concerned. While states must also be sensitive to such issues, local governments—and especially large, older central cities—are particularly subject to this constraint on policy responsiveness. Moreover, even if localities might have wished to increase revenues to compensate for federal cuts, to do so by increasing existing taxes, or establishing new ones, often requires the concurrence of state government.

Interpretations

What determined the differential behavior of states and localities? First, state and local replacement efforts were conditioned by the interaction between a jurisdiction's fiscal capability and its dominant political ideology. Politically liberal jurisdictions in good fiscal condition would, thus, be expected to replace more of the federal cuts than poorer conservative ones.

But it wasn't quite as simple as this. Liberal ideology alone, or lack of fiscal pressure alone, didn't lead to replacement funding. One factor must be strong while the other is at least of intermediate strength. That is, a liberal state under only moderate fiscal stress, or one in good fiscal shape which is at least politically moderate, were most inclined to substantially replace lost federal dollars. In fact, the highest state "net replacement" of federal cuts occurred in Oklahoma (politically moderate, little fiscal pressure), Massachusetts and New York (politically liberal, moderate fiscal pressure), and New Jersey (politically liberal, little fiscal pressure). More liberal states, but not cities, still did something to replace some of the federal cuts regardless of fiscal pressure. One example was California, a politically liberal state, then under extreme fiscal pressure (Nathan, Doolittle, and Associates 1983). Perhaps an even better example was the politically liberal state of Michigan. Here, despite the fact that in 1982 and 1983 the state was under probably the greatest fiscal stress of any state in the nation, it nonetheless provided some replacement funding for Alcohol, Drug Abuse, Mental Health, and Maternal and Child Health programs (Elling 1988).

Why did health programs fare better than programs in other substantive areas? One reason is that these particular health programs were not generally perceived to be, although in fact they are to some extent, redistributive programs. They were not viewed as "public assistance," as "handouts," as programs which only benefit have-nots. This is important because programs that were perceived as redistributive generally fared least well as candidates for replacement funding (Nathan, Doolittle, and Associates 1983).

Second, programs that had a long history of state and local involvement, especially those antedating the federal role, or in which the state or local role was substantial, fared particularly well. Alcohol and drug abuse programs, mental health services, and many maternal and child health programs are generally programs in which state or local involvement are either longstanding, substantial, or both.

Critics of categorical grants typically argue that one of their undesirable qualities is that they include matching requirements that "seduce" states into spending more for an aided function than they "really" want to spend. Hence, block grant proponents have typically tried to eliminate such requirements. Indeed, neither the ADAMH nor PHHS block grants contained matching requirements. Yet it doesn't appear that elimination of these requirements has led to the kind of state or local funding reductions which the critics of categorical programs expected. One observer accounted for this surprise by arguing:

> Most states already are spending more than the amount necessary to capture the maximum federal contribution. At the margin, therefore, their spending is no longer being subsidized by federal matching incentives. For these cases, the conversion to block grants cannot be counted on to restrain state and local program spending. An asymmetry is at work. It may well be true, as the Reagan theory of grants hypothesizes, that the categorical matching grants offered by the federal government helped induce state-local expenditure growth in the first place. But it does not follow that the process can now be arrested by reversing the grant structure. The state programs are in place. They involve expenditures beyond the federal categorical grant ceiling. The structure of price incentives for most grants cannot be altered by block grants (Peterson 1984, 243).

In health, unlike some other program areas, the states were typically spending far more than required under categorical matching requirements.

A final factor conditioning the degree of state or local funding replacement was fundamentally political. Programs with a politically mobilized clientele, or which had a well-organized network of service providers, tended to fare better. One group of observers noted: ───────────

> The larger the stake providers have in a given social service, the more likely it is to win support in periods of retrenchment. . . . A number of operating grant programs that were cut in fiscal 1982 benefitted from organized lobbying by the providers of the services being funded. This was especially important for health programs. . . . Many of the providers of these public health. . . . services are skilled professionals, and in many states they have well-organized and politically strong "trade" associations (Nathan, Doolittle, and Associates 1983, 201).

Comparison of ADAMH Spending
and Other ADAMAHA Spending, FY81–88 ****

Fiscal Year

Program	1981*	1982	1983	1984	1985	1986	1987	1988
ADAMH	585	428	468	462	490	469	672	679
Other ADAMHA	541	343	344	388	439	461	640	757

TABLE 10–5

****SOURCE: Budget of the United States, Appendices, (FY84–90).

*FY81 is the spending for the predecessor programs now in each block grant.

The degree to which program supporters are mobilized also interacts with the history or degree of state involvement. Thus, the same scholars contend that the organization of health service providers:

> tends to have the greatest effect where a parallel state program exists. For some health and social services aided by federal grants, state financial support often exceeds federal aid, so the service providers involved are accustomed to lobbying at the state level (Nathan, Doolittle, and Associates 1983, 201).

For those who opposed block grants because they did not believe that the states had either the means or the will to even partly sustain health programs, the experience with the Reagan health block grants has to constitute surprisingly good news. But in trying to make this important point, we would be remiss not to note evidence which is bad news for those who desire to see public spending increased for the programs aided by the various health block grants. First of all, while the magnitude of federal cuts varied, there were always cuts *in constant dollars*. From the point of view of the Reagan administration, which pushed for such cuts, this was success. From the point of view of those who believe that the federal government should play an important role in providing the funding for health programs, this change from annual real increases of some magnitude under the old categoricals was a serious setback.

The federal cuts that did occur, while neither as substantial as in nonhealth areas, and ameliorated as they were in various ways, hurt. Block grant proponents were often inclined to argue that elimination of categorical constraints, simplification of administrative procedures, and unleashing of states and localities from close federal supervision would have benefits sufficient to allow fewer federal dollars to go farther (Williamson 1981). While it is indeed true that there were significant improvements in the administrative capacity of the states in the 1970s and 1980s (Thompson 1986), no disinterested observer believes that possible increases in programmatic or administrative efficiency associated with the transition from health categoricals to block grants were sufficient to counterbalance the cumulative reductions in real federal dollars that occurred.

One final point. Readers of table 10–3 will be easily persuaded that the PHHS block grant was "starved." Upon seeing that the MCH block grant grew from $455 to $527 million and the ADAMH block grant increased from $585 to $692 million, however, they may question the specific conclusion that shrinking dollars required program cuts and therefore also the general theory that Congress for political reasons resists funding block grants. The seeming paradox between the numbers and theory is, however, easily explained. First, as has previously been mentioned, the key issue is trends *in constant dollars,* and in these terms the block grants are still funded at a lower level than the previous programs.

More interestingly, there is also some important, albeit indirect, evidence that block grants continue to be unattractive as a programmatic form to Congress. Contrast the real, but minor, growth of the MCH block grant in recent years with the dramatic expansions of Medicaid to cover pregnant women and infants traced in other chapters of this book (Lipson Ch. 9; Fraser Ch. 16). Even more tellingly, as shown by table 10–5, funding for the ADAMH block grant has *fallen* relative to other federal programs administered by the Alcohol, Drug Abuse, and Mental Health Administration. This occurred despite the previously mentioned greater cut in other ADAMHA programs between FY81 and FY82. Recent growth of the MCH and ADAMH block grants demonstrates the heightened importance of these *subjects*—not an increased appreciation of the benefits of block grants by Congress.

REFERENCES

Conlan Timothy. 1988. *New federalism: Intergovernmental reform from Nixon to Reagan.* Washington, DC: The Brookings Institution.

Elazer, Daniel. 1984. *American federalism: A view From the states.* New York: Harper and Row. 3rd edition.

Elling, Richard. 1988. Federalist tool or federalist plot? Michigan responds to the Reagan block grants. In *The Midwest Response to the New Federalism,* edited by Peter Eisenger and William Gormley. Madison: University of Wisconsin Press.

Grodzins, Morton. 1966. *The American system: A new view of government in the United States.* Chicago: Rand McNally.

Ingram, Helen. 1977. Policy implementation through bargaining: The case of federal grants-in-aid. *Public Policy* 25:499–526.

Kettle, Donald. 1980. The management squeeze: Centralization and federal grants. Paper presented at the Annual Meeting of the Midwest Political Science Association. Chicago, Illinois, April 1980.

Nathan, Richard, Fred Doolittle and Associates. 1983. *The consequences of cuts: The effects of the Reagan domestic program on state and local government.* Princeton: Princeton Urban and Regional Research Center.

Niskanen, William. 1971. *Bureaucracy and representative government.* Chicago: Aldine Publishing Co.

Peterson, George. 1984. Federalism and the states: An experiment in decentralization. In *The Reagan record,* edited by John Palmer and Isabel Sawhill. Cambridge, MA: Ballinger.

Peterson, George E., Randal R. Bovbjerg, Barbara A. Davis, Walter G. Favis, Eugene C. Durman, and Theresa A. Gullo. 1986. *The Reagan block grants: What have we learned?* Washington, DC: Urban Institute Press.

Peterson, Paul. 1981. *City limits.* Chicago: University of Chicago Press.

Peterson, Paul, Barry Rabe and Kenneth Wong. 1986. *When federalism works.* Washington, DC: The Brookings Institution.

Radin, Beryl A. 1972. *Implementation, change and the federal bureaucracy.* New York: Teachers College Press, Columbia University.

Reagan, Michael, and John Sanzone. 1981. *The new federalism.* New York: Oxford University Press. 2nd edition.

Riker, William. 1964. *Federalism: Origin, operation, significance.* Boston: Little Brown and Co.

Robins, Leonard. 1974. *The conversion of categorical into block grants: A case study of the 314(d) Block Grant in the Partnership for Health Act.* Unpublished doctoral dissertation, University of Minnesota.

Stenberg, Carl. 1980. Federalism in transition: 1959–79. In *The future of federalism in the 1980s.* Washington, DC: Advisory Commission on Intergovernmental Relations.

Stenberg, Carl and David Walker. 1977. The block grant: Lessons from two early experiences. *Publius, The Journal of Federalism* 7:31–60.

Sundquist, James. 1969. *Making federalism work: A study of program coordination at the community level.* Washington,DC: The Brookings Institution.

Thompson, Frank. 1986. New federalism and health care policy: States and the old questions *Journal of Health Politics, Policy and Law* 10:657–669.

U. S. General Accounting Office. 1984. *Maternal and child health block grant: Program changes emerging under state administration.* Human Resources Division Report #84–35. Washington, DC: U. S. General Accounting Office, May 7.

U. S. General Accounting Office. 1984. *States have made few changes in implementing the alcohol, drug abuse, and mental health services block grant.* Human Resources Division Report #84–52. Washington, DC: U.S. General Accounting Office, June 6.

U. S. General Accounting Office. 1984. *States used added flexibility offered by the preventive health and health services block grant.* Human Resources Division Report #84–41. Washington, DC: U.S. General Accounting Office, May 8.

U. S. General Accounting Office. 1985. *Block grants brought funding changes and adjustments to program priorities.* Human Resources Division Report #85–46. Washington, DC: U. S. General Accounting Office, February 11.

Williams Walter. 1980. *Government by agency: Lessons from the social program grants-in-aid experience.* New York: Academic Press.

Williamson, Richard. 1981. Block grants: A federalist tool. *State Government* 54:114–117.

Wright, Deil. 1982. *Understanding intergovernmental relations.* 2d ed. Monterey, CA: Brooks Cole.

Part Three

The Role
of Interest Groups
and Public
Opinion

Chapter 11

Health Associations and the Legislative Process

Paul J. Feldstein

Many studies have been conducted to evaluate the effectiveness of U.S. federal subsidy programs in the medical care sector.[1] In examination of federal manpower subsidies to increase the number of dentists, it was found that an equivalent number of dental visits could have been produced, at less than one-tenth the cost, if the federal subsidies had been provided in a different manner, namely, if the wages of dental auxiliaries had been subsidized (Feldstein 1977). Evaluations of the federal Nurse Training Act revealed that an increase in the number of employed registered nurses could have been achieved at between one-fifth and one-tenth the cost had an alternative approach been used, namely, if the wages of registered nurses had been subsidized, thereby increasing their participation rate in the market (Feldstein 1977). These analyses of the federal manpower subsidy programs have questioned the justification offered for such programs, based, as it was, on the use of health-manpower-to-population ratios to indicate a "need" or "shortage." The method used to distribute the subsidy funds is also open to question. A possible conclusion is that further economic analysis is needed if governmental programs are to be cost-effective. The assumption is that with additional information, policymakers would generate better legislation. However, another interpretation of the type of health legislation that results from the legislative process is that the resulting legislation is actually what is intended. Under this hypothesis, the participants in the legislative process are assumed to have rational goals and to be aware of the effects of the legislation that is proposed. If the resulting legislation is not cost-effective, it is because it was not meant to be cost-effective.

An examination of the beneficiaries of such

---

[1]This chapter is based on the author's chapter, The Political economy of health care, in *Health Care Economics* (Feldstein 1988), and is based upon his earlier work, *Health Associations and the Demand for Legislation: The Political Economy of Health* (Feldstein 1977).

legislation lends support to this hypothesis. The major beneficiaries of health manpower legislation were the health professional schools, because they were the recipients of the vast majority of funds distributed.

If the legislation that results is the outcome intended by a rational and knowledgeable group of participants, then the prospects for improving the cost effectiveness of future health legislation by merely providing additional economic analyses of its intended effects is uncertain. To predict legislative outcomes, it becomes necessary to develop a model, not of the most cost-effective approach to achieving the stated objectives of the legislation, but rather of the supply and demand for legislation. In other words, a model of the political economy of health care is required (Feldstein 1988). A theoretical framework to explain the outcome of the legislation would include the following participants in the legislative process: legislatures and/or the particular legislative committee with jurisdiction over the proposed legislation; the health interest groups affected by the legislation, such as the American Hospital Association (AHA) and the American Medical Association; the bureaucracy that will administer the legislation; the executive branch of the federal government; and other interest groups such as industry and unions. Those who may be affected by the proposed legislation undoubtedly would like to influence it so that it coincides with their particular interests. For example, legislators favor (or propose) particular legislative actions because they improve their chances of being reelected: If the legislation is viewed favorably by their constituents or other proponents, support will be forthcoming to the legislators—in the form of campaign funds, volunteers for helping in the election campaign, or simply votes. The health interest organizations have a demand for legislation because it benefits their members. The demand for legislation by these interest groups, which is an indication of how much a group would be willing to "pay" for those legislative benefits (in terms of campaign funds, etc.), depends upon benefits the legislation provides beyond the legislative benefits the members of the group already possess. The cost of obtaining these legislative benefits, as determined by the direct monetary and nonmonetary outlays necessary to achieve them, depends,

among other things, on the action of other interested parties to the legislation. The greater the adverse affect of the legislation upon other interest groups, the greater will be their willingness to "pay" to forestall or defeat the proposed legislation, which in turn increases the cost of having such legislation passed. The cost of obtaining the legislation may well exceed the positive benefits to members of a group favoring the legislation, in which case they will be unsuccessful in achieving their legislative program.

Another interested participant in the legislative process is the bureaucracy that is to administer the legislation. Bureaucrats wish to see their own bureaucracies survive and grow, thereby justifying their larger salaries as both the size of their agencies and their responsibilities increase. The particular bureaucracy administering the legislation can promise benefits to legislators or to particular interest groups if the legislature increases the agency's budget. The executive branch of government, which has overall responsibility for the government budget, may have an interest in the legislation because of its effect on total government expenditures. The executive branch of government would like to start new programs so as to increase its own reelection chances. To do so, it may be interested in constraining expenditures on old programs, since new legislation would require additional dollars, which could come either from politically unpopular higher taxes or from underfunding current programs.

These are some of the participants in the legislative process. Other possible participants are industry and labor unions, who would be affected in their costs of production and in number of workers employed or wages, respectively. A complete model to explain the actual outcome of legislation would have to quantify the perceived benefits and the costs of the proposed legislation to all of these participants.

This chapter examines the legislative behavior of one of the participants in the legislative process: the health interest groups. The reason for selecting them is that in the past much of the health legislation at both state and federal levels has been strongly influenced by these groups. In fact, the structure of the U.S. health care system is, in many respects, the result of legislative activity by these health associations. Health interest groups often provide the only testimony on legislation; their positions are well publicized and are presented as being synonymous with that of the public interest. All legislation is complex and requires knowledgeable people to understand it. In the past, the public has been inclined to believe that health legislation is best understood by health professionals and, therefore, has been willing to accept the politics of health as espoused by health professionals.

The potential impact of health interest groups is enormous. From 1965 to 1985 state and federal expenditures on personal medical care rose from $7.7 billion to $148 billion a year. Total personal expenditures on medical care increased during this same period from $36 billion to $371 billion. Had the health legislation that was passed during this period been written in a different fashion—less to the liking of the health interest groups—health expenditures would likely have risen at a slower pace. This massive redistribution of income from patients and taxpayers to health professionals during this same period is an indication of the legislative success of health professionals. Yet few people would maintain that these massive increases in medical expenditures represented the most efficient means to increase health levels in the United States.

The belief that legislation can confer large monetary benefits to interest groups is not new. Nearly 200 years ago, in *The Federalist,* James Madison expressed this idea (Madison 1787). The reason special-interest legislation is enacted is that the economic interests of producers are concentrated whereas the economic interests of consumers are diffused over the many areas of economic activity. The benefits to special-interest groups from legislation are potentially so large as to provide them with ample incentive to secure legislation on their behalf. The cost to each consumer from special-interest group legislation is relatively small, since the costs are spread over a great many consumers. The proponents of such legislation are rarely so bold as to admit that their incomes will be increased by imposing what is the equivalent of a tax on all consumers of their products. Instead, such legislation is presented as being in the public's or country's interests.

Whereas producers often receive their entire incomes from the products they produce, consumers rarely spend more than a small portion of their income on any one product; thus, their economic interests are considered diffuse. Further, for consumers to learn of the special-interest legislation that is being proposed, to ascertain the effects of such legislation on the prices they must pay for the affected products, and to inform other consumers and mobilize them against such legislation is clearly more costly to the consumer than any monetary benefits that would be derived from having the legislation defeated.

The beneficiaries of special-interest group legislation have been documented in a number of studies: Milk producers benefit from milk marketing boards, domestic producers benefit from tariffs on imported goods, maritime workers benefit from maritime subsidies, and northern industrial workers benefit from federal minimum wage legislation. A less obvious but no less important interest group that has benefited from legislation is health associations. The activities of such associations and their success in the legislative marketplace have been virtually unnoticed.

Because expenditures for medical care are a relatively small percentage of consumers' incomes, it is to their advantage to allocate their time and efforts to other activities that have a greater impact on their budgets and incomes. For health professionals, however, health legislation may affect a good share of their income. It is, therefore, in their interests to be involved in the legislative process by contributing money and time to political campaigns, testifying at legislative hearings, and providing information to legislators and the public on their positions.

Most health legislation that is of importance to health associations has been at a state level. This is to the advantage of the health associations, since opponents would have to organize and bear the necessary costs of becoming involved in the legislative process 50 times rather than once. What makes it even more difficult for the consumer to become involved in health legislation at a state level is that such legislation does not outwardly appear to affect the consumers' dollars. State practice acts, which define the tasks to be performed by different health professionals and set the requirements for licensure, and state appropriations for medical, dental, and other health professional educational institutions, are policy decisions that appear to be too remote to affect the consumers' pocketbooks.

Demand for Legislation By Health Associations

To gain a better understanding of the type of health legislation that exists in the United States, it is necessary to develop a model of the demand for legislation by health interest groups. Such a framework should indicate the type of legislation different health associations would favor or oppose. If the framework presented is a fairly accurate predictor of the political behavior of different health associations, then it should also be possible to anticipate future legislative changes and the form that such legislation might take. The political behavior of two types of health associations will be examined: first, those health associations that represent the interests of health manpower professions, such as the American Medical Association, the American Dental Association, and the American Nurses' Association and, second, those associations that represent nonprofit providers, namely, the American Hospital Association, the Blue Cross Association (BCA), and the Association of American Medical Colleges (AAMC).

A framework of the demand for legislation will be presented to describe the specific types of health legislation that the various health associations desire. The necessity for having a framework is twofold: (1) It is not possible merely to state that health associations act in their own interests without first defining their interests, and (2) a model is required to indicate how particular legislation works to achieve those interests. Without such a framework, it is not always obvious how legislation promotes the interests of the health associations. The test of the validity of the proposed approach is how accurately the proposed framework predicts the political positions of the health associations. Finally, the implications of such a framework for explaining the political behavior of the health associations with regard to the structure, organization, and financing of medical care will be presented.

Several Caveats

Before discussing the economic model of political behavior, however, it is important to clarify certain situations in which the model would predict that an association would take a certain political position on legislation but it clearly ends up taking a different position. Before concluding that the economic framework is inaccurate, it must be determined whether the association's preferred position is no longer politically possible. For example, no health association favors reexamination for licensure. Some of its members may not be able to pass the exam. If the examination is made so simple that all members can pass, then nonmembers would claim that they should be allowed to enter the profession since they could pass the examination. If there is a great deal of pressure from the media for reexamination, the profession may propose a less costly alternative—continuing education. The association would not normally propose continuing education, since it imposes some costs on its members. However, to forestall an even more costly policy, the association comes out in favor of it. Thus the association's policy on continuing education, while not its preferred position, is consistent with the model's predictions.

Another example where it may appear that the political position of an association diverges from its members' interests occurs when the cost of taking a position exceeds its potential benefits. An association may be fearful that its continually negative position on legislation may be a greater cost to its members than any possible benefits to be derived from opposing it. An example of such a situation is the American Hospital Association's position on applying the minimum wage law to hospital employees. Minimum wage law can increase the cost of labor to hospitals. For many years, the AHA was successful in exempting hospitals from such legislation. When such legislation was once again proposed to include hospital workers, the AHA decided not to take a position. One reason is that hospital workers were being paid in excess of the minimum wage and so its effect on hospitals would have been small. More importantly, however, the AHA could see that this time such legislation was going to pass, and, therefore, it would be a needless loss of political capital to oppose the legislation. Similarly, in more recent years, the AMA has been muted in its opposition to certain legislation because of its concern that a continually negative position may be a greater cost to its members' interests than any possible benefits from opposing the legislation.

There are two other minor situations in which it may appear that the political positions of a health association diverge from the self-interest of its members. The first is when there has been a change in the perceived self-interest of the association's members. Such a change in self-interest would occur when the organization's very survival is threatened. An example of such a situation is Blue Cross's relationship to hospitals. Hospitals started Blue Cross to ensure payment for their services. In many cases, hospitals provided initial capital for Blue Cross, controlled the board of directors, and, until very recently, owned the Blue Cross emblem. One would therefore expect Blue Cross's self-interest to be synonymous with that of hospitals. However, during the last several years Blue Cross has come under attack for not performing its intermediary function adequately, that is, for not monitoring hospital costs or being an innovator in containing the rapid rise in hospital costs. Such behavior is not unexpected because hospitals controlled Blue Cross. But if Blue Cross is to survive as an intermediary under any national health insurance program, then it must demonstrate that it can do more than merely reimburse hospitals. In order to create a new image for itself and survive, Blue Cross has become an adversary of hospitals. Blue Cross's political positions have shifted during the last several years as it has had to redefine its self-interest in order to convince a skeptical group made up of government officials, legislators, unions, and industry that it can perform as an intermediary and should not be replaced in this function by a government agency. A similar situation has occurred with Blue Shield and its relationship to organized medicine.

The second example of an association not opposing legislation that is inimical to the interests of its members occurs when it decides to go along with the desires of other health associations in hopes of receiving their support for legislation that is of greater importance to its members' interests. Such trade-offs would not be a

refutation of the model's prediction that health associations act in their members' interests regardless of the effect on the "pubic" interest.

Definition of Health Association Members' Self-Interest

Since the predictions made by the economic framework are based on the premise that the health association will demand legislation according to the self-interest of its members, it is necessary to define more precisely the self-interest of the different health associations to be analyzed.

Whether legislation has a positive, negative, or neutral effect on the association members' self-interest depends upon what the members perceive their interests to be.

When defining self-interest for a large number of health professionals such as physicians, dentists, and nurses or for organizations that may be quite diverse even though they are considered to be one type of institution such as hospitals, there is a natural tendency to make the definition complex so that it encompasses the diversity. If, however, the self-interest goals are complex or if new goals are specified for each separate piece of legislation, then it is not possible to develop a good predictive model. However satisfying a complex goal statement may be, it is easier to evaluate the effect of legislation using a relatively simply defined goal. Besides, unless the goal that the association is pursuing is easy for its membership to understand, the members may be distressed over the activities on which the association is spending their dues. The true test of whether the specified goal of the association is an accurate measure of the self-interest of its membership is how well the model is able to predict the legislative behavior of the association.

For purposes of this discussion, it is assumed that the legislative goals of the association are maximization of the incomes of its current members. Although health professionals have many goals, income is the only goal that all the health professionals in an association have in common. (Increased autonomy and control may be another goal, but it is highly correlated with increased incomes. Income is thus a more general goal.)

The goals or "self-interest" of the associations representing the nonprofit institutions (AHA, BCA, AAMC, and American Association of Dental Schools—AADS) must differ from those of the health professional associations, since such organizations cannot retain any "profits." Hospitals and medical and dental schools are assumed to be interested in maximizing their prestige. Prestige for hospitals is seen in terms of their size and the numbers and types of facilities and services. The availability of a full range of facilities and services also makes it easier for a hospital to attract physicians to its staff. Administrators of large prestigious hospitals are held in esteem by their peers and earn high incomes. Prestige for a medical school is usually defined as having students who wish to enter one of the specialties, most probably to become teachers and researchers themselves, having a faculty that is primarily interested in research, and having a low student-faculty ratio. Little prestige accrues to a medical school that trains students to enter general practice or practice in a rural area.

Blue Cross plans have a goal other than that of profit or prestige: It is assumed that Blue Cross seeks to maximize its growth in enrollment and revenues. A larger organization provides management with greater responsibility, which justifies greater management incomes. It is further assumed that prestigious hospitals and medical schools and large Blue Cross plans also have some form of satisficing behavior as a goal. For example, a Blue Cross plan with a high percentage of the health insurance market in its area can afford to be less concerned with efficiency. In prestigious hospitals and medical schools, the return to efficiency similarly falls as the organization approximates its prestige goals.

Although there are differences in the objectives of the health associations, the members of these associations all try to make as much money as possible, either to retain it themselves, as in the case of health professionals, or to expend it to achieve either prestige or growth goals. Thus, the model of demand for legislation is the same for all health associations. Basically, each health association attempts to achieve for its members through legislation what cannot be achieved through a competitive market, namely, a monopoly position. Increased monopoly power and the ability to price as would a monopolist seller of services is the best way for associations to achieve their goals.

Health Association Legislation

Specifically, there are five types of legislation a health association will demand. Four of these legislative actions have the effect of increasing the association members' revenues whereas the fifth should decrease the members' costs of operation. Legislation to increase revenues is legislation that does the following: (1) increases the demand for the members' services, (2) causes an increase in the price of service that substitutes for those services produced by the members, (3) limits entry into the industry, and (4) enables the providers to charge the highest possible price for their services, such as by preventing competition based on prices and by charging different prices according to different purchasers' willingness to pay (i.e., price discrimination). Legislative policies that lower the provider's cost of operation are as follows: (1) subsidies to the inputs used in the production of the providers' services and (2) changes in the state practice acts that allow for greater productivity of the inputs used in production. Each of these legislative policies will be discussed in more detail, and illustrative examples of legislative behavior of the various health associations will be given.

Demand-Increasing Legislation

An increase in demand along a given supply curve will result in an increase in price, an increase in total revenue, and, consequently, an increase in income or net revenue. The most obvious way of increasing the demand for the services of an association's members is to have the government subsidize the purchase of insurance for the provider's services. But rather than government coverage for all persons in the population, such as is done in the British National Health Service, the demand for insurance subsidies in the United States is always discussed in relation to specific population groups in society, namely, those persons with low incomes. The reason for selective government subsidies is twofold: First, those persons with higher incomes presumably have private insurance coverage or can afford to purchase the provider's services. The greatest increase in demand would result from extending coverage to those currently unable to pay for the services. Second, extending government subsidies to those currently able to pay for the services would greatly increase the cost of the program to the government. Greater commitment of government expenditures would result in greater government control over the provider's prices and use. Thus, for the purpose of increasing the demand for the provider's services, government subsidies are always requested in relation to specific population groups rather than for the population at large.[2] A related point is that health associations always want an intermediary between the government and the provider of services. The reason is the fear that the government would otherwise interfere in the setting of prices.

An example of such demand-increasing policies is the AMA's program for national health insurance (NHI), which proposed demand subsidies for low-income groups. A further example of what is preferred by the health professional associations is the AMA's Blue Shield plan. The AMA initially started and controlled Blue Shield. Blue Shield only provided coverage for physician services and covered the patient's entire bill only if the patient's income was below a certain level. The physician was able to charge patients with higher incomes an amount above the Blue Shield fee. In this way, the physician was able to price discriminate, a factor that will be discussed in the following section.

Similarly, the ANA, whose members must work for other providers, has favored demand-increasing proposals that increase the demand for those institutions in which registered nurses work. Increased demand for hospital care will result in increased demand for registered nurses. The ANA has also favored policies that would increase the demand for registered nurses (RNs) directly, such as requiring increases in the use of RNs in hospitals and nursing homes. Another demand proposal favored by nurses is one that would increase their roles, that is, increase the number of tasks they would be permitted to per-

form. If they are successful in this strategy, the demand for nurses will increase because their value will have increased in that they will be able to do more renumerative tasks. Because nurses will be able to be used more flexibly than before, one nurse can then perform the tasks that might have required the hiring of two different types of health professionals. As nurses and other health professionals try to increase their roles, they also wage a struggle in the legislative marketplace to prevent other health professionals from competing with them. One example is the attempt by optometrists to increase their role at the expense of ophthalmologists and restrict ophthalmologists to surgical tasks. The health professional association that is successful in enabling its members to increase their role while preventing other health professionals from encroaching upon that role will assure an increased demand for its members' services and, consequently, higher incomes.

A major attempt by the AHA to increase its demand has been the establishment and control of the Blue Cross Association. Blue Cross originally paid for the costs of hospital care only, thereby lowering the costs of hospital care to consumers and increasing their demand for such services. Blue Cross also reimbursed hospitals in a manner preferred by hospitals. Later, the AHA favored government subsidies for the aged under Medicare, which would have increased the demand for hospital care by a high user population with generally low incomes. In doing so, the AHA sought government payment for such services through an intermediary (their own Blue Cross Association) rather than directly from the government, which would have gotten the government more directly involved with the hospitals' charges for Medicare patients.

Securing the Method of Highest Reimbursement

Whether the association members' goal is income, prestige, or growth, the method by which the provider is reimbursed is crucial to the attainment of that goal. High prices, netting larger revenues and increased incomes, facilitate the achievement of institutional objectives through the expenditure of those revenues. There are two basic approaches to being able to secure the

---

[2]Even when demand subsidies are requested for a particular population group, it is proposed that such demand subsidies be phased in gradually. If the increase in demand is too large, this might create dissatisfaction among the patients because of the limited supply; prices and waiting times would tend to increase rapidly, possibly resulting in pressure on the government to enter the market. If the increase in demand is large, it may result in pressure to cause a greater increase in the number of providers than the association believes is in the best economic interests of its members.

highest possible reimbursement for services. The first is to charge different patients or payors different prices according to their ability to pay. This method of pricing (price discrimination) results in greater revenues than will a system of charging all patients the same price. The second approach is to preclude price competition among competing providers. Essential to price competition is the provider's ability to advertise differences in prices and any other measures of differences in service, such as availability and competency. Price competition is most important for new practitioners or firms entering the area who must let potential patients know they are available and be able to attract them away from established providers. To prevent such competition from occurring, health professional associations banned advertising and other forms of competition in their practice acts and sanctioned such "unethical" behavior by suspending practitioners' licenses and assessing penalties. Since such competitive behavior is not necessarily related to low quality, the inclusion of competitive behavior as part of the unethical practices for which a practitioner can be penalized can only be interpreted as a means of preventing price competition among providers.

Physicians and dentists have a strong preference for "usual, customary and reasonable" (UCR) fees. Such a method of pricing essentially lets the providers charge what the market will bear. Patients with higher incomes (who would be willing to pay more) can thus be charged higher fees than those with lower incomes, as has been the case with the use of Blue Shield income limits. In Kessel's (1958) classic article, "Price Discrimination in Medicine," he describes how county and state medical societies attempted to forestall the development of prepaid group practices, which are a form of massive price cutting since they offer to provide medical services at the same price to all people regardless of income. Similarly, Blue Shield in Spokane, Washington, boycotted physicians if they offered their services through a health maintenance organization (HMO). It ended its boycott only when ordered to do so by the Federal Trade Commission (FTC), acting on its belief that it was an anticompetitive tactic. The method that is proposed for payment of providers under proposed legislation is often

crucial to its acceptance by the provider association.

The fee-for-service approach, based on UCR fees and used so successfully by the AMA, is being imitated by other health professional associations. Registered nurses are striving to become nurse practitioners who will be able to bill the patient directly under the fee-for-service approach. The ANA has attempted to secure such an amendment to the Medicare law. Other health professionals have also tried to gain the authority to bill according to fee-for-service. Such an approach, using UCR fees, which in most cases are reimbursed by the government or other third party payor, is the most direct route for a health profession to increase its income.

The methods of reimbursement favored by the AHA for its members are ones that either discourage or do not provide consumers with any incentive to compare prices among different hospitals and methods that enable the hospitals to charge different payors different prices for their services.

When hospitals started the Blue Cross Association, Blue Cross plans were required to offer consumers a service benefit plan. A service benefit provides the hospitalized patient with services rather than dollars. In so doing, it actually provides the consumer with an incentive to enter the most expensive hospital, since the services at such a hospital, which are presumably of higher quality, will not cost the consumer anything extra. Thus, under a service benefit policy, hospitals cannot compete for patients on the basis of prices.

If hospitals are to be able to generate sufficient funds to expand their facilities and services, then they must be able to set prices in excess of their costs. The manner in which this is done is to charge different prices to different payors and to set prices for different services according to what the market will bear, that is, according to price elasticity of demand. Hospitals thus prefer multiple sources of payment, rather than one major purchaser of their services, so that they can charge some payors higher prices for the same services. An example of this pricing behavior is to charge commercial insurers and patients responsible for their own bills higher rates than those charged to Blue Cross (which receives a discount) or to Medicare (which pays on the basis of fixed prices per admission). Another method by which the hospital is able to use price discrimination in its rate setting is to set higher price-cost ratios for those services for which the demand is believed to be more price inelastic, such as ancillary services, than for services that are price elastic, such as obstetrics. That hospitals have used their pricing strategy to their benefit can be seen by the large increase in net revenues after Medicare was instituted. This resulted both from the favorable payments terms and from the inclusion in their reimbursement structure of previously unreimbursable expenses, such as unfunded depreciation.

The use of community rating, which was originally used by Blue Cross as a means of setting premiums, may also be viewed as a method of price discrimination. Under community rating, all groups are charged the same premium regardless of their utilization experience. High-user groups are thus subsidized by low-user groups. High-user groups were also, in many cases, large unions, such as the UAW, who could switch to other insurers or even self insure if they were not provided insurance at low premiums. This method of pricing resulted in the largest enrollment for Blue Cross.

Medical and dental schools, as stated earlier, would prefer to receive large unrestricted government subsidies rather than charge their students the full educational costs. The government, for one reason, has a much greater ability to pay than does the individual student. Further, unrestricted operating subsidies allow the school to produce the type of education the faculty prefers without having to respond to the demands of students. That the schools have been relatively successful in charging the government a monopoly price for their services is an observation supported by data that indicate that public medical schools receiving state support have higher per student costs than do private schools. Medical and dental schools are opposed to the government's providing those same subsidies directly to the student. If government subsidies went directly to the student, the student would be able to select the school and the schools would have to compete for students.

Under the current system of providing subsidies, the student can receive a subsidy only by attending a subsidized school. The current system guarantees the survival of the schools and requires the students, not the schools, to compete. Similar to their preference for receiving operating subsidies, the schools prefer to distribute loans and scholarships themselves rather than having the students apply directly to the government for such financial assistance.

Legislation to Reduce the Price and/or Increase the Quantity of Health Manpower Complements

In medical care it is difficult to know when an input, such as a nurse, is a complement or a substitute based just on the task to be performed. A nurse may be as competent as a physician to perform certain tasks; if the nurse works for the physician, however, and the physician receives the fee for the performance of the task, then the nurse is a complement and will increase the physician's productivity. If, however, the nurse performs the same task and is a nurse practitioner operating and billing independently of the physician, then the nurse is a substitute for the physician in providing that service. The essential element in determining whether an input is a complement or a substitute is who controls the use of that input and who receives reimbursement for the services provided by that input.

The legal authority for the different tasks each health profession can perform and the source of stipulations defining under whose direction health professionals must work are the state practice acts. A major legislative activity for each health association is to seek changes in the state practice acts; health associations representing complements attempt to have their members become substitutes, whereas other health associations whose members currently control complements seek to retain the status quo. For the physician, almost all of the health professions and health institutions are complements; nurses and optometrists are examples of professionals who desire to expand their scope of practice and to practice independently of physicians.

With an increase in the demand for health services, providers can increase their incomes if that increased demand is met through greater productivity on their part rather than through an increase in the number of competing providers. The providers' incomes can be increased still further if their productivity increases are subsidized and if they do not have to pay the full cost of increasing their productivity. Examples of legislation that would have the effect of subsidizing increased productivity are educational subsidies, capital subsidies, and changes in the state practice acts to permit greater delegation of tasks. The AHA, for example, has favored the Nurse Training Act (NTA), which in subsidizing the training of RNs resulted in a greater supply of nurses. With a greater number of nurses, nurses' wages would be lower than they might otherwise have been. The AHA has favored both the Hill-Burton program, which provided capital subsidies to modernize hospitals, and educational subsidies to increase the supply of allied health professionals. The AHA has opposed legislative actions that would have increased the hospitals' costs of inputs. It opposed the extension of minimum wage legislation to hospital employees and has called for a moratorium on the separate licensing of each health professional. (Separate licensing of each health professional would limit the hospital's ability to substitute persons and to use such persons in a more flexible manner.)

The AMA has similarly favored both subsidies to hospitals, because hospitals are inputs to physicians, and increases in the supply of RNs under the Nurse Training Act. However, the AMA has opposed the increased educational standards that the ANA wanted to impose on nursing institutions as a condition for receiving funds under the Nurse Training Act. Higher educational standards for nurses do not necessarily increase the productivity of nurses, but they do limit the supply of nurses and increase the nurse's qualifications as a potential substitute for the physician.

An interesting example of the AMA's attitude toward a new complement was its position on the physician's assistant (PA). Physician's assistants are potential substitutes for the physician if they practice independently. Thus, the AMA wanted to ensure that the fee from services rendered by the PA always went to the physician. In fact, whether there was direct or indirect supervision of the PA was less important to the AMA in determining its political position toward this new category of health professionals than was who received the fee. Another important characteristic

of the AMA's attitude toward the use of PAs was whether or not the introduction of such personnel in an area would have created excess capacity among physicians in the community, resulting in greater competition among them for patients. If the physician did not have sufficient demand to keep as busy as he or she would have liked, then the introduction of inputs that increase the physician's productive capacity would be against the interest of those physicians who want to be busier. The tendency by the health professions to permit productivity changes to occur have been more related to changes in the demand for their services than to issues related to quality.

One would expect to find those state practice acts with the least delegatory authority in those states in which there is the lowest level of demand per practitioner. The introduction of new types of health professionals and methods to increase productivity has been related more to local demand conditions than to the competence of such personnel to perform the tasks for which they were trained.

The AAMC has been relatively successful in its demands for input subsidies. Medical schools have received subsidies for construction, research (which has been used to subsidize teaching programs), teaching hospitals, and the cost of education. The subsidies received from state governments are unrestricted; however, to receive federal capitation grants the schools had to provide for small enrollment increases. The enrollment increase requirement was later changed and instead the medical schools had to ensure that a certain percentage of their graduating class practiced in underserved areas. The schools have opposed all conditions attached to receiving government subsidies. It is not surprising that the schools have been more successful in their legislative efforts at a state level than at a federal level, where it is relatively easier for opponents to lobby against the schools with Congress.

In the 1970s pressures for cost containment began to increase. However, instead of directly attempting to lower the price of its major input-hospital costs, Blue Cross's main political activity was directed toward the development and strengthening of hospital planning agencies. Because Blue Cross reimbursed hospitals according to their costs, hospitals had an incentive to add facilities and services and merely pass those costs on to Blue Cross and its subscribers, who then had to pay higher health insurance premiums. In a number of cases, the addition of facilities and services, and even bed capacity, was duplicative in the community in which they were built. Hospitals competed among themselves for physicians and patients. (And since the hospitals were reimbursed on an individual cost basis and the patient had no incentive under a service benefit policy to select the lowest-cost hospital, the process of adding duplicate beds and facilities could continue.) Blue Cross's premium consisted almost entirely of the costs of hospital care. To remain competitive against commercial insurance companies whose premiums were based upon a smaller portion of hospital care and whose policies did not reimburse patients for the complete costs of their hospitalization, it was in Blue Cross's interests to keep the cost of hospital care (both hospital use and the cost per unit) from rising.

Because of the traditional relationship Blue Cross had with hospitals, it was difficult for Blue Cross to control hospital costs directly. An alternative, indirect approach to restraining the cost of the Blue Cross premium, and one that would not have been opposed by the major hospitals served by Blue Cross, was to prevent the development of new hospitals and the expansion of beds and facilities in smaller existing hospitals. The existing large hospitals either had the latest facilities and services or would have been the likely candidates to receive the planning agency's approval to add such facilities. As a means of restraining competition, these large hospitals favored the strengthening of planning agencies. Limiting the increase in hospital beds and the addition of services, whose costs Blue Cross would have had to pay even if they were duplicative, would have held down both hospital use and Blue Cross premiums. Although Blue Cross was a strong advocate of limiting hospital use and duplicative facilities and services, its efforts had not been very successful in limiting the rise in hospital costs.

Legislation to Decrease the Availability and/or Increase the Price of Substitutes

Any health association will attempt to have the price of a service increased (or its availability de-

creased) that is considered to be a substitute for the services delivered by its members. If it is successful in doing so, then the demand for services provided by its members will be increased. Three general approaches are used in the legislative arena to accomplish these goals. The first is to have the substitute service declared illegal. If substitute health professionals are not permitted to practice or if substitutes are severely restricted in the tasks they are legally permitted to perform, then there will be a shift in demand away from the substitute service. The second approach, usually used when the first one is unsuccessful, is to exclude the substitute service from payment coverage by a third party, including any government health programs. This latter policy raises the price of the substitute to a person who is eligible to purchase that service under the third-party coverage. The last approach is to try and raise the costs of the substitute, thereby causing the substitute to increase its prices. The following examples illustrate the political behavior of health associations in each of these areas.

For many years, the AMA regarded osteopaths as cultists. It was considered unethical for physicians to teach in schools of osteopathy. Unable to prevent their licensure at a state level, however, the AMA attempted to deny osteopaths hospital privileges. A physician substitute is less than adequate if that substitute cannot provide a complete range of treatment. As osteopaths developed their own hospitals and educational institutions, the medical societies decided that the best approach to controlling this potential increase in the supply of physician substitutes was to merge with the osteopaths, make them physicians, and thereby eliminate any future increases in their supply. An example of this approach, which was used in California until it was overturned by the California Supreme Court, was to allow osteopaths to convert their Doctor of Osteopathy degree to a Doctor of Medicine degree on the basis of 12 Saturday refresher courses. After a merger between the medical and osteopathic societies occurred in California, the Osteopathic Board of Examiners was no longer permitted to license osteopaths.

Optometrists and chiropractors are potential substitutes for ophthalmologists and family practitioners. One approach used by the AMA toward such substitutes has been to attempt to raise their price relative to that of physicians. Medicare, which reduces the price of physician services to the aged under Part B, has been the vehicle for much legislative competition. The AMA has long fought to prevent both the optometrists and chiropractors from qualifying as providers under Part B, thereby effectively raising their price to the aged relative to that of physicians, whose services are reimbursable.

An example of the legislative behavior of dental societies toward substitute providers is illustrated by dentistry's actions toward denturists. Denturism is the term applied to the fitting and dispensing of dentures directly to patients by persons who are not licensed as dentists. Independently practicing denturists are a threat to dentists' incomes, since they offer dentures at lower prices than do dentists. Dentists have, however, been successful in having denturism declared illegal. (Denturists are legal in seven out of Canada's 10 provinces. As a result of their success in Canada, denturists in the United States have become bolder by attempting to have certain state practice acts changed to permit them to practice.) Occasionally, denturists illegally sell dentures to patients. To combat this potential competition, local dental societies, such as those in Texas, responded in two ways: First, they offered to provide low-cost dentures to low-income people, and, second, they pressured state officials to enforce state laws against illegal denturists.

A special ADA commission set up to study the threat of denturists reported that the number of people who are edentulous is much greater in the lower-income levels, and it is among these people that the denturists have met with great success in selling low-cost dentures. An editorial in the Journal of the American Dental Association (1976, 665) commenting on this special study commission's report proposed the following:

> Organized dentistry should set up some system for supplying low-cost dentures to the indigent or the near indigent all over the [United States], but especially in those states where the legislatures are considering bills that would allow dental mechanics to construct dentures and deliver them directly to the patient. . . . This is the type of program that would have a favorable impact on the public—not to mention legisla-

tors. . . . The supplying of dentures to low income patients by qualified dentists at a modest fee (or even at no fee in special cases) and in quantities meeting the public demands would go a long way toward heading off the movement for legalized denturists.

It is only the threat of competition that results in the dental profession's offer to provide low-cost dentures to the indigent or near indigent. If this competitive threat by denturists is eliminated through dentistry's successful use of the state's legal authority, the net effect will be to cause the public to pay higher prices for dentures.

One of the most important substitutes for registered nurses training in this country is the foreign-trained RN. Because nursing salaries are considerably higher in the United States than in many other countries, there is a financial incentive for foreign nurses to come to the United States. The manner in which the ANA has tried to decrease the availability of a low-cost substitute for United States trained nurses has been to make it more difficult for foreign nurses to enter the United States. The ANA has attempted to have the Department of Labor remove the preferential status of foreign nurses from the immigration regulations. The ANA has also proposed that foreign nurses who wish to enter the United States be screened by examination in their home country before being allowed to enter. The ANA's advocacy of screening before admittance to the United States, where the nurses would again be screened by having to pass state board examinations, is consistent with a policy of reducing the inflow of foreign nurses. If the screening examination were administered in the United States, then foreign nurses could still work in some nursing capacity even if they did not pass the examination, and they could then retake it in the future. Establishing an additional screening mechanism before nurses emigrate erects another barrier to nurses' entering the United States; if they do not pass the examination, they are unlikely to emigrate.

Another legislative tactic used by the ANA is to prevent other personnel from undertaking nursing tasks performed by RNs. The ANA has opposed policies that would have permitted physicians to have greater delegatory authority over which personnel can perform nursing tasks; the ANA has opposed permitting licensed practical nurses to be in charge of skilled nursing homes, since this would cause substitutions for RNs who currently perform such functions; the California Nurses' Association opposed a bill that would have authorized fire fighters with paramedic training to give medical and nursing care in hospital emergency departments; and the ANA, as a means of preventing PAs from moving into a role that the ANA would like to see reserved for RNs, has favored a licensing moratorium. Such a moratorium would prevent any new health personnel from being licensed to undertake tasks that RNs perform or would like to be permitted to perform.

Examples of the approach used by the AHA to raise the price of substitutes has been to oppose free-standing surgicenters and to attempt to raise the relative price of for-profit hospitals to patients. Surgicenters are outpatient surgical facilities and, therefore, low-cost substitutes for hospitals. Any increase in the use of surgicenters will decrease the demand for inpatient care. In order to limit the availability of such low-cost substitutes, hospitals have argued that surgicenters should be permitted only when they are developed in association with hospitals. In this manner, hospitals would be able to control the growth of a competitive source of care, and they would be able to benefit (since presumably they would operate the substitute service) as such surgicenters develop. Hospitals also favored including surgicenters under certificate-of-need legislation. If such substitutes were subject to the approval of planning agencies, which are heavily influenced by the hospitals in the community, then it is unlikely that a low-cost substitute would be permitted to develop. Existing hospitals have claimed that the growth of these institutions would leave them with excess inpatient surgical facilities, which, under cost-based reimbursement, the community (through Blue Cross) would have to pay for anyway.

Methods used by nonprofit hospitals to raise the cost of a substitute are to oppose the granting of tax-exempt status to for-profit hospitals, thereby raising their costs, and to oppose granting Blue Cross eligibility to for-profit hospitals or even to new nonprofit hospitals when the existing nonprofit hospitals claim that there are sufficient beds in an area. Denying third-party reimbursement to potential or actual competitors in effect precludes the use of the facilities by patients whose costs of hospitalization would be reimbursed if they entered a hospital that was eligible for Blue Cross reimbursement.

The political position of Blue Cross with respect to substitutes is similar. Blue Cross has been in favor of excluding, by law, the Social Security Administration (SSA) from being able to compete with Blue Cross and Blue Shield as intermediaries under any government payment program. Further, Blue Cross opposed granting to commercial insurers the tax-exempt status that Blue Cross plans once enjoyed, which caused their competitors' costs to be increased.

Legislation to Limit Increases in Supply

Essential to the establishment of a monopoly position are limits on the number of providers of a service. The justification given by health associations for supply-control policies is that they ensure high-quality care to patients. At the same time, however, these health associations oppose quality measures that would have an adverse effect upon existing providers. This apparent anomaly—stringent entry requirements and then virtually no quality-assurance programs directed at existing providers—can be consistent only with a policy that seeks to establish a monopoly position for existing providers. If the health associations were consistent in their desire to improve and maintain high-quality standards, they should favor all policies that ensure quality, regardless of the affects on their members' incomes. Quality control measures directed at existing providers, such as reexamination, relicensure, and monitoring of the care actually provided, would adversely affect the incomes of some providers; more importantly, such "outcome" measures of quality assurance would make many of the entry and process requirements unnecessary, thereby permitting larger numbers of providers into the industry.

The following examples illustrate measures to assure quality that are in the economic interests of the members of a health association and those that are not and are, therefore, opposed by the association. The health professions are always in favor of licensing. The profession ends up controlling the licensure process by setting the necessary requirements for licensure and having members of the profession itself comprise the licensing board. Once licensing requirements have been legislated at a state level, the profession, through its representatives on the licensing board, imposes additional requirements. The major requirement is that before any person can take a licensing examination, he or she must have had a specified education, usually of a minimum number of years (which keeps increasing), and this education must have taken place in an educational institution approved by the profession or its representatives. The number of educational institutions is always limited so that, as in medicine and dentistry, there is continually an excess demand by applicants for admission. Limiting the number of educational spaces and specifying an educational curriculum that imposes training requirements in excess of the skills required to practice in the profession reduces the number of people who can take the licensing examination. If licensure merely required passing an examination, then potential practitioners could secure the necessary knowledge in a number of different ways, in different lengths of time, and in different institutions. In such a situation, the number of people who could potentially take the examination and pass it would be much greater than if the number of those applying to take the examination were limited by the number of approved educational spaces.

The foregoing policies have been successfully developed in medicine and dentistry. Nursing is also moving in this direction through attempts to require that nursing education take place only in colleges that offer a baccalaureate degree. Previously, the predominant place of education for a nursing degree was in a diploma school, generally operated in conjunction with a hospital. By proposing that the educational requirement for nursing be increased, the ANA must be well aware that fewer nurses will be trained since the costs of training have increased. The ANA also must be aware that with the additional training it would presumably be easier to justify having nurses perform additional tasks, thereby increasing nurses' incomes.

At times the professions impose requirements on new entrants into the profession that are blatant barriers to entry. Examples were U.S. citizenship requirements for foreign medical and dental graduates in order to practice in some states and a one year residency requirement if a duly trained and licensed professional, such as a dentist, wished to practice in another state, such as Hawaii. These requirements cannot be remotely related to a concern for quality. The current method of quality assurance for health professionals is aimed solely at entry into the profession rather than at monitoring the quality of care provided by health professionals. The inadequate performance of state licensing boards in disciplining their members is evidence of this practice. The public is less protected against unethical and incompetent practitioners than it has been led to believe.

Hospitals, medical and dental schools, and Blue Cross plans are also advocates of supply-control policies, since they provide these institutions with a monopoly position in their market. Since such institutions cannot achieve a monopoly position through the normal competition of the marketplace, they seek to achieve it through legislation. Large hospitals favored certificate-of-need (CON) legislation. The CON agencies, which were often controlled by the administrators of the large existing hospitals, have used their legislative authority to limit the growth of potential hospital competitors. With fewer providers in a community, patients have less choice among providers and the existing providers are more easily able to increase their costs and prices. The survival of existing hospitals is more likely to be assured, since competing hospitals will have been excluded. Larger hospitals are likely to be favored over smaller hospitals in their requests for the addition of specialized facilities. Because many specialized facilities are useful to a limited number of patients in the community, it is likely that a larger hospital will be able to justify having the facility more easily than will a smaller one; also, larger hospitals are more likely to have complementary facilities that may be required for new specialized services. The CON legislation did not control the increase in hospital costs; it merely restricted expansion and additions to capacity and facilities.

Concluding Comments

Because the members of each health association cannot achieve a monopoly position through the normal competitive process, they seek to achieve it through legislation. They then attempt to improve their monopoly position by further demanding legislation that will increase the demand for their services, permit them to price as would a price-discriminating monopolist, lower their costs of doing business, and disadvantage their competitors, either by causing them to become illegal providers or by raising their prices. Health associations have been relatively successful in the legislative arena, as is indicated by the large sums of money being spent on their services and by their members' positions in society's income distribution. What are the costs or implications to the rest of society of the success of these interest groups in the legislative marketplace?

The Outlook for Legislative Change in Medical Care

The incentive and reason for the legislative success of health associations is that the benefits to their members are greater than the costs imposed on individual consumers. Proposed legislative changes that would remove the monopoly protection that members of health associations currently enjoy would be difficult to achieve. Because the members of the health associations have more to lose than the individual has to gain from such legislative changes, they will be more involved in trying to prevent such legislative changes.

Are there alternative approaches to structural change in the delivery system that will achieve the twin goals of quality assurance and minimum cost? One proposal that has been suggested is to place consumers on health institutions and licensing boards. This is a false panacea. Even assuming that consumer representatives would know the most efficient manner of structuring the delivery system (which is unlikely), it is improbable that they would be effective. Consumers are currently represented on all the boards mentioned. To date, consumer representatives have not made Blue Cross plans more aggressive in their monitoring of hospital costs, they have not been able to deter their hospitals from establishing duplicative facilities and services, nor

have they moved licensing boards to become more active in disciplining their errant members. Consumers are usually nominated by the professions or administrators of the institutions themselves, and it is far easier to remove a particular board member than for a particular board member to change the performance of the profession. Consumers also do not have all the necessary information; they must rely on the professionals and administrators themselves for the appropriate information. Thus it is difficult to conclude that improved performance of an institution or a profession will be related to the number of consumers on their boards.

Another approach that has been suggested to improve the performance of the delivery system is to have greater government intervention and regulation of the industry or profession. When one examines the performance of regulatory agencies in other fields, it can be observed that these agencies rarely perform in the consumer's interests. Such agencies are either captured by the industries they are meant to regulate or respond in a manner that seeks to minimize outside conflict. There is no reason to believe that health care regulatory agencies would perform any differently. A growing body of evidence with regard to certificate-of-need agencies and state agencies responsible for regulating nursing homes has not produced the hoped for accomplishments. It is unlikely that additional government regulation would succeed any better.

Certain other developments may have some beneficial effects in the legislative marketplace. The first of these is the involvement of a greater number of interest groups in the legislative process. The success of the AMA and the ADA has not gone unnoticed by other health professional associations. Greater competition among health associations in the legislative process is occurring. As more health associations attempt to increase the benefits to their members through changes in the various state practices acts, the cost to the AMA and ADA of preventing such changes increases. The possible gains to these other health associations from becoming substitutes for, rather than complements to, the physician and dentist are very large. They are becoming more willing to assess their members the necessary costs to compete for legislative changes.

Other interest groups that are becoming more active are industry, unions, and the federal and state governments themselves. As the costs of health care continue to rise at a rapid rate, such costs, when embodied in wage agreements as fringe benefits, are passed on to the worker in terms of lower wages (since the cost of the fringe benefits have increased) and to the consumer in terms of higher prices for manufactured goods (since the wage costs of producing these goods and services have increased). Unions, to receive higher wages for their members, and industry, so as not to have to raise the prices of its products, have become more concerned with the rise in costs of medical services. In the past, certain large unions have attempted to resolve this problem by proposing to shift the costs of medical care to the federal government through national health insurance. It is increasingly being recognized, however, that the costs of health care cannot be completely shifted to other taxpayers and that a significant part of that cost will be borne by industry and labor (ultimately, by consumers) through various payroll taxes. Because both industry and labor are affected by the rise in medical costs and because the costs to each of them of gathering the necessary information and participating in the legislative process are much less than the possible benefits of reducing the rise in medical costs, they are becoming active participants in the legislative process.

Many states have experienced large increases in their share of Medicaid expenditures. Increased Medicaid expenditures mean that these funds are no longer available to meet the demands of other interest groups within a state, such as for education and welfare programs. To continue paying such large amounts for Medicaid, without cutting back on expenditures for other politically popular programs, would necessitate an increase in the state income tax, which is also not politically popular. Given their limited choices, states are seeking legislative changes to reduce their Medicaid costs. States have become much more receptive to using competitive approaches for reducing their Medicaid expenditures.

In the past, the states have delegated their responsibility for protecting the public from unqualified practitioners to the separate health professions. The states should not be allowed to abrogate their responsibilities in this manner. The state agency responsible for this function should be required to develop performance measures to determine how well it performs its monitoring function. Further, the legislature should hold annual oversight hearings on the performance of the responsible state agency. If this were to occur, interested people, as well as organized interest groups, would be able to participate (at a low cost) in the process of structuring the delivery system and in quality assurance. To further ensure that the responsible state agencies perform their tasks of quality assurance, patients and consumers should have recourse to the courts. Greater publicity and accountability in the area of quality assurance should permit changes and innovations in the delivery system that have in the past been inhibited by health associations whose members' monopoly position would have been adversely affected.

The federal government has also developed a concentrated interest in holding down the increase in medical expenditures. The federal government is responsible for funding the Medicare program and for one-half of Medicaid expenditures. Faced with the alternatives of reducing benefits for the aged, raising taxes to provide more funds for these programs, or becoming more aggressive toward health providers, the federal government appears to have concluded that it will lose less political support by being tougher on health providers.

It is possible that because of the rise of new health interest groups—industry, unions, and the federal and state governments themselves— there will be greatly increased competition in the legislative process. As a result of this competition, more information will be provided by the different interest groups regarding the cost, quality, and efficiency of different systems of delivery for medical services. The Supreme Court decision that upheld the applicability of the anti-trust laws to the health field is also likely to ensure that previous anticompetitive actions by health providers will no longer be permissible.

The political power of health interest groups is likely to decline with the rise of opposing groups with a concentrated interest in health care costs and with the applicability of the anti-trust laws to health providers.

REFERENCES

Feldstein, Paul J. 1988. *Health care economics.* New York: John Wiley & Sons.

Feldstein, Paul J. 1974. A preliminary evaluation of federal dental manpower subsidy programs. *Inquiry* 11:196–206.

Feldstein, Paul J. 1977. *Health associations and the demand for legislation: The political economy of health.* Lexington, Mass.: Ballinger Publishing Co.

Feldstein, Paul J. 1988. *The politics of health legislation: An economic perspective.* Ann Arbor, Mich., Health Administration Press.

Journal of the American Dental Association. 1976. Action urgently needed on denturist movement. (editorial), *Journal of the American Dental Association* 92:665.

Kessel, Reuben. 1958. Price discrimination in medicine. *Journal of Law and Economics* 1:20–53.

Madison, James. 1787. *Federalist* No. 10.

Chapter 12

A Political Analysis of the Political Behavior of Health Interest Groups

Bette S. Hill
Katherine A. Hinckley

How do health interest groups behave in the political arena, and why do they act as they do? Although these are apparently simple questions, like most simple questions they are far easier to ask than to answer. In fact, since they have not been answered very well for any set of interest groups, we need to begin this study with a short review and a bit of theoretical exploration.

In answer to the first question—how groups behave politically—we may distinguish between tactical and strategic actions. Tactics typically refer to fairly narrow, short-range activities in pursuit of some specific, pre-established goal. Providing political campaign contributions is one example. Strategies, on the other hand, are normally longer-range and broader in scope, and sometimes very close to the goals themselves. For instance, a decision to help elect as many liberal or conservative candidates as possible is clearly a strategic decision; how one goes about it constitutes the tactics.

Most interest group studies concentrate on tactics rather than strategies, probably because they are easier to define and locate. Every textbook includes a list of such tactics—grassroots mobilization, committee testimony, providing research data, endorsing candidates. Although we will provide some information on health group tactics here, our primary interest is in strategic behavior, which is at least as important but has received less attention.

Interest groups make a variety of strategic decisions, though no typology of them has ever been developed. We know for example, that different groups select different arenas in which to work; some concentrate on the federal courts, while others choose state legislatures. They also make different decisions about which issues deserve top priority for their attention (Smith 1984). But one pair of interlocking strategic decisions is absolutely central: How a group defines the issues, and what stance it takes on them.

The way in which an issue is defined pushes toward a particular type of solution. For instance, if the primary health issue is defined as making sure that the quality of care is never compromised, one set of options comes to mind—building well-equipped hospitals and training better personnel. If, however, cost is the primary issue, quite another set of options comes under consideration. So as interest groups offer different issue definitions to decision-makers, they are simultaneously advocating different policy directions.

Groups also need to decide how strong and uncompromising a stance they will take with regard to their definitions and preferred solutions. If they do not admit other possibilities, they may win big. They may also lose big. The amount of flexibility a group displays is thus a vital aspect of its strategic behavior, and may have a lot to do with its success.

Sources of Strategic Behavior

Now, what kinds of factors might account for differences in these two central aspects of group strategy? We suggest four major possibilities: Group resources, the character of the organization itself, the nature of the target system it seeks to influence, and the nature of the current issue agenda. As we note below, these four factors often interact with each other in determining group strategies.

Group Resources

These have generally been examined for their tactical rather than strategic possibilities. If we think of resources as items that may be directly deployed in seeking influence, then their relationship to tactics is clear. Money, for example, is vital for everything from campaign contributions to data gathering, whereas membership size and commitment are central to grassroots lobbying. Because of the emphasis on tactics in most interest group studies, resources have been fairly well studied; some writers almost seem to equate a group's resources with its ultimate success (Schattschneider 1960).

Organizational Character

On the other hand, we would argue that organizational character is more closely related to strategy. Under this general classification we include such attributes as degree of internal cohesion, centralization and complexity of decision-making processes, locus of leadership, ideological proclivities, and even the organization's age. While many of these are cited in textbooks, they are rarely used in explanation, probably because they do not appear very important in explaining immediate tactical choices. However, they are vital in explaining many strategic (broader) choices, particularly with regard to issue definitions and stances. An interest group suffering from internal divisions may find it difficult to reach any clear-cut position at all on an issue, much less communicate it forcefully to politicians. Leadership processes dominated by professional Washington staff may produce quite different strategies than those dominated by the broader membership. Some strategies (and tactics) may come to be habitually favored as the organization ages (Hayes 1981). So a group's political behavior is determined not just by its resources, but also by its general way of doing things.

Target System Characteristics

The importance of target system characteristics is widely recognized in the classic interest group literature (Truman 1951; Ziegler 1964). Any given system may offer very expansive or very limited opportunities for different groups. Congress, for example, has generally offered a rich set of strategic and tactical opportunities to interest groups in comparison with those afforded by the federal courts and even the White House.

While it has generally been thought that interest groups are highly skilled at matching strategies to these opportunities, we are not so sure. After all, political systems are moving targets, not stationary ones. They change—sometimes rather rapidly—with "windows of opportunity" for groups, legislators and bureaucrats opening and shutting in an irregular way (Kingdon 1984).

Whether groups in fact respond by altering their issue definitions and stances strikes us as very much an empirical question. We suspect the answer will depend at least in part on their own organizational character. That is, some groups, because of their decision processes, leadership or internal situation, may not change their strategies very much despite changes in the target system situation.

Nature of the Agenda

Much the same argument could be made concerning the nature of the agenda, the last class of variables that potentially affects interest group behavior. Of course, groups themselves have a hand in setting agendas. But prominent issues arise from other sources too—executive or legislative entrepreneurs, the media, judicial action, and especially, unexpected or unplanned-for developments in the outside world. We are interested in how groups "read" the political agenda at any given moment, and to what extent they alter their behavior in response. Again, we expect that for the organizational reasons discussed earlier, different groups will not only take different readings, but adjust their strategies in different degrees.

Study Design

Health interest groups provide an admirable subject for investigating the impact of all four of these classes of variables—group resources, organizational character, target system characteristics and nature of the agenda—on group strategies. To permit some detail in analysis, we have limited our investigation to the dealings of four health interest groups with Congress (and to some degree, the executive branch) on health cost containment policy from 1977 through 1986.

The four groups analyzed here are all provider groups. Two—the American Medical Association and the American Nurses Association—are professional manpower groups, while the American Hospital Association and the Federation of American Hospitals represent hospitals as insti-

tutional providers. The 1977–1986 time span covers continuing changes in both Congressional and Presidential systems. It also covers the transformation of health care costs from a nagging worry to a top agenda item, intertwining with the near-obsessional issue of deficit reduction.

Health Interest Groups: Resources and Organizational Character

We begin our consideration of the four health provider interest groups with an examination of their resources and organizational character. As will be seen, they differ from each other in a variety of interesting ways.

American Medical Association. The AMA is composed of approximately 255,000 physician members—about 44 percent of all U.S. physicians—and fifty-four state groups (*Encyclopedia of Associations* 1986; Locin 1985). The AMA's monetary and political resources are quite impressive. Its total annual budget is approximately $122 million Although the national headquarters is in Chicago, a slight disadvantage for federal lobbying, about $2.4 million is provided for its permanent Washington office. In 1986 the Association employed a lobbying staff of forty persons headed by Dr. John Zapp, a dentist and former federal Health, Education and Welfare official (Pear 1986).

The AMA's political action committee, AMPAC, was founded in 1961. Each year AMPAC ranks among the top five contributors to national political campaigns (Weinberger and Greevy 1982). In 1986 it gave almost $2.1 million in contributions, 61.7 percent of which went to Republican candidates (*Federal Election Commission Reports* 1985–1986). It has also become a leader in developing and testing new campaign techniques. For example, Federal Election Commission rules treat surveys as a type of in-kind contribution to candidates, and estimate their cash value as a function of time. So when AMPAC releases the results of a survey conducted for a favored candidate after sixty days, it reports only 5 percent of the original cost as a contribution. It can thus provide more services within the federal campaign contribution limits of $5000 per candidate per election (Pressman 1984). AMPAC not only has large total contributions but spreads them broadly. In 1986, it made direct contributions to 465 Congressional candidates (Sorauf 1988). It is also one of a half-dozen PACs that make large independent expenditures (i.e., outside of candidate contributions). Such independent expenditures serve as both a supplement to candidate contributions and a way of putting issues directly to the public (Sorauf 1988). AMPAC spent over $1.5 million in 1986 on independent expenditures; in fact, AMPAC was the only one of the PACs of our four groups to make any independent expenditures at all (*Federal Election Commission Reports* 1985–1986).

The AMA is able to mobilize influential members to testify before Congress. But its grassroots resources are limited because its members, though of high status, are often too busy to exert widespread political pressure. Furthermore, its massive approach to election contributions has sometimes backfired. Congressmen for example may vote against AMA-backed legislation to show their independence, especially when media attention has been focused on the issue (Pressman 1984, 19). In general, though, the AMA is extraordinarily rich in resources.

On the other hand, its organizational characteristics are not quite so impressive. For one thing, its governing structure presents something of an obstacle to effective action. Final authority to take policy stands rests with a 371-member House of Delegates. The Board of Trustees, which governs the organization on a day-to-day basis, can adopt positions in the interim between meetings of the House of Delegates. The Board, however, tries to match these positions to "the tenor of past and current action" of its parent body (AMA *Reference Guide to Policy and Official Statements* 1985). As a result of these decision processes and the organization's distinctly conservative bent, AMA positions on legislative proposals tend to be rather inflexible, leaving its lobbyists very little room for the give and take necessary in the drafting of legislation (Pressman 1984, 17). A former AMA lobbyist has admitted that one of the big problems he faced was "Chicago headquarters' unyielding opposition to legislation" (Rhein 1978). In the 1980s the AMA has tried to adopt a strategy of keeping changes to a minimum rather than simply stonewalling. But

its image is still one of rigidity rather than compromise.

Another set of potential problems concerns the AMA's internal cohesion. High cohesion was not difficult to sustain in an age when most members were like small businessmen, engaged in individual practices or partnerships. Today, however, with the rise of group practices and other new financial structures, political consensus among physicians becomes more problematic. Rep. William Gradison (Rep., Ohio), a member of the House Ways and Means health subcommittee, noted that the AMA (and AHA) have a problem as "umbrella organizations trying to represent a diverse membership" (Pear 1986, A24). Insofar as they cannot cope fully with such diversity, they face competition from new groups claiming to speak for physicians. We will examine this competition in detail as we look at the Congressional target system a little later.

The AMA's membership problem is in turn connected to an image problem. Many young doctors are apathetic about joining the AMA, perhaps partly because it is seen in some quarters as not especially forward-looking and more concerned with doctors' pocketbooks than the nation's health (Pear 1986; Pressman 1984). This problem was highlighted in the AMA's 1982 fight to seek exemption for physicians from Federal Trade Commission regulations prohibiting price-fixing and deceptive advertising. The AMA "pulled out all the stops" on this issue and in turn created a negative backlash, with opponents accusing doctors of wanting to be "above the law." This fight cost the AMA a significant amount of credibility, especially in terms of representing broader health issues for the public rather than, as Henry Waxman (Dem., Calif.) noted, "narrower issues that concern doctors economically" (Locin 1985, 16).

American Hospital Association. The AHA consists of a combined membership of approximately 42,000 individuals, hospitals and other institutions. Its member hospitals include urban and rural, non-profit and investor-owned, secular and religious facilities (Pear, 1986), representing considerable diversity in geography, services offered and patient mixtures (AHA *Annual Report* 1985). This diversity provides representation in all types of congressional districts, and as Rep. Paul Rogers (Dem., Fla.), former chairman of the

House Commerce health subcommittee noted, "hospitals are often a major industry" in a congressman's community (Rhein 1978, 81). As in the case of the AMA, however, the range of membership also creates problems for the AHA's organizational cohesion.

The fiscal resources of AHA include an annual budget of $82 million, with $3 million for its Washington offices. There are about 900 employees in its Chicago headquarters (Pear 1986). In Washington, it maintains a lobbying staff of thirty-seven people headed in 1986 by Jack Owen, former president of the New Jersey Hospital Association. Its political action committee, P.A.C. of A.H.A, was only founded in 1976, but by 1979–80 had grown from 2044th to 160th in terms of total contributions. In 1986 it contributed $347,981 to 317 congressional candidates, with 59 percent of this going to Democrats (*Federal Election Commission Reports* 1985–1986). The vast majority of these won, according to the AHA 1986 *Annual Report,* but it should be remembered that interest groups classically "pad" their success rate by not endorsing very many likely losers.

Like the AMA, the AHA has a complex and rather cumbersome governing structure. While a Board of Trustees governs on a day-to-day basis, a 218-member House of Delegates is the highest authority for approving A.H.A. policy. Below that is a complex set of regional advisory boards, which debate policy stands at length at the grassroots level before they even come to the House of Delegates. Because of this sizable structure and the diverse interests it represents, the AHA has some problems in maintaining organizational cohesion and credibly representing a membership majority (Rhein 1978). The diversity issue is potentially a greater problem for the AHA than for the AMA, because the differences in hospitals have been accentuated by cuts in the budget that force them to compete for limited federal funds (Pear 1986). However, some observers have noted that in spite of this difficulty, the AHA is adept at reinforcing its message with appeals from state associations and local hospitals (Pear 1986).

Federation of American Hospitals (now Federation of American Health Systems). Originally formed in 1966 by a small group of hospitals in a few states, the Federation of American Hospitals

evolved into a major health care organization representing 1,300 investor-owned hospitals and some sixty parent companies, primarily located in the South and Southwest. The Federation changed its name in 1986 (from FAH to FAHS) to reflect the diversification of its members into areas of health care besides hospitals.

The organization's offices are located in Washington, D.C., and Little Rock, Arkansas. Legislative and regulatory activities are performed by the national office in Washington, while daily administrative functions (e.g., publications and membership) are functions of the Arkansas office (F.A.H. *Report to the Membership* 1985, 10). The FAH's political resources include a political action committee, FED PAC, organized in the early 1970s. FED PAC's role has grown in tandem with the Federation's increasing responsibility in tracking government decisions that affect the industry. During 1986 FED PAC contributed $165,267 to 166 congressional candidates, attempting to insure support for the role of private, investor-owned hospitals in the health care delivery system. Not surprisingly, Republican candidates received the bulk of the money—54.7 percent (*Federal Election Commission Reports* 1985–1986).

Professional leadership is a key asset of the FAH. Executive Director Michael Bromberg, a lawyer and former congressional aide, is sometimes rated as the best health lobbyist in Washington (Rhein 1978; Pressman 1984). Highly knowledgeable about health policy-making processes, he gets credit for having developed an excellent staff and particularly for being able to generate strong grassroots pressure from members. Of course, he is greatly helped in the latter by the fact that many FAH hospital board members are prominent people with good access to lawmakers (Pressman 1984, 18). Both the FAH and AHA mobilized such members in Congressional hearings on President Carter's hospital cost containment legislation.

The organizational structure of the Federation consists of an executive committee, board of directors, board of governors, standing committees, special committees, and occasional task forces. Its organizational resources are more streamlined and business-oriented than those of the AMA or AHA. With a smaller size and more homogeneous membership, the FAH has a high level of cohesion, representational credibility and the flexibility needed for quick negotiations. Observers have noted that Bromberg can make compromises and can bring them quickly to his group's membership for ratification. He once was quoted as saying, "I can call 10 people [representing large corporate members] and get a decision" (Rhein 1978, 78). In contrast, the AMA House of Delegates might take six months to approve (or reject) a Washington lobbyist's compromise—far too late for most "horse trading."

The FAH is probably the highest of the four provider groups in prestige with Congress, largely because of the leadership skills of Bromberg. But it has also gained status by piling up a number of small wins, by taking an honest approach to the proprietary hospitals' image (they admitted "skimming" the best patients) and by showing support for broader, sometimes liberal, health issues such as health planning, which was strongly opposed by the AMA (Rhein 1978).

American Nurses Association. The ANA, established in 1896, is organized into fifty-three state nurses associations and 900 district associations. Its 188,000 members represent about 12.5 percent of the 1.5 million *employed* nurses. In 1985 the operating budget was $13.1 million, with $600,000 going towards lobbying efforts. The headquarters in Kansas City, Missouri, maintains a staff of 185 persons (126 professionals), but there is also a Washington, D.C., legislative office with a staff of twenty-six (ANA *Annual Report* 1985).

ANA sponsors an affiliated policial action committee called N-CAP (Nurses Coalition for Political Action), but now renamed ANA-PAC. It stands out among the PAC's of the four groups studied for several reasons. First it is the only one of the four classified as a labor PAC; the other three are listed among trade/membership health committees. Second, it is the most partisan of the four in its contribution patterns. Of the $292,703 ANA-PAC gave to 183 congressional candidates in 1986, 88.4 percent went to Democrats (*Federal Election Commission Reports* 1985–1986). Such heavily Democratic giving is standard for labor union PACs, but does distinguish ANA-PAC from the others in this study. ANA-PAC also is one of the few national PACs that make special efforts to contribute to women candidates (Symons 1984). Finally, ANA-PACs

recent contributions to incumbents show a different pattern from those of the other groups examined. Only 40.8 percent of its 1986 contributions went to incumbents, even lower than the overall 57.6 percent average for labor PACs. In contrast, each of the other three PAC's channeled at least 70 percent of their contributions to incumbents—close to the 69 percent normal figure for all PACs in that year (*Federal Election Commission Reports* 1985–1986; Sorauf 1988).

The ANA also has increased its grassroots lobbying efforts through the establishment of a network of Congressional District Coordinators (CDCs)—in 326 districts as of 1985—whose function is to develop campaign organizations for nurses within their districts, register nurses to vote, and distribute literature on endorsed candidates. Motivating more members to become active in politics is the goal of a special project, "Nurses Visible in Politics (N:VIP)" which has developed a National Nursing Agenda and held regional workshops (Symons 1984).

Over the last decade, therefore, the ANA has become considerably more active in the political process. By 1980, one of its top four priorities was to "continue to enlarge the influence of the nursing profession in the determination and execution of health policy" (Carlin 1980, 17). And its lobbying efforts show some sophistication. In 1978 the ANA's Deputy Executive Director for Government Relations explained to its national convention the importance of a newly created position of policy analyst and a lobbying staff which could "remain flexible and switch fast when we have to" (Holleran 1978, 20). The ANA has also expanded its lobbying efforts to reach the political parties; it was one of fifteen women's organizations caucusing together as Women's Central each day at the 1988 Democratic National Convention (Freeman 1988). Thus, although nurses mobilized somewhat late politically, they learned at least the basics rather quickly—organize grassroots efforts, target your financial resources and be adaptive to the legislative environment.

According to its national headquarters, the ANA adopted its federated structure of state, territorial, and district associations in 1982. It claims the move has resulted in a growth of the organization through more action at the state level. But such a structure can create problems for effective national leadership. The nursing profession is still divided over a central issue—the educational credentials necessary for professional entry. The ANA has sought since 1965 to make a bachelor's degree the minimum requirement for licensing registered nurses, arguing that those with less training should be designated "technical nurses." But there is still disagreement on the matter among members, and lack of consensus has "contributed to a widespread belief that nursing is unable to get its own house in order" (Inglehart 1987, 649). However, nurses have demonstrated an ability to unite on other issues. For example, in 1979 the ANA, along with three other nursing groups, successfully lobbied to restore funds the Carter administration wanted rescinded from nursing education grants and to obtain a one- year reauthorization of the Nurse Training Act (Isaacs 1979–80). They have also been united in their opposition to the AMA on several issues involving their ability to practice in independent community-based settings and to receive direct reimbursements from third-party payers for such services (Inglehart 1987). Beginning with their support *for* Medicare/Medicaid (and other national health insurance proposals), and continuing through their opposition to the AMA's stance on being exempted from FTC regulation, the ANA has long been on the more liberal side of the question of government involvement in health care.

Target Systems: Congress

Congress has always been regarded as a splendid target for interest groups, and not just because of its vital role in the policy process. The electoral sensitivity of its members means that groups are quite welcome on Capitol Hill, especially if they represent important constituencies. Moreover, the jurisdictions of many Congressional committees and indeed their very names—Agriculture, Education and Labor, Commerce, etc.—invite such interest group activity.

The first requirement for interest groups, then, has long been access to the committees and especially to their powerful chairmen. Generally speaking, chairmen in the past controlled the committees, and the committees controlled floor action. Without committee approval, it was al-most impossible to get a bill before the whole membership of either House or Senate; and, once there, both chamber procedures and general deference to expertise gave the committees an immense advantage which even party leaders could only rarely overcome.

The whole process was really highly conservative. If a group could stop legislation at the committee level in either chamber, it could generally stop it entirely. Should that fail, there were still so many other potential barriers to action in the long, complex Congressional process that outcomes showed a decided tilt to the status quo. It is no wonder that interest groups were once referred to as "veto groups" for their power in stopping legislation (Riesman, Glazer and Denney 1950; Safran 1967).

In recent years, however, a great many changes have taken place in the Congressional system that affects the groups' situation. Among those most relevant for health care interest groups are the following:

Level of Group Competition. One of the most startling changes in Washington in recent years is the tremendous increase in interest groups hovering about Congress (Schlozman and Tierney 1986). In consequence, older groups face more and more competition for Congressional access. Furthermore, some of, this competition is very close to home. The AMA, for instance, long laid claim to being "the" representative of organized medicine. But specialty physician groups such as the American Society of Internal Medicine have expanded their offices in Washington or moved there to improve their political clout (Rhein 1978). Increasingly these groups are contacting Congress directly rather than allowing the AMA to assume leadership. Moreover, in 1984 a small group of doctors formed a new (and presumably more liberal) general medical organization, Health USA. Though the AMA viewed this group as a "gnat on an elephant" (Pressman 1984, 19), it cannot so easily dismiss the claims of the physician specialty organizations. Similarly, the hospital lobby has become more divided over strategies and goals as government control over health costs has increased. There are now a number of different types of hospital associations representing particular interests—for example, the National Council of Community Hospitals and the American Protestant Hospital

Association. These groups emerged because their member hospitals felt that the AHA with its diverse membership could not speak forcefully enough for their specific interests (Inglehart 1977).

Indeed, entire sectors of organized medicine have come into conflict with each other as increasing budget cuts put pressure on old alliances. For instance, the AMA and AHA, "the longtime standard bearers of organized medicine," found themselves on opposite sides of the issue in 1983 debates on prospective payment system reforms, in part because the AMA was not directly affected whereas hospitals were. Some observers contend that the two have come to take quite different approaches to Congress, with "the AHA attempting to position itself as a midwife to change, and the AMA preferring to resist" (Kosterlitz 1986).

Committees. For current health legislation, two sets of committees are central, and their jurisdictions overlap. General health legislation typically goes to the House Energy and Commerce Committee and the Senate Labor and Human Resources Committee. But any revenue legislation—and therefore anything involving a payroll tax such as Medicare—must go to the House Ways and Means Committee and the Senate Finance Committee. To complicate matters further, House Energy and Commerce has complete jurisdiction over Medicaid and joint jurisdiction with Ways and Means over Medicare Part B, while Senate Labor and Human Resources lacks jurisdiction over either.

The important thing to note is that these committees not only differ from each other in their approaches to health issues, but also change over time. The two revenue committees tend to be conservative compared with their more program-oriented counterparts; but all four committees experienced considerable membership turnover and at least one change of chairman during the period we are examining. Moreover, all were less controlled by their chairmen, more diverse in ideology and more dependent on committee staff than had been the case before the mid-1970s. Interest groups today thus face a wide variety of committee situations in planning strategy. While this gives less well-established groups more chances for access, it has disturbed the comfortable long-standing relationships that older groups once enjoyed.

Floor Action. Further contributing to some interest groups' difficulties have been changes in the handling of bills once out of committee. Groups must now consider more seriously than before the attitudes of party leaders and junior members; for the power of the Speaker of the House, and the tendency of members to offer floor amendments rather than to just accept the committees' work, are both on the rise (Sinclair 1983, 1986). Equally important is that as the press of issues in Congress has become overwhelming, leaders have increasingly resorted to a two-track system of legislation, with urgent business on the "fast track" receiving expedited treatment. Under these circumstances interest groups with limited organizational flexibility are particularly disadvantaged.

The Budget Process. Finally, the arena for health interest groups was deeply affected by the changes in the Congressional budget process set in motion by the Budget and Impoundment Control Act of 1974. Under this act, the newly created House and Senate Budget committees were to develop each year a concurrent resolution setting targets for revenues, expenditures, and the overall deficit for the coming fiscal year. Other committees were then to complete their normal activities. But shortly before the October 1 beginning of the new fiscal year, the sums of their individual bills were to be "reconciled" with a second, binding resolution of the budget totals.

In their first few years of existence, the budget committees performed largely an accounting and compiling function, sometimes bargaining with authorizing, revenue or appropriations committees over "budget-busting" actions (Schick 1980). But in the face of huge budget deficits, they ultimately became more sensitive. Beginning in 1980 they moved toward including reconciliation *instructions* in the *first* budget resolution, forcing if necessary the authorizing and revenue committees to change federal law in order to meet their targets.

Interest group lobbyists were originally not much concerned with budget reform; but its long-run implications were potentially devastating. For one thing, the process eventually reduced the autonomy of non-Budget committees, so that access to them was in a sense worth less; the committees were bound by the strictures of the reconciliation instructions. Moreover, as

Fuchs and Hoadley (1987) note, many reconciliation meetings were closed to public and press, and thus interest groups often could not tell what was happening to them until a completed package emerged.

The overall effects of all these changes are hard to characterize simply; different ones tug in different directions for different groups. Querying group representatives on a list of changes somewhat similar to ours, Schlozman and Tierney (1986) found that most groups felt their lives had on balance been made harder. Yet citizen groups, in contrast to business and labor organizations, found their lives easier in the new system. Perhaps the best overall conclusion is that these changes have considerably heightened the level of strategic uncertainty for any group dealing with Congress.

Changing Agendas

Related to the Congressional changes described above (and in fact, one major source of some of them) is our fourth type of independent variable, the nature of the agenda. This can best be examined in terms of the three types of problems that have historically dominated the health agenda: quality, access and cost.

Much post-war health legislation centered on improving health care quality. The Hill-Burton Act for hospital construction and various acts subsidizing medical training represent responses to this type of problem. As these tended to increase provider incomes, they were generally vigorously supported by provider groups.

In the early 1960s, however, the national agenda came to be dominated by concern for those left behind in the race for wealth and progress, as evidenced by the "War on Poverty." Not surprisingly, the health agenda shifted too. Medicare and Medicaid, passed in 1965 to ensure access to care for the elderly and poor, were the results. Though the AMA opposed these programs as dangerous to quality of care, it ultimately realized that such programs could be very profitable for physicians.

The implementation of Medicare and Medicaid, however, led directly to rising concern over a third issue—cost. "Within two years of the pas-

sage of Medicare, policy makers were astonished by the steep rise in the costs" (Kingdon 1984, 111). As a result, despite the efforts of such liberals as the AFL-CIO and Senator Edward Kennedy (Dem., Mass.) to keep access on the agenda, cost increasingly became "the" health issue.

Once again, health and more general national agendas became linked. With the rise of inflation and the federal deficit in the 1970s, the size of the federal budget itself became the central issue for both President and Congress. In fact, by the early 1980s the Congressional agenda had become *primarily* a budget control agenda, with other problems redefined in budgetary terms or simply crowded out. Health care was inexorably drawn into this vortex—especially as it was an increasing share of the ballooning federal expenditures.

Health care policy was simply becoming one part of budget policy. For health interest groups, this was a disturbing change. To begin with, some groups would become more vulnerable because they had a vested interest in high-cost programs like Medicare. Big budget cuts would probably center on "their" programs. Further the groups would now be fighting over a differently defined issue, with the same committees assuming different roles. For example, groups would have to deal with the Ways and Means Committee not just as the authorizer and funder of Medicare, but also as a tax-raiser and budget-cutter under reconciliation. Strategies that had worked well in the past might not work well at all when the major issue was defined as cost control rather than program access and quality.

Of course there were differences within Congress, between Congress and President, and between Presidents in approaches to health cost controls. These in turn related to differing program priorities and ideological inclinations. For President Carter, the cost problem seems to have been largely one of controlling hospital prices, the most inflationary area of the economy; for President Reagan, it was an essential element in cutting domestic budgets and shifting programs back to the private sector while increasing defense expenditures. Congress generally lagged in willingness to cut costs until after 1980; even then there were distinct differences between the priorities of the House and Senate, as well as those of the revenue committees and the more program-oriented House Energy and Commerce Committee and the Senate Labor and Human Resources Committee.

These agenda shifts and differences emerge clearly in the health policy actions taken from 1977 to 1986. We can only briefly chronicle these actions here as a background for the strategic stances groups took at different times.

With hospital inflation rates running at 15 percent—over twice the Consumer Price Index—Carter in 1977 proposed legislation to limit hospitals' price increases and capital expenditures nationwide (*CQ Weekly Report* April 30, 1977, 787). The proposal, developed without any input from the hospital lobby or organized medicine, quickly ran afoul of Senate Finance's health subcommittee chairman, Herman Talmadge (Dem., Ga.), who had his own plan for some reform of the basic retrospective payment system. To stave off action, the hospitals developed a voluntary cost containment plan, further complicating the situation. Though the Senate actually passed a watered-down version of the Carter bill in 1978, no action was taken in the House. In early 1979, Carter submitted a compromise plan resembling the previous year's Senate bill, but even that ultimately failed. It was replaced in Senate Finance by the Talmadge plan, and was completely torpedoed on the House floor by the "Gephardt amendment" which merely called for a study commission on hospital costs. The President's reaction was reported to be "unprintable" (*CQ Weekly Report* Nov. 17, 1979, 2575).

In 1980 Congress began attaching reconciliation instructions to the first budget resolution; the initial result was the Omnibus Reconciliation Act (ORA). From then through 1986, most major health legislation was contained in reconciliation bills rather than separate acts.

The merger of the budget and health agendas was clearly demonstrated in 1982 with the passage of the Tax Equity and Fiscal Responsibility Act (TEFRA). This act imposed $15.5 billion in Medicare cuts and another $1.1 billion in Medicaid—about 15 percent of the total tax and reconciliation package. Clashing priorities among the Reagan administration, House, Senate, and various committees were evident throughout TEFRA's passage. Nonetheless,, the act reflected consensus on the need to control hospital costs, which amounted to about 70 percent of all Medi-

care expenditures and had long since outstripped the "voluntary" standards of 1978. TEFRA imposed among other things, strict annual caps on hospital reimbursements. Ironically, these provisions were at least as stringent as the Carter proposals that had failed three years earlier. Though Part B premiums for the elderly were also increased to cover 25 percent of program costs, and hospital-based physician reimbursements reduced, almost two-thirds of the TEFRA cuts fell on hospitals.

TEFRA also directed the Department of Health and Human Services (DHHS) to submit within five months a prospective payment system for reimbursing hospitals by set amounts for each type of illness, or Diagnostic Related Group, rather than by retrospective payment of costs. A fundamental and radical change in the way government did business with hospitals, PPS represented a first attempt to slow the swift movement of Social Security's Hospital Insurance Trust Fund toward bankruptcy. It was therefore attached to the 1983 revamping of the Social Security old age program, and passed Congress with remarkable speed (Fuchs and Hoadley 1987).

With hospitals in transition to the PPS system, attention turned to controlling physicians' fees. In 1983 President Reagan proposed for the first time a freeze on physician payment increases under Medicare. Deep disagreements in Congress over this and other proposals delayed passage of any reconciliation bill until 1984, but the Deficit Reduction Act (DEFRA) of that year did impose a fifteen-month freeze. (Doctors willing to accept "assignment" of Medicare reimbursements as full payment were offered expedited payment procedures and higher post-freeze rates.)

Almost two years elapsed before another reconciliation act was passed, as Congress and President struggled over whom to target in the fight against burgeoning health costs. The Consolidated Omnibus Budget Reconciliation Act (COBRA) of April, 1986, was actually a belated revival of the previous year's bill. It did extend the physician fee freeze through December for all but "participating" physicians who accepted Medicare reimbursements as full payment for all elderly patients.

Finally, the 1986 Omnibus Budget Reconciliation Act (OBRA), passed only months later, more or less concludes the six-year trend of reconciliation bill cuts in health. Reductions in services and payments were only minor; physicians were released from the freeze; and hospital reimbursement rates were slightly increased. Both elderly and poor benefited, too. OBRA capped the swiftly-rising deductible under Part A, indexing future rises to hospital reimbursement rates. OBRA's increases in health programs thus considerably outweighed its cuts. For all the "easy" cuts had now been made, and other health agenda items were being asserted. With this shift would come another set of strategic conditions for interest groups to face.

Group Stances and Issue Definitions: The AMA

The four groups we have chosen to study displayed quite interesting strategic differences on these issues. They varied not only in their definitions of the issues and in the strength of their stances, but also in the breadth and depth of their comments on legislative proposals.

The AMA began this period holding to its traditional rejection of government interference in health care and opposition to new initiatives on anything but a small scale—a stance many critics have characterized as "do nothing now, wait and see, keep the status quo" (see Locin 1985; Kosterlitz 1986). It strongly opposed Carter's hospital cost containment proposals, testifying that though an AMA commission was studying the problem, there was "not enough information . . . present to draw up appropriate legislation at this time" (Senate Human Resources, Health and Scientific Research Subcommittee May 24–26, 1977, 319). When specifically asked by subcommittee chairman Kennedy about the Talmadge bill, the AMA said that while some provisions were more appropriate than the Carter bill, even the Talmadge approach should be tried only on an experimental, geographically limited basis. Unlike the FAH or AHA, the AMA did not endorse a specific alternative and gave no date for producing one.

But in 1979 in the final set of hearings on this legislation, the AMA began to show more specificity in its responses to congressional questioning and admitted that physicians had not in the past been trained to pay attention to cost matters (Hill and Hinckley 1988, 19). Along with the AHA and FAH, the AMA demonstrated excellent coalitional politics in the development of the health industry's "Voluntary Effort" strategy to demonstrate to Congress that costs could be contained without federal regulation—though this effort had only temporary effect.

Thus while the AMA's stance on the Carter bill continued its long opposition to government involvement, its approach to issue definition in conjunction with coalitional politics was gradually broadening. For example, in the struggles over Medicare in the 1960s, and HMOs in 1973, the AMA had concentrated on labeling proposals "socialized medicine" or "a return to contract medicine." But in 1977–1979, its representatives argued, along with the hospital lobbies, that the Carter bill unfairly singled out the health care industry for controls. All three interest groups attempted to drive home the idea that the Carter plan would have serious effects on quality of care and would actually penalize efficient hospitals the most. But the AMA preferred no legislation at all, while we will see that the AHA and FAH offered alternate suggestions for other ways to control costs.

The 1982 TEFRA and 1983 PPS proposals marked a transition phase both for Congress and the AMA. The health industry's voluntary cost control effort of 1978 soon withered, and by 1982 there was little disagreement in Congress that something must be done to control this increasingly important part of the budget. In addition, 1982 was the first time that the groups appeared before the tax committees for hearings on a range of health budget matters, not just a limited topic. It is also at this point that the AMA was treated to a lesson on the virtues of specificity, courtesy of Senate Finance Committee chairman Robert Dole (Rep., Kans.), one of the most vigorous Republican advocates of deficit reduction.

In March, 1982, ten days before its Finance testimony, the AMA testified before Ways and Means with a formal statement that was not only strikingly short, but also remarkably aloof. It apparently was trying to take the "high road" approach, as the following excerpt demonstrates:

We have been asked to appear today to comment on changes in the Medicare program . . . designed to generate approximately $3 billion in Federal budget savings. Respectfully, we do not intend to address those cuts today . . . because we believe that addressing individual items and particular programs does not provide the direction and leadership necessary to chart a course for the delivery of health care . . . for this and future decades. . . . Now is the time to set priorities for the future and not continue to deal with crises on an annual basis. . . . There is a need for evaluation of long-term health policies. . . . We are undertaking such an evaluation and will make recommendations. . . . (House Ways and Means, Health Subcommittee March 2, 1982, 87–89).

The Ways and Means members reacted in fairly mild fashion, though they did note that the voluntary cost containment efforts of physicians (and hospitals) had not been successful and some action was forthcoming. But absent serious negative feedback to the tone of the statement, the AMA apparently thought it safe to present this same testimony to Finance ten days later. This time, however, there was a reaction, and a most emphatic one. As chairman, Dole opened the committee responses to the AMA testimony:

> It looks like a clear signal to me that you don't want to do anything, to be very frank about it. If we are going to do something short term—we've got short-term budget problems. We cannot wait two or three years for some long-term change. And I'm disappointed that you are not willing to help us come to grips with the budget right now. . . . So I am not very excited about your testimony (Senate Finance March 12, 16, 1982, 6).

This evidently had a sobering effect on the AMA. In its second round of budget testimony before Ways and Means three months later, its rhetoric was much more conciliatory and its representatives were definitely willing to address particular items under consideration. For example, they stated that the AMA now "empathizes with the committee as it addresses the budget dilemma. . . . We have identified short-term budgetary savings in the Medicare program to recommend to you" (House Ways and Means, Health Subcommittee June 15, 1982, p 466) In fact, they supported eleven of the Administration's budget proposals and only opposed three, presenting five pages of formal statement. They fur-

ther expanded their testimony in hearings before Energy and Commerce the following month, adding rather specific criticisms of many of the Finance committee's proposals. In spite of the Association's new-found candor and specificity, however, TEFRA passed.

In 1983, the AMA opposed continuation of the TEFRA limits but, unlike the AHA and FAH, flatly opposed the DHHS prospective payment system "unless [it] is first proven through limited demonstration projects to be effective in both cost savings and retaining of health care" (House Ways and Means, Health Subcommittee February 14–15, 1983, 183). This stance is reminiscent of the organization's position on earlier bills that since insufficient research was available, Congress should "wait and see." The AMA claimed that previous demonstrations and state-level experiments had not adequately evaluated prospective payment for its effects on quality and access but only on program costs. In their view, such a "radical restructuring" using an untried system of prospective pricing could reduce the quality of health care.

Nonetheless, the AMA had apparently learned a lesson from its confrontation with Dole. Rather than attempting to stick to the "high moral ground," it took a multifaceted approach to the issue and provided more specific objections. Indeed, it voiced some of the same concerns as did the hospital associations, that the proposal failed to.

1. specify the methodology to be used
2. recognize some of the legitimate differences between hospital costs
3. recognize variations in the intensity of illness, and complications within DRG's
4. incorporate any appeal process.

But the AMA was not adamant on the subject of PPS. Though it recommended that Congress authorize only demonstrations of the program, it was not really active in its opposition. In part this was because physicians were not *directly* affected (CQ Weekly Reports Jan 29, 1983; Congress and The Nation 1985, 539); it may also have been because major segments of their hospital industry allies favored it. One of their lobbyists admitted, "we will not try unilaterally to prevent its passage" (CQ Weekly Reports March 5, 1983, 455–57).

In hearings on physician reimbursements and health budget proposals from 1983 through 1986, the AMA generally opposed most legislation, but also continued its trend towards broader concerns and greater specificity. In the 1983 House and Senate budget hearings, the AMA kept some of its old rhetoric about the problems of government intervention, yet added quite specific pros and cons of proposed budget changes. For example, its testimony noted positive actions the Association was taking to eliminate "inappropriate expenditures" (Senate Labor and Human Resources May 19, 25, 1983, 166). Although these actions probably did not lead to large immediate savings, the testimony represented a milestone in the AMA's use of cost-effectiveness language.

In 1985, when the Administration proposed extending the freeze on physicians' fees beyond the fifteen months originally enacted in DEFRA, the AMA adopted another strategy—pointing up promises made by government in the past. An AMA representative told House committee members in joint hearings:

> Adoption of the proposal would mean that the Congress has reneged on its promise to physicians that reimbursement for services would be allowed to increase on October 1, 1985, and the duration of the freeze would last no more than 15 months (House Energy and Commerce, Health and Environment Subcommittee; House Ways and Means, Health Subcommittee April 26, 1985, 647–648).

This rhetoric of failed promises by Congress was repeated in several hearings in 1985–86 with increasingly strong language, as illustrated below with the commentary in sequence from April, 1985, to April, 1986:

> An extension of the freeze would be particularly discriminatory as *only* physicians would be subjected to a *two-year freeze* (House Energy and Commerce, Health and Environment Subcommittee; House Ways and Means, Health Subcommittee April 26, 1985, 649); a continued freeze will not only discourage physicians from accepting assignment, it may discourage physicians from treating Medicare beneficiaries (House Energy and Commerce, Health Subcommittee July 17, 1985, 520); . . . [We] are appalled by the cavalier and discriminatory actions of the Congress in failing to adhere to previously made prom-

> ises. . . . quite concerned with the almost adversarial attitude of the Federal government toward the nation's physicians. . . . increasingly frustrated by a program that is in constant change where one cannot rely on rules. . . . [These actions] will result in a loss of faith by physicians in the Medicare program (House Ways and Means, Health Subcommittee April 14, 1986, 78–82).

The AMA exhibited similar reactions to the Participating Physicians Program initiated in the 1984 DEFRA, which provided financial incentives to physicians for accepting assignment, that is, government reimbursements as payment in full for all Medicare claims. It objected strongly to proposals for raising fees only for participating physicians, claiming that while only 30 percent of physicians elected participating status, 69 percent of all claims were accepted under assignment (Senate Finance September 11–13, 1985, 32). In a 1986 request for repeal it argued that the act "has made it possible for beneficiaries of substantial means to receive medical care services at reduced costs while . . . expenses . . . are shifted to non-Medicare patients" (House Ways and Means, Health Subcommittee June 10, 1986, 34).

This last argument suggests that by 1986 the AMA was starting to define the issue even more widely in terms of "inter-generational fairness." In March of that year they pointed out that unless Congress and the President stopped "ignoring the major issue of the future of this program . . . the coming generation of Americans will have paid into [it] their entire working lifetimes only to discover that Medicare is no longer able to meet their needs" (House Ways and Means, Health Subcommittee March 6, 1986, 158). Thus the AMA sought to use many types of appeals in fighting health care cuts directed at them. It is especially interesting that they sought to point out that the cuts would affect not just their own members, but the young and poor as well.

In addition to offering a range of objections to these cuts, the AMA also revived the classic tactic of providing expertise in a highly technical field. One example involved its criticisms of an "anti-dumping" provision which would have made it a criminal violation to transfer a patient from one hospital to another without determining that an emergency medical condition existed. The AMA agreed with the intent of the legislation but noted that it would hold physicians liable for failure to admit a patient even if they did not have admitting privileges at that hospital, which is often the case for emergency room physicians. Similarly, the AMA pointed out the problems a proposed DRG system of physician payments would pose for doctors who:

> . . . see patients with the most severe illnesses. Since the DRG methodology is based on 'averages' and individual physicians (unlike hospitals) do not ordinarily have a large enough patient population with identical diagnoses to enable costs to be spread over a larger base, a DRG system could operate as a disincentive for physicians to accept critically ill patients and could discourage necessary use of consultants (House Ways and Means, Health Subcommittee April 14, 1986, 87).

All of these strategic adjustments, however, still left the AMA's stance basically oppositional in nature—opposed to payment freezes, DRGs, and the Participating Physicians Program. In view of Congressional determination to reduce the deficit *somehow,* a purely oppositional strategy was bound to be inadequate. So the AMA finally moved toward some positive suggestions for action. It urged Congress to examine a wide range of alternatives from new taxes on cigarettes and liquor to across-the-board spending cuts and many possibilities in between, such as a relative value scale (RVS) payment method for physicians and/or a voucher system for beneficiaries (Senate Finance, Health Subcommittee December 6, 1985). While many of these ideas might seem to lack broad political appeal, they do indicate an important addition to the AMA's strategic arsenal.

In sum, then, the AMA gradually broadened its strategies against federal legislation deemed hostile to its members. It moved from defining Carter's Hospital Cost Containment proposals as unnecessary federal control which would jeopardize quality of care to defining Reagan's Participating Physician Program and Medicare/Medicaid budget cuts as not only unfair to physicians but as potentially damaging to future generations. While continuing strongly opposed to most legislation, it began to provide more positive alternatives in light of the new budget agenda.

FAH Strategies

Like the AMA, the FAH was adamantly opposed to Carter's Hospital Cost Containment proposals. In May, 1977, FAH Executive Director Michael Bromberg defined the issue in highly emotional terms. He said that if Congress passed the Carter bill with its ceiling on hospital revenues and technology, it would be voting to become "the moral judge of the dollar value of increased lifespans, fewer fatal heart attacks, reduced infant mortality . . . and every other lifesaving device or technique." He characterized the Carter ceiling on hospitals' revenues as "price controls on a single industry" amounting to "nothing more than a more stringent version of [Nixon's] phase IV hospital price control mechanism," and further claimed that the flat ceiling approach would only reward existing inefficiencies because the cap was based on current revenues. He objected to the bill's failure to provide for restraints on expenses "uncontrollable" from the hospital's viewpoint (e.g., expenses required for government compliance, malpractice insurance, and supplies such as fuel and food). Further, FAH claimed that the haste with which the Carter plan was supposed to be implemented ignored important "complexities and start up problems" like acquiring and training the necessary government and hospital personnel (House Ways and Means, Health Subcommittee; House Interstate and Foreign Commerce, Health and Environment Subcommittee May 11–13, 1977, 262–266).

According to Bromberg, the Carter proposal also would reduce the hospitals' potential for acquiring needed new medical technology. He avowed support for reducing duplication of hitech equipment, but felt planning and authorizing of new technology should be determined locally rather than by HEW. His arguments about perpetuating inefficiencies while failing to address uncontrollable costs seemed to have made the biggest impact on the congressmen who questioned the witnesses.

The FAH's stand on the Carter bill was therefore at least as adamant as that of the AMA. But unlike the AMA, the FAH offered both specific objections to the Carter bill and several alternatives. For example, it supported, with modifications, the Talmadge bill (establishing prospective Medicare target rates) and adequate funding for the Health Planning Act.

With the rising budget pressures of the 1980s, however, the FAH found it difficult to maintain such an adamant stance. In the 1982 TEFRA hearings the FAH followed its usual course of specificity in opposing the Administration's 2 percent across-the-board cuts in Medicare hospital reimbursements. But it also tried to redefine the cost control issue in much broader, market-based terms. For example, Bromberg claimed that the whole regulatory approach to health failed to provide incentives to increase efficiency, foster competition and restrain utilization—the real bases of cost control (House, Ways and Means, Health Subcommittee March 2, June 15, 1982). This emphasis on efficiency formed the basis of the FAH's support for several legislative proposals as well as the later PPS bill.

The strictures eventually passed under TEFRA were so onerous that it was not surprising the FAH and other hospital groups were rather desperate to replace them. They immediately cooperated with DHHS and Congress to develop the prospective payment system legislation. The FAH and AHA took similar overall positions on the DHHS plan, supporting immediate enactment but with several modifications. The FAH particularly wanted to (a) require DHHS to publish the DRG price list in advance, (b) incorporate a formula in the legislation for updating payment rates, and (c) give hospitals the right of judicial and administrative review. The main difference in the AHA and FAH positions was that the former wanted hospital-specific rates and the latter did not. Since the FAH's for-profits hospitals are mainly in the South and Southwest, where labor costs are lower, they would benefit from a national average rate. Thus, the FAH targeted its modifications of the Administration's PPS to those procedures most favorable to its members.

In 1983–86 hearings before the revenue committees, the FAH primarily concentrated on administration efforts to freeze the newly enacted PPS payments to hospitals. In 1985 testimony, it labeled these freeze proposals unfair and arbitrary. Bromberg said:

> . . . we think we have kept our part of the contract and the bargain that was implied when we

supported this [PPS] legislation before Congress 2 years ago. And a freeze would not reward those managers who have taken the hard actions they have taken by laying off workers, cutting costs, postponing modernization of plant and equipment. And if they have to do those things again, one day it will impact quality . . . We are doing fine under this program [PPS], but you can't keep freezing our rates and expect that to continue (Senate Finance September 11–13, 1985, 392).

The FAH further suggested that the hospital industry's support for PPS could be undermined if Congress responded to expenditure-reducing efforts by a freeze in future payments. It continued to lobby for market place strategies and ways of restraining demand for "free" health care. It also continued to argue strongly against the "command and control" regulatory approach, often with rather sophisticated data analyses. For example, in 1983 FAH presented results of a regression analysis that showed no significant savings in hospital spending from state rate-setting programs, except at the expense of hospital modernization (Senate Labor and Human Resources May 19, 25, 1983, 194). In addition, it offered quite detailed analyses of the profits and reinvestment practices of privately-owned hospitals. This emphasis on hard evidence and frank discussion of their industry has been and continues to be a hallmark of the FAH. But its strategy also incorporates an approach of reasoned discourse whenever possible, reminders of past cooperation, and a push toward redefining the issue of health costs in terms broader than simple budget control.

Stance and Issue Definitions: AHA

Along with the AMA and FAH, the AHA adamantly opposed Carter's Hospital Cost Containment bills in 1977–79. But it took a less emotional and more educational tone than the FAH in its testimony. It attempted to define the issue as a misunderstanding about factors which had contributed to hospital cost increases and which it felt the Carter bill did *not* effectively address. These included (1) inflation in general, (2) increased demand stemming partly from Medicare/Medicaid legislation and new treatments, (3) intensification of hospital services, (4) maintenance and modernization expenses, (5) manpower development, especially more physicians adding to intern and residency program costs, and (6) more government regulation of hospitals. It also echoed the quality of care theme cited by the other groups, claiming that the Carter bill would limit hospitals' necessary growth and development.

This educational focus was continued in the particular objections the AHA raised. The controls would unfairly tie hospitals to the GNP deflator (meant for the economy as a whole), penalize those hospitals that had already become cost effective, be "impossible to administer," and require new and extensive data collection on costs, revenue and admissions (House Ways and Means, Health Subcommittee; House Interstate and Foreign Commerce May 11–13, 1977, 657–658). In addition to this "educational" stance, the AHA (like the FAH) also offered some alternative suggestions for cost control, including public disclosure of hospital costs, better utilization reviews and a prospective payment system (such as that in the Talmadge bill).

This unity of opposition to the Carter bills by the AMA, FAH, and AHA was carried through to the 1982 TEFRA legislation. In its testimony before the Senate Finance Committee on the Administration's TEFRA proposal, the AHA again emphasized that reimbursement caps would penalize efficient hospitals and would adversely affect those serving a higher proportion of Medicare patients. However, its opposition failed this time, and the outcome was to escalate the AHA's difficulties in appeasing its diverse membership.

With the 1982 battle on TEFRA lost, the AHA (like the FAH) saw PPS as a much preferred alternative to the serious financial hardships created by TEFRA. It claimed that its Council on Finance had already concluded in 1981 that a PPS approach was the only viable strategy for the hospital field and that in 1982 it had actually proposed an interim PPS plan as an alternative to the TEFRA limits. However, in developing its proposal the AHA ran into serious internal disagreements over a hospital-specific rate versus a national rate, finally settling for the former. As noted earlier, the AHA is an umbrella organization representing a wide range of different hospitals. This heterogeneity makes it impossible to please "all the people all the time." When asked

about the degree of support for its PPS plan in 1982, AHA President Alex McMahon said, "my guess is that it would not be a unanimous agreement and that a number of hospitals would not like it at all" AMA News May 7, 1982, 21). For-profit hospitals were not the only ones opposed to the AHA's position on this matter; some state hospital associations (e.g., the Washington state association) claimed they were already more efficient and therefore would receive smaller payments. These members sought relief in the form of alternatives for small rural hospitals, safeguards for teaching, inner city or high volume Medicare hospitals, and safeguards to "provide equity and limit price distortions if prices are based on a national average" (Lefton Feb. 11, 1983, 28). The AHA at least partially addressed such concerns in its final proposal, which requested a phase-in transition period and the option of nonassignment (the ability to charge patients the difference in payments not received from the government). While it lost on the issues of nonassignment and hospital-specific rates, it did succeed in getting a transition period. However, this later became another source of conflict among hospitals, as some sought to delay the transition while others sought to push it forward.

These differences within the hospital lobby were exacerbated when hopes for relief under PPS from budget-cutting pressures were dashed in 1984. Under DEFRA that year, hospitals' rate increases (in both the old and new payment systems) were limited. And in 1985, the Reagan administration proposed to freeze DRG rates in the FY86 budget, overriding an existing provision for a "hospital market basket" increase plus .25 percent. However, unlike the Carter and TEFRA cases, there was no longer a united front opposing the administration. In fact, FAH's Bromberg accused hospitals of "squabbling over side issues" such as the one-year extension of the PPS transition, an area wage index and capital reimbursements, instead of concentrating on opposition to the DRG freeze (Baldwin and Fackelmann 1985, 26). The FAH's ability to concentrate on a single issue versus the AHA's need to represent its diverse membership is highlighted in the stances the latter took in asking for not only a "market basket" increase in rates plus 1 percent, but also rate differentials for rural and urban hospitals with heavy caseloads of poor people, reimbursement for teaching hospitals' indirect education costs, and regional differences in wage indexes. In the final legislation hospitals won a .5 percent reimbursement increase, though this actually became a .5 percent reduction because of automatic cuts under the Gramm-Rudman deficit reduction requirements. The AHA also got the requested rate differentials and a one-year delay in the transition to a national DRG rate, but it lost the indirect payments for medical training (Hinckley and Hill 1988). What hospitals could have won with a completely united front can of course never be known.

In 1986, the AHA again testified against the Administration's proposals to cut the Medicare hospital budget. It stated that because of past cuts, Medicare hospital payments had lost 8 percent against inflation, requiring hospitals to deliver the same service for less money (House Ways and Means, Health Subcommittee March 6, 1986, 122). It again defined the issue in terms of quality of care, with complaints that patients were being discharged "quicker and sicker." With the support of senior citizen and other consumer groups, such as the American Association of Retired Persons, these concerns were at least partially heard. Though hospitals received payment increases of only 1.15 percent and were required to develop safeguards for patient rights, DHHS was directed to submit legislation removing at least part of the problem by allowing for severity of illness and case complexity (Hinckley and Hill 1988, 13). These 1986 compromises gave the AHA a little breathing room, but there is no doubt that overall, this new era of government regulation in health care has had a splintering effect on the hospital lobby. As the government stepped up its cost-cutting efforts in the 1980s, the AHA was often caught between the proverbial "rock and a hard place" in attempts to satisfy all its members all of the time.

Issues and Stances: The ANA

The strategies of the ANA in this period differ in some basic ways from those of the other groups we have examined. We believe the reasons for this revolve around the fact that the ANA is a less *well-established* group than the others,

in three senses. First, its resources are fewer and its national lobbying experience less extensive. Second, the ANA represents a profession that is itself less well-established in terms of status; nurses have never had the professional cachet of physicians or hospital administrators. Third, and most important for this study, nursing interests are less well-entrenched in the budget; and, as we have seen, the budget agenda was very nearly *the* health agenda from 1978 through 1986.

As a result, the strategies of the ANA seem to have been aimed less at protection from broad health budget cuts, and more at becoming fully established professionally and politically. For instance, the ANA did not actively lobby Congress on Carter's hospital cost containment efforts in 1977–79. It focused instead on reauthorizing the Nurse Training Act and restoring funds Carter had wanted rescinded, as described earlier. These efforts, in fact, represented one of the first major successful uses of the ANA's new grassroots lobbying operation. The staff director of the House Energy and Commerce health subcommittee noted that "it was the number [of nurses] we heard from when a vote was coming up on the House floor that really determined the fact that the rescission was beaten back . . . the critical element was to have data and statistics so the floor debate could be well informed. The nurses' groups were able to give us that data immediately" (Isaacs 1979–80, 91–92).

On the otherhand, the ANA did testify regarding the PPS proposal in 1983. It joined the AMA in opposition, arguing that PPS did not adequately reflect differences in intensity and variety of care. But unlike the AMA, the ANA was also concerned that PPS failed to encourage non-surgical treatments. So its proposed alternatives for cost control were therefore different; it suggested loosening the medical profession's control over statutory restrictions on nurses in order to let them independently provide less expensive health services (Bauknecht 1983).

In the 1983–86 debates over cutbacks and reforms in the Medicare program, the ANA continued to pursue this strategy of emphasizing the need for some nursing independence from the medical community in order to develop less costly alternatives in health care delivery. It waged this battle on several fronts: Requesting more nursing education funds to train nurse practitioners; lobbying for FTC authority to address anti-competitive practices in the health care market; and pushing the right of nurse anesthetists who accept assignment to be paid directly by Medicare Part B rather than through hospitals. The latter was achieved in the 1986 OBRA (Inglehart 1987; Michels 1986). Most of these efforts are, of course, opposed by the AMA.

But like the other groups examined, the ANA's lobbying efforts do not simply effect its own members' interests. It has, in fact, been a strong proponent of federal health insurance for the elderly dating back to the original Medicare legislation. In the 1980s, the ANA was adamantly opposed to Reagan administration proposals to control costs by increasing the elderly's out-of-pocket expenses—for example, through co-payments for home health care and indexing the Part B deductible to the CPI. It testified that these cuts were "grossly unfair" and represented serious financial burdens on senior citizens (House Ways and Means, Health Subcommittee March 2, June 15, 1982). From the nursing profession's viewpoint this emphasis on fairness to Medicare beneficiaries is part of their obligation to protect patient rights, although, of course, it is also consistent with nurses' economic interests in supporting services such as home health care.

Conclusions

Our original question was how and why these four health provider interest groups behave, particularly during a period of environmental changes. We defined our dependent variable, the groups' strategic behavior, as involving how they defined each policy issue, the stances they took and the degree of flexibility exhibited. We noted four independent variables which we believed would explain their strategies: group resources and organizational character (both internal), and target system characteristics and agenda changes (both external). We now would like to briefly review these variables for each group and then conclude with a general discussion of the overall pattern we see.

The external independent variables, target system characteristics and agenda changes, had approximately the same import for all groups. In

Congress the primary changes involved alterations in the role and composition of committees and increasing use of the budget reconciliation process to determine health program content and funding. Overall these changes tended to decrease the interest groups' access to key decisions. With regard to the agenda, the budget deficit (and the need to limit costs) became the overriding issue, seriously decreasing the groups' maneuvering room.

For the internal variables, resources and organizational character, we found wide differences. The AMA continued to be number one in terms of financial and membership resources. The other manpower group, the ANA, also had a sizeable membership but much more limited financial resources, although its grassroots lobbying efforts appear to be stronger than the AMA's. The two hospital groups, the AHA and FAH, had moderate-sized financial and institutional membership resources. But the greatest differences among groups were in their organizational characteristics. The AMA and AHA, as large umbrella organizations with highly structured internal decision making processes, demonstrated less flexibility in responding quickly to changing policy options. In addition, the AMA's conservative ideology and "status quo" orientation limited its flexibility. The AHA displayed, especially in the post-PPS period, serious difficulties with internal cohesion. But its more moderate ideology and recognition of the need to adapt to coming changes helped to compensate for its internal problems. In contrast to both of these groups, the FAH's more business-like structure, its very homogeneous membership, its moderate ideology on selected issues (e.g., support for health planning), and particularly its highly respected leader, Michael Bromberg, helped increase its flexibility and credibility with Congress. The ANA, on the other hand, has no highly prominent leadership, and it has a fairly awkward decision-making structure as well. Yet its liberal attitude toward less expensive alternative health systems, such as community-based nursing services, brought it more in line with Congress's determination to keep the lid on costs.

In its issue definition and stances, the AMA did demonstrate, albeit reluctantly, changes in behavior from the 1977 Carter proposals to the 1984–86 Medicare budget cuts. But to really see how it changed, we need to remember the organization's behavior when Medicare and Health Maintenance Organizations were being developed. Back then the AMA generally defined the issue as one of unnecessary and unwanted government intervention into the private physician-patient arena. It also cited insufficient information and threats to quality of care as reasons for opposing these "new" policies. These themes continued in AMA testimony on the Carter, TEFRA, PPS, and physician payment freeze bills, but new themes were also added. Proposals were attacked for unfairly singling out the health industry or physicians, being administratively difficult to implement, and/or being unfair to future generations. Although it continued to oppose most of the legislation we examined and preferred a "wait and see" position (after its *own* research was available), the AMA gradually exhibited more flexibility in its strategic behavior over time. It was not adamant about PPS, and it began making positive suggestions for alternative cost cutting measures (e.g., "sin taxes" and RVS payment reforms). But it still seems reluctant to move too far from traditional positions, probably because of its membership's conservatism and its own internal dynamics.

The AHA agreed with the AMA (and FAH) in defining the Carter and TEFRA bills as unfair to hospitals, but it also sought to define the issues in educational tones; for example, Congress did not sufficiently understand the factors causing health cost inflation and did not appreciate the problems of giving too much administrative discretion to DHHS. In addition, it often defined Congress' budget cutting as seriously impacting access and quality for persons unable to afford health insurance. But except for these themes, the AHA generally appeared to be more reactive than proactive. It appears to have understood the changing agenda more than the AMA, but was hampered in its efforts to respond because of conflicting demands within its organization. After PPS, it appeared to have a strategy of "putting out brush fires," trying to fine-tune the new system through such "micro issues" as extending the PPS transition period.

The FAH, on the other hand used a combination of strategies—sometimes highly emotional (as in Bromberg's 1977 criticism of the Carter bill's implications for who lives and dies), and

sometimes very business-like, as in its pro-market, anti-regulatory approaches. It almost always seemed ready to provide "hard" data to support its positions when asked. Overall, it appeared to change the least, primarily because it began with a more flexible strategy.

Finally, the ANA is still in a period of building resources and experimenting with tactics. As noted, its more liberal positions on alternative health systems are more in tune with the current agenda of Congress, but it does not yet appear to have positioned itself to develop a concentrated strategy and become a major player on issues outside those most relevant to its members.

Overall, what have we learned about the relative importance of our four independent variables in explaining organizations' strategic behavior? When viewed over a short time period, the internal variables of resources and especially organizational character seem more relevant. The AMA and AHA, with less homogeneity and internal decision-making flexibility, have had obstacles to their organizations' ability to respond to change, while the FAH's cohesion and leadership give it greater flexibility. But when viewed over a long time period, it is clear that the external variables of changes in target system characteristics and agenda (especially the budget deficit), have forced all organizations to adapt as best they can in order to survive.

REFERENCES

AHA backs prospective reimbursement. 1982. *AMA News* (May 7):1, 21.

American Hospital Association. 1985. *Annual report.*

American Medical Association. 1985. *Reference guide to policy and official statements.*

American Nurses Association. 1985.*Annual report.*

Baldwin, Mark and Kathy Fackelmann. 1985. Hospital squabbles over 'side issues' could pave way for medicare freeze. *Modern Health Care* 15:26–27.

Bauknecht, Virginia. 1983. ANA opposes using diagnostic groups for calculating payment. *The American Nurse* 15:1, 14.

Carlin, Diane. 1980. ANA a politically oriented organization. *Kentucky Nurses' Association Newsletter* (June/July): pp 17–18.

Congress and the nation. 1985. Washington, D.C.: Congressional Quarterly, Inc.

Congressional Quarterly weekly report. 1977–1986. Washington, D.C.: Congressional Quarterly, Inc.

Encyclopedia of associations. 20th Edition. 1986.

Federation Election Commission reports on financial activity. 1985–1986. Volumes III–IV.

Federation of American Health Systems. 1985 and 1986. *Report to the membership.*

Freeman, Jo. 1988. Women at the 1988 Democratic convention. *PS* 21:875–881.

Fuchs, Beth C., and John F. Hoadley. 1987. Reflections from inside the beltway: how Congress and the president Grapple With Health Policy. *PS* 20:212–220.

Hayes, Michael T. 1981. *Lobbyists and legislators.* New Brunswick: Rutgers University Press.

Hill, Bette S., and Katherine A. Hinckley. 1988. Changing health policy and the AMA: Adaptation and resistance to change. Presented at the annual meeting of the Midwest Political Science Association, Chicago, IL.

Hinckley, Katherine A., and Bette Hill. 1988. Biting the bullet: Congressional processes and Medicare/Medicaid decisions in the 1980s. Presented at the annual meeting of the American Political Science Association. Washington, D.C.

Holleran, Constance. 1978. Nursing unity-political power. *Washington State Journal of Nursing* 50:18–21.

Inglehart, John K. 1977. The hospital lobby is suffering from self- inflicted wounds. *National Journal* 9:1526–1531.

Inglehart, John K. 1987. Health policy report: problems facing the nursing profession. *The New England Journal of Medicine* 316:646–651.

Isaacs, Marion. 1979–1980. Nurse political action: Interview with Marge Colloff. *Advances in Nursing Science* 2:89–95.

Kingdon, John W. 1984. *Agendas, alternatives, and public policies.* Boston: Little, Brown and Company.

Kosterlitz, Julie. 1986. Organized medicine's united front in Washington is showing more cracks. *The National Journal* January 11.

Lefton, Doug. February 11, 1983. AHA backs DRG-based prospective pay plan. *American Medical News,* pp. 1, 27.

Locin, Mitchell. 1985. Medicine men: Working to cure the ills of the American Medical Association. *Chicago Tribune Magazine* (August 25): 10.

Michels, Kathleen. 1986. Advanced nursing care is focus of ANA lobbying. *The American Nurse* 18:11–19.

Pear, Robert. 1986. The medical lobbies: Differing opinions. *New York Times* (August 19): A24.

Pressman, Steven. 1984. Physicians' lobbying machine showing some signs of wear. *Congressional Quarterly Weekly Report* (January 7): 15–19.

Rhein, Reginald W., Jr 1978. Health lobbyists: Clout in the corridors of power. *Medical World News* (June 12): 19:65–81.

Riesman, David, Nathan Glazer, and Reuel Denney. 1950. *The lonely crowd.* New Haven, Conn.: Yale University Press.

Safran, William. 1967. *Veto-group politics: The case of health-insurance reform in West Germany.* San Francisco: Chandler Publishing Company.

Schattschneider, E. E 1960. *The semisovereign people.* New York: Holt, Rinehart and Winston.

Schick, Allen. 1980. *Congress and money.* Washington: The Urban Institute.

Schlozman, Kay Lehman, and John T. Tierney. 1986. *Organized interests and American democracy.* New York: Harper & Row.

Sinclair, Barbara Deckard. 1983. *Majority party leadership in the U.S. House.* Baltimore: Johns Hopkins University Press.

Sinclair, Barbara Deckard. 1986. Senate styles and senate decision-making, 1955 to 1980. *Journal of Politics* 48:877–907.

Smith, Richard A. 1984. Advocacy, interpretation, and influence in the U.S. Congress. *American Political Science Review* 78:44–63.

Sorauf, Frank J. 1988. *Money in American elections.* Glenview, Ill: Scott, Foresman.

Symons, Joanne L. 1984. Political education—political action. *Nursing Administration Quarterly* 8:32–36.

Truman, David. 1951. *The governmental process.* New York: Alfred A. Knopf.

U.S. Congress, House. Joint Hearing, Subcommittee on Health, Committee on Ways and Means, and Subcommittee on Health and the Environment, Committee on Interstate and Foreign Commerce. 1977. *President's hospital cost containment proposal* (May 11–13). 95th Cong., 1st sess. Washington: USGPO.

U.S. Congress, Senate. Hearings, Subcommittee on Health and Scientific Research, Committee on Human Resources. 1977. *Hospital Cost Containment Act of 1977* (May 24–26). 95th Cong. 1st sess. Washington: USGPO.

U.S. Congress, Senate. Hearings, Committee on Finance. 1982. *Administration's FY83 budget proposal, part 2* (March 12, 16). 97th Cong. 2nd sess. Washington: USGPO.

U.S. Congress, House. Hearings, Subcommittee on Health, Committee on Ways and Means. 1982. *Administration's proposed budget cuts affecting the Medicare program* (March 2; June 15). 97th Cong. 2nd sess. Washington: USGPO.

U.S. Congress, House. Hearings, Subcommittee on Health, Committee on Ways and Means. 1983. *Medicare hospital prospective payment system* (Feb. 14–15). 98th Cong. 1st sess. Washington: USGPO.

U.S. Congress, Senate. Hearings, Committee on Labor and Human Resources. 1983. *Health care cost: defining the issues* (May 19, 25). 98th Cong. 1st sess. Washington: USGPO.

U.S. Congress, House. Hearings, Subcommittee on Health and Environment, Committee on Energy and Commerce and Subcommittee on Health, Committee on Ways and Means. 1985. *Medicare and Medicaid issues* (April 26). 99th Cong. 1st sess. Washington: USGPO.

U.S. Congress, House. Hearings, Subcommittee on Health and Environment, Committee on Energy and Commerce. 1985. *Health financing* (July 17). 99th Cong. 1st sess. Washington: USGPO.

U.S. Congress, Senate. Hearings, Committee on Finance. 1985. *Budget reconciliation parts 1 & 2* (Sep. 11–13). 99th Cong. 1st sess. Washington: USGPO.

U.S. Congress, Senate. Hearings, Committee on Finance, Subcommittee on Health. 1985. *Reform of Medicare payments to physicians* (Dec. 6). 99th Cong. 1st sess. Washington: USGPO.

U.S. Congress, House. Hearings, Subcommittee on Health, Committee on Ways and Means. 1986. *1987 Medicare budget issues* (March 6). 99th Cong. 2nd sess. Washington: USGPO.

U.S. Congress, House. Hearings, Subcommittee on Health, Committee on Ways and Means. 1986. *Medicare reimbursement for physician services* (April 14). 99th Cong. 2nd sess. Washington: USGPO.

U.S. Congress, House. Hearings, Subcommittee on Health, Committee on Ways and Means. 1986. *Out-of-pocket costs for physician services under medicare Part B* (June 10) 99th Cong. 2nd sess. Washington: USGPO.

Weinberger, Marvin and David Greevy. 1982. *The PAC directory, a complete guide to political action committees.* Cambridge, MA: Ballinger.

Wilson, James Q. 1973. *Political organizations.* New York: Basic Books, Inc.

Ziegler, Harmon. 1964. *Interest groups in American society.* Englewood Cliffs, N.J.: Prentice-Hall.

Chapter 13

Public Opinion and Health Policy[1]

David A. Rochefort
Paul E. Pezza

Consider the following three episodes in health care policymaking:

In March of 1985 in the town of Portsmouth, Rhode Island, a group of local residents organized to oppose a new group home for the retarded in their neighborhood. A petition for closure of the facility was signed by 38 persons, some of whom also presented their demand in person before the Town Council. One complained, "These people go out in the back yard and rock back and forth and make yelling noises. I don't need that." The Council voted to ask the state Department of Mental Health, Retardation, and Hospitals to assess the group home residents for possible need for institutionalization and to erect a fence around the home (*Providence Journal* March 31, 1985). Similar public resistance to the establishment of community residences for the developmentally and emotionally disabled has occurred in numerous states nationwide, at times preventing the development of planned facilities (Maypole 1981).

In November of 1987, voters in Washington State rejected by a margin of 63.9 percent to 36.1 percent a ballot initiative making it a consumer protection violation for physicians to charge more than Medicare's reasonable fee (Keith 1988). In effect, the proposal would have compelled all physicians in the state to accept Medicare patients on an "assignment" basis. Opinion poll results gathered early in the campaign over the initiative showed 58 percent of the public in favor, 28 percent opposed, and 14 percent undecided. Ensuing months leading up to the actual vote saw a determined effort by the Washington State Medical Association (WSMA) to turn voters against the initiative by means of extensive radio and television advertising, direct mailings, and personal conversations between physicians and their office patients. More than $600,000 in funds from the WSMA and donations from physicians and organizations was expended.

[1]The authors are grateful to Ann E. P. Dill, Department of Sociology, Brown University and William J. Waters, Office of Health Policy, Rhode Island Department of Health for their helpful comments on an earlier draft of this chapter.

In January of 1989, the nation's most distinguished medical journal, the *New England Journal of Medicine,* published two proposals for a national health program in the United States (see also, *Boston Globe* January 12, 1989). Advanced by the progressive Physicians for a National Health Program, the more radical alternative recommended a Canadian-style overhaul of the existing system of U.S. health care financing that would provide coverage of basic medical services for the entire population and do away with private health insurance. In support of the political feasibility of its controversial proposal, the physicians' group cited opinion poll findings that a majority of Americans consistently have given support to the idea of "a universal, comprehensive, publicly administered national health program." The group concluded by observing that "If mobilized, such public conviction could override even the most strenuous private opposition" (Himmelstein et al. 1989, 107).

Major differences in context distinguish the above situations from each other. The matters at stake, actors involved, action arena, and time and place are variable. Yet one element is common—all display the crucial relevance of public opinion to the realm of health politics, policy-making, and administration.

It is a subject that, despite its importance, has so far escaped sustained scholarly inquiry. Articles and books regularly appear discussing the interests, stratagems, conflicts, and relative strength of visible and well-organized members of the health policy community, including hospitals, health insurers, physicians, public officials, and (the latest entrants) business executives. Relatively little attention, however, has been given to the relationship between what the average citizen thinks about the health system and its problems and the political process.

This chapter examines public opinion on health care issues and its influence upon government decision-making. Over the past couple of decades, popular views of major health care problems and policy proposals have become a leading interest among pollsters and other survey researchers. Accordingly, the following section provides a summary of the rich data base they have assembled. This is followed by three case studies that explore the role of public opinion, variously activated and expressed, in selected discrete health policy-making episodes.

We conclude with some general analytical statements.

Contemporary Public Opinion on Health Care

The American public has had a longstanding interest in health issues and the manner in which health care is provided for in the United States. In the last two decades this interest has been heightened by several developments. Among these are recognition of the role of behavioral risk factors in the etiology of health problems; the application of new technologies with outcomes both astounding and ethically challenging; a dramatic increase in the commitment of this nation's resources to the provision of health care; the appearance of new modes of health care delivery; the "corporatization" of medicine evidenced by the increased presence of for-profit providers; and the advent of an expanded role for government in paying for care and ensuring its quality.

A series of polls conducted over the past twenty-five years provides insight into public opinion as an element of the sociopolitical environment for health care policy-making. Considered here are surveys on national, state, and local levels by major polling organizations (Gallup, Harris, Roper, etc.), government, university centers, private institutes, and the media. (An earlier summary of these data appears in Rochefort and Boyer (1988).)

The Cost of Health Care

A substantial segment of the American public has for some time perceived the cost of health care as high and rising. Of eight national issues ranging from government deficits and high interest rates to public education and job opportunities, the high cost of health care was ranked first, second, or third in importance by 43 percent of a national sample in 1983 for the American Association of Retired Persons (AARP), with 13 percent of all respondents ranking it first (Hamilton and Staff 1983). In the same year, a Harris poll of New York City residents determined that the cost of health care was second only to police protection as a serious concern (*New York Times* January 30, 1983).

In a 1988 study by the American Medical Association (AMA), cost was mentioned six times more frequently than the second cited concern as the "main problem confronting health care and medicine in the United States today" (Harvey and Shubat 1988). A succession of surveys confirms the persistent saliency of this issue since the late 1970s (American Medical Association 1979; Shapiro and Young 1986). With a specific focus "on your area," 63 percent felt that the cost of medical care was "much too high given the quality of care provided" in the AARP survey. More than half shared this opinion in all age-groups. In another study in November of 1987, six out of ten people expressed the opinion that fees charged for medical care were less reasonable than they were five years prior (Pokorny 1988).

The impact on low-income Americans of cost as a barrier to health system access appears to have increased during the 1980s. Responses from large samples queried in 1982 and 1986 indicate that while the mean number of physician visits made annually diminished for the non-poor as well as the poor, the decline was greater for the poor. For respondents in fair to poor health, physician visits by the non-poor actually increased by 42 percent, while the poor made 8 percent fewer visits. In the same four-year period, the gap between black and white physician-visit rates in this same subgroup widened (Freeman et al. 1987).

Turning to public opinion about societal investment in health care, eleven National Opinion Research Center (NORC) polls spanning fifteen years indicate that a near constant 60 percent of the public felt we were spending too little on improving and protecting the nation's health, while 8 percent or less believed we have been spending too much (Shapiro and Young 1986). A minority of 46 percent of those responding to a 1983 survey for the Equitable Life Assurance Society would oppose limiting the use of expensive technologies for patients with "virtually no hope of recovery" (Taylor 1983). In a survey by the Harvard Community Health Plan in 1987, a large majority held that "Health insurance should pay for any treatments which will save lives even if it costs 1 million dollars to save a life." It has

been suggested that such generous views may be tied to the present vigor of the economy and, therefore, are susceptible to change (Blendon 1988).

Right to Health

Most Americans believe that everyone should be guaranteed as much health care as he or she needs (Pokorny 1988). Seventy-three percent of the public favors a constitutional amendment assuring every American "a right to adequate health care if he or she cannot pay for it" (Gabel, Cohen, and Fink 1989).

Although a large majority of the population (84.5 percent) has some insurance coverage (National Center for Health Services Research and Health Care Technology Assessment, 1989), the number of uninsured persons lately has been on the rise, and many of those with insurance suffer gaps or interruptions in coverage. Therefore, it is not surprising that many persons are concerned about access to care. In one study, while 70 percent were generally satisfied with their health insurance benefits, only 42 percent were satisfied with their out-of-pocket costs for health care (Taylor 1983). A third of those interviewed in a nationwide poll for the *New York Times* in 1982 said they had foregone needed care in the previous year because they could not afford it (*New York Times* March 29, 1982). Almost half were apprehensive about coverage as they grow older. Even those earning in excess of $40,000 annually reported uncertainty about paying for hospital visits and nursing home stays in their old age. Twenty percent said that their families had already been "seriously hurt by medical bills."

Availability of Care

For most people the availability of care, as distinct from its affordability, is not a concern. In a 1983 survey, 13 percent reported dissatisfaction with the availability of medical care when they needed it, a decline from the 21 percent holding similar views ten years earlier (Shapiro and Young 1986). In a 1988 survey of residents of the United States, Canada, and Great Britain, 13 percent of those in the U.S. stated that at some time in the previous year they did not get care they felt was needed. The corresponding figures in Canada and Great Britain were only 4 percent and 5 percent, respectively (Blendon 1989).

What had been a longstanding, rural/urban differential in mean physician visits virtually disappeared by 1986 (Freeman et al. 1987), and most recently, only 5 percent of Americans reported encountering non-economic barriers to needed care (Blendon 1989). Nevertheless, nearly half of black respondents (47 percent) believed that there are too few doctors in the community (Harvey and Shubat 1988). Moreover public concern over the availability of health care to the poor and the elderly persists. In the 1988 AMA survey, only one in three agreed that "poor people are able to get needed medical care," and four of ten agreed that the elderly could get the care they needed.

Quality

In five Roper polls over the period from 1973 to 1983, 83 to 87 percent of the public was satisfied with the quality of the medical care they received (Shapiro and Young 1986). One-third of those asked by the AMA in 1988 about the quality of care they personally received stated that it had improved "over the last few years," while half felt that it had not changed. Moreover, quality of care was rated as a very important influence on the choice of where to seek care by 94 percent of the respondents. By contrast, only 47 percent considered cost very important. Yet despite a largely favorable opinion of the quality of health care, only 27 percent of respondents in the 1988 AMA poll said that "we get our money's worth," when asked to judge the cost of health care against its perceived quality.

Health Care Providers

The central role played by physicians and hospitals in the provision of health care warrants consideration here. Physicians have long been the primary source of professional medical care, and hospitals have been the locus of much of

that care. Physician numbers, location, choice of specialty, and modes of practice are fundamental determinants of the availability, quality, and cost of care. These factors are, therefore, of particular interest to health policy analysts.

The proportion of individuals viewing "the health care industry, including physicians and hospitals" favorably steadily increased from 46 percent in 1979 to 59 percent in 1984 (Shapiro and Young 1986). Nevertheless, polls have discerned some areas of unhappiness. A pair of 1988 surveys found one-eighth to one-quarter of respondents dissatisfied with their most recent visit to the doctor (Harvey and Shubat 1988; Blendon 1989). In the latter study twice as many younger people were dissatisfied as were older ones, and an unsatisfactory experience was reported more frequently by blacks.

Several polls conducted by the AMA in the 1980s have delved more deeply into public perceptions of physicians (Freshnock and Shubat 1984; Harvey and Shubat 1986; Harvey and Shubat 1988). The results of those surveys reveal that one-third of the patients perceived doctors as acting "like they are better than other people," that one-half felt that they should be involved by doctors to a greater extent in treatment decisions, and that the proportion of patients describing doctors' fees as "usually reasonable" has declined from 42 percent to 33 percent over the last six years. In addition, two-thirds of the public believe that most physicians are "too interested in making money," and 49 percent agree with the statement that "doctors don't care about people as much as they used to." Still, three-quarters felt that most doctors are "genuinely dedicated to helping people."

The multinational survey of public opinion by Blendon (1989) already cited places the U.S. experience in comparative context. In that survey, 54 percent of those in the United States reported being very satisfied with their most recent doctor's visit, whereas in Great Britain the figure was 63 percent, and 73 percent in Canada.

Interestingly, there is an "image gap" between how the public sees its personal physician versus physicians in general (Freshnock and Shubat 1984). Responses to twelve questions on subjects ranging from availability and fees to knowledge of medicine and humility revealed differentials no smaller than 13 percent (dedication) and as large as 51 percent (faith in doctors/my doctor). This illustrates to some extent the "paradox of personal satisfaction and perceived crisis" noted by some health system observers (Robert Wood Johnson Foundation 1978).

Opinion sampling of the general public and of "physician leaders" (physicians who head local, state, and specialty medical societies) permits comparison of the views of these two groups on various health system issues. As noted by Rochefort and Boyer (1988, 652; Jeffe and Jeffe 1984), "striking disparities emerge." Each group tends to account for the inflation of health care costs by blaming the other's lack of cost-consciousness. Not surprisingly, while a majority of the public finds government price controls on doctors' and hospital fees acceptable, nine of ten physicians do not. Physician leaders are three times more likely than the general public to agree with the statement that "On the whole the health care system works pretty well, and only minor changes are necessary to make it work better."

Cost-Control Strategies

Price controls for hospitals, medical centers, and drugs were identified as a means for reducing the cost of health care by 70 percent of those polled for the American Board of Family Practice in 1985 (Pisacano 1985). Almost as many (64 percent) believed that fixing doctors' fees would reduce costs. Opinion favoring such limits is not surprising since, according to other surveys, 77 percent of the public feel that "there is no real competition among doctors, hospitals, and nursing homes to keep prices down" (Taylor 1983), and only 21 percent say that doctors are active in trying to hold down the cost of medical care (Freshnock and Shubat 1984). Tight control of health care costs on the other hand was not expected to adversely affect the quality of care according to 53 percent of those responding to the AARP poll in 1983 (39 percent said it would). Five years later, however, a plurality in one survey believed that cost-containment efforts were hurting the quality of care (Harvey and Shubat 1988). In the interest of ensuring medical care which is cost-effective and of high quality, public

trust in government (16 percent) to regulate the medical profession ranked above trust in individual physicians (11 percent) to do so, but below that placed in physician associations (AMA, etc.) (29 percent). Independent public affairs groups inspired the most confidence (34 percent) (Harvey and Shubat 1986).

Public opinion appears open to some modifications in medical practice in pursuit of cost-containment. In the Equitable Healthcare Survey of 1983, for example, the requirement of a second opinion for nonemergency surgery was acceptable to nearly all people (88 percent), as was a system which promotes testing and minor surgery in clinics and doctors' offices (83 percent). Same-day surgery was acceptable to 63 percent. Encouraging the use of non-physican providers (63 percent) and discouraging regional duplication of expensive hospital equipment and specialists (62 percent) were also generally acceptable. Similarly, two-thirds viewed employee copayment of health insurance premiums and larger patient copayment of medical bills as effective cost-containment strategies, although smaller proportions (58 percent and 52 percent) approved of adopting these strategies.

In general, practice arrangements that limit an individual's choice of doctor or hospital are not favored (Blendon and Altman 1984; Gabel, Cohen, and Fink 1989). Also, practice arrangements that limit patient access to care have only modest appeal. In the 1982 *New York Times* poll just 34 percent found longer waiting periods for a doctor's appointment acceptable. About the same number would agree "to limit the opportunities for people to use expensive modern technology." Thus, while majority opinion backs changes in existing methods for delivering care, levels of support vary with the approach proposed, and there are limits to what is deemed acceptable.

It should be noted that small variations in question wording from survey to survey that are perhaps indicative of sponsorship effects produce different levels of support for specific cost-control options (Rochefort and Boyer 1988). Thus it is not surprising that the Equitable survey item on deductibles—which included the qualifying clause that the purpose of deductibles was "so that people become more cost-conscious when seeking medical services"—elicited a degree of popular approval 13 percentage points higher than another question on deductibles by the *New York Times,* which did not use this phrase.

Government and Health Care Policy

Public opinion of government in its role as third-party payer for health services and as regulator of private service provision is ambivalent. The 1984 AMA survey showed that only one in five respondents thought that government does a good-to-excellent job of advocating their interests as health care consumers. Non-physician professionals (46 percent), hospitals (34 percent), and physicians (27 percent) all fared better. Yet, while public confidence in the leaders of government is low relative to that placed in the leaders of eight other major institutions including medicine, expectations of "government" are high (Rochefort and Boyer 1988).

Data gathered over a period of 17 years indicate as much support in 1982 (69 percent) as in 1965 (67 percent) for more government activity on "health measures" (Shapiro and Young 1986). These data show that two-thirds of those interviewed would prefer increased activity even if higher taxes were necessary. Widespread antagonism toward public welfare in the United States notwithstanding, strong support exists for health care assistance for the poor and needy (Rochefort and Boyer 1988). A series of polls from 1960 to 1978 revealed steadily increasing agreement (from 75 percent to 85 percent) with the idea that government ought to assume responsibility for seeing to it that health care is provided at low cost. Not surprisingly, there has been a parallel increase in the proportion of people who favor government regulation of doctor and hospital charges (Shapiro and Young 1986). In New Jersey, where an approach to hospital reimbursement based on diagnosis-related groups (DRGs) was already in place, 56 percent of the residents polled in 1983 said that hospital costs should be subject to "considerable" regulation by government (New Jersey Hospital Association 1983).

Among those who favor limits on provider charges, 59 percent believe such limits should be set by either state or federal government (Hamilton and Staff 1983). When asked what impact less governmental regulation of health care would have on the quality of care, 43 percent said quality would decline at least somewhat, while 22 percent said quality would improve (Shapiro and Young 1986). Half of all polled felt that the good effects of regulation outweighed the bad. Public approval of regulatory strategies aimed toward health care cost-control was sampled nationwide in 1986 by Cambridge Reports, Inc. (Byers and Fitzpatrick 1986). Respondents were evenly split on the employment of DRGs, with 43 percent in favor and 43 percent opposed; 62 percent favored a freeze on Medicare payments to physicians; and 61 percent approved the establishment of professional review organizations.

Little support exists for curbing health care costs by restricting Medicare eligibility and coverage (Schneider, 1985). Reducing Medicare benefits by 10 percent is thought of as desirable by only 13 percent of persons polled. Raising the age of eligibility for Medicare to 67 years (29 percent) and increasing the deductible on medical bills to be paid by Medicare recipients (32 percent) are favored to a somewhat greater extent but are not supported by most. Eight out of ten people believe that expenditures for health care programs for the elderly should be raised, while nearly sixty percent say they would accept a small tax increase to pay for long-term care for the elderly (Blendon 1988). Support for care of the aged is not without limit, however. Most people do not approve reducing payments to doctors and hospitals for Medicare (and Medicaid) patients if this would result in cost-shifting to those with private insurance and paying more out-of-pocket (Taylor 1983). Also, when forced to choose, the public ranks care for premature children over that of the elderly (Gabel, Cohen, and Fink 1989). It would appear that attitudes towards increased expenditures for health care entitlement programs depend on how the additional cost burden is to be spread and who the beneficiaries are to be.

National Health Insurance

Several polls have indicated support for some form of national health insurance, ranging from 49 to 64 percent of all respondents (Shapiro and

Young, 1986). In 1982, 59 percent of those interviewed had positive attitudes toward such a program even if implementation required a tax increase (Health Insurance Association of America 1982). Yet only 19 percent in 1987 expressed a willingness to pay more than $50 annually in additional taxes for such a program (Pokorny 1988). Nine Roper surveys from 1973 to 1983 required respondents to make an explicit choice between the current system of private health insurance and a national plan provided for by government (Shapiro and Young 1986). In each case, nearly equal proportions chose the government plan and the current system.

As for quality of care under a national insurance program, a 1987 *Health Management Quarterly* poll found expectations to be mixed, with 24 percent anticipating an improvement, and 34 percent expecting a decline (Pokorny 1988). Nonetheless, most Americans (80 percent) feel that government should be making at least "some effort" to "set up a national health insurance system" (Shapiro and Young 1986). Finally, the international comparative survey by Blendon (1989) found that Americans' dissatisfaction with their current system is so high that a majority would want to change it for that of Canada (but not Great Britain). In neither Canada nor Great Britain did a majority of citizens want to replace their system.

The Challenge of AIDS

Acquired Immune Deficiency Syndrome (AIDS) emerged in the 1980s as a health problem of great concern to the American public. Uncertainty about this newly recognized disease entity has been reflected in public opinion about AIDS. Opinion remains in flux as public education efforts and media coverage convey an evolving understanding about the impact of AIDS on individuals, on populations, and on social systems.

Awareness of AIDS is virtually complete, with 99 percent of those polled by the Gallup organization in 1988 saying they had read or heard about the disease (*Gallup Report* June 1988). When asked what is the most serious health problem facing the country today, respondents in two polls conducted in 1986 ranked AIDS second,

behind cancer and ahead of heart disease (Singer, Rogers, and Corcoran 1987; *New York Times* March 25, 1987). The Gallup poll found 68 percent of people of the opinion that AIDS was the "most urgent health problem in this country."

While awareness of AIDS is very high, self-assessed knowledge about the condition is not. From 1987 to 1988, among those queried on behalf of the AMA, the proportion holding the belief that they "have a lot of information" about AIDS increased from 19 to 29 percent. This outcome ranged from 40 percent of those with a college education to 18 percent of those without a high school diploma. Responses to specific questions about risk factors for AIDS reinforce the impression that some people are misinformed and others are uncertain. For example, of 3,248 adults responding to the National Health Interview Survey (NHIS) in July of 1988, 45 percent believed that blood transfusions are safe, whereas 26 percent did not, and 29 percent were not sure (Dawson 1988). This was so despite the fact that 67 percent reported that they believed that donated blood is screened for the AIDS virus. On the other hand, insect bites, use of public toilets, sharing of kitchen utensils with AIDS-infected individuals, and being coughed or sneezed on by those infected were correctly ruled out as likely modes of AIDS transmission by 60 percent or less of respondents in all cases. Still it is of interest to note that only 27 percent of those sampled in another national poll said that they had a "great deal" of trust in "current scientific knowledge about AIDS" (*New York Times* May 22, 1987). Similarly, 34 percent of those interviewed for the NHIS, were either doubtful of or didn't know if they could believe information about AIDS provided by federal health officials.

Measures for dealing with the AIDS epidemic have had various and varying degrees of public support. A poll conducted for the *Los Angeles Times* in 1985 (Field 1986) found that 51 percent of a nationwide sample of 2,308 favored quarantine of those diagnosed with AIDS; 48 percent felt that those infected should have to carry an identity card indicating their affliction; and 15 percent felt that a tatoo would be an effective means of identification (*New York Times* December 20, 1985). A more recent poll found 29 percent favoring quarantine and 39 percent opposed

(Steiber 1988). Moreover seventy-seven percent of those responding to the *Los Angeles Times* survey said they would favor criminalizing blood donation by members of groups at high risk for AIDS and 51 percent would favor criminal penalties for an AIDS patient who engages in sexual activity with someone.

According to a 1986 poll in which 86 percent of respondents favored sex education in the schools, among those holding this opinion, 38 percent said that courses for children aged eight should include AIDS education and 93 percent said that courses for twelve-year olds should include AIDS content (Singer, Rogers, and Corcoran 1987). Finally, data from the National Health Interview Survey indicated that seven out of ten people would, with assurances of privacy, submit to a blood test for AIDS infection status in order to assist in determining the prevalence of infection in this country (Dawson 1988).

Public opinion about the regulation of school and work environments in order to control the transmission of AIDS has been sampled several times. According to the *Los Angeles Times* survey, (Field 1986) 55 percent of all respondents would allow their children to attend a school where a student with AIDS was present. An ABC survey also in 1985 tested public confidence in government by asking if school attendance by AIDS patients should be allowed, given assurances of no danger by "health officials." The policy was favored by nearly two-thirds (Singer, Rogers, and Corcoran 1987). In another study, twenty-four percent of those opposed to such a policy were unsure about the risk of casual contact (*New York Times* April 17, 1986). On the other hand, a diagnosis of AIDS is not seen as a disqualification for employment by most people. Two-thirds of respondents to an NBC poll in 1985 said that those with AIDS should be retained in their jobs, while one-fifth felt that employers should have the prerogative of firing such individuals (Singer, Rogers, and Corcoran 1987). Uncertainty about the risk posed by affected coworkers remains, however. Although 84 percent of those sampled by the Gallup organization in 1988 said that working near someone already affected is not a way of getting AIDS, only 65 percent said that they "would not refuse to work along side someone who has AIDS."

Finally, slightly more than half (53 percent) of the public is not satisfied with government's past level of activity in combatting the AIDS epidemic (*Gallup Report* January/February 1988), and 59 percent feel that government should pay for the medical care of uninsured AIDS victims (Blendon and Donelan 1988).

Patterns and Implications

The American public's views on health care issues are complex and, in some respects, difficult to fathom. Concerned about rising costs of care and problems of access and distribution, the public is hampered in its choice of a remedial course by the contending values of compassion vs. self-interest, efficiency vs. convenience, change vs. stability, and private vs. public control. While believing that the system may be approaching some kind of crisis, many citizens are reluctant to entertain the idea of limits on technology or heroic medical intervention. This is perhaps not surprising, given how these very issues divide experts in the field. At the same time, a majority of the public is generally satisfied with their own health care experience, including their relationships with personal physicians.

Indications are mixed, as well, when it comes to the subject of government policymaking and regulation for health care. Most citizens want government to act more effectively to resolve contemporary health system problems, and recent government innovations such as DRGs have gained considerable, though not universal, acceptance. Yet the public has little confidence in government protecting its interests within the health arena, even as compared to special interests such as physicians, hospitals, and insurance companies. Moreover, support for regulatory strategies depends on where, how, and by whom their impact is to be felt.

Existing entitlement programs—especially Medicare—enjoy solid backing. Eligibility and benefit reductions in these programs are not generally acceptable as a means of health care cost containment, notwithstanding certain recent policy changes of this nature. Many people assert that the nation should be spending even more on government health programs. The difficulty arises when such an expansion is linked specifically to increased tax burdens, as inevitably, in practice, it would have to be. With respect to national health insurance, one of the most pressing health policy issues of the day, a majority of the public seems committed in principle to the idea. It remains to be seen, however, whether an actual program with specified costs and benefits can be crafted that will garner a clear popular mandate.

Until such time as a major breakthrough of this kind may be accomplished, public officials will likely have to stick to their present course of a "multipronged approach" to health care policy-making (Rochefort and Boyer 1988; Blendon and Altman 1984). Rather than a single, comprehensive reform strategy, decisionmakers are constrained to pursue a heterogeneous program of policy and administrative techniques spanning the areas of planning, regulation, and competition. Sizeable segments of the public seemingly are disturbed enough about the present health care cost problem and access issues to go along with a variety of measures ranging from new constraints on hospital and physician behavior to modifications in traditional health insurance arrangements. But the dominant perception is that these actions will both be more effective and more legitimate to the extent that they emerge from a coordinated public-private partnership rather than a one-sided increase in governmental interventionism.

Many citizens' health care views rest on a foundation of superficial information and understanding. Glaring gaps in popular knowledge exist concerning government's present regulatory activities in the health care sector, not to mention the distinguishing features of alternative delivery systems. Even on subjects where there is general awareness, such as AIDS, many people have not absorbed correctly the basic facts about disease transmission which have been very broadly disseminated by the media. Unquestionably, the health care field is becoming more, not less, specialized and technical, serving only to further strain the public's ability to appreciate and contribute effectively to the ongoing health policy debate. The varying circumstances under which such influence actually is exercised is the topic to which we turn in the remainder of this chapter.

Public Opinion and Health Policymaking: Three Cases

Having sketched the portrait of contemporary health care opinion within the United States, three case studies will illustrate variations of the linkage between public opinion and the health policymaking process. The selected cases deal, in turn, with federal, state, and local levels of government, and with salient health policy issues of the 1960s, 1970s, and 1980s.

The Community Mental Health Centers Act of 1963: Agenda-Setting through Convergent Voice

The transition from one policy orientation to another inevitably engenders resistance. Careers, jobs, program benefits, and belief systems all are at stake. Overcoming this barrier requires a strong commitment to innovation, the kind that frequently depends on the emergence of a new ideological consensus (Cameron 1978).

This conceptual framework offers a useful approach for understanding the emergence of a national community mental health program in the United States during the 1960s.[2] Representing the status quo in public mental health care was a 150-year-old hospital based system under state government control. The Community Mental Health Centers Act of 1963 (CMHC Act) ushered in an alternative delivery system focusing on outpatient rather than inpatient facilities, primarily dependent on federal dollars, and answerable to federal operational guidelines. This shift, one of the most dramatic in the history of post-war health policymaking, was made possible by the crystallization of new social views concerning the nature and extent of mental illness. Opinion change among scholars, professionals, and political elites in this period paralleled and reinforced shifts within the general public, as both, together, influenced a redirection in policy-making.

Several concurrent historical developments and social forces underlay this process. The rejection on psychiatric grounds of thousands of military inductees during World War Two, combined with large numbers of mentally disabled veterans, broadcast the extensiveness of mental health problems in American society. Studies in the nascent field of psychiatric epidemiology during the 1950s and early 1960s provided confirming data through surveys of the general pop-

---

[2]This case study is based on the more detailed version that appears in Rochefort (1986, chapter 2).

ulation and other scientific methodologies. Also in this period, new group and social therapies and drug treatments were applied with unprecedented effectiveness, giving fresh hope in the treatment of the most severe disorders. Mental illness's traditional stigma as an isolated social problem best handled through long-term, custodial institutionalization began to be challenged.

A series of mental hospital exposés in the mass media and critical studies by social scientists further undermined the legitimacy of the existing system. Overcrowded, understaffed, decrepit facilities with deficient treatment programs seemed to exacerbate the disorders they were supposed to treat. At this same time, vigorous debate proceeded within the mental health professions between adherents of the traditional "medical model" for mental health care and advocates of a community-based, prevention-oriented, "public health" approach. The National Institute of Mental Health, established by Congress in 1946, became a powerful proponent of the latter point of view, which it helped diffuse through the kinds of research and services its grant programs funded.

Adding to this social ferment, public opinion toward mental illness and the mentally ill underwent its own transformation in this period. A growing popular audience, for example, demonstrated interest in the coverage of mental health topics in the daily press and other media (Ridenour 1961, 110–113). Voluntary mental health organizations, too, experienced striking growth around the country (Ridenour 1961, 124–130, 137). The mental hygiene movement founded by Clifford Beers in 1908 had about fifty state and local societies by the 1930s. In the late 1940s, close to 200 were in existence. In 1960, the National Association for Mental Health, established ten years earlier through the merger of the National Committee for Mental Hygiene and two other national mental health organizations, claimed more than 800 local and state chapters. Members and volunteers were estimated to be in excess of 1 million.

Poll results in the early post-World-War II era documented the existence of negative attitudes toward the mentally disordered as well as low levels of information on mental illness and mental health services. In a study in Louisville, Kentucky in 1950, most respondents did not under-

stand the benefits of outpatient mental health care nor the role of psychiatrists in treating milder forms of mental illness (Woodward 1951). Relatively few of those surveyed in a national sample in this same year could recognize schizophrenia as a form of mental illness when it was described to them in a case story. Three-quarters, on the other hand, could recognize an instance of paranoia as indicative of disturbance (Rochefort, 1986, 43, Table 2.1). A review of published and unpublished studies in this area by the Joint Commission on Mental Illness and Health, a body created by the U.S. Congress in 1955, observed that "a pervasive defeatism" colored attitudes toward psychiatric treatment (Joint Commission on Mental Illness and Health 1961, xix).

Yet public opinion on these subjects was in transition. Compared to earlier studies, surveys of the 1960s recorded important changes both in information levels and attitudes regarding mental illness and the mentally ill. For example, answers to the same questionnaire items used in previous research suggested an increased ability among respondents to recognize mental illness. In a major survey in Baltimore in 1960 which sampled 1,736 persons, 78 percent correctly identified schizophrenic behavior as symptomatic of mental illness, and 91 percent did the same for paranoia (Lemkau and Crocetti 1962). Studies in other locales produced comparable results (Dohrenwend, Bernard, and Kolb 1962; Meyer 1964). Further, when measured in terms of a standard "social distance scale," fewer respondents in these surveys than in earlier investigations personally expressed views rejecting individuals who had been mentally ill (Rochefort 1986, 44, Table 2.2). On the basis of a broad-ranging examination of studies conducted in the post-war period, a 1963 federal government report concluded: "The overall impression one unmistakably gets from a review of these surveys is that there has been forward motion during the past decade in terms of better public understanding of mental illness and greater tolerance or acceptance of the mentally ill. It appears to be reasonably clear that the American public does not universally reject the mentally ill nor is it thoroughly defeatist about the prospects of treating mental illness" (Halpert 1963, 19).

Along with new information on the scope of the problem of mental illness, treatment innovations, and the shortcomings of the state hospital system, awareness of a changing public opinion figured directly in policy-makers' deliberations on national community mental health legislation. For example, in congressional testimony on the Community Mental Health Center bill, the president's special assistant for health and medical affairs linked the medical and social impacts of recent discoveries in psychopharmocology as follows: "The tranquilizing drugs have made quite an impact on the management of mental illness, and I think people are increasingly coming to the viewpoint that mental illness is an illness, and not a result of a scourge or condemnation for which the individual is responsible" (Rochefort 1986, 50). In response to a question as to whether citizens would be disinclined to use the new community centers being considered for creation, the special assistant stated, "I think the opposite is true . . . I think the American public now has a much more enlightened attitude toward mental illness than was true even ten years ago" (Rochefort 1986, 171, note 104). Another central participant, Robert Felix, at the time director of the National Institute of Mental Health, which was primarily responsible for drafting the CMHC program, later recalled that after World War II, "the arousal of the American people was rapid and dramatic. Much of the stigma of mental illness, which had been prevalent since time immemorial, began to fall away. Mental and emotional disorders were spoken of much more frankly, and the need for increased knowledge, more skilled manpower, and facilities of all types was increasingly accepted" (Felix 1967, 50–51). For their part, House committee members and their staff also appreciated "that the Joint Commission [and the president] . . . had alerted the electorate" on the community mental health issue (Foley 1975, 62).

Granted the relevant influence of public opinion within this policymaking episode, some have cast it in terms of a top-down manipulation by activists who molded or manufactured the views needed to suit their programmatic ends (Foley 1975; Scull 1977). That certain community mental health partisans inside and outside of government desired such an outcome is clear. But their unique responsibility for changes in public thinking on mental illness is doubtful, and in any case impossible to determine, operating as they did

within the context of a larger, more spontaneous socio- professional shift in understandings of the problem. Research has shown how deliberate attitude change in this area is notoriously difficult to achieve (Cumming and Cumming 1957; President's Commission on Mental Health 1978). Moreover, in considering public receptivity to numerous newspaper columns, magazine articles, books, radio and television programs, and movies on mental illness in this period, the distinction between opinion leaders and opinion followers is nebulous, for publishers, broadcasters, and film producers all depended on pleasing their audiences by responding to perceived interests (Rochefort 1986, 68). Cook's (1981, 126) "convergent voice" model of agenda-setting, in which a given issue in society is "independently and similarly articulated by several different groups at the same time," best describes this case in national policymaking. As part of the emerging consensus for change, public opinion thus contributed to the culminating pressure that impelled government to undertake community care as an important mental health policy innovation.

Health Planning in Rhode Island: Public Mobilization through Conflict Expansion

The idea of "health planning as a technical exercise conducted outside of the political arena" has been described as a myth shattered by the experience of federally sponsored health planning in the United States under Public Law 93-641 (P.L. 93-641) (Lipschultz 1980, 3). The recent history of health planning in the state of Rhode Island bolsters this view. Insofar as the health planning program initiated by Congress in the 1970s provided for the negotiation of diverse interests, it was inherently political. The enabling legislation established a forum for the consideration of the often competing agendas of a variety of health care provider groups, consumer representatives, and governmental entities, each with its own values and vested interests. The very definition of problems to be addressed, their prioritization, the elaboration of strategic solutions, and proposals for their implementation and evaluation were all activities taking place in a political environment. P.L. 93-641 was a mandate for planned change in the provision of health care, prevention of disease, and promotion of health in the United States. Change necessarily meant moving toward a system more expressive of the values held by some constituents and away from those important to others. That the planning process engendered conflict was to be expected. In Rhode Island, that conflict produced a dynamic, surprising in its character and intensity to participants and observers alike.

This case examines the manner in which intergroup conflict was choreographed by health care provider interests during the development of the smallest state's first Health Systems Plan. Providers, perceiving a potential disadvantage in the debate over planning goals and a threat to their long-term interests, effectively mobilized public opinion to influence health policy formulation in their own favor. The Rhode Island experience illustrates Schattschneider's (1960) concept of the "contagiousness of conflict," specifically as refined by Cobb and Elder's (1983) work on conflict management and the dynamics of issue creation and expansion. According to this approach, when a conflict arises between two groups it will often initially be limited in scope, involving small numbers of organized and unorganized individuals. In all probability, both sides of the conflict will not be equal in terms of the political power that can be brought to bear in negotiating a solution. It is to the advantage of the weaker side to expand the scope of the issue by recruiting additional participants for "it is extremely unlikely that both sides will be reinforced equally" (Schattschneider 1960, 3). This can be achieved by simply broadcasting news of the conflict. The issue may also be defined, or redefined, in ways calculated to excite or appeal to an expanded audience (Cobb and Elder 1983, esp. ch. 6 and 7). As Schattschneider asserts, "Theoretically, control of the scope of the conflict is absolutely crucial" to its outcome (Schattschneider 1960, 5). Coverage by the *Providence Journal* of events occurring just before, during, and after public hearings in 1980 on the first *Rhode Island Health Plan* provide evidence for the effective employment of these strategies by provider interests (*Providence Journal* October 28, December 2, 20, 21, 22, 23, 27, 28, 1979; January 1, 2, 3, 4, 9, 11, 17, 18, 27, 1980).

The National Health Planning and Resources Development Act of 1974 required each state to prepare a Health Systems Plan. The primary objective of this legislation was to foster the "achievement of equal access to quality health care at a reasonable cost." Community involvement in the development of the Plan was to be accomplished by gubernatorial appointment of volunteer health care "consumers" and "providers" to a Statewide Health Coordinating Council (SHCC). Consumer members were to represent the demographic composition and geographic regions of each state. Within every state, population blocks of from 500,000 to 3,000,000 persons were designated as Health Service Areas, each served by a Health Systems Agency (HSA) (Koff 1988). The HSAs were charged with the responsibilities of identifying the health needs of the Area and for developing the Health Systems Plan (HSP) and Annual Implementation Plan (AIP) for their Areas. The federal planning legislation also created a state-level entity, the State Health Planning and Development Agency (SHPDA), to consolidate the Area HSPs into a coordinated State Health Plan for submission to the SHCC for review and approval. Comprised of professionals, the SHPDA provided technical assistance to the SHCC and was responsible for plan implementation as well. As a prelude to SHCC approval of the State health Plan, P.L. 93-641 and its amendments set forth a requirement for public hearings to allow for citizen commentary on the Plans as input into the planning process.

In Rhode Island the SHCC consisted of thirty volunteers. Because of this state's small size and concentration of population and health services, it was exempted from having individual Health Service Areas and Health Systems Agencies. The functions of the Health Systems Agency were assumed by the SHPDA (Rhode Island Department of Health 1981).

The first draft of the *Rhode Island Health Plan*, as approved by the SHCC, was far-sighted and far-reaching. Noting demographic changes within the state, the emergence of chronic illness as the major source of morbidity and mortality, rising health care costs, and the absence of competition in the health care "marketplace," the draft made numerous recommendations for disease prevention, alternative types of health care, and cost-control measures. Specific strategies for health promotion and disease prevention included a prohibition on advertising of alcohol, tobacco, and drugs aimed at children; a sales tax on harmful foods; elimination of the sale of junk food in all schools; and handgun control. Among the health service goals articulated by the plan were reductions in general and psychiatric hospital use, inappropriate nursing home use, overall nursing home use, and total physician visit capacity. Strategies aimed at bringing health facilities into line with community needs featured an overall reduction in the number of short-stay hospital beds, the application of minimum size standards for acute-care hospitals and their obstetrical, pediatric, and medical-surgical services, and a curb on nursing home construction. Limits on the total number of physicians, particularly pediatricians and surgeons, were advocated, as was the institution of salaried versus fee-for-service payment of hospital-based radiologists, pathologists, and anesthesiologists. Restriction of the number of practicing registered nurses and the closure of at least one nursing education program in the state were proposed as well. Increases were recommended in the ratio of primary care physicians-to-population and in occupational health manpower. Savings to be realized by system cost control measures would be reallocated, augmenting support of health education, community mental health programs, alcohol and drug abuse services, primary health care, and home health services.

Clearly, the plan as originally drafted and presented for public commentary challenged the state's institutional and professional status quo. Most inflammatory regarding provider concerns, were the recommended elimination of 25 percent of the state's hospital beds and of hospital services so small as to be considered inefficient and incapable of providing sufficient experience to maintain professional skill. The prospect of government regulating the number, specialty, and location of professionals practicing within the state also rankled.

Provider groups organized statewide in opposition to those components of the plan deemed threatening to their interests. The hospital association, state medical societies, and the presidents of hospital medical staffs formed an umbrella organization, the Voluntary Committee of Health Providers, to represent their constituen-

cies. The committee engaged a major Boston-area consulting firm, at a cost of $40,000, to evaluate the plan. The consultant's report challenged the SHCC's "incorrect" use of statistics, took issue with several plan elements, and speculated about possible negative impacts should the plan be implemented. Raised was the spectre of "queuing" for care, an exodus of "quality, hospital-based physicians," and an inequitable and inconvenient situation wherein patients who could afford to would be leaving the state for care, with others having attention to their needs delayed or denied. The consultant's report provided a technical basis for the strident and emotional assertion, made by one hospital executive, that the plan would "destroy access to health care of the poor and the elderly."

Individual institutions also organized responses to the state planning effort. In one hospital, a special task force was assembled which sponsored a full-page newspaper advertisement urging local residents to turn out for the hearing scheduled in their area and protect their "freedom of choice." The ad offered transportation to and from the hearing site. The ambulance corps serving this and neighboring communities mounted a drive at area shopping malls to warn the citizenry that local health services were "in jeopardy" and to encourage attendance at the upcoming hearing. A trustee of another hospital formed "Citizens for Community Care" to "mobilize opposition" and to promote a widespread public response. Still another hospital established a speakers bureau to broadcast its opposition to the plan and conducted a petition drive to register negative public sentiment.

A spate of newspaper items appearing in the weeks prior to the commencement of hearings on the plan gave some hint of what was to take place. The first of several allusions to an Orwellian regime appeared, and the credibility of state officials was challenged. Various provider sources offered the opinions that the planning effort was "a rigid, top-down approach," one which promoted a "dangerous, centralized and governmentally controlled" system. It was asserted that "doctors know what's in the best interest of Rhode Island patients." One Chamber of Commerce publicly characterized the health plan as an "unwarranted intrusion by government into the free enterprise system." Despite assurances offered by the governor and health department officials that the plan was an advisory document only, without the force of law, the administrator of the state's smallest hospital was quoted as saying that it would be a "dangerous practice" for communities to accept the governor's "informal assurances." The administrator of another small hospital in an outlying area described the plan as "very dangerous," a mandate for facility closings and the rationing of care. He drew an analogy to the British health system with its "six week wait for surgery and 20 year pause in hospital construction." This area's town council passed a resolution urging changes in the plan and attendance at the upcoming hearing. Less than one week earlier, the state's senior senator had publicly acknowledged a "firestorm of protest and concern," which elicited his promise that the health plan would not close hospitals. Officials of two hospitals in the northern part of the state, while acknowledging that the 800-page document approved by the SHCC did not specify that either of their institutions must close, nonetheless pledged to rally public opposition to the plan. Expressing concern that the plan posed a threat to the economy of his area, the state legislator from this region claimed that the closing of just one of its hospitals would cost some 500 jobs.

During January of 1980, seven evening hearings were conducted throughout Rhode Island, making the public review process accessible to virtually everyone. A sampler of headlines accompanying newspaper accounts of the hearings conveys something of the character of these events and the atmosphere that prevailed: " 'Big Brother' label cheered by foes of state health plan"; "Marathon hearing ends at 1:10 A.M."; "Doctor tells health-plan drafters they were 'duped by bureaucrats.' "

The first of the hearings, held in a town of 18,000, drew an estimated 3,000 residents. Eight hundred people marched in a candlelight procession from town hall to the hearing site and were accompanied by a dozen fire engines, sirens sounding, and two high school bands. An East Bay community was the site of the second hearing. There, a capacity crowd of 1,200 shouted their disapproval of the health plan when prompted by the city hospital's former trustee board chairman. "Upstaters" and "bureaucrats"

were blamed for the plan that would "hurt" the local facility after its president communicated the fear that it would be reduced to "little more than a first-aid receiving station" (Rosenberg 1980, 42). The hospital's auxiliary supplied refreshments to those attending the hearing and invited signatures upon a petition against the plan. This scenario was essentially repeated with an overflow crowd of 1,700 at the next hearing, held in the northern part of the state. An estimated total of 10,000 people turned out for all seven hearings. The populace had been effectively aroused and engaged as an ally in an expansion of the provider conflict with government.

Following the first two hearings, with their often raucous proceedings and sometimes caustic input, a member of the SHPDA and a principal author of the draft plan cast the best possible light on the events by offering the opinion that the public and professional reaction had been "healthy." He went on to predict that the planning program would "eventually receive widespread community support." But after the seventh and final hearing, the chairman of the SHCC was moved to remark that the council had "failed in its perception of what the people of Rhode Island would find acceptable." The lone private medical practitioner serving as a SHCC member concurred, stating that "the preliminary draft was too far out in front of public opinion to be acceptable or implementable" (Rosenberg 1980, 51).

Others had different interpretations. A spokesman for the AFL-CIO charged that the hospital association had misled the public by generating rumors about the health plan. And a news report attributed to one state planner the view that "hospital officials had stirred up city residents with statements charging falsely that the plan would dismantle Newport hospital 'brick by brick.' " The planner believed, further, that "hospital officials went so far as to write many of the speeches delivered in Newport by local residents."

No basis for judging the validity of such accusations is provided here. Whatever the facts of the matter, however, health care providers in Rhode Island plainly succeeded in broadcasting their concerns so as to enlist thousands of people in support of their cause. Planning issues were defined to tap strongly held popular values regarding limited government and the protection of personal freedoms. Moreover, provider activists wisely portrayed the health plan battle as a crusade to protect valued community resources. Significantly, a national survey in 1978 on attitudes toward health planning under P.L. 93-641 found that 71 percent of respondents felt all existing beds in hospitals serving their area were needed (Mick and Thompson 1984). Sixty-five percent were opposed to "a policy which could reduce costs by reducing the number of hospital beds in the community if this means that, on occasion, people would have to wait to get a bed in the hospital." And regulatory action limiting choice of hospital, increasing travel time for non-emergency care, or increasing waiting time for such care would make majorities of individuals "very" or "somewhat" unhappy.

Hospital and physician interests in Rhode Island were also able to exploit the "image gap" and the "paradox of perceived crisis and personal satisfaction" described earlier. This they did by focusing public attention on the individual's relationship to his doctor and community institutions. Limited citizen knowledge of the planning process made Rhode Islanders all the more open to persuasion by the providers' arguments. As noted by one analyst, while the state health plan was "technically sound," there had been no local community involvement in its development; thus, "the information obtained from the opposition became the basis of the residents' understanding of the plan's impact" (Lipschultz 1980, 6).

When the dust settled, statewide health planning in Rhode Island had a decidedly different look about it. The SHCC requested from the U.S. Department of Health, Education, and Welfare an extension of its deadline for submission of a final plan. With this granted, the council went to work revising the draft to reflect the realities of health planning in a political environment. In the plan's final form, the number of practicing physicians specified as appropriate for the state was raised from 1,480 to 1,800; specialty-specific limits no longer appeared; and the original proposal to eliminate 25 percent of all hospital beds was replaced by the recommendation that a voluntary effort be made to reduce beds.

Anderson (1977, 188) has written that "Planning for health has been constrained for too long by the specific structures of a health care delivery system. Priorities have been constrained by the policy of preserving a specific delivery system, or at least that portion which employs personnel." This observation aptly describes the initiation of federally-sponsored health planning in Rhode Island in the late 1970s, a situation of conflict in which one side successfully mobilized public opinion to tip the balance of power in its favor. Provider interests, heavily invested in the status quo and facing a sudden threat to their traditional control over the health care system, enlarged the audience for their contest with government and galvanized local community action. Public opinion was effectively molded by provider definition of the issues in such a way as to elicit popular reaction against comprehensive health planning and its attendant strategy of resource allocation. The existing apparatus for health care delivery in Rhode Island was maintained.

Boston's Sterile Needles Debate: Elite-Mass Dissensus

The third case study concerns a recent proposal in the city of Boston to distribute sterile needles to intravenous (IV) drug users as a means of fighting the spread of AIDS. It illustrates how a fundamental opinion dissensus, among political elites and the organized and unorganized public, complicated consideration of a policy put forward on pragmatic grounds and ultimately determined its defeat. The Boston Globe's careful chronicling of the dispute, which occupied the first six months of 1988, provides the basis of our narrative (Boston Globe January 10, 13, 17, February 24, 25, 26, 28, 29, March 1, 2, 5, 23, 30, April 7, 11, 12, 13, 14, 15, 27, 29, May 1, 5, June 9, 10, 19, 26, 27, 28).

The issue was initiated in January, when Boston Mayor Raymond Flynn sent Dr. George Lamb, director of Boston's Department of Health and Hospitals, to Liverpool, England and Amsterdam, the Netherlands to gather information on those cities' operating needle-exchange programs. Following a favorable report by the director, Mayor Flynn formally proposed to the City Council that Boston undertake a similar effort. The recommendation was for a 180-day pilot program, under medical supervision, to hand out clean needles and syringes to drug addicts who turn in their used "works." A maximum of 200 IV drug users would be served, primarily those uninterested in entering rehabilitative treatment. Projected costs were between $60,000 and $70,000.

Massachusetts prohibits the dispensing of syringes without a doctor's prescription. To mount the experimental needle exchange, therefore, Boston would need to be exempted from state law through a home rule petition. The procedure involved approval by the City Council, followed by the state legislature, then governor.

From the outset, the sterile needles proposal touched off an intense political controversy. Early opponents included Governor Dukakis and his public health commissioner, Dr. Deborah Prothrow-Stith. Immediate strong support was given to Flynn from the Massachusetts AIDS Action Committee, an advocacy group. Within a short while, numerous other individuals and state and local organizations joined the fray. To appreciate the resulting debate and its underlying value dimensions, it is useful to consider the instrumental versus expressive aspects of public policy (Rochefort 1986; Gusfield 1981; Elder and Cobb 1983). The former refers to policy's means-ends nature, its purpose as a strategic solution to the given social problem. The latter refers to policy's symbolic uses as a collective statement of social views toward the underlying nature of the problem and the individuals affected by it. Perceptions of causality, need, and deservingness are involved. This distinction goes far in explaining the pattern of support and opposition crystallized by the sterile needles issue.

Spokesmen in favor of the plan emphasized an intrumental view of the situation. For them, the severity of the AIDS problem was paramount. Any measure promising effective counteraction of the disease was worth pursuing. Dr. Lamb, for example, drew attention to the inadequate number of drug treatment slots in the state and the unwillingness of some addicts to enter treatment. In view of these realities, he explained, a needle exchange represented one practical approach for helping to protect such individuals from AIDS. Another top advisor to the mayor affirmed: "We have the twin tragedies of AIDS and drug addiction and we have to address them simultaneously and in dramatically new ways. We cannot look for *the* answer regarding AIDS prevention because, other than a vaccine or cure for the disease, no one strategy can contain the spread of the disease. . . . We cannot accept the status quo." Throwing its support behind the mayor's plan, the *Boston Globe* shared this sense of urgency. In calling for a broad-based attack on AIDS that included, but was not limited to, a needle-exchange program, the editorial writer quoted the chairman of the president's commission on AIDS, who warned of officials getting bogged down in debates of this kind "while the forest behind us is burning."

The case for sterile needles as a pragmatic intervention directly relied upon facts and figures documenting the objective magnitude of the AIDS problem in the Commonwealth. Information appearing in the *Globe* in this period included the following. As of early 1988, the Massachusetts AIDS caseload was 1,235. Of these, 516 lived in Boston. One out of every fifty-six babies born in Boston City Hospital is infected with the AIDS virus; many of the mothers of these AIDS babies used IV drugs. Boston has about 14,000 needle-using drug addicts. In March of 1988, officials upgraded the previous year's estimate of the percentage of this population that might be infected with the AIDS virus from 25 to 39 percent. At the beginning of this controversy, only 2,000 slots existed in all the methadone treatment programs in the state, 90 percent of them under private auspices. Statewide waiting lists stood at about 1,000. Finally, the costs of caring for one AIDS patient in the city of Boston was estimated at $50,000.

Opponents of the needles plan were hardly unaware of the mounting public health crisis described by these data. Many, however, questioned on moral grounds the appropriateness of the government adopting the mayor's idea, irrespective of its promised efficacy as a method of combatting the AIDS epidemic. For them, it was difficult to justify public participation in the commission of an illegal act. In January, following his announcement of a planned increase of $2.65 million in state funds to fight AIDS among drug addicts, Governor Dukakis said he would oppose a needle exchange even if data were to show such programs effective in slowing the transmission of AIDS without increasing drug abuse. Articulating a theme soon echoed by many others, he asserted on another occasion: "I don't believe we ought to be encouraging people to shoot up with heroin." Public Health Commissioner Prothrow-Stith stated her point of view simply, "[I]t's a bad message. It says we don't care what is really their [IV drug users'] primary problem, we just don't want them to spread AIDS around." A Boston city councilor also voiced his concern over the policy's symbolic significance: "It's so improper for the city to entertain this. It gives the appearance that we condone drug use, excuse it, and that it's part of everyday living. That sends the wrong message to young people."

In February, Boston's Cardinal Bernard F. Law came out against the sterile needles proposal in a column in the Catholic Archdiocese's newspaper. Quoting scripture, Law admonished drug addicts to "Reform your lives. Now is the acceptable time. Now is the day of salvation." That same day, a group of leading black ministers held a press conference to add to criticism of the mayor's plan. In turn, little more than a week had passed before representatives of 16 Protestant denominations in the state joined in support of the mayor. One of the most trenchant anti-needles statements came from the executive director of the Massachusetts Chiefs of Police Association, who declared, "[Drug abuse] is a violation of law. Are we going to go along with a program that violates the law? I don't believe we should." The executive director called for stepped-up efforts to arrest drug addicts.

Not just politicians, public health experts, and clergymen were at odds on this issue. Drug users themselves could not agree on the mayor's proposal. For example, one anonymous addict interviewed by the *Globe* thought the needle-exchange plan "would lower the count of people dying from this disease. It's saving somebody's life, I figure." "It's a great idea. Go for it," another said. "It's hard to get needles out there. Giving out clean needles would stop shooting galleries." But a third interviewee felt uncertain, interpreting the program to mean that "it's OK to kill yourself, just don't spread AIDS to anyone else." A former addict who became a drug counselor explained his opposition by saying, "I'm selling treatment. I'm selling hope. I can't condone needle exchange and sell treatment at the same time."

After receiving the sterile needles plan from the mayor, the Boston City Council referred it for review to its Committee on Substance Abuse and Neighborhood Crime Prevention. Three four-hour public hearings were scheduled in April. As perceived by the mayor and his top policy advisers, the hearings offered a two-fold opportunity. First was the chance to counteract, through open discussion, the fears and disapproval of the plan's adversaries, both in the council and on the state level. Second, the hearings would provide a forum for public education on the sterile needles issue. This, the mayor more than once acknowledged, might be an uphill battle: "It is not a very good political solution; it does not have the support of the people of this country, but I am thoroughly convinced it is the right thing to do. I am thoroughly convinced it will have the acceptance of the public in due time. When that time comes, I don't know."

Once the hearings convened there were political fireworks, as both the instrumental and expressive definitions of this issue were propounded. On the one side were representatives of the mayor's office including Flynn himself, medical authorities arranged by the administration to appear, a spokesman for the Massachusetts Council of Churches, and selected private citizens, among others. Flynn argued, "Quite frankly, we can't wait for a medical solution and I can't wait for a better political environment to introduce this legislation." The other side of the debate was pressed by other religious leaders, recovering addicts, and many community residents, one of whom stated: "The junkies don't need nobody to help them do bad, because they do enough of that on their own. I don't think we should encourage them to do bad. We should educate people. . . . The name of the game is saving lives, not taking lives." A representative of the Lyndon LaRouche organization, which staged a protest outside City Hall, characterized the plan as "a surrender. We've got to always be against drugs, and government has to represent that. This is like saying drugs are all right." In all, the *Globe* counted about equal numbers of people speaking in favor of and against the proposal.

Although local polls on this issue are lacking, selected national data help account for the vehement negative reaction that greeted the needles proposal in many quarters—despite the mayor's and other respected figures' attempted leadership on the matter. In May of 1988, drugs were the top-most rated items in a national survey asking respondents an open-ended question about "the most important problem facing this country today" (*Public Opinion* 1988). The 16 percent naming drugs was double that for the same question thirteen months earlier, probably due, in part, to the heavy attention given the issue in the ongoing presidential campaign. In a 1987 poll, 97 percent correctly believed that sharing hypodermic needles was a way for people to catch AIDS, more than for any other single method of transmission (*Gallup Report* January/February 1988). Undoubtedly related to this awareness, 51 percent in this survey felt that people who get AIDS are personally to blame. As to the specific idea of a needles-exchange program, a *New York Times* /CBS News poll, also in 1988, found 40 percent in favor and 53 percent opposed (*New York Times,* October 14, 1988). Support was found to be a function of the respondent's views about the nature of drug addiction. Of those who thought of addiction as an illness, 52 percent favored the distribution of needles; only 26 percent who saw addiction as a crime backed the measure. While 75 percent of repondents expressed sympathy for people in general with AIDS, only 26 percent said they had a lot or some sympathy for "people who get AIDS from sharing needles while using illegal drugs" (*New York Times* October 14, 1988).

In an 8–5 vote, the Boston City Council approved the needle-exchange proposal on April 27. A slim majority in opposition in early February was turned into a majority in favor in April as two previously undecided councilors were swayed by medical testimony at the hearings, and another councilor changed his position following a tour of the AIDS pediatric ward in Boston City Hospital. An important hurdle, the Council vote was but a preliminary step in the home-rule petition process, which next involved consideration by the Massachusetts State Legislature.

Within the legislature, the proposal was doubly disadvantaged by the same deep division of opinion already seen at the city level plus the promised veto of the governor. The *Globe,* commenting on Boston's representatives to the state legislature, concluded: "If there is any consensus among members of the Boston delegation at the

State House regarding the city's proposed needle exchange program, it is that there is no consensus." Another round of public hearings, this time before the Joint Health Care Committee of the State Legislature, evoked the by-now familiar point-counterpoint, with many of the same players involved. In addition, this time around some opponents, including Commissioner Prothrow-Stith, various health care providers, and a faculty member at Boston University's medical school, endeavored to score points on pragmatic as well as moral grounds by challenging the health merits of the needles plan and the validity of the European data introduced in evidence of the efficacy of needle-exchange programs there.

On June 28, in a packed hearing room, the Joint Health Care Committee rejected Boston's home-rule petition. The vote was 10 to 5. In a following news conference, Mayor Flynn once more referred to the unpopularity of his proposal: "In my opinion, it came down to issues of politics and medical information, and politics won out." He vowed to reintroduce his legislation when there was "a more calm political environment."

Summary and Analysis

Following a description of recent trends in health opinion poll data, we explored empirically the influence of public opinion within the health policymaking process through three case studies. Plainly, no single model emerges for predicting future decisionmaking situations, for the dynamics involved are highly variable. As illustrated in these three episodes, public opinion can be a potent force compelling or obstructing change. It can help lead the way or it can be strategically mobilized to one group's relative advantage. Much depends on the situation at hand, particularly the method of issue origination, how issues are defined, and the relationship between these definitions and pre- existing popular values and beliefs.

In health as in other areas of public policy, the impact of public opinion cannot be assessed in isolation from other pressures simultaneously bearing on the decisionmaking process. Policy outcome is always multiply determined. Nonetheless, it is possible to identify certain general conditions under which public opinion is likely to have greater as opposed to lesser influence.

Structure of the decisionmaking situation counts. Policy decisions that are framed for public approval or rejection by means of popular referenda or within electoral contests offer the greatest possibility of direct citizen influence. At the other extreme are decisions made out of the public spotlight by regulatory and other bureaucratic bodies or by legislative committees and subcommittees. Between the two are decisionmaking processes requiring at least a minimum of public notification and comment, such as through public hearings. It is often in this context that the formal appearance of public input turns into a reality as media coverage and group activism expands the scope of the issue.

Public opinion is more likely to be influential in dictating general policy directions than policy particulars. We have noted how polls show that the public is limited in its understanding of current issues, even with so publicized a problem as AIDS. Government officials do not expect the citizenry to be deeply involved in the deliberation of legislative details or in the application of technical standards. On the other hand, the nitty-gritty work of policymaking often flows from a broader value position that the public is instrumental in establishing. A serious problem for democratic theory can occur, however, when there is a discrepancy between what goes on at the public and elite levels, that is, when behind-the-scenes policymaking produces outcomes inconsistent with popular will and the general welfare, while the public is symbolically reassured that its interests are being protected (Edelman 1964; Elder and Cobb 1983). The difficulties faced by the general citizenry in monitoring the day-to-day execution of public policy are great and obvious.

Public opinion is also probably going to have greater impact on policy questions that do not turn on specialized, expert knowledge or on questions which divide the experts. For example, if the response to some emerging public health crisis is a medical intervention that public health professionals uniformly agree upon—such as mass immunization with an existing safe and effective vaccine—then policy action is likely to proceed directly, without significant public en-

gagement. Policymaking situations this clear-cut are extraordinarily rare, however, and can still generate widespread debate over the best means to implement the consensual solution.

The variables of scope and intensity also help to predict when public opinion will succeed in stimulating decision-makers' responsiveness. To risk stating the obvious, all other things being equal, issue positions supported by constituencies of greatest scope and intensity are those most likely to prevail in the political process. Of course, no iron law dictates that these qualities of opinion need go together, and intense minorities in politics commonly stymie or defeat opponents more numerous in size. Something of this threatens to take place in the abortion controversy in the United States, fueled in recent years by an increasingly activist pro-life movement. In 1989 the Supreme Court, with the Bush administration's urging, undertook consideration of overturning or revising the 1973 Roe vs. Wade decision, despite clear and consistent poll findings that most Americans support the policy of legalized abortion that this case established.

In conclusion, much work remains to be done in building upon these general propositions and evaluating where they are most applicable. In addition, analysts interested in the public opinion-health policy nexus must examine the role of various intermediating mechanisms of influence not discussed here, such as political parties and interest groups. More case studies are needed, as well as quantitative data investigating the correspondence between elite and mass attitudes on salient health policy concerns. Longitudinal analyses are essential to track the evolving relationship between public opinion and health policymaking over time. For in this as in other areas, the vacillating nature of popular concern with specific social issues is better documented than it is understood. And the success or failure of newly-enacted programs may shape subsequent citizen demands for public action. Only by careful exploration of these and related questions can we begin to illuminate the intricacies of democratic governance in the health policy field.

REFERENCES

American Medical Association. 1979. *Health Care Issues: Physician and Public Attitudes.* rev. ed. Chicago.

Anderson, Donald O. 1977. Priorities and planning. in *Epidemiology and health,* edited by S. Gilderdale and W. Holland, 174–196. London: Kimpton.

Blendon, Robert J. 1988. The public's view of the future of health care. *Journal of the American Medical Association* 259: 3587–3593.

Blendon, Robert J. 1989. Three systems: A comparative survey. *Health Management Quarterly* 11:2–10.

Blendon, Robert J. and Drew E. Altman. 1984. Public attitudes about health-care costs: A lesson in national schizophrenia. *The New England Journal of Medicine* 311:613–616.

Blendon, Robert J. and Karen Donelan. 1988. Discrimination against people with AIDS. *The New England Journal of Medicine* 319:1022–1026.

Boston Globe. 1988. City explores needle-exchange plan to fight AIDS. January 10.

Boston Globe. 1988. The sterile-needles debate: Governor opposing distribution to addicts. January 13.

Boston Globe. 1988. The sterile needles debate: Program in Britain impresses hub doctor. January 13.

Boston Globe. 1988. Give clean needles to the drug addicts. Anonymous Letter to the Editor. January 17.

Boston Globe. 1988. Dukakis, 7 councilors oppose Flynn needle exchange plan. February 24.

Boston Globe. 1988. Pro and con, addicts react sharply. February 24.

Boston Globe. 1988. A drug program that needs action, not preaching. Column by Robert L. Turner. February 25.

Boston Globe. 1988. Mayor's needle plan is sent to council study panel. February 25.

Boston Globe. 1988. Religious leaders oppose needle plan. February 26.

Boston Globe. 1988. Beyond a needle program. Editorial. February 26.

Boston Globe. 1988. Cardinal assailed in needle dispute. February 28.

Boston Globe. 1988. Flynn invites leaders to drug summit : Defends needle exchange plan; Cardinal maintains opposition. February 29.

Boston Globe. 1988. Treating the addict: Help can be hard to get. March 1.

Boston Globe. 1988. Treating the addict: Needle plan called risky. March 1.

Boston Globe. 1988. Koop doubts harm if needles sold. March 2.

Boston Globe. 1988. Needle plan worth a try. Column by Robert A. Jordan. March 5.

Boston Globe. 1988. Needle proposal is backed by Protestant Leaders. March 5.

Boston Globe. 1988. Police chiefs spurn Flynn's needle plan. March 23.

Boston Globe. 1988. AIDS risk seen rising for addicts. March 30.

Boston Globe. 1988. Some see council shift toward needle plan. April 7.

Boston Globe. 1988. 2 ex-addicts fault needle swap plan. April 7.

Boston Globe. 1988. Flynn's needle-exchange plan heads for hearings. April 11.

Boston Globe. 1988. Details on needle plan. April 11.

Boston Globe. 1988. Citing rapid AIDS spread, doctors urge passage of clean needle plan. April 12.

Boston Globe. 1988. Tackle AIDS, help addicts, speakers urge city council. April 13.

Boston Globe. 1988. Council seen leaning toward needle plan. April 14.

Boston Globe. 1988. Needle-swap plan gets final council hearing. April 15.

Boston Globe. 1988. City council expected to approve needle plan. April 27.

Boston Globe. 1988. Odds tipping tenuously toward needle exchanges. April 29.

Boston Globe. 1988. Boston delegation divided on needle plan. May 1.

Boston Globe. 1988. Legislature to receive needle swap plan. May 5.

Boston Globe. 1988. Hearings open on needle exchange. June 9.

Boston Globe. 1988. Words fly at hearing on needle plan. June 9.

Boston Globe. 1988. Needle trial set in Oregon. June 10.

Boston Globe. 1988. Lawmakers delay clean needle vote, but back study. June 19.

Boston Globe. 1988. Health panel leaning against needle plan. June 26.

Boston Globe. 1988. An AIDS counterattack. Editorial. June 26.

Boston Globe. 1988. Flynn presses needle plan on eve of vote. June 27.

Boston Globe. 1988. Legislative panel rejects hub plan for needle swap. June 28.

Boston Globe. 1988. Medical journal opens debate on health coverage. January 12.

Boston Globe. 1988. Health care fairness. Editorial. January 12.

Byers, Edward and Thomas Fitzpatrick Jr. 1986. Public's concern about benefits for elderly rises. *Hospitals* 60:41.

Cameron, James M. 1978. Ideology and policy termination: Restructuring California's mental health system. *Public Policy* 26:533–570.

Cobb, Roger W. and Charles D. Elder. 1983. *Participation in American politics: The dynamics of agenda-building.* 2d ed. Baltimore: The Johns Hopkins University Press.

Cook, Fay Lomax. 1981. Crime and the elderly: The

emergence of a policy issue. In *Reactions to Crime,* edited by D. A. Lewis, 123–147. Beverly Hills, CA: Sage Publications.

Cumming, Elaine and John Cumming. 1957. *Closed ranks: An experiment in mental health education.* Cambridge, MA: Harvard University Press.

Dawson, Deborah A. 1988. AIDS knowledge and attitudes for July 1988: Provisional data from the National Health Interview Survey. *Advance Data From Vital and Health Statistics* No. 161. DHHS Pub. No. (PHS) 89–1250. Hyattsville, MD: National Center for Health Statistics, Public Health Service.

Dohrenwend, Bruce P., Viola W. Bernard, and Lawrence C. Kolb. 1962. The orientations of leaders in an urban area toward problems of mental illness. *American Journal of Psychiatry* 118:683–691.

Edelman, Murray. 1964. *The symbolic uses of politics.* Urbana: University of Illinois Press.

Elder, Charles D. and Roger W. Cobb. 1983. *The political uses of symbols.* New York: Longman.

Felix, Robert H. 1967. *Mental illness: Problems and prospects.* New York: Columbia University Press.

Field Institute. 1986. *The California poll.* San Francisco.

Foley, Henry A. 1975. *Community mental health legislation: The formative process.* Lexington, MA: D.C. Heath.

Freeman, Howard E., Robert J. Blendon, Linda H. Aiken, Seymour Sudman, Connie F. Mullinix, and Christopher R. Corey. 1987. *Americans Report On Their Access to Health Care. Health Affairs* 6:6–18.

Freshnock, Larry and Stephanie Shubat. 1984. *Physician and public opinion on health care issues: 1984.* Chicago: American Medical Association.

Gabel, Jon, Howard Cohen, and Stephen Fink. 1989. Americans' views on health care: Foolish inconsistencies? *Health Affairs* 8:103–118.

Gallup, George. 1988. *The Gallup Poll: Public opinion 1987.* Scholarly Resources: Wilmington.

Gallup Report. 1987. Public expresses compassion for AIDS victims but holds them responsible for contracting disease. 263 (August):12–19.

Gallup Report. 1988. Special report on AIDS. 268/269 (January/February):2–49.

Gallup Report. 1988. AIDS: 35 nation survey. 273 (June):2–73.

Gusfield, Joseph R. 1981. *The culture of public problems: Drinking-driving and the symbolic order.* Chicago: University of Chicago Press.

Halpert, Harold P. 1963. *Public opinion and attitudes about mental health.* Washington, D.C.: U.S. Department of Health, Education, and Welfare. USGPO.

Hamilton & Staff. 1983. *A Nationwide survey of opinions toward health care costs and Medicare.* Chevy Chase, MD.

Harvey, Lynn and Stephanie Shubat. 1986. *AMA sur-veys of physician and public opinion 1986.* Chicago: American Medical Association.

Harvey, Lynn K. and Stephanie C. Shubat. 1988. *AMA surveys of physician and public opinion on health care issues, 1988.* Chicago: American Medical Association.

Health Insurance Association of America. 1982. *Health and health insurance: The public's view.* Washington.

Himmelstein, David U., Woolhandler, Steffie, and the Writing Committee of the Working Group on Program Design. 1989. A national health program for the United States: A physicians' proposal. *The New England Journal of Medicine* 320:102–108.

Jeffe, Douglas and Sherry Jeffe. 1984. Losing patience with doctors: Physicians vs. the public on health care costs. *Public Opinion* 7:45–55.

Joint Commission on Mental Illness and Health, 1961. *Action for mental health.* New York: Basic Books.

Keith, Donald M. 1988. Mandatory Medicare assignment: How Washington State Doctors Battled It and Won. *Consultant* 28:92–97.

Koff, Sondra. 1988. *Health systems agencies.* New York: Human Sciences Press.

Lemkau, Paul V. and Guido M. Crocetti. 1962. An urban population's opinion and knowledge about mental illness. *American Journal of Psychiatry* 118:692–700.

Lipschultz, Claire. 1980. *Political action in health planning: Building a consumer constituency.* Bethesda, MD: Alpha Center for Health Planning.

Maypole, Donald E. 1981. Fears about the development of A group home. *Administration in Mental Health* 9:67–75.

Meyer, Jon K. 1964. Attitudes toward mental illness in a Maryland community. *Public Health Reports* 79:769–772.

Mick, Stephen S. and John D. Thompson. 1984. Public attitudes toward health planning under the health systems agencies. *Journal of Health Politics, Policy and Law* 8:782–800.

National Center for Health Services Research and Health Care Technology Assessment. 1989. New survey confirms 37 million live without health insurance. *Research Activities.* No. 115. Rockville, MD.

New Jersey Hospital Association. 1983. We asked New Jerseyans what they thought about their hospitals . . . here's what they told us. Princeton, N.J.

New York Times. 1982. Majority in survey on health care are open to changes to cut costs. March 29.

New York Times. 1983. Medical-care spending found a major concern within city. January 30.

New York Times. 1985. Poll indicates majority favor quarantine for AIDS victims. December 20 .

New York Times. 1986. Poll finds support for pupils with AIDS. April 17.

New York Times. 1987. AIDS overtakes disease of heart as No. 2 worry. March 25.

New York Times. 1987. Study finds doctors back AIDS patients in schools. May 22.

New York Times. 1988. Poll finds apathy towards some AIDS victims. October 14.

Pisacano, Nicholas J. 1985. *Rights and responsibilities: A national survey of healthcare opinions.* Lexington, KY: The American Board of Family Practice.

Pokorny, Gene. 1988. At issue: Americans rate their health system. *Health Management Quarterly* 10:2–9.

President's Commission on Mental Health, 1978. Vol. IV. *Task panel reports: Report of the task panel on public attitudes and use of media for promotion of mental health* IV. Washington, D.C.: U.S. Government Printing Office.

Providence Journal. 1979. Major changes proposed in Rhode Island's health care system. October 28.

Providence Journal. 1979. Holman calls plan a rigid approach. October 28.

Providence Journal. 1979. Dr. Hill against limit on physicians. October 28.

Providence Journal. 1979. Equal access to quality care at a reasonable cost. Supplement. December 2.

Providence Journal. 1979. R.I. health officials: Hospitals won't close. December 20.

Providence Journal. 1979. Despite denial, some fear state would close hospitals in N. Smithfield, Woonsocket. December 21.

Providence Journal. 1979. Garrahy tells health plan foes that no hospital will be closed. December 22.

Providence Journal. 1979. Pell: Plan won't close hospitals. December 23.

Providence Journal. 1979. Bill would require legislative approval of state health plan. December 27.

Providence Journal. 1979. Garrahy words draw skepticism. December 28.

Providence Journal. 1980. 3000 are expected at health care hearing. January 1.

Providence Journal. 1980. Hospital head favors most of health plan. January 2.

Providence Journal. 1980. Health plan goes on the road, runs into westerly buzzsaw. January 3.

Providence Journal. 1980. Aquidneck dwellers turn out in force to defend hospital. January 4.

Providence Journal. 1980. Newport hits health plan as 'upstate' concoction. January 4.

Providence Journal. 1980. A bright future seen for state health plan despite controversy. January 9.

Providence Journal. 1980. Health plan may be in for major surgery January 9.

Providence Journal. 1980. Doctor tells health-plan drafters they were 'duped by bureaucrats.' January 9.

Providence Journal. 1980. Ambulance corps asks hearing attendance. January 11.

Providence Journal. 1980. Hospital size hearing last in state series. January 17.

Providence Journal. 1980. 'Big brother' label cheered by foes of state health plan. January 18.

Providence Journal. 1980. Health care planner head hears mixed signals from aroused public. January 27.

Providence Journal. 1985. The neighbors at 95 Linda Terrace. March 31.

Public Opinion. 1988. Opinion roundup: Most important problems. 11:34–35.

Ramsey, Glenn V. and Melita Seipp. 1948. Attitudes and opinions concerning mental illness. *Psychiatric Quarterly* 22:428–444.

Rhode Island Department of Health. 1981. *Planning for health in Rhode Island,* Providence.

Ridenour, Nina. 1961. *Mental health in the United States: A fifty-year history.* Cambridge, MA: Harvard University Press.

Robert Wood Johnson Foundation. 1978. A new survey on access to medical care. *Special Report* No. 1. Princeton, NJ.

Rochefort, David A. 1986. *American social welfare policy: Dynamics of formulation and change.* Boulder, CO: Westview Press.

Rochefort, David A. and Carol A. Boyer. 1988. Use of public opinion data in public administration: Health care polls. *Public Administration Review* 48:649–660.

Rosenberg, Charlotte. 1980. These doctors headed off a health planning debacle. *Medical Economics* 27 (October):33–51.

Schattschneider, E. E. 1960. *The semi-sovereign people: A realist's view of democracy in America.* Hinsdale, Illinois: The Dryden Press.

Schneider, William. 1985. Public ready for real change in health care. *National Journal* March 23:664–665.

Scull, Andrew T. 1977. *Decarceration-Community treatment and the deviant: A radical view.* Englewood Cliffs, NJ: Prentice-Hall.

Shapiro, Robert Y. and John T. Young. 1986. The Polls: Medical Care in the United States. *Public Opinion Quarterly* 50:418–428.

Singer, Eleanor, Theresa F. Rogers, and Mary Corcoran. 1987. The polls—A report: AIDS. *Public Opinion Quarterly* 51:580–595.

Steiber, Steven. 1987. Public supports AIDS education, research. *Hospitals* 61:67.

Steiber, Steven. 1988. AIDS: Explosive growth in public awareness. *Hospitals* 62:96.

Taylor, Humphrey. 1983. *The Equitable healthcare sur-*

vey: Options for controlling costs. Louis Harris and
Associates.

Woodward, Julian L. 1951. Changing ideas on mental
illness and its treatment. *American Sociological Review* 16:443–454.

Part Four

Health Policy and the Political Process

Chapter 14

The Politics of Health Care Reform[1]

James A. Morone

The American health policy agenda is crowded with reform proposals. National health insurance schemes continue to attract attention, though that elusive ideal has been pursued for more than seven decades. Less ambitious programs promise solutions to a wide array of perceived problems, though there is considerable controversy over which problems need solving. This chapter analyzes the evolving political dynamics that frame our health policy debates. It traces the traditional biases of the American polity, the implications of past policies for current proposals, and the political prospects for health care reform in the 1990s.

Problems

Political scientists have long contended that the issues on the political agenda are, in themselves, a political matter. Different interests compete to turn their concerns into national priorities. Naturally, objective conditions (rising health care costs) set the parameters of the debate. However, the political key is how those conditions are interpreted. (Kingdon 1984; Stone 1988)

Today, the American health policy agenda is especially crowded with issues competing for attention. Perhaps the most important are rising costs, uninsured citizens and accountability for the medical system as a whole. Consider each in turn.

Rising health costs have been a fixture in American health policy for more than two decades. The usual perception is that when Medicare was implemented in 1966 costs began to soar. In fact costs were already rising. In the five years preceding Medicare, health care costs rose 13 percent as a proportion of Gross National

[1]An earlier version of this paper, beyond the Words, was prepared for the New York Academy of Medicine. I wish to thank Marvin Lieberman for his helpful comments and suggestions.

Product while in the five "cost crisis" years that followed they rose 20 percent (computed from Wattenberg 1976, 74) However, before Medicare, policy makers simply interpreted rising costs within the framework of the dominant issue; inflation was one more barrier to access. After Medicare, inflation was suddenly being financed partially through tax revenue, and costs swiftly became the major health policy concern.

Twenty years later, costs continue to rise. In 1965, health spending consumed 6 percent of GNP, in 1975 8.4 percent, in 1980 9.1 percent, and in 1988 11.1 percent. Despite a steady tattoo of cost containment efforts, the overall rate of growth has not even been slowed. In 1986, for example, costs rose .3 percent of GNP, exactly the average since 1980; the hospital and physician sectors grew at annualized rates of 10.2 percent and 11.9 percent while general inflation rose just 1.1 percent (Anderson and Erickson 1987, 96–101). Moreover, the health sector consumes a larger portion of the economy in the United States than in any other member of The Organization for Economic Cooperation and Development (OECD). The nearest competitor is France, thirteen percent lower at 9.4 percent of Gross Domestic Product (GDP). Between 1982 and 1986, the health sector grew more rapidly in the United States than it did in all but three OECD nations (Finland, Iceland and Switzerland). In fact, in those four years, most industrialized nations saw a decline in the health sector's portion of their GDP (Schieber 1987, 105–112). Such figures suggest the unambiguous failure of American cost control policy. Nevertheless, the entire matter—still a problem by any objective measure—has diminished somewhat as a policy issue. Although the United States is spending more, and 73 percent of its citizens label medical fees "unreasonable" (Blendon and Altman 1987), cost control has lost its monopoly on top of the American health care agenda.

The new policy problem is the roughly 38 million Americans who have no health insurance. Many of the poor, near poor, and low wage earners cannot pay for their health care. Their sheer number places enormous pressure on medical providers who treat them. The problem has become visible largely as a result of programs designed to deal with rising costs.

Until recently, Americans dealt with indigent care in two ways. Medicaid paid directly for many poor and near poor patients. Perhaps more importantly, loose private funding arrangements (partially subsidized by the tax code) permitted providers to treat indigent patients and shift the costs to their properly insured patients. Public welfare programs were, in effect, backed by an elaborate private network of cross subsidies. In response to the cost problem, however, both public and private payers began restricting reimbursements to providers. States began to cut back their Medicaid programs until, by the mid-1980s, they covered less than 40 percent of the population under the official poverty line. Worse, private payers such as commercial insurers began to cut back their own payments, jeopardizing the traditional cross subsidies for the poor.

For a long time, the United States could have it both ways—limited government programs and relatively widespread access to care. For reasons which are explored in the next section, Americans have always preferred implicit solutions (such as the private cross subsidies) to public relief programs (such as Medicaid). The unravelling of the former now places an enormous access problem squarely on the public agenda. Demands for reform come not just from the poor, who often find it difficult to control the policy agenda, but from the more politically weighty medical institutions that are being pushed into the red by patients who cannot pay. Solutions to the new problem are complicated by the failure to resolve the old one—steadily rising medical costs.

Finally, while the related problems of inflation and indigent care dominate contemporary discourse, a host of secondary issues compete for attention: long term care in an aging society, medical education, prenatal care, the AIDS epidemic, and malpractice suits to name a few. A large array of changes—mostly designed as cost control devices—have been set into place with little concern for their cumulative effect or their impact on medicine. It is not clear what the American stew of regulatory controls, financial incentives, and reimbursement innovations is adding up to. However, it raises a profound underlying question: who is accountable for American medicine?

Various models of accountability are, of course, available. We can look to government, to citizen planning boards, to large corporate capitalists, to individual consumers or—as is the case in most nations—to the profession itself. However, the United States is trying all the models at once, diffusing responsibility and driving the medical sector in unpredictable, perhaps dangerous, directions. Whatever the cumulative effect, one clear upshot is an enormous encroachment on physician-autonomy. The entire range of innovations ultimately shares a common ideal: reshaping provider behavior to some murky standard of efficiency. As a result, a vague sense of gloom has developed among many physicians, especially younger ones. The general public seems to concur. Three quarters of them believe that the "health care system requires fundamental change" while only a fifth agree that "it works pretty well" (Blendon and Altman 1987). The matter of accountability—which raises such fundamental questions as what kind of medical system we are to have, and the nature of the physicians role within it—constitutes perhaps the most significant and intensely felt problem lurking just off the contemporary policy agenda. Though it complicates almost all our policy debates it is a difficult problems to articulate, much less address. And, like the issue of indigent care, it is the kind of problem which the American political system is especially maladroit at reforming.

Solutions

The solutions available to American policy makers are comparatively limited and tend to repeat a set of distinctive patterns. These limits flow from a familiar ideology: Americans do not like government. Perhaps because, in de Tocqueville's celebrated phrase, Americans "were born free without having to become so" (1966, 9), they have traditionally distrusted governmental activity, socialist enterprises, or welfare policies. Each is viewed more as a threat to individual liberty than as a mechanism for achieving the public good. Infused by this wariness of their state, Americans have designed a government with relatively weak powers and studded it with checks and balances designed to thwart unwanted actions far more easily than to undertake desired

ones. Fragmented political authority—attenuated parties, the separation of political branches, federalism—creates barriers to any reform. More generally, there are at least three interrelated consequences for political reformers.

First, since Americans distrust both politics and politicians, they tend to seek solutions which do not rely on either. Rather than empowering leaders to make political choices (say bargaining over medical prices), they restlessly seek out mechanistic, self enforcing, automatic solutions which can be set in place without further politics or even self conscious deliberation. For over a century, reformers have sought permanent policy fixes. The benign, invisible hand of a properly functioning market is the paradigmatic case. However, markets are only the most often repeated expression of an ideal deeply embedded in American political culture.

The same ideal animates a broad range of contemporary health care reforms. Whether HMOs, DRGs, capitation, regional health planning or medical vouchers, all share the Progressive aspiration that with a bit of tinkering and a few new incentives, the problems of the health care system can be solved without politics. The health care system will, it is imagined, run itself without the intrusion of government regulators making choices sullied by politics. Each policy proposal promises some kind of magic fix.

Second, and relatedly, the emphasis on policy gimmicks leads to a devaluation of good public administration. If hard choices are to be automatic ones, there is no need to find public officials who are capable of making difficult judgments. The recruitment patterns, social standing, and reward structures of public service all reflect this low priority. The result is both less effective administration and a reliance on implicit or covert solutions.

For example, public administrators are, in effect, empowered to negotiate with hospitals under the technical cover of DRGs. Effective administrators might actually employ the device to make thoughtful choices about which medical services to reward or restrain—essentially setting social values on different services. (Veatch 1985) More often, those values are set by default. In either case, the reality of administrators setting hospital prices is obscured by the politically useful illusion that DRGs are "scientifically" derived.

The search for a magic fix results both in less concern about effective administrators and a reliance on implicit policy choices. The two consequences are analytically distinct. Competent administrators can expand their scope of authority by making conscious but hidden choices. Nevertheless, burying their deliberations retards the development of an effective public service.

Third, the distaste for government action is articulated most forcefully in the well known reaction against welfare programs. The United States is, as Rodwin puts it, "commonly regarded as a welfare laggard" (1987, 120). European leaders such as Bismarck or Lloyd George offered welfare benefits in a bid for working class support; Americans worried more about prompting laziness than promoting loyalty. (Starr, 1982, 237) Despite their relatively large numbers, poor people are unpopular clients for public programs. The social welfare programs that have flourished have been those that mix the less needy into the clientele, for example, social security, disability insurance, Medicare.

Reformers searching for solutions to contemporary American problems are bound by these parameters of American reform: the faith in gimmicks, an ascetic's stance toward public administration, a penchant for implicit solutions, and a marked preference for respectable clients. These tendencies have shaped past programs: they constrain current possibilities and are likely to characterize the fate of future policies. The next sections trace the evolution of American institutions within this broad ideological rubric. Focus falls upon the popular, admittedly sketchy, distinction between markets and government—the settings that respectively elicit the most enthusiasm and the most scepticism in the United States.

Institutions: Politics and Markets

Solutions must be set in institutions. In the broadest general terms, Americans value private sector competition and are wary of governmental intervention. However, the health care politics of the past two decades have significantly altered both the symbols and the realities associated with these categories. This section examines some of the changes and speculates on the implications for contemporary health care reform.

Markets

Free market competition offers a powerful image and a politically effective solution. Over time, different political interests have infused it with entirely different meanings and advanced it as an answer to all kinds of troubles. The recent difficulties of the market approach changes the politics of health system reform—essentially shifting the action into the government sector.

Originally, free medical markets meant deferring to providers. In effect, the market was a circumlocution for professional autonomy and power. The profession claimed control over both medical practice and health care policy. The frequent invocation of market capitalism did not rule out government action. Rather, a broad range of policy programs which ceded public authority to professional judgments were enacted with the enthusiastic support of provider groups. (Licensure regulations, The Hospital Construction Act popularly known as Hill Burton, and the National Institutes of Health all illustrate the pattern.) On the other hand, reforms such as National Health Insurance which were perceived as threats to professional autonomy were loudly decried as tyrannical, usurpatory and socialistic. Physicians warned against the destruction of free markets as a way to muster political allies against government incursions onto their political and professional turf. In effect, they mobilized precisely the political biases described in the preceding section.

As long as the issue on the political agenda was insuring access to care, deferring to providers was a plausible policy. After all, Americans thought their medicine was the envy of the world—the only problem was seeing to it that everybody shared its benefits. Professionals could claim to know how best to do so. However, the politics of deference ended when Medicare authorized massive public funding with minimal public control. The effort to fit a new kind of program into the old institutional forms swiftly changed the dominant health policy problem from access to cost control.

The new problem prompted a revision of the old solution. Deferring to providers was an unlikely way to cut costs. The same free market symbol that the profession had long used in its struggle for autonomy was now turned against it. The free market ideal had a new meaning. Now it was a way to discipline providers, to force them to behave more efficiently. The task, argued the new market advocates, was to tinker with the incentives in the medical system until each actor was responding to the proper cues. Consumers would get incentives to shop for high quality at a low price; payers would also shop for the best deal. Providers would race to win customers. Either they would become more efficient or lose their customers and go broke.

There were many variations of the free market argument. Almost by definition, they evinced the classic characteristics of policy solutions in the United States: they avoided government (and the dead hand of regulatory administration) and instead promised a set of automatic, mechanistic answers that, once set in place, would operate more or less permanently.

Ironically, setting the solution into place was complicated by the same ideology that promoted the solution in the first place. Much of the appeal stemmed from its reliance on private initiative rather than public intervention; yet introducing a comprehensive market system required carefully coordinating a wide array of government actions (including HMO regulations, adjustments in the tax law, changes in anti-trust policy, and so on). After the Nixon, Ford and Carter administrations tinkered with these changes on the political margins, the Reagan administration finally appeared to give full head to what was soon known as the competition revolution. Crucially, it did not introduce the many regulatory innovations required to launch a comprehensive competitive effort. Instead, the administration encouraged each health care actor to harness competition in whatever manner it saw fit. A wide range of devices—competitive, quasi-competitive, even non competitive—were unleashed on the health care system in the name of free markets and efficiency.

The result was a fierce effort among health care payers to constrain their own costs. Although each took a different fiscal tack, all introduced their efforts with the rhetoric of competition and efficiency. Corporations offered their employees the option of enrolling in HMOs. Many left traditional insurance carriers and insured themselves; some negotiated special deals with health care providers through Preferred Provider Organizations (PPOs). Blue Cross tried to restrain its own premiums with its highly touted "managed care," then hedged its bets by sponsoring HMOs. Commercial insurors responded with their own cost controlling schemes, in many cases promising lower premiums in exchange for higher patient cost sharing. Medicare introduced its complex DRG price setting scheme as a form of competition. Medicaid and Medicare (Part B) simply froze fees.

Perhaps what is most remarkable about all this activity is the extent to which it has failed. Indeed, the competition revolution has exacerbated the major dilemmas of contemporary health care policy.

In the first place, the managerial innovations have not controlled costs. As noted above, health care inflation quickened relative to GNP during the Reagan years. Moreover, the competition among payers may have contributed to the problem. It has forced enormous administrative costs on health providers. Worse, the very notion of multiple payers may have an inflationary bias. After all, many of their cost control strategies (from DRGs to PPOs) are simply institutional devices through which payers negotiate with providers—one of the keys to Western European cost control strategies as well. However, Americans undermine the bargaining strategy by establishing a multitude of bargainers (in the name of competition and choice). Providers seek to maintain their income by shifting costs from the payers who are most effective at controlling their own costs (notably, Medicare and Medicaid) to those who are least effective (business corporations have proven notoriously ineffective). (Etheridge 1986, 311) In effect, providers are offered a multiplicity of safety valves through which to escape from tough cost control programs. Ultimately, many payers, each competing to keep their own costs down, facilitate the continued inflationary pressure on everybody's costs.

A second distressing consequence is the rise of the uninsured. This follows logically from the competition among payers whose incentives are to pay as little as possible for their own clients and nothing at all for anybody else. Increased patient cost sharing and declining health care insurance coverage are partially responsible. However, the still more fundamental problem, noted above, is that an elaborate system of cross subsidies is coming to an end. The problem is complicated by an increasing fragmentation of the risk pool.

Since a relatively small number of patients consume a large portion of medical resources, the most effective way to reduce payments is not through tough negotiating or efficient managerial devices but, rather, avoiding poorer risks. The incentives for competing payers are clear: (1) pay as little as possible for your own clients, (2) insure the healthiest possible market segment, and, (3) above all, do not bear anybody else's costs. Providers in turn, face a corresponding set of incentives: (1) find patients whose payers pay relatively more, (2) shift costs from the payers who pay less to those who pay more, (3) seek less sick patients (who are less costly to treat), and, (4) above all else, avoid non payers (who will demolish your reputation for efficiency.) Thus, everyone's market incentives are similar: seek the healthy and shun the sick. The result is a fast erosion of the medical commons, a destruction of the very notion of community.

What is not fully recognized yet is the great size of the policy task that confronts us as a result. Americans have traditionally had political trouble converting previously implicit solutions—solved behind the political scene with limited government action and funding—into explicit programs. Now that the old system of hidden cross subsidies has ended, we face the problem of designing programs that will extend some sort of medical coverage to over thirty-seven million people. The sheer numbers of uninsured are staggering. To put them in perspective, the number of Americans without health insurance today is more than twice the size of Medicare's constituency when that program was first implemented. (Compare Marmor 1973, with Schwartz 1988)

Throughout the 1970s, policy makers looked hopefully to the promises of competition. Here was an efficient, apparently painless solution to the problem of health care costs which fit traditional American ideologies as well as the increasingly conservative temper of the time. By the middle of the 1980s a raft of new policies had been (not completely honestly) introduced and celebrated as forms of competition. As the troubles of the health care sector worsened and multiplied, the image of an efficient, painless, competitive solution began to vanish. It is becoming clear that Americans will have to solve their medical sector dilemmas without the hidden, automatic, non governmental gimmick implicit in the magic of competitive markets.

Government

The difference between health politics in the United States and those in other industrialized nations is usually taken to be a question of financing—Americans don't have national health insurance. There is another, often overlooked difference which is every bit as important for the politics of reform: the comparative incapacity of American government.

The general reluctance to develop competent public administration has been particularly disabling for health care policies. Negotiating with a well organized, highly interested, highly trained profession requires skill and competence. Relying instead, on pluralism, gimmicks, and implicit solutions (honored as choice, competition and proper incentives) may conform to the American spirit of reform, but it offers little opportunity to control the medical sector or manage its problems.

However, as the market solution has declined, American government has slowly developed its capacity for sustained administrative action within the health arena. The progress has been slow, hesitant, obscure and often contradictory. Nevertheless, what appears, at first blush, to be a random succession of programs can also be interpreted as the government's slow progress from deference to control.

To illustrate the point, consider the evolving political and administrative realities that underlay the major post-war health policies. The Hill Burton Act, for example, included elaborate legislative precautions designed to proscribe any administrative meddling in medicine; the federal government promised financing without controls. Almost twenty years later, Medicare appeared to carry on in the same traditions—the legislation opened with stern prohibitions against any governmental "supervision or control over the practice of medicine" (Social Security Act 1965, Section 101). However, in this case, Congress protested so loudly precisely because it had broken with a half century of deference and passed the entitlement over the bitter objections of organized medicine. When funding without "supervision or control" proved inflationary, the federal government inched further into the medical sphere. The Peer Review program (PSROs, passed in 1972) appeared to be a timid capitulation to organized medicine in the face of the cost crisis. Although it created local boards which were mandated to constrain physician practice, the boards were not permitted to use national standards, collect national data or place non-physicians in decision making roles. On the political surface, the federal government appeared to avoid the prospect of building up its administrative authority or competence. However, the reality was a new, albeit timidly asserted, mission; for the first time, public agencies were seeking to reverse the practice patterns of the profession, to encourage physicians to do less.

The National Health Planning Act, signed in January 1975, turned the attention of health policy analysts to local boards mandated to write health plans and oversee capital expenses in medical facilities. The local boards, Health Systems Agencies (HSAs) derived their authority largely from state "Certificate of Need" Laws, and they sought legitimacy not by deferring to physicians, but by turning to the public. The politics of these health agencies depended, in large measure, on the apparently bizarre effort to get citizens, "broadly representative" of their communities, to constrain capital expenditures. The entire episode still baffles most observers. What was the purpose of asking lay people to face aroused hospital administrators in packed meeting halls and vote on whether to grant exceptions to incomprehensible bureaucratic standards which ostensibly forbade more beds or machines? Once again, the federally designed effort seemed to go out of its way to avoid competent national administration. However, something important was happening.

Most observers look at the long, late night, HSA meetings and ask the apparently sensible questions: Did the HSAs stick to their tasks and say "no" to providers? Did doing so reduce health care costs? The answers are occasionally and no. But the wrong questions are wrong. For what is important about those late night meetings is not that the providers usually won but that they had to argue their case before lay people in the first place. Those arguments took place in communities across the country. They broke the long tradition of deferring medical matters to medical providers. In many communities, new constituents—community leaders, businessmen, public officials—continued to play an active role in medical politics even though the health agencies soon faded from the scene. It is no coincidence that the first American laymen to cross the boundaries of professional dominance and cast judgments about medical matters were not public administrators. They were citizens "broadly representative" of the people. New kinds of controversial government action are often introduced by the latter, rarely by the former. In short, reformers nervous about the legitimacy of their reforms have often made progress against the American scepticism about the role of government with a call to "the people" (Morone 1990, ch. 8).

While the Health Systems Agencies did not transform American health politics, they were a critical step in the progress from the deference of Hill Burton to the development of an independent public capacity to shape health policy (even to the point of significantly altering the practice patterns of the profession). To note just a few examples of the programs that soon followed: In a handful of states, public officials set the prices for all hospital services, regardless of payer. In states like New Jersey and Massachusetts, broad government programs approximate the publically mandated health insurance schemes that have long been decried as "socialistic." Medicare's hospital reimbursement method (DRGs) was designed to affect the way physicians practice medicine. By the late 1980s, federal officials were proposing changes in Medicare physicians payment as a mechanism for promoting some medical specialties over others.

This is not to deny that governmental health policies remain inchoate and contradictory. Reforms such as the ones just noted are rarely administered in a fashion that inspires confidence in the American public sector. However, in the larger historical perspective, they are the latest steps in a steady progress away from the deferential politics that once typified American health policy. Governmental capacity has grown on both the state and the national level; so has the range of interventions that the public sector can legitimately attempt (when it finds the political will—no small caveat, of course).

The lesson for reformers is clear. Americans are most comfortable with their market cure. However, a decade of complication has harmed, perhaps ruined, the appealing market image of a simple, painless, democratic solution which can reduce inflation while making providers more responsive without the meddling of government. Even under the Reagan presidency (indeed, especially under Reagan), the government continued a long trend toward assuming a central role in medical policy. The host of new problems created by old policies is likely to continue the trend. Unfortunately, there is a problematic tension between the politically simple and the policy sensible: more gimmicks, hidden solutions, middle class clients and weak administrators are likely to win approval. Simple, carefully designed administrative programs might be more effective; however, they remain politically difficult to win. The tension between the politically possible and programatically sensible remains the central conflict for political reformers, as what Victor Fuchs (1987, 54) calls the counterrevolution—the backlash against payer reforms—gets under way.

Into the 1990s: Contemporary Reform Proposals

The following section considers four types of reform proposals in the context of the problems, solutions, and changing institutional frameworks described above. On the surface', at least, the reforming task is complicated by shifts in each one of these dimensions.

Health systems problems have become interrelated: continuing inflation is now linked to an enormous access problem and relatively widespread anxiety about the rapidly changing nature of the medical sector. Proposals which seek to address one trouble while exacerbating another are apt to be politically unstable and relatively short lived. Moreover, the most facile solution is gone, at least for the moment. Calling for free market competition in health care no longer evokes the same clear, easy, political resonance. At the same time, the role and capacity of the government has continued to evolve. However, the underlying political instincts that led Americans to celebrate the former and doubt the latter remain. Reform proposals continue to embody the faith in automatic solutions, implicit rather than explicit policies and hostility towards the "undeserving" poor.

Pluralism

A host of different perspectives march under the amorphous banner of pluralism. Essentially, the pluralists argue that Americans should keep their options open. Since no obviously correct solutions have emerged, Americans should encourage diversity and experimentation. States can each pursue reforms that fit the local political and medical cultures (thus restoring an old ideal of American states as laboratories, where many different experiments can be tried before policies are thrust on the nation as a whole). At the same time, private payers and entrepreneurs can continue their own effort to promote efficiency and cut costs. The key to the pluralist argument is simple: the federal government should avoid any bold new departures; it should avoid constraining future choices; indeed, it would do best by doing nothing at all.

The pluralist view rests on a mix of perceptions and prejudices. It begins with the perception that a systematic effort to introduce market principles has fallen from political favor—tainted by the current public and private programs that were sold as competition. Consequently, current reforms are likely to involve active government. The related prejudices are familiar ones and reflect all the usual patterns in the American reforming mindset. The pluralists feel a deep and hostile scepticism towards the government, particularly national government. They believe that private sector solutions (derived, somehow, from business principles) will ultimately work. They constantly refer to the better management and improved efficiency that emanate from corporate benefits officers or for-profit medical enterprises. And they place their faith in the scattershot of largely payer efforts to induce efficiency through such mechanisms as managed care, capitation, or "a new generation of insurance products" (Boland 1987, 75; *New York Times* 1988, d2)

Clearly, the political image of health care competition has been reconstructed once again, and now appears in the call for national government restraint along with private and local initiatives. Many of the old market images are present: avoid government coercion, maximize free choice and flexibility, seek incentives for efficiency, be pragmatic, and trust in business principles. And in deference to the academic proponents of this view, a new argument has attached itself to the list: study the consequences of the many options.

Like the original proponents of free market medicine, this new generation takes comfort in the usual reluctance to press big new government programs when there is no major crisis at hand. And as the pluralists see it, there is no major crisis in medicine. On balance, they view the pastiche of public and private forces that are currently transforming medicine as a reasonably good thing. Pluralists point out that the length of stay in the nation's hospitals is falling. New medical care settings (even sectors) are proliferating. Ultimately, this perspective is rooted in what might be called a business school faith— all this activity, all this innovation, all these new forms of private sector administration and management must be (on balance) a good thing.

In fact, not only is the pluralist view wrong, but it is precisely the mindset that created the current problems in the medical system. First, a multiplicity of public and private regulators are less likely to constrain costs, regardless of their many innovative gimmicks. These devices amount to a host of different ways of negotiating with providers. By opting for a large number of them. Americans invite their medical providers to shift costs from more effective regulators to the less effective (and from more effectively regulated health care settings to those which are less carefully constrained). The image of choice is powerful. But the choice in this context is illusory. It is choice among many inefficient efforts to control costs—indeed, they are inefficient precisely because there are so many. As Eli Ginzberg puts it, an "open ended" third party pay-

ment system is invariably an inflationary one (1987, 1151–1154).

Secondly, the pluralist mode is hard on the poor. In theory, relatively healthy groups that work their way out of the general risk pool stand to profit: the corporations that self-insure; the new closed panel medical plans that select a healthier than average population, the insurance company that effectively manages its beneficiary. However, this leaves a weaker, sicker pool less protected by classic insurance principles. The pluralistic ideal—let each payer worry about its own costs—gives each the same incentive: avoid the weak, the sick, and the poor. Harvey Sapolsky terms it a race to "beggar thy neighbor" (1988, 32–37). These are not unfortunate side effects. They are the direct result of incentives structured into a health care system that sets aside ideals of community—of a single communal insurance pool—for notions of individualistic competition.

The problem of the poor is made far more complicated by the American view of welfare. Fragmenting the communal pool and exposing the poor creates a situation that is conceptually uncomplicated but politically almost impossible. It requires large public expenditures towards groups who are very unpopular program clients in an era of large budget deficits.

Finally, the pluralist ideal of multiple payers each pursuing efficiency in its own way is apt to make life increasingly miserable in the medical sector itself. Foreign observers are already astonished at the diminished autonomy of American physicians. A wide multiplicity of gimmicks and incentives is now designed to reshape their behavior. Taken individually, most are not yet particularly powerful, but their cumulative effect is another matter. As Vladeck points out, the lack of public financing creates more rather than less invasive regulations, from both public and private sources (1986, 100–107).

Fixing Medicaid: The Rationalist Perspective

On the face of it, the sensible solution to the problem of indigent care is an expansion of Medicaid. Of course, we could fiddle with many of the details, even change the name. However, now that the system of hidden private subsidies has come apart, many thoughtful observers are calling for the public sector to pick up the slack. Indeed, proponents range from liberals who are horrified at the size of the indigent population to pluralist corporate executives who are frustrated by their inability to avoid having the indigent costs shifted to them.

However, in politics the most direct route between two points is often not a straight line. A new national effort in welfare medicine may be good logic but it is poor politics. Before considering how to fix Medicaid, consider why it is broken.

Welfare medicine is difficult to legislate in the United States. And unlike most other areas—where winning the legislation poses the most political difficulty—welfare medicine is even more difficult to maintain. The poor, as noted above, make a politically unpopular clientele. Their unpopularity is only partially offset by the indirect beneficiaries, the medical profession. When health care costs rise more quickly than general inflation, government officials face a difficult choice. They can spend relatively more on Medicaid (perhaps at the expense of a more popular constituency), or they can cut the program back. The record of the past two decade is unambiguous—officials chose the latter (Etheridge, 1986, 310)

These are predictable political consequences as long as medical inflation runs faster than general inflation. In effect, public officials are asked to steadily increase the size of a program aimed at an unpopular constituency. The pressure of deficits, intermittent tax revolts and competing priorities exacerbates the problem. And Medicaid (even along with Medicare) does not permit public policy makers a large enough lever to control health system costs. The predictable result is a succession of freezes, cuts, and cost control devices that restrict the growth of the Medicaid program in the face of medical inflation. Over time, government officials seek to control their own costs and, as a consequence, induce either cost shifting or bad debt.

In short, restoring Medicaid—making it as it should have been made from the start—is an important task and an appealing reform. However, if it is attempted without a simultaneous (and successful) assault on general medical inflation,

advocates should be prepared for the same painful political treadmill of the past two decades—a steady erosion of benefits and beneficiaries in an effort to control program costs.

The political lesson is not a new one. Programs for the poor tend to be poor programs in the United States. This is especially exacerbated in a problem area with a high rate of inflation. Protecting the health care of the poor requires containing the health care costs of everyone else. Public programs aimed only at the poor do not have the leverage with which to do so. Instead, they leave public officials with incentives to cut back the programs in order to control their own costs—effectively shifting the problems of the poor to the providers and the private payers. If pluralists think too much about the costs to private payers, many rationalist liberals do not worry about them enough. Reformers will need to think in global health system terms if the reforms they manage to win are to be maintained.

The New Jersey Model: Semi-Implicit, Semi-Global

The conundrum for reformers is clear: how to address both costs and access in a political system that is sceptical of government intervention and welfare programs. A third category of contemporary proposals seeks to do so, essentially by tailoring programmatic details to political necessity. One example is the New Jersey model,[2] although all sorts of variations are possible. The key is to focus equally on both the proposed program and its political effects.

In New Jersey, public officials used DRGs to set prices for all payers. At the same time, they established an uncompensated care pool, essentially taxing each payer (public and private) to assist the hospitals that served the uninsured. Thus, the program addressed both the problems of inflation and indigents.

The crux of the cost containment effort was not the use of DRGs but the introduction of a single negotiator empowered to set prices

---

[2]For more on the New Jersey experience. see Dunham and Marone, 1983; Morone and Dunham, 1986; Sapolsky, 1988; Windman and Light, 1988.

throughout the system. In effect, this limits the cost shifting and provides state officials with a reasonably powerful lever against rising costs. Of course, the extent to which they actually use their negotiating leverage is a function of both the will and the skill of the state health officials. The related problem of indigent care was addressed, essentially, by taking each hospital's uncompensated care load and dividing it among the major payers (very roughly according to their proportion of the total hospital bill). There is plenty of dispute about the merits of the New Jersey system; opponents claim that it stifles innovation, retards new forms of health service delivery, and rewards inefficient management. However, no one doubts its role in assisting (perhaps saving) the inner city hospitals which serve the poor.

The details, however, are less important than the political effects. Here is a program that appears incremental, obscure, pragmatic and technocratic; at the same time, it seems to avoid welfare, administrative interventions and new taxes. Although none of these impressions is entirely accurate, they are crucial nevertheless. They substantially reduce the political barriers to the reform. Consider the political pieces one at a time.

First, "extending DRGs from Medicare to all payers and factoring the costs of uncompensated care into the prices" is incremental. American policy makers are always wary of bold new policy ventures. American institutions are designed to deflect them. Extending DRGs is an incremental step. It takes a price setting mechanism in place for one payer and extends it to others.

Second, it sits easily in the nation's reforming tradition. Rather than explicitly empowering public officials to jawbone prices with providers, it offers an apparently scientific, self equilibrating mechanism designed to force efficiency on the medical sector. Here is a gimmick that "objectively" sets a price; efficient providers do the work for less and make money, the inefficient won't and don't. As noted above, this can be seen as a somewhat devious way to introduce the centrally negotiated prices that characterize many European systems. However, it does so in a thoroughly American fashion. It relies on an efficiency gimmick while avoiding the appearance of active intervention by public administrators.

Third, it does not look like welfare. "Factoring the costs of uncompensated care into DRG prices" hardly sounds like a liberal effort to sneak a free lunch to the poor. On the contrary, the direct beneficiaries are not poor people but the hospitals that serve them. In short, the program establishes a thoroughly respectable institutional client, entitling the poor only in an indirect—and politically obscure—fashion.

Fourth, the program buries much of the tax hike for covering indigents in the premiums of the private sector. Each payer carries a portion of the burden. Although economists are often critical of such "hidden taxes," poor economics often make good politics. No doubt the program's budget projections will annoy the economists still further when cost increases in Medicare and Medicaid are ofset by projected savings resulting from the all payer system, thus rendering the whole enterprise budget-neutral in "the long run."

Finally, the politics of this proposal are obscure. They are difficult to explain, hard to turn into a cause, and unlikely to harm a legislative career. Reforms that stay out of the political limelight are more likely to win. This is especially true of reforms directed (albeit, indirectly) at the poor. By avoiding broad symbols, the proposal reduces the likelihood of bureaucrat or welfare bashing. Such relative obscurity is a significant political advantage for a program designed to address the twin health sector problems of inflation and poverty.

The model presented here, patterned on the New Jersey case, is just one possibility. The policy proposal does not need to turn on DRGs—any other mechanism will do, as long as it is technical, is apparently automatic, seemingly provides incentives for efficiency, and is reasonably obscure. And while there may be other ways to treat the health care problems of the poor, the trick is to keep it from looking too much like welfare. This is not an ideal model; on the contrary, it is full of problems. For example, it focuses only on the acute care hospitals, ignoring ambulatory, chronic, and long term care settings. Moreover, the complexity of the system may be a political advantage, but it is likely to pose difficulties for both patients and providers.

Still, in the end, something like this will emerge. The problems of medical inflation and indigents are too pressing to ignore over the long run. Action, when it comes, is likely to be designed for political ease as much as programmatic logic. The key for political reformers—and medical leaders—is to help see that these imperatives are balanced. Too much emphasis on political factors results in poorly designed programs; too little emphasis results in irrelevance.

Beyond the N Words: The Changing Politics of NHI

Finally, there is national health insurance. Reformers have tried to win this policy, off and on, for seventy years. Their failure is one of the most distinctive features of the American welfare state. Note, however, that the reform itself has evolved, changing, to fit new problems and achieve entirely different ends.

Twenty years ago, national health insurance was about an egalitarian health care system, "a right to health care." Today, the old reform is infused with a new content. The new national health insurance is about cost control. The medical system, we are told, will remain inflationary until a single, unitary mechanism is set in place to control the level of resources that we allocate to health care. Now the key to this policy proposal turns on providing American government with the institutional capacity to set a global medical budget. Egalitarian outcomes are merely happy side effects.

Advocates make the argument today, not by referring to conceptions of justice, but by comparing American medical inflation to that of other nations. The Canadian health care experience has become a fixture in debates over American health care financing. As Robert Evans has argued, American and Canadian health expenditures were almost identical (as percentage of GNP) until Canada implemented its national health insurance program, known as Medicare. In the fifteen intervening years, our costs have continued to rise while theirs remained more or less level. By 1987, Americans were spending two percent more of their GNP on health care than the Canadians (Evans 1986; Evans et al. 1989).

The key point is not that the comparative data is beyond dispute. It is not. Rather, it is that the dispute over national health insurance now turns on how to effectively control costs. American medicine has no global budgeting mechanism and by far the highest rate of inflation. The new policy question is whether those two matters are related. Does the absence of political mechanisms implicit in national health insurance programs contribute to our continuing inflation? Uwe Reinhardt was answering precisely this question when he told the New York Academy of Medicine: "Americans spend two percent of their gross national product for nothing more than the privilege of making the following statement: 'we have no national health insurance' " (Reinhardt 1987).

If the foreign comparisons are instructive, then rising costs may eventually drive us in the direction of a government centered health system. Significantly, the usual retort is not that the American system is superior for the additional expenditure. The braggadocio with which Americans once made international comparisons has melted before the enormous number of uninsured and the relatively pervasive sense of gloom that permeates American health care. Rather, national comparisons are now set aside for being misleading in unpredictable ways. After all, argue the sceptics, American institutions, political culture, and regulatory mores are different, even peculiar. Bargaining arrangements that work well in a nation which respects public administration (not to mention polite queues) might be a mess in a nation of bureaucrat bashers (and queue jumpers).

If foreign comparisons are only partially instructive, we need a comparable American industry. Harvey Sapolsky (1987) argues that there is an obvious case: the American defense industry. Here is another highly technical industry performing services that are simultaneously vital and baffling to the laymen. In both cases, we must often rely on the same providers: a few high tech-defense firms, the local hospital. Moreover, we set impossibly conflicting values before producers in both sectors. Health providers are asked to square the circle between high quality, broad access and low costs; likewise, defense contractors are asked for timeliness, high performance objectives and low cost. In each case, the other values are important enough that costs are apt to spin out of control. However, the two industries are funded differently. Health care, of course, relies on "open ended" funding from a variety of public and private sources. Defense is funded—like the classic national health insurance schemes—by the government.

The differences in cost experiences are remarkable. Health care, as a percentage of GNP, has continued its steady upward spiral stopping only for a very occasional year (such as 1984). In contrast, defense has been kept under political control. Despite occasional rises (1965–7, 1974–5), it consumed a steadily diminishing portion of the American economy until the Reagan administration. The Reagan defense build-up illustrates the syndrome of government controlled expenditures: a popular politician articulates a new demand for spending; a large increase in funds is allocated; spending rises relative to other national priorities; however, the growth soon runs up against competing national goals, programs, and tax resistance; before long, the growth ends. After the growth of the early and mid-1980s, defense spending flattened out and then began to decline as percentage of GNP.

No comparison "proves" anything. But mounting evidence suggests that global budgets are the most likely way to take control of rising sectoral costs. What is most significant, in political terms, is the growing discussion of just this point. It is not often that Americans look abroad for a policy fix to anything.

Of course, despite these intimations of cost control, few policy entrepreneurs are interested in pushing a proposal that has been defeated as often as this one. It is hard to even imagine where the advocates would come from, at least in the immediate future. Still, there are at least two political constituencies apt to fare somewhat better in a Canadian style system—one is obvious, the other not.

First, obviously, are the poor. As argued above, the current incentives are to avoid sick and poor people. The old national health insurance logic was based on a desire to even out the medical differences among classes. That logic has not changed as the class differences have grown. Only the blindest hostility to the public sector would lead to the conclusion that poor Americans would be made worse off by a national health care system. Enfolding the poor into a national (Social Security style) system is likely to give them better health care and set into

place the political coalitions that would protect their gains. Modeling the American system on that of Canada might very well reduce inflation as it rescues the poor.

Secondly, physicians themselves might find relief in a national system. To be sure, it would likely end the steady transfer of national resources to the medical sector. However, it would also end the steady diet of new bureaucratic and economic techniques, designed to push and pull American physicians into practicing more "efficiently." Most nations with a fixed medical budget defer to providers over how to allocate those funds. They do not need to change the practice of medicine, for they control total costs more directly. In contrast, Americans abjure a budgetary limit and try instead their array of gimmicks—PROs, DRGs, PPOs, and on and on. Ironically, nationally financed medicine is likely to mean more professional autonomy over medical matters. It is, of course, an unlikely political deal. However, American physicians could do far worse than supporting a national health plan in exchange for increased autonomy, that is, in exchange for an end to the long series of manipulative policies designed to change the way they practice medicine.

A national health plan might be both popular and effective. It might substantially ameliorate the problems of the health care system described above. However, it is radically at odds with the kinds of solutions which have typified American politics. In the short run, it is difficult to imagine how Americans could get there, from where we are today—short of some genuinely ghastly crisis (for which AIDS is the most frequently nominated current candidate). Barring that, all three of the policies noted above are more likely than this one.

And yet, liberals ought to take heart. If we are still a long way from Harry Truman's ideal, we are nevertheless far closer than we were a decade ago. This is so for two reasons: first, the decline of competition and deregulation as the American panacea, and, second, the reconstruction of national health insurance from an avowedly liberal device aiming at equity, to a strategy for promoting cost control. Cost control is more politically respectable, for its clients are the middle class. Politically savy liberals will emphasize the evolution. The imperatives of cost control may eventually prove harder to resist than the ideal of equity.

REFERENCES

Anderson, Gerald and Jane E Erikson. 1987. National medical care spending. *Health Affairs.* 6:96–101.

Blendon, Robert and Drew Altman. 1987. Public opinion and health care costs. In *Health care and its costs,* edited by Carl Schramm 140–158. New York: Norton.

Boland, Peter. 1987. Trends in second generation PPOs. *Health Affairs.* 6:75–81.

Dunham, Andrew and James A Morone. 1983. *The politics of innovation,* Princeton, NJ: HRET Press.

Etheridge, Lynn. 1986. Ethics and the new insurance market. *Inquiry.* 23:311–318.

Evans, Robert. 1986. Finding the levers, finding the courage: Lessons from cost containment in North America. *Journal of Health Politics, Policy and Law* 11:585–615.

Evans, Robert et al. 1989. Controlling health expenditures—the Canadian Reality. *New England Journal of Medicine.* 320:571–577.

Fuchs, Victor. 1987. The counterrevolution in health care financing. *New England Journal of Medicine.* 316:1154 ff.

Ginzberg, Eli. 1987. A hard look at cost containment. *New England Journal of Medicine* 316:1151–4.

Kingdon, John. 1984. *Agendas, alternatives and public policies.* Boston: Little Brown and Co.

Marmor, Theodore. 1973. *The politics of medicare.* New York: Aldine Publishing Co.

Morone, James A. 1990. *The democratic wish.* New York: Basic Books.

Morone, James A. and Andrew Dunham. 1985. Slouching to national health insurance. *Yale Journal of Regulation* 2:263–291.

New York Times. 1988. Honeywell's push to track doctors. Feb, 23, D2.

Reinhardt, Uwe. 1987. The incentives of physician payment. Presentation before the 1987 annual meetings of the New York Academy of Medicine, May 7.

Rodwin, Victor G. 1987. American exceptionalism in the health sector: The advantages of backwardness in learning from abroad. *Medical Care Review* 44:119–154.

Sapolsky, Harvey. 1986. Prospective payment in perspective. *Journal of Health Politics, Policy and Law.* 11:640–652.

Sapolsky, Harvey. 1988. An evaluation of the New Jersey DRG hospital payment system. *New Jersey Medicine.* 85:32–37.

Schieber, George. 1987. Trends in international health care spending. *Health Affairs.* 6:105–112.

The Social Security Act. Title 18. Washington D.C.: USGPO.

Starr, Paul. 1982. *The social transformation of American medicine.* New York: Basic Books.

Stone, Deborah. 1988. *Policy paradox and political reason.* Boston: Little Brown.

Swartz, Kathleen. 1988. A statistical portrait of the medically uninsured," Washington DC: Urban Institute, unpublished.

Thompson, Frank. 1981. *Health politics and the bureaucracy.* Cambridge: MIT University Press. 1981.

DeTocqueville, Alexis. 1966. *Democracy in America.* Garden City, New York: Doubleday.

Veatch, Robert. 1987. The implicit ethics of DRGs. Paper prepared for the Seton Hall Conference on the New Jersey All Payer System. Seton Hall University, June.

Vladeck, Bruce. 1986 America's hospitals: What's right and what could be better? *Health Affairs.* 5:100–107.

Wattenberg, Ben J. 1976. *The statistical history of the United States.* New York: Basic Books.

Windman, Mindy and Donald Light. 1988. *Regulating prospective payment.* Ann Arbor, Michigan: Health Administration Press Perspectives.

Chapter 15

Life and Death, Money and Power:

The Politics of Health Care Finance

Robert G. Evans

The Universality of Collective Finance

In all developed societies, the financing of health care is a collective process. Pools of funds are assembled through more or less compulsory levies on the general population, within or outside the formal tax system. These funds are then transferred to the providers of care through institutional structures and processes which vary considerably from one country to another. But in no society does direct payment by the user of services, at time of service, account for more than a small fraction of the total cost of health care.

Care is not, of course "free"; the residents of each country must pay, one way or another, the cost of that country's health care system. But who pays, and how much, is largely or wholly unrelated to the pattern of health care utilization. It is in this context, and through the management of these collective processes, that the political struggles are played out, and compromises struck, over who gets what, when, where, and how.

The United States is a partial exception to this generalization, in that the proportion of direct, out-of-pocket payment by patients for the services they receive is well above that in all the other member countries of the OECD.[1] But even in the United States, direct payment accounts for only about one dollar in three (Maxwell 1981). Two-thirds of all health care expenditures, even in the United States, flow through collective channels, and have done so for over two decades.

This fact, though well known or at least well documented, is often obscured by emphasis on an alternative distinction, that between "private" and "public" finance. (The latter is often characterized as "socialized medicine," a term which has long lost any clear meaning but remains no less politically potent.)

In the United States, roughly 40 percent of

---

[1] Organization for Economic Co-operation and Development, essentially Western Europe, Canada, the United States, and Japan.

health care financing is labelled as coming from the "public" sector, which includes the public programs for the elderly and some members of the low income population, Medicare and Medicaid, but also services for the military and their dependents, public health, and a variety of subsidies to research and education in the health sciences. This proportion is by far the lowest in the OECD where the average percentage for all OECD countries is just under 80 percent. Austria and Switzerland have the next lowest share of health spending with two-thirds, reported as in the public sector (Scheiber and Poullier 1988).

The difference between this 40 percent, and the total of two-thirds paid "through collective channels," is "private" insurance. But how private is private? The United States is clearly more private than, say, Canada, where health care is also provided by private medical practitioners, reimbursed by fees for service, and with admitting privileges in not-for-profit hospitals under the direction of boards of trustees, just as in (much of) the United States. But the fees are entirely paid by provincial ministries of health, and hospitals negotiate their annual operating budgets with the same ministries.

In essence the insurance function—but not the delivery of care—is completely "socialized," integrated into the line responsibilities of provincial governments. In Canada, although about 95 percent of the expenditures for hospital and medical care are paid through the public sector, the latter pays for only about three-quarters of all health care expenditures, because there is still considerable direct payment for dentistry, drugs, and long-term care.

In the Federal Republic of Germany, on the other hand, insurance is provided by a number of separate *Krankenkassen,* sickness funds, which might be based on an industry, a region, or an individual industrial enterprise. They are organized on a non-profit basis, and sufficiently tightly regulated by the federal and regional governments as to justify their treatment by the OECD statisticians as essentially "public" finance. Germany is reported as providing 78 percent of its health care finance through the "public" sector (Scheiber and Poullier 1988).

A similar pattern is found in several other countries of Western Europe. Expenditures flow through a large (Switzerland) or small (France, Belgium, the Netherlands) number of health insurers which are non-profit and closely regulated. Such organizations occupy a middle ground between the strictly "private" (for-profit, commercial) and strictly "public" (line civil service) sectors.

The OECD categorizes the funds flowing through all such organizations as "public" funding, while the non-government insurance sector in the United States is entirely labelled "private." Yet the "Blues" are non-profit, and are certainly subject to a high degree of public regulation.

Nonetheless, the OECD distinction is probably justified. The Blues are more similar to private commercial organizations, and have become increasingly so over time, while European insurers have been subjected to increasing public accountability as pressures on costs have mounted. The key point, however, is that the difference in labels is a cut across a spectrum or a continuum, not a sharp distinction. Even the private, for-profit insurance sector (in and out of health care) is heavily regulated, in a variety of ways.

Furthermore, the notion that "private" insurance coverage is a commodity bought over the counter by individual American consumers, along with boxes of soap flakes or cans of beans, is at variance with reality. In the first place, private insurance in the United States is heavily subsidized through the income tax system. Premiums paid by an employer are deductible as a part of wage and fringe benefit costs, but unlike ordinary wages, they are not then taxable in the hands of the employee. The "private" system thus receives a substantial, if slightly indirect, infusion of public funds through this form of tax expenditure.[2]

This, in turn, strongly encourages the establishment of work-related health insurance programs, partially or fully employer funded out of before-tax dollars. Under such circumstances, to treat the decision of the worker to participate as "voluntary" is absurd. Such coverage is not of course "free"; employer-paid fringe benefits have a wage cost at the bargaining table even if public

[2]This form of subsidy provides the largest benefits to people in the highest tax brackets, while those with no taxable income receive no support at all from the general taxpayer. The "reverse Robin Hood" feature no doubt accounts for the political popularity of this form of tax expenditure.

subsidies reduce that cost. But no *individual* worker can avoid the wage cost by opting out of coverage.

This tax incentive is further reinforced by the problems of information flow in insurance markets, the well-known process of "adverse selection." Individuals who know or suspect, on any number of grounds, that they are at greater than average risk of health care expenditures, have an above-average incentive to purchase coverage. Insurers respond in three ways. They require medical examinations, whose costs must be borne directly or indirectly by the would-be purchaser; they escalate the premiums charged to individual buyers, to compensate for the higher expected outlay and the greater risk; or they refuse to cover individuals entirely (Fein 1986).

Health care insurers prefer to concentrate instead on the employee group market, making coverage conditional on some minimum number of group members signing up. This way they can guarantee both a relatively healthy risk pool— the sicker members of society are less likely to be employed—and most important, a group which is not self-selected on the basis of illness. Thus the interests of the insurer, like the tax system, militate strongly against individual purchase.[3]

Persons left out of work-based "private" health insurance are picked up by the residual public programs for the elderly or poor, or simply left out entirely. Currently about 15 per cent of the United States population, almost all below the age of sixty-five, have no coverage at all (Short et al. 1988). This exclusion does not appear to have any parallels in any other developed society. The proportion with coverage inadequate to meet the costs of any major illness or injury has been estimated as another 5 to 10 percent, although obviously standards of adequacy vary.

Thus the American worker who belongs to an employer-sponsored health insurance plan may appear to have more "choice" than the Canadian worker who pays for the public system through taxes. The national and international statisticians may treat the former as purchasing a private ser-vice while the latter is taxed to pay for a public service. But if the American employer is paying the premiums—which is strongly encouraged and assisted by the tax system—and the worker's take-home wage reflects this, then the real difference is remarkably small.

The "public/private" distinction is not meaningless; it really does make a difference how a society organizes the institutions through which it assembles and distributes the funds destined to pay for health care services. The experience of the United States, compared to the other OECD countries, and particularly to the otherwise very similar country of Canada, right next door, is most instructive in this regard. An outlier with respect to both the extent of direct charges to patients, and the proportion of overall funding flowing through the public sector, the United States health care financing system has also become an outlier (on the downside) on several important performance measures as well.

Even as an outlier, however, the United States conforms to the general rule. Developed societies channel the bulk of their health care funding through collective institutions. These may be government agencies, as in Canada, Sweden, or the United Kingdom, or closely regulated "quasi-public" non-profit insurance agencies, as in Germany, France, Belgium, or the Netherlands, or the unique American blend of different forms of insurance—direct government (Medicare, Medicaid), regulated non-profit (the Blues), and regulated for-profit (the commercial industry). The politics of health care finance is expressed through the creation, modification, and control of these collective institutions.

Planes of Cleavage: Providers versus Payers

The fundamental mathematical identity of health care finance is that total expenditures on health care are, always and by definition, exactly equal to the total incomes earned from its provision. Those incomes may be salaries or professional fees; they also include interest on hospital bonds or dividends from private pharmaceutical or equipment companies. They are earned by doctors and nurses, dentists and pharmacists, but also by employees of firms writing health in-

---

[3]There is a market for individual coverage, but in these contracts only about one dollar in two is actually paid out in benefits. Marketing expenses eat up much of the rest, since bad products take a lot of selling.

surance or providing management consulting services to hospitals or ministries of health.

The channels through which funds flow may be multiple and complex, but at the end of the day every dollar that someone has paid out must have been received by someone else. And if the goods or services which that dollar of expenditure bought were defined (albeit somewhat arbitrarily) as health care, then the corresponding dollar of income was by the same definition earned by providing health care.

This elementary fact of accounting underlies the primary political conflict in every health care system, that between the payers for care, and the providers of care.[4] There are also secondary conflicts on each side of this divide, among providers and among payers. Still the most prominent division follows the income/expenditure distinction.

This political struggle is most commonly and simply presented in the universal discussions, even lamentations, over "cost containment." In political rhetoric, "cost explosions" in health care are commonly presented as if they were some elemental force of nature, like tides or earthquakes, against which all those concerned with health policy struggle as best they can. This image is false.

Those who *pay* for care are to a greater or lesser degree concerned to limit the escalation of costs. But those who *are paid* for care are engaged in discouraging or avoiding such controls, and in trying to keep the costs rising, for a variety of motives. For the sake of political credibility, they may wish to be seen to share in the general hand-wringing about the relentless pressure of health care costs. But in actual fact, many if not most providers of health care believe that the adoption of appropriate priorities would lead to *more* spending, not less.

Their motives are not particularly mysterious when one considers the factors which determine health spending. At a highly aggregated level, these are three in number. First and most obvious is the level of care, quantity and quality,

which is provided to the people of a society. All else held equal, more care costs more and less care costs less.

But all else is *not* equal. The second factor influencing the costs of health care is the relative incomes of providers, compared with the rest of the population or labor force. Countries vary in the generosity or parsimoniousness with which they treat providers of care. The United States is particularly good to its physicians, for example, as is Germany. The United Kingdom and Belgium are more niggardly. Canada is, as usual, in an intermediate position. These international differences correspond to differences in the institutional structures through which physicians are paid, and contribute to differences in the share of national income going to health care, quite independently of the amount or effectiveness of the care provided (OECD 1987, ch.6).

These two components, the amounts and types of care provided and the rates at which people or organizations are paid for providing it, represent the "quantity" and "price" terms in the health care expenditure equation, and in an accounting sense, their product determines total health expenditures. There is a third factor, however, that is receiving increasing policy attention in a number of countries—the relative efficiency and effectiveness with which care is provided.

Unnecessary or harmful services add to costs—and generate employment and incomes—without yielding any corresponding health payoff. Health care is, after all, valued not for itself but for its anticipated (positive) impact on health. Absent this payoff, most health care services are "bads", not "goods." Furthermore, effective or ineffective care may be provided at different levels of technical efficiency. One country may spend more, not because it is getting more health benefits, or even more health care, but simply because its institutions for providing care are less efficient, more wasteful of human and physical resources.

Meeting Needs of Marketing Services—How Much Care Is Enough?

In their quest for more resources from the rest of society, and in resisting pressures for cost containment, providers and their spokesmen tend to emphasize the first point. This is the classic "Your money or your life!" argument; if enough

---

[4]Not "buyers" and "sellers"! The dominance of collective funding, combined with professional self-regulation and external public regulation, and rooted ultimately in the obvious fact that most users of health care are not able to define their own needs without professional help, implies that the images of the "free market," with voluntary exchange of goods/services for money, between fully informed, self-interested, autonomous and unconstrained transactors, exist only in the dreamworld of neoclassical economic theory.

resources are not forthcoming people will die, or at least suffer, unnecessarily. We must "meet the needs," which are alleged to be continually expanding due to such factors as the aging of the population, advances in technology, and "other and unspecified."

Such an argument is probably as old as medicine itself. At the individual level, it is the standard method whereby the therapist exerts power over the patient—which may well be in the patient's best interest. "Doctor's Orders" are combined with references to the ill effects of non-compliance. The relationship has a fundamental political dimension—"orders" are the exercise of power backed up by the perception of superior knowledge, and thus the ability to make credible, if not always specific, threats.

As noted above, in developed societies the financing of health care is collectivized. Thus providers must influence the controllers of those collective funds, inducing them to spend more and on more different types of services. Political pressure is therefore brought to bear, by convincing the relevant constituency (voters, employees, or premium-payers) of the adverse consequences of refusal. "Heartless" bureaucrats, politicians, employers, (even economists) are placing dollars above peoples' lives! Such claims, supported by human-interest anecdotes, are politically very powerful, and also sell newspapers.

Of course, as Williams (1978) has pointed out, if there is no natural limit to the scope of medicine, and if there is always *some* small benefit that might be gained, through sufficiently large expense, then logically it is impossible for *any* society to "meet all the needs" in a technical sense. Needs are infinite. It is then an essentially political question as to which needs are "worth" meeting. Technical expertise may be necessary to determine what the payoffs to further expenditure in a particular situation might be, but the expert is no more qualified than any other citizen to state whether the benefits are worth paying for. In a democratic society everyone gets one vote.[5]

Providers accordingly seek to persuade their fellow citizens that the benefits of further expenditures are large, that is, more "medical miracles." But they emphasize especially the catastrophic consequences, in health and human happiness, of any (successful) attempt to restrain the escalation of costs. In other fields of endeavour this activity would be recognized as marketing. In the United States, in particular, the technique has been refined into the spectre of "rationing." Ever-advancing technology is portrayed as constantly enhancing the ability to extend life and maintain function, but at ever greater cost. Sooner or later, it is argued, we shall be forced to "ration"—deny people access to effective services, let them die—for sheer lack of the necessary resources (the "Painful Prescription" of Aaron and Schwartz (1984). But in the meantime, and to postpone the evil day—send more money.

This specter may become reality at some time in the future, but is by no means a certainty. There is, at present, no direct linkage between levels of expenditure on health care, and the achievement of health outcomes, in any health care system in the industrialized world.[6] We are all a long way from the grim trade-off of "Your money or your life."[7] But emphasis on this possibility plays the very important political role of diverting public attention from the other two major factors which also interact to determine health expenditures. Most obviously, it avoids

---

[5]Some might wonder why the question of "What is worth paying for?" is treated as political rather than economic. For many commodities we appeal to the principle of Consumer Sovereignty, and rely on individuals to indicate, in the marketplace, what commodities each of them believes is worth paying for. The choice process is decentralized. But the decision to leave that process to the free market—where among other things peoples' preferences are weighted by their wealth, not by their

needs—is itself a political choice. For a variety of reasons, no country in the world has seen fit to do this for health care. In the United States, however, the very strong ideological commitment to free markets as ends in themselves is in continuous tension with powerful humanitarian values. These make citizens very uncomfortable with the inevitable results generated by markets in health care. The result has been a form of schizophrenia in health policy, and a lurching back and forth from one approach to another.

[6]Maynard (1981, p. 145) puts it bluntly, "It is foolish to believe that increases in health care inputs and throughputs lead to increases in health status outcomes". But it is not at all foolish to try to persuade others to this belief, if one can thereby enhance the willingness to pay for one's own services, or avoid awkward questions about efficiency or effectiveness.

[7]A 1989 proposal considered by the Oregon legislature to establish explicit rationing criteria for Medicaid services and to deny funding for certain life-prolonging but very expensive procedures, does not reflect resource constraints on the United States system as a whole, but only on the funds which the American political system is willing to make available for the care of the lowest income groups. Such explicit rationing can coexist with over-funding, and over-provision, for other segments of the population.

questions about the relative incomes of health care providers.

The Struggle Over Relative Incomes—How Much Are Providers Worth?

The costs of health care depend, not only on how much is provided, but on how much is paid to those who provide it. In Reinhardt's (1987) arresting phrase, much of health policy is taken up with "the allocation of life-styles to providers," or the determination of their levels of income, relative to the rest of the community.

In a competitive marketplace, relative incomes are determined by "demand and supply" and are not amenable to political bargaining. In the reality of health care, however, the boundaries set by market forces tend to be broad and indistinct, and to leave a wide band of discretion. International comparisons of physicians' incomes, for example, show that their skills and long education periods lead to correspondingly high incomes everywhere, just as "demand and supply" would predict. But the *size* of their income advantage relative to the rest of the community is quite variable, both from country to country, and over time within countries (OECD, 1987).

In most systems, the political process of bargaining over provider incomes takes place "in the open," in negotiations over the level of fees or salaries that will be paid by public or quasi-public insurers, and over the opportunities physicians in particular will or will not have to increase their incomes by charging patients directly. In the United States, however, there is still great political conflict over the design of the institutions through which provider incomes will flow. In most other countries this issue has been largely settled (at least for the moment).

Current political attention in the United States is focused on whether the federal government or some coalition of insurers should *develop* a uniform fee schedule for paying physicians, rather than permitting physicians to set their own fees.[8] From time to time, direct political action has been taken to freeze fees and incomes of health

care providers, but no institutional structure has been established for on-going negotiation on this issue.

As a result, providers in the United States have been relatively successful in maintaining and enhancing their relative incomes, and this has contributed to the continuing escalation of health care costs. In contrast, such costs have for the past decade been more or less contained—though often with bruising political struggles—in most of the other OECD countries. In 1986, the United States spent 11.1 percent of its Gross Domestic Product (GDP) on health care, up from 9.2 percent in 1980 and 8.4 percent in 1975. For the OECD countries as a group, the corresponding average ratios were 7.3 percent, 7.1 percent, and 6.7 percent—an average that includes the United States (Scheiber and Poullier 1988).

More detailed comparisons with Canada, a country in many respects comparatively similar to the United States, have shown quite clearly that the centralization of bargaining over physicians' fees resulted in a slowing in the escalation both of fees, and of overall outlays on physicians' services (Barer et al. 1988; Evans 1987). This slowing is observed both relative to previous patterns in Canada, prior to the establishment of the public universal insurance plans, and relative to contemporaneous experience in the United States.

The shift of the political debate from *how* physicians were to be paid, to *how much* they were to be paid, ended the tendency for fee increases to outrun the general rate of inflation, year after year, and contributed to the stabilization of overall health care costs (as a share of national income) after 1971. In the United States, despite nearly a decade of "pro-competitive" health policies intended to control costs through market forces, fees and costs are escalating in real terms, after adjusting for the general inflation rate, as fast as ever (United States 1987; Levit and Freeland 1988).

The terms of the political debate over how much providers should be paid encompass three aspects—appeals to fairness, concerns for system integrity, and simple threats. Providers, whether salaried or self-employed, try to convince the rest of the community that they deserve more money, by emphasizing the sacrifices

---

[8]There is, of course, a fee schedule for services paid for by Medicaid, but this is generally viewed as "welfare medicine," outside the American mainstream.

made, the difficulty of the task, and the various economic and non-economic burdens they carry.

The second line of argument is that if higher incomes are not forthcoming, either the quantity or the quality of services will fall. People will leave the field, or emigrate, or (over the long haul) will choose other professions. Those in the field will become demoralized and depressed, and the quality of their work will suffer. Finally, there is always the threat, and sometimes the reality, of "job action"—strikes, slow-downs, study sessions, and other forms of collective withholding of services.

Once again the United States appears to be the outlier, but the difference is only in the degree of decentralization. The individual American physician expresses dissatisfaction with, for example, Medicaid fees, by withholding services from Medicaid patients. The same process, withdrawal of services to get higher fees, is at work, but on a one-to-one basis, not collectively. Physicians and their spokesmen also make the same types of political argument as in other countries, about the deleterious consequences of measures to limit physicians' incomes (e.g., Baumol 1988; Feldman and Sloan 1988). But these arguments are made to fend off political action, institutional change which might permit collective fee negotiation, rather than to influence the outcomes of such negotiations.

Controlling the Practice of Medicine—Which Services, and How Provided?

The concerns of providers of care go, however, well beyond simply their own incomes. The third major factor influencing the costs of health care, the total quantity of resources allocated to the health care system by the rest of society, is the relative efficiency and effectiveness of that system. This, in turn, is connected with the process of management and the locus of power and control.

Traditionally the payers for care, whether public or private, have avoided "the practice of medicine," They have not inquired into the details of servicing patterns, or how or why providers made their diagnostic and therapeutic decisions. Political and administrative negotiations or conflicts have focused on fees and salaries.

Payers in virtually every country have also tried to exert some control over the total capacity in the health care system, particularly hospital and major equipment capacity. There is general understanding that utilization of health care is predominantly capacity-driven, heavily influenced by the availability of facilities and personnel, independently of the "needs" however defined of the populations served.[9]

Capacity control contributes to, but is not sufficient for, overall cost control, as American health planners have learned. Culyer (1988) argues that Canada and the European countries have been more successful because they have also placed global restraints on total financing rather than relying on controls of "demand," "supply," or capacity.

Such global controls leave the maximum scope for provider autonomy, within the overall physical and financial limits. They do, however, leave the determination of those limits rather arbitrary. Providers can always allege that the limits are too tight, and that serious needs are going unmet—people dying on the waiting lists. Payers counter with the rhetoric of cost explosions—more than the country can afford. The general public, in its various roles as actual or potential patient, taxpayer, or voter, is unlikely to find the facts of the case significantly clarified by either side.

For a number of years, however, researchers have been observing that there are large and unexplained variations between patterns of practice and servicing rates, between countries, or regions in the same country, or between practitioners, which seem to bear no identifiable relation to the needs of the populations served (Bunker 1970; Vayda 1973; McPherson et al. 1982; Roos et al. 1986; Chassin et al. 1986; Ham 1988). These variations show up in the fine structure of care—in particular procedures, not just aggregate utilization rates.

At the same time, a considerable proportion of diagnostic and therapeutic interventions is carried on in the absence of any scientific evidence

---

[9]This virtually universal observation provides another refutation of the "Your money or your life" proposition. If current levels and patterns of care are significantly influenced by factors other than patient needs, then changes in those levels or patterns have no necessary connection, either way, with health outcomes.

that they actually benefit patients, and in a nontrivial number of cases have been shown to do actual harm. A still more important problem, quantitatively, are those interventions which *have* been shown to benefit certain patients with particular conditions, but which are offered to a much wider range of patients for whom no such evidence is available (Banta et al. 1981; Feeny et al. 1986).

Such observations have for a long time indicated that there was considerable potential for containing or reducing health care costs, with no harm or even benefit to patients. Realization of this potential for both lower costs and better health outcomes depends, however, on improving the management of the health care system. More specifically, the system must be managed explicitly to achieve health outcomes, and to identify and eliminate ineffective and wasteful practices and procedures, rather than just to sustain traditional practices plus whatever other new ideas attract the attention of clinicians (Wennberg 1984, 1988).[10] But only very recently has this realization begun to emerge in serious political debate (*The Economist* 1988; Roper et al. 1988; Andersen and Mooney 1989).

The principal reason for virtually universal political inaction on this issue, up till now, may be that such management would directly challenge the professional prerogatives of providers. Practitioners have always insisted that the "best" medicine was practiced by trained and experienced clinicians relying on their own clinical judgment. The threat of accountability to others, who will draw on statistical and experimental evidence in evaluating and even directing their performance, strikes directly at professional autonomy. It is likely to excite even more severe political counterattacks than attempts at economic control, and to elicit substantially less support among the general public. "Cost control" and fee/income bargaining are viewed as legitimate roles for payers. But it is not clear whether there is sufficient political support for more detailed intrusion into the way care is provided. Even if there is widespread and very solid evidence that a great deal of inappropriate and unnecessary care is being provided, members of the general public are not familiar with that evidence. As users of that care, they believe their needs are being met.

Thus it is probably not accidental that in the United States the political debate has most clearly turned to the evidence of specific inefficiencies in the provision of health care, and the need for detailed utilization review (Roper et al. 1988). Other countries have managed to contain their overall costs at an acceptable level, without taking on the political dangers inherent in appearing to attack professional autonomy. But the United States has thus far completely failed to achieve such control, while simultaneously failing to provide adequate coverage for its population. There appears to be widespread agreement among the American population that major reform is called for (Blendon 1989).

Desperate times call for desperate measures. In these circumstances the United States may be able to establish a degree of sophistication in health care management that is politically impossible in better functioning systems. The result could be a substantially better match between the needs of the population served, and the types and numbers of procedures performed. But there is, unfortunately, no necessary connection between this, and the objective of overall cost control. Whatever level of resources *is* devoted to health care may, however, be better spent.

But perhaps not. Who guards the guardians? Patients trust physicians and other professionals to make decisions on their behalf. The evidence on utilization patterns suggests that there is a good deal of identifiable room for improvement in this process. But if governments or private payers—employers, insurance companies—begin to take a more active role in determining what shall be done for particular patients, designing treatment protocols, for example, how can we ensure that *they* do not subvert patient interests, in the direction of underuse?

The answer may be that the vigilance—and economic and professional interests—of providers, combined with the natural emotional bias against those who "sacrifice lives for dollars," will provide sufficient check on the niggardliness of payers. But it is by no means necessarily so.

---

[10]Such evidence provides further reasons to reject the politically powerful, but totally unsupportable, allegation that cost containment at present levels must lead to "rationing" of effective care, and an increasing load of potentially avoidable morbidity and mortality. "Rationing" of *ineffective* care may well occur; but that is a solution, not a problem.

There may be a real need for "political entrepreneurship" to design institutions and assemble coalitions capable of offsetting payer interests, if the balance of power should swing in their direction.

Conflicts among Payers

The more immediate problem for the United States, however, is to find ways of organizing payers so that they can match the influence of providers, and establish some control over the global system. Most other OECD countries have passed this stage, and have either a unitary payment system, or tight regulation and coordination of payment agencies.

That unity or coordination, however, is not a once-and-for-all achievement. It must be maintained in the face of continuing pressures from providers who recognize very clearly the connection between "sole source funding" and overall cost control. In the debates over "privatization" which have been going on in Canada and Western Europe, providers are quite explicit in their attempts to expand the flow of resources to health care systems which they claim to be "underfunded," by diversifying the sources of funding (Weller and Manga 1983).

The assembly or maintenance of coalitions is made difficult not only by the efforts of providers, but also by the natural conflicts of interest among payers for and users of services. However a society determines the share of economic resources to be given to the providers of care, it must still allocate that burden among its various members. At the same time, the terms and conditions of access to the health care goods and services provided, that is, "Who gets what, when and how," will also depend on the structural and administrative framework.

In a fully tax-financed system, the distribution of economic burden will be generally related to ability to pay, as indicated by income, wealth, or consumption. It will be more or less progressive, depending on the overall tax structure. European-style payroll taxes or "social insurance" premiums result in a regressive distribution of burden, since they take a higher proportion of lower incomes and exempt income from non-labor

sources. Canadian-style finance from general tax revenue tends to be more or less proportionate to income from all sources. Some might regard this as fairer—a political value judgment. But in either case the allocation of total health care cost bears no relationship to health status.[11]

Private insurance systems, by contrast, set premiums on the basis of expected losses, usually as indicated by past experience. People with chronic illnesses, or elderly people, will carry a larger share of health expenditures, in the form of significantly higher premiums for coverage. Competition among insurers dictates this result; a company that tried to cover all comers at the same premium ("community rating") would find that it attracted all the worst risks.[12] Direct charges to patients distribute costs according to actual illness/care experience, rather than prior expectation of expense.

Since illness and income are strongly negatively correlated, both direct charges and private insurance result in the largest share of cost being borne by those with the least resources. But it is manifestly impossible to finance a modern health care system solely on the basis of such a distribution. Hence the universality of public payment. In the United States this takes the form of both public programs for those with the greatest needs and least resources (Medicare and Medicaid), and indirect public subsidy (through income tax exemptions) of the private insurance system.

In such a mixed system, however, there is still room for much debate over the extent of reliance on direct charges or private insurance. Great political and intellectual energy is devoted to struggles over the marginal adjustments of burden distribution, whether by ability to pay, expectation of illness, or actual care use. This serves to divert attention from the primary questions of

---

[11]Total outlays on health care services are, however, only one component of cost. Being ill or injured is a significant burden in itself; it may also result in loss of income and/or other additions to living expensee. The direct burden is inevitably borne by the patient; other economic losses are partially compensated at best.

[12]The non-profit "Blue" plans in the United States began in the 1930s by community rating, with exactly this result. Competition from the for-profit sector eventually forced a shift to experience rating, or charging different premiums to different groups on the basis of estimated risk (Fein 1986).

how much to spend, and on what. It is as if a group of diners at a restaurant, greatly disturbed at the size of the bill (and very suspicious) nevertheless spent all their energy debating who was to pay what share, rather than calling in the manager to demand an accounting for the overall cost.

Needless to say, the restaurant manager would prefer that the guests argue among themselves, rather than present a united front. The simplest summary explanation for the complete failure of cost control in the (dis?)United States, in contrast with the experience everywhere else, is that the institutional framework of health finance in the United States makes it easy and natural for the payers to argue among themselves, to try to pass the costs on to someone else, and very difficult for them to confront providers directly.

The intellectual framework provided by the rhetoric of the marketplace also tends to focus attention on the distribution among payers. The American economic literature perpetuates endless discussion of "deterrent charges," and the almost universal conviction that cost escalation results from low or zero "prices" to "consumers" at point of service, in spite of the obvious counter-examples in the rest of the world. Thus the recent efforts by employers to shift the burden of health care costs from their balance sheets to those of their workers—an understandable but unhelpful response to unchecked escalation—are applauded as "welfare-improving" despite their obvious lack of effect on overall costs (Manning et al. 1987).[13]

Tax-financed systems, in which the principle of universal coverage has long been accepted, are less vulnerable to these diversions. They do, however, show increasing conflict over access to care. If the community as payer controls outlays by limiting its overall "willingness-to-pay," there will remain individuals who, perhaps encouraged by their physicians, perhaps not, want more. Or

they may want care on more favorable terms, for example, shorter waiting lists, more convenient bookings, and nicer surroundings. Pressure from unsatisfied users generates cleavages of two kinds, between users and payers, and among users themselves.

The split between users and payers is quite straight-forward. As noted above, payers are ultimately responsible to some user constituency, whether it be voters, premium-payers, or workers. (In the final analysis, in a democratic society, they are always responsible to voters.) If the relevant constituency comes to believe that payers' efforts to limit cost escalation are threatening their own health, the controls will fail.

A delicate balance must be maintained between the voter-as-payer and the voter-as-patient. Much of the political activity by both payers and providers is intended to elicit from voters the identification favorable to their cause. People who think of themselves as actual or potential patients are likely to support increased health care spending; people who think of themselves as taxpayers or premium-payers are more likely to support efforts to control costs.

Another important, and perhaps even more interesting question concerns the treatment of those who want more services, even though there is a well-established political consensus for restraint. Should they be able to pay for more, separately from the collective system?

The affirmative argument is usually presented as an alleged "natural" right to spend one's own resources as one sees fit, spiced with anecdotes of patients dying for lack of care. But the issue is, in reality, more complicated. Very few people are really willing or able to cover the full costs of medical care for serious illness out of their own pockets. Rather, those who are relatively healthy and wealthy are more likely to favor "moderate" deterrent charges, co-payments, which enable them to purchase better access by screening out some of those with lower incomes. They would like the right to buy their way to the front of the queue, not to pay the full price of additional services.

And providers, of course, would like the power to enhance their incomes by charging additional amounts for preferential treatment, as has been the practice in the United Kingdom for years. Very few, if any, providers imagine that they

---

[13]There is also a very strong ideological component to the conflict among payers and users (Weller and Manga 1983). Since illness is inversely correlated with social class, whether measured by income or education, or by looser measures of status, the detachment of economic burden from either actual or expected illness results in a corresponding redistribution of income from higher to lower levels in the social hierarchy. To some this egalitarian effect is offensive *per se*, even if it is associated with a lower overall burden.

could survive in a system where more than a small minority of users had to pay the full cost of their own care. But a "multi-class" system not only enables providers to charge extra for preferred access to care which is predominantly collectively financed, it also permits them to "whipsaw" payers and undermine global restraints. A perception that those who pay a bit extra are getting *therapeutically* superior care, that is, better outcomes, not just better amenities, will in a democratic society eventually lead to "more" for everybody.

All of this discussion sidesteps the critical question of whether additional services are worth buying, or whether additional expense is required to buy them. As emphasized above, the more fundamental issue is whether the services currently provided are medically necessary, or efficiently produced. As noted, there is substantial evidence that the short answer is "No," and that even the health care systems of Canada and Western Europe are in fact *overfunded.* In these circumstances, further expenditures whether individual or collective would seem ill-advised, to say the least.[14]

But the specter of "rationing," the threat that some will be denied "needed" services, is a very potent mechanism for undermining the unity of users or payers. The least sick, and most well off, whether as voters or as patients, can be persuaded that they might fare better in a fragmented financing system with a greater element of user-pay. And indeed some of them would. But the much larger losers will be those, whether poor or moderately well off, who have the misfortune to become seriously ill. And the winners, at least in the short run, are the providers. Their long run position, however, is less clear.

Conflicts among Providers

The fragmentation of financing systems, under various justifications, is a common objective of

providers the world over, because it enhances their ability to negotiate increased resources from the rest of society, and to protect their own autonomy from external accountability for the use of those resources. From a professional perspective, a multiplicity of funders with deep pockets and few questions represents the ideal environment both for doing good and for doing well. But can it last? Here, the United States experience is critical, though the results are by no means all in yet, and may not be for years. Certain generalizations, however, seem secure.

First, economic success brings competitors. Large and rapidly growing pies attract others who would like to share. The normal reaction of a competitive marketplace to a "growth industry" is that new suppliers offer the same or better products/services at lower prices. The customer benefits from improved quality and falling costs—consider personal computers. But health care is not and has never been a competitive marketplace. The growth of the "total revenues" of the industry—health expenditures and incomes—has indeed drawn in new sharers, but the process and the results have been quite different from the predictions of hypothetical models of the "competitive marketplace."

The first form of potential competition, starting in the 1960s, came from substitute personnel—nurse practitioners, midwives, dental therapists, chiropractors, denturists, etc. In a number of cases these practitioners could offer the same or better services at lower cost; in others the question of quality and servicing patterns was more open. But extensive research (e.g., Record 1981; Spitzer 1984) has left no room for doubt that, technically, such persons could significantly reduce the costs of health care services by substituting for the services of the peak professionals, physicians and dentists.

Unfortunately they would in the process also reduce the income streams of such personnel— the expenditure-income identity again. Accordingly during the 1970s professionals in all countries, including the "highly competitive" United States, used their political control of the self-regulatory process to suppress the development and deployment of their potential competitors. As a result, a major form of inter-provider conflict never emerged; the victory of the peak professionals was swift and complete (Spitzer 1984).

---

[14]Rachlis and Kushner (1989) have written a comprehensive and very accessible survey of that evidence for the Canadian system. The Western European systems show a similar pattern (Maynard 1981; Enthoven 1985, Culyer et al. 1988). Yet Canada and the major European nations spend between 8 and 9 percent of their national income on health care; the United States spends over 11 percent.

At the same time, however, two other groups in the United States were steadily expanding their shares of the growing health income stream. By the end of the 1980s, they have become established as the most potent new competitors for health incomes. But they will be difficult if not impossible for the providers themselves to deal with, because they have successfully integrated their services with the delivery of health care. Their relationship is not competition, but a complex combination of symbiosis and parasitism. These are, of course, payment administrators and lawyers (Lee and Etheredge 1989).

Physicians in particular are intensely aware of the claim which lawyers have established to a share of their gross revenues through malpractice litigation.[15] Generally they are very hostile to this process, and often attribute rising health care costs to the pressures placed on them by the tort system. They emphasize the addition to servicing made necessary by "defensive medicine," a cost several times greater than malpractice premiums themselves. Such an argument implicitly concedes that a considerable proportion of servicing is "medically unnecessary," and would not be provided in the absence of the malpractice threat.

Less frequently do physicians consider how they could maintain their incomes if they were *not* providing, and being paid for, the additional services which make up "defensive medicine." In an environment in which physician supply is growing much faster than population, either per capita servicing or fees must rise, or incomes must fall. The lawyers provide a justification for the increase in servicing, even as they skim off a share of the gross revenue and subject physicians to the miseries of litigation.

Even more significant is the role of the payment administrator. The fragmented funding system, which permits the continued escalation of overall expenditures, also costs a great deal to administer. The difference between premium or tax payments *to* insurance agencies, public or private, and claims or benefits paid *by* such agencies, is the overhead cost of the payments system. It is the cost of pushing paper rather than of providing services. Some such cost is unavoidable; complex institutions are not self-administering. But these costs in the United States are much larger than anywhere else for which data is available, and add literally tens of billions of dollars to American health care costs. They are also rising rapidly (Evans 1986).

Corresponding to these costs of the insurance and prepayment process, are large and increasing administrative costs within care institutions—hospitals and physicians offices—made necessary by the process of complying with an increasingly complex payment system. These internal costs, which appear to be part of the cost of providing care but again are simply "paper-pushing," add further tens of billions to expense without corresponding benefit to patients (Himmelstein and Woolhandler 1986).

No other country incurs administrative costs on this scale, to support what Reinhardt (1988) has identified as a huge private bureaucracy. Yet the simplified payment systems of other countries also permit direct negotiations between providers and payers, and resulting overall control of expenditures.

In terms of our restaurant analogy above, the embattled American diners have each called in their own accountants and lawyers to support their attempts to minimize their share of the bill. The total cost of the meal is predictably escalating even more rapidly, and the restaurant is now quite noisy and crowded. The manager is becoming somewhat nervous. These new participants in the discussion are disturbing the smooth functioning of the restaurant—and they do not order anything to eat! Furthermore, they are taking a share of the customers' money, threatening to reduce the amount available to pay the bill.

American providers are caught in a dilemma. The financing system which by its diversity and complexity protects them from external financial control, is absorbing a larger and larger share of health system incomes just to keep it running. And to add insult to injury, pressures from payers are leading to greatly increased attempts to influence the practice patterns of individual physi-

---

[15]The lawyer's fees are paid from the plaintiff's award, which is paid by the malpractice insurer, who in turn collects an increasing share of the physician's gross receipts as malpractice premiums. The physician passes on this cost in higher fees, and/or increased rates of servicing, to the patient or the patient's insurer. The latter, government or employer, passes the cost to taxpayers or customers. At no point is there an agency with the authority or the incentive to control the process.

cians. Physicians' autonomy is under threat from the payment system itself. Their allies are becoming increasingly expensive, and are even threatening to grab the levers of power (Webber and Goldbeck 1984; Roper et al. 1988; Lee and Etheredge 1989). Machiavelli would have appreciated the situation.

Beyond Conflict?

The politics of health care finance has been presented as a tale of continuing conflict, particularly between providers and the rest of society. This conflict is less clearly focused in the United States than in other countries, because this country has not as yet developed institutions to limit the expansion of the health care sector. When, or if, it does so, it will experience the same process of a struggle, waxing and waning in intensity, but never disappearing. It comes with the territory.

The very persistence of the struggle, however, and its universality, carry an important message. The conflict is legitimate, and necessary. Both providers and payers have important roles, based on fundamental but in this case opposing principles of authority (Evans 1984, ch. 14). Neither can be dispensed with. On another level, they need each other. Payers cannot provide services; providers would starve without collective funding.

The political art is thus to design institutions and administrative structures which focus and contain the conflict where it is inevitable—over relative incomes, for example—and inhibit it from spilling over into areas where there might be considerable common interest. As Marmor (1983) emphasizes, these structures and processes matter enormously for the quality of health system performance. Permanent conflict of interest is not the same as permanent open warfare; and the latter is a poor environment for providing health care.

Nor, at the end of the day, should one be too completely drawn into the intellectual landscape of health *care* politics. It is inevitable, and understandable, that providers should for bargaining purposes insist on the strength of the connection between health care and health—"Your money or your life!" That connection is, after all, their

primary *raison d'etre*. Furthermore payers must implicitly accept the same relationship, at least in principle. Determining what is and is not reimbursable requires a distinction between health care and "other things" which is administratively if not conceptually sharp. More generally, the whole apparatus of special institutions which each society has developed for both delivering, and paying for, "health care," presupposes that this label corresponds to a relatively well-defined sub-set of goods and services whose use is a fundamental determinant of health.

The reality, however, is that "health" in a broad or even a narrow sense depends on much more than the provision of health care services. Seen in the long perspective such services may be among its less important determinants. The current international emphasis on the measurement and evaluation of the "outcomes" of health care services, their contribution to the health of recipients, is a natural step towards the much larger question of the other and perhaps more important determinants, and how *they* might be influenced. The really fundamental political challenge for the next generation will be to expand the politics of health care finance into a serious politics of health.

REFERENCES

Aaron, Henry J. and William B. Schwartz. 1984. *The painful prescription: Rationing in health care.* Washington: The Brookings Institution.

Andersen, Tavs Folmer and Gavin Mooney, eds. 1989. *The challenge of medical practice variations.* London: MacMillan.

Barer, Morris L., Robert G. Evans and Roberta J. Labelle. 1988. Fee controls as cost control: Tales from the frozen north. *The Milbank Quarterly* 66:1–64.

Banta, H. David, Clyde Behney and Jane S. Willems. 1981. *Toward rational technology in medicine: Considerations for health policy.* New York: Springer.

Baumol, William J. 1988. Price controls for medical services and the medical needs of the nation's elderly. Paper prepared with the financial support of the American Medical Association and presented before the Physician Payment Review Commission (Feb. 11). Washington, D.C.

Blendon, Robert J. 1989. Three systems: A comparative survey. *Health Management Quarterly* 11:2–10.

Bunker, John P. 1970. Surgical manpower. A comparison of operations and surgeons in the United States and in England and Wales. *New England Journal of Medicine* 282:135–144.

Canada, Health and Welfare Canada. 1987. *National health expenditures in Canada, 1975–1985.* Ottawa: Minister of Supply and Services.

Chassin, Mark R., Robert H. Brook, R.E. Park, et al. 1986. Variations in the use of medical and surgical services by the Medicare population. *New England Journal of Medicine* 314:285–290.

Culyer, Antony J. 1982. The NHS and the market: Images and realities. In *The public-private mix for health: The relevance and effects of change,* edited by G. McLachlan and A. Maynard, 23–55. London: Nuffield Provincal Hospitals Trust.

Culyer, Antony J. 1988. *Health expenditures in Canada: Myth and reality, past and future.* Toronto: Canadian Tax Foundation.

Culyer, Antony J., J.E. Brazier and Owen O'Donnell. 1988. *Organizing health service provision: Drawing on experience.* Working paper No. 2. Working Party on Alternative Delivery and Funding of Health Services. London: Institute of Health Services Management.

Economist, The. 1988. Fallible doctors. Patient's dilemma. 309:19–21.

Enthoven, Alain, C. 1985. *Reflections on the management of the national health service.* London: The Nuffield Provincial Hospitals Trust (Occasional papers No. 5).

Evans, Robert G. 1984. *Strained mercy: The economics of Canadian health care.* Toronto: Butterworths.

Evans, Robert G. 1986. Finding the levers, finding the courage: Lessons from cost containment in North America. *Journal of Health Politics, Policy and Law* 11:585–616.

Evans, Robert G., Jonathan Lomas, Morris L. Barer, et al. 1989. Controlling health expenditures—The Canadian reality. *New England Journal of Medicine* 320:571–577.

Feeny, David, Gordon Guyatt and Peter Tugwell. 1986. *Health care technology: Effectiveness, efficiency and public policy.* Montreal: Institute for Research on Public Policy.

Fein, Rashi. 1986. *Medical care, medical costs: The search for a national health policy.* Cambridge, Massachusetts: Harvard University Press.

Feldman, Roger and Frank A. Sloan. 1988. Competition among physicians revisited. *Journal of Health Politics, Policy and Law* 13:239–262.

Ham, Chris, ed. 1988. *Health care variations: Assessing the evidence.* London: The King's Fund Institute (Research Report No. 2).

Himmelstein, David U. and Steffie Woolhandler. 1986. Cost without benefit: Administrative waste in U.S. health care. *New England Journal of Medicine* 314:441–445.

Lee, Philip R. and Lynn Etheredge. 1989. Clinical freedom: Two lessons for the UK from US experience with privatisation of health care. *The Lancet* (February 4):263–266.

Levit, Katherine R. and Mark S. Freeland. 1988. National medical care Spending. *Health Affairs* 7:124–136.

Marmor, Theodore R. 1983. *Political analysis and American medical care: Essays.* Cambridge: Cambridge University Press.

Manning, Willard G., Joseph P. Newhouse, N. Duan et al. 1987. Health insurance and the demand for medical care. *American Economic Review* 77:251–277.

Maxwell, Robert J. 1981. *Health and wealth: An international study of health-care spending.* Lexington, Massachusetts: Lexington Books.

Maynard, Alan. 1981. The inefficiency and inequalities of the health care systems of western Europe. *Social Policy and Administration* 15:145–163.

McPherson, Klim, John E. Wennberg, O.B. Hovind and P. Clifford. 1982. Small area variations in the use of common surgical procedures: An international comparison of New England, England and Norway. *New England Journal of Medicine* 307:1310–1314.

OECD. 1987. *Financing and delivering health care: A comparative analysis of OECD countries.* Social Policy Studies No. 4. Paris: OECD.

Rachlis, Michael and Carol Kushner. 1989. *Second opinion: What's wrong with Canada's health-care system and how to fix it.* Toronto: Collins.

Record, Jane Cassels, ed. 1981. *Staffing primary care in 1990: Physician replacement and cost savings.* New York: Springer.

Reinhardt, Uwe E. 1987. Resource allocation in health care: The allocation of lifestyles to providers. *The Milbank Quarterly* 65:153–176.

Reinhardt, Uwe E. 1988. On the b-factor in American health care. *Washington Post August* 9:20.

Roos, Noralou P., G. Flowerdew, Andre Wajda and Robert B. Tate. 1986. Variations in physicians' hospitalization practices: A population-based study in Manitoba, Canada. *American Journal of Public Health* 76:45–51.

Roper, William L., W. Winkenwerder, G.M. Hackbarth and H. Krakauer. 1988. Effectiveness in health care: An initiative to evaluate and improve medical practice. *New England Journal of Medicine* 319:1197–1202.

Scheiber, George J. and Jean-Pierre Poullier. 1988. International health spending and utilization trends. *Health Affairs* 7:105–112.

Short, Pamela Farley, Alan Monheit and Karen Beauregard. 1988. *Uninsured Americans: A 1987 profile.* Rockville, Maryland.: National Center for Health Services Research and Health Care Technology Assessment.

Spitzer, Walter O. 1984. The nurse practitioner revisited: Slow death of a good idea. *New England Journal of Medicine* 310:1049–1051.

United States, Health Care Financing Administration, Division of National Cost Estimates. 1987. National health expenditures, 1986–2000. *Health Care Financing Review* 8:1–36.

Vayda, Eugene, 1973. A comparison of surgical rates in Canada and in England and Wales. *New England Journal of Medicine* 289:1224–1229.

Webber, Andrew and Willis B. Goldbeck. 1984. Utilization review. In *Health care cost management: Private sector initiatives,* edited by P.D. Fox, W.B. Goldbeck and J.J. Spies, 69–90. Ann Arbor: Health Administration Press.

Weller, Geoffrey R. and Pran Manga. 1983. The push for reprivatization of health care services in Canada, Britain and the United States. *Journal of Health Politics, Policy and Law* 8:495–518.

Wennberg, John E. 1984. Dealing with medical practice variations: A proposal for action. *Health Affairs* 3:6–32.

Wennberg, John E. 1988. Practice variations and the need for outcomes research. In *Health Care Variations . . . q.v.,* edited by C. Ham, 32–35.

Williams, Alan. 1978. Need: An economic exegesis. In *Economic Aspects of Health Services,* edited by A.J. Culyer and K.G. Wright, 32–35. London: Martin Robertson.

Chapter 16

Health Policy and Access to Care[1]

Irene Fraser

Financing health care for poor Americans, particularly since the inception of the Medicare and Medicaid programs has been an intergovernmental, and shared public/private, responsibility. The federal government finances health care through Medicare, the Veterans Administration and a variety of other federal programs, and through a tax policy that subsidizes employer provision of group health insurance. State and local governments provide a variety of health care programs and services, including support for public hospitals and clinics, while the private sector supports care for the working poor through sponsorship of group health plans and subsidizes health care for the uninsured poor by absorbing the costs of free care. Finally, the federal government and the states share responsibility for Medicaid.

In the 1980s, increases in the number of people living below the poverty level, greater competition in the health care industry and concerted cost containment efforts in the public and private sectors have led both to a growing indigent care problem and a disruption of traditional ways for financing it. From 1980 to 1987 alone, the number of uninsured grew by 25 percent to reach 37 million people (Gramlich 1987; Swartz 1989; Short, Monheit and Beauregard 1988). Millions more are underinsured, either because their private coverage omits essential benefits—maternity care or mental health services, for example—or because the public programs for which they are eligible have reimbursement rates so low that the beneficiary has little purchasing power in the health care marketplace.

Access Issues

This deterioration in coverage creates two access problems—one indirect, and one direct. The

[1]Opinions expressed are those of the author and do not necessarily represent the views of the American Hospital Association. The author would like to thank Thomas A. Granatir, Lawrence Hughes and Ellen Pryga for their comments on an earlier draft of this chapter.

indirect threat is that the surge in the ranks of uninsured, and the resultant increase in the volume of uncompensated care, is occurring at a time when changes in the medical care financing system are dismantling long-standing mechanisms for financing this care and threatening the ability of traditional "safety net" hospitals to continue to serve the poor. The direct threat is that those without health insurance are less likely to seek care at all.

Indirect Threats to Access

Because of their mission, the vital nature of their product, and community expectations, hospitals historically have provided care to some patients without charge or at reduced charges. These reductions can take many forms, ranging from negotiated discounts for particular insurer or employer groups, to less voluntary reductions for public payers, to what traditionally has been termed charity care or bad debt—care for individuals who are unable to pay or from whom the hospital has been unable to collect. State studies in Florida (Duncan, Colbert, and Pendergast 1986) and North Carolina (Duke University 1986) indicate that most uncompensated care, whether labelled "charity care" or "bad debt," results from care to those who are poor or near-poor and uninsured.

In recent years, the volume of uncompensated care has been increasing rapidly and, because the burden is unevenly distributed among hospitals, threatens the very survival of some of those which have traditionally served as the provider of last resort. As shown in figure 16–1, uncompensated care costs for hospitals rose from $3.5 billion in 1980 to $8.8 billion in 1987, rising from 4.6 percent to 5.8 percent of total hospital costs. Although some uncompensated care costs are defrayed by state and local tax appropriations, these allocations have been growing much more slowly than the cost of uncompensated care, with the result that a greater and greater proportion of the care remains truly "unsponsored"—not paid for by the patient or insurer, and not covered by state and local tax appropriations. In 1980, for instance, unsponsored care totalled $2.8 billion. By 1987, it reached $7.2 billion.

These rising levels of unsponsored care would indicate serious financing and access problems even if the burdens were evenly distributed among hospitals. For reasons having to do with location, mission, and a myriad of other factors, however, the burdens are not evenly distributed. In 1986, for example, unsponsored care represented five percent of hospital costs nationwide, but 1,400 hospitals provided unsponsored care exceeding 6 percent of their costs, and almost 300 of these provided unsponsored care totalling more than 11 percent of their costs (American Hospital Association 1986 Annual Survey Data).

The indirect threat to access comes from the fact that hospitals have declining ability to shift costs, and those with high indigent care burdens have less ability than others. Traditionally, hospitals—and, in particular, those hospitals serving large numbers of uninsured patients—have been able to subsidize the cost of care provided to the medically indigent by increasing charges to privately insured patients and to those able to pay their own bills. But changes in reimbursement under public and private insurance programs are making this arrangement more and more difficult to sustain. The principal sources of government financing, Medicare and Medicaid, provide no subsidies for costs incurred by indigent non-beneficiaries (and, in many cases, fail to cover the costs of their own beneficiaries). Insurers or large employers often are able to negotiate reduced rates and thereby exempt themselves from cost shifts as well. The growth, and uneven distribution, of unsponsored care is occurring within an increasingly competitive system; hospitals that continue to provide large amounts of unsponsored care are at a competitive disadvantage in an increasingly price-driven payment environment.

Direct Threats to Access

But these trends in uncompensated and unsponsored care, no matter how serious, are only a part of the broader indigent care problem. The $7.2 billion in unsponsored care does not include, for example, the undoubtedly sizable amount of uncompensated care provided outside of the hospital setting (American Medical Associ-

Uncompensated*

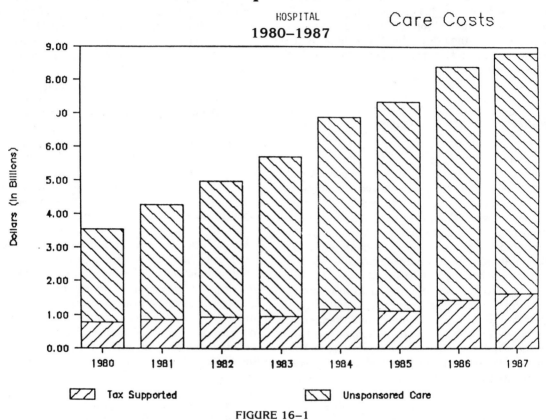

HOSPITAL
1980–1987

Care Costs

FIGURE 16–1

Source: American Hospital Association, forthcoming.

*Uncompensated care cost figures include the cost of charity care and bad debt, but not contractual allowances or Medicare/ Medicaid payment shortfalls. Most Uncompensated care, whether labelled "charity care" or "bad debt", results from care to those who are poor or near-poor and uninsured. (Duncan, Colbert, and Pendergast 1986; Duke University 1986)

ation 1988; Kilbane and Blacksin 1988). It also does not include out-of-pocket expenditures by the poor and middle class uninsured who do manage to pay at least part of their bills.

Finally, and most important, unsponsored care figures only take account of care that *was* received, and therefore do not reflect the enormous human, social and economic costs resulting from unmet needs—care that the uninsured either did not seek or did not receive. Study after study (Robert Wood Johnson Foundation 1987; Davis and Rowland 1983) has shown that the uninsured are less likely to seek and receive timely and appropriate care. While they eventually receive care, they tend to seek too little, too late. They go to hospitals to deliver their babies, but often without benefit of prenatal care; they arrive in hospital emergency rooms with serious illnesses that could have been treated less expensively, and more successfully, a year earlier. For example, a recent survey of uninsured patients admitted to Washington, D.C. hospitals found that 23.5 percent of the admissions could have been prevented through appropriate and timely primary care (District of Columbia Hospital Association 1988). Because the human, social and financial tragedy of medical indigence is broader and deeper than the uncompensated care problem, most efforts to address the issue have focused on covering the uninsured rather than reimbursing providers.

The 37 million uninsured are a diverse group, but most of them share three characteristics. Almost two thirds are poor or near poor, about two thirds are women and children, and almost all are in working families (Swartz 1989). Taken together, these facts say a great deal about the origins of the problem, and also about where one should look for solutions. Assuming the continued lack of a comprehensive National Health Insurance program, any real reduction in the number of uninsured is going to require an overhaul of the Medicaid program, a substantial boost in employer-based health insurance, or both. In the short term, to solve the indirect threat to access, such actions may also have to be coupled with direct efforts to prop up financially stressed "safety net" hospitals who serve large numbers of uninsured.

Because the indigent care problem's recent growth has occurred during a period of at-

tempted federal disengagement from many domestic policy problems under the "New Federalism" banner, much of the responsibility for designing and financing a solution is being borne by the states—sometimes willingly, and sometimes in response to federal mandates. During the past several years, states have seen a quantum increase in their opportunity, and their responsibility, to extend health care protection to targeted groups of the poor. State and local experimentation and innovation in private sector programs has also been extensive.

But while the levels of state and local energy and activity are impressive, it is too soon to tell whether they represent momentum or simply movement. Given the precarious condition of state finances and the fiscal reluctance of the federal government, it is not at all clear that the sum total of these state actions will be sufficient to restrain the seemingly inexorable growth in the number of uninsured, and to neutralize the indirect and direct threat to access that the uninsured and the underinsured are facing.

Medicaid

Ostensibly, Medicaid is the public program designed to address the health care needs of the poor, just as Medicare serves the elderly, blind and disabled. In reality, however, Medicaid does an increasingly bad job of insuring the poor and, in particular, of protecting the indigent non-Medicare population (Fraser 1989; American Hospital Association 1987). During the past decade, the program has exhibited three significant trends which, in combination, bode ill for the uninsured. First, the program covers a small and declining percentage of the poor. In the last decade, Medicaid coverage of the poor has dropped from 65 to 40 percent (U.S. Department of Health and Human Services 1983, 1987; Smith 1984; Swartz 1989).

Second, Medicaid eligibility levels tend to vary considerably from state to state. In January 1989, the eligibility ceiling for a family of three was $4,792 in an average state, but in six states this same family would have to earn less than $3,000 a year in order to qualify. Finally, in terms of expenditures, Medicaid increasingly has become a secondary insurance program for the elderly, blind and disabled, rather than a primary insurance program for the poor. About three quarters of all Medicaid expenditures are used to pay long-term care costs and other expenses generated by Medicare enrollees, leaving about one fourth for the growing number of non-elderly, non-disabled poor (U.S. Department of Health and Human Services 1987).

Problems of this magnitude are not likely to be resolved through minor tinkering: Those studying the Medicaid problem over the past decade have agreed that the program will need to be radically overhauled if it is to serve its original purpose of insuring health care for the poor (The National Study Group on State Medicaid Strategies 1984; Holahan and Cohen 1986; American Hospital Association 1986; Health Policy Agenda for the American People 1989).

There have, in fact, been some substantial positive changes in the program during the past few years—although, as Debra Lipson points out elsewhere in this book (Chapter 9), there also have been some significant contractions. For instance, the 1986 and 1987 Omnibus Budget Reconciliation Acts (OBRAs) gave states options to expand Medicaid eligibility for the very vulnerable—poor mothers and young children. Subsequently Congress mandated such coverage for all pregnant women and infants below the federal poverty level. In addition it required Medicaid programs to pay the Medicare premiums, copayments and deductibles—including the sizable beneficiary share under the drug benefit—for the elderly and disabled poor. Finally, it also established new "spousal impoverishment" rules which made it easier for the elderly and disabled to "spend down" and become eligible for Medicaid-sponsored nursing home care without depleting the assets of a non-institutionalized spouse.

These most recent changes have been in the direction long recommended by critics. The OBRA 1986 and 1987 expansions took the significant step of beginning to unlink Medicaid and welfare eligibility, and the targeting of pregnant women and infants certainly made sense from both a financial and political, as well as a moral and philosophical, perspective. But because the reforms have been incremental, and in particular because they have not been accompanied by a federal commitment to significantly increased funding, these reforms leave an important part of the Medicaid agenda untouched, and may even exacerbate some existing strains in the Medicaid program.

Eligibility

Despite recent expansions of state options, the Medicaid program fails to cover many of the most vulnerable groups. For instance, even if all of the states were to enact the maternal and infant care options contained in OBRA 1986 and OBRA 1987, some very serious eligibility gaps and state-to-state inequities would remain. In Alabama, for example, a single mother of two earning $1,417 a year still would be covered only if she were pregnant, and then only for pregnancy-related care. Her children would be covered only if they were under age eight. A nine-year-old in this family would be too old for inclusion under the OBRA options and too rich for inclusion under the traditional program. Moreover, a nine-year-old living with both parents in Alabama would lack coverage even if the family income were *below* $1,417, because Alabama does not cover two-parent families.

Eventually, we as a society must come to terms with the core problem: Medicaid eligibility ceilings are linked to Aid to Families with Dependent Children (AFDC) payment levels, and these AFDC payment levels, in turn, show both tremendous interstate variation and a steep decline over time. In twenty-one states, eligibility levels are now at or below 50 percent of the poverty line, meaning that dependent children and their mothers in three-person families earning more than $4,650 a year do not qualify.[2] In addition, because Medicaid eligibility for the most part still hinges on eligibility for welfare programs (SSI and AFDC), people who do not meet the demographic profile required to receive welfare payments can't get health insurance protection either, no matter how poor they are. Unless they are elderly or disabled, for example, single adults and childless couples are ineligible at any income level and in any state. Until categorical re-

---

[2]Medically needy programs in some of these states raise the income ceiling somewhat but never by more than one-third.

quirements are eliminated and a minimum national eligibility floor is established at 100 percent of the federal poverty level or above, the Medicaid program will continue to exclude large numbers—perhaps most—of the poor.

The reason these reforms have not taken place, of course, is that they cost money, and at least half of the funds would come from the federal government. The numbers are not huge by federal budget standards. For example, current estimates are that raising the eligibility ceilings for those groups eligible under current categorical requirements would cost about $1.4 billion (Long and Rodgers 1988), and simultaneously eliminating the categorical requirements would raise the total cost between $9.05 and $11.7 billion depending on how many people with individual coverage moved over to the Medicaid program (Thorpe, Siegel and Dailey 1989). But at a time of intense concern about the federal deficit, even expenditures of this size are not likely to occur. Instead, what has been happening in each of the past several years has been incremental eligibility expansions for those groups most politically attractive and inexpensive to serve, and for whom the best long-term cost savings arguments can be made, that is, pregnant women and children. However welcome these expansions might be, the longer term impact will be to leave a substantial, and still growing, number of uninsured poor who are less attractive politically, and therefore for whom creating the political environment for change will be more difficult.

Enrollment

A second important avenue for Medicaid reform is to increase the program's "market penetration." At present, although data are scant, Medicaid researchers agree that a sizable number of people eligible for Medicaid coverage are not in fact enrolled (Hill 1988; Brown 1988; Rosenbaum and Hughes 1986; Rymer 1984). This gap exists even for the welfare-linked groups, and it can be very large for newer, state-option groups. For example, the short-term "work transition" eligibility program for people moving off of welfare tends to have very low enrollment levels, despite the fact that most people leaving wel-

fare do not obtain group insurance at work (Hill 1986).[3] Individuals who are eligible but not enrolled may incur sizable out-of-pocket costs, generate uncompensated care costs for hospitals, or delay necessary care.

For pregnant women, the presumptive eligibility program authorized as a state option under OBRA 1986 affords a partial solution. Under this program, pregnant women can receive a temporary card valid for ambulatory pregnancy-related care while their application is being processed. Elimination of the assets requirement for pregnant women, a second state option under OBRA 1986, also can facilitate enrollment by enabling states to design a shorter, more error-proof application, easier to administer and less susceptible to subsequent federal challenges and financial penalties.

Making major inroads into the enrollment problem, however, would require changing the incentive system for states. At present, faced with major expansions in the number of people who are eligible, and changes in financial responsibility for those already eligible states are already having great budgetary difficulties. An active and aggressive program to expand enrollment of those already eligible would add to these financial problems.

Current federal quality assurance rules provide an added reason for states to be very conservative in making eligibility determinations. Eligibility rules are very complex—in part because each expansion adds a new layer of eligibility rules onto an already Byzantine system. Applicants must not only meet income and categorical criteria, but must pass a rigid assets test as well. If, as they work their way through this cumbersome process, states make too many errors in favor of applicants and thereby enroll too many people later determined to be ineligible, a stiff penalty can be levied, reducing the federal matching portion of the entire Medicaid budget. States, how-

---

[3]Since the beginning of AFDC, a portion of a family's earnings has been disregarded in calculating AFDC eligibility. However, OBRA 1981 severely limited the extent to which this work incentive would apply, forcing many families off cash assistance and Medicaid. In 1984, Congress passed a "work transition" provision requiring states to provide Medicaid for nine months to families disqualified from AFDC because of this change. States have the option of providing an additional six months of coverage.

ever, are not penalized for excluding people who are eligible.

Eliminating the assets test for some or all groups would be one important way to reduce the enrollment-eligibility gap because it would remove the major opportunity for error and therefore the major justification for a lengthy application form. While little data on the subject exists, there is considerable reason to believe that the main function of the assets test is to serve as a procedural hurdle. Applicants fail the test, or drop out, not because their assets are too great but because they cannot successfully document how few possessions they actually have (Shuptrine and Grant 1988).

In addition, there are several things the federal government could do to change the current incentive structure for states in a more direct way. These range from changing the way current error rates are computed to providing more direct financial incentives for increasing program participation. For example, the federal matching rate for states could vary in accordance with state success in achieving targeted "market penetration" rates, or improved enrollment levels could be part of the performance objectives for Medicaid staff. The private sector has many long established individual and institutional incentives to encourage "sales," and there is every reason to believe that public agencies could respond to these as well, if increasing program participation really were an agency goal.

Other proposals to facilitate enrollment might be to mandate state presumptive eligibility programs (or other state programs designed to achieve these same objectives), extend such programs to groups other than pregnant women (children, for example), and mandate automatic enrollment of Supplemental Security Income (SSI) beneficiaries. Potentially, hospitals could play an important role to help close this enrollment/eligibility gap through on-site enrollment, participation in presumptive eligibility programs, and outreach activities, and many hospitals have begun to fill this need (American Hospital Association forthcoming).

The political difficulty with all of these solutions is that, in a time of strong budget concerns at the federal as well as state levels, finding the money to extend eligibility to new politically photogenic groups such as young poor children or near-poor pregnant women is easier than finding the funds to assure greater enrollment of groups that presumably already have been taken care of.

Financing and Reimbursement

Finding the money to assure adequate reimbursement is an even more difficult political feat. Medicaid programs already are staggering under the burden of financing existing health care services excluded under Medicare. Care for the elderly and disabled, particularly long-term care services, already accounts for three-fourths of Medicaid expenditures. In some states, programs also are absorbing a large and growing share of expenses for people with AIDS. Medicaid currently pays for the care of about 40 percent of the nation's people with AIDS, and in some areas the percentage may be as high as 65 to 70 percent (Institute of Medicine and National Academy of Sciences 1988).

In the past several years, states have been struggling to finance Medicaid expansion or, in some cases, straining simply to maintain the current level of commitment. Sometimes they fail. In Illinois and Michigan, for example, hospitals and nursing homes have gone for months at a time with no Medicaid reimbursement because the state Medicaid agency ran out of funds well before the end of its fiscal year (Fraser 1989).

One way states have reacted to the financing problem is by holding down provider reimbursement—an opportunity ushered in by the 1981 Omnibus Budget Reconciliation Act. In the past, state Medicaid programs were required to reimburse hospitals based on Medicare reasonable cost criteria. Under OBRA 1981, states are free to establish their own reimbursement methodologies, as long as the rates they pay are reasonable and adequate to meet the costs that must be incurred by efficiently and economically operated facilities to provide care and services in conformity with applicable state and federal laws, regulations, and quality and safety standards. In addition, payment must be reasonable and adequate enough to ensure that individuals eligible for medical assistance have reasonable access to inpatient hospital services of adequate quality

(Section 1902(a)(13)(A) of the Social Security Act). Section 1902(A)(30) of the Act requires that payments be consistent with efficiency, economy, and quality of care.

In their Medicaid plans, states are required to provide satisfactory "assurances" to the Health Care Financing Administration (HCFA) that these conditions have been met. But federal regulations provide no details concerning what states must do to meet minimum reimbursement requirements; that is, what kinds of evidence states must submit to prove that their rates are, in fact, adequate to ensure access to care, and adequate to meet the costs of efficiently and economically operated facilities. Thus far, HCFA has not shown an inclination to challenge state reimbursement rates, despite state proposals to reduce reimbursement rates by as much as 46 percent, and despite a proliferation of lawsuits by hospital associations and other interested parties on this issue (*West Virginia University Hospitals, Inc.* v. *Casey* 1988; *AMI SUB (DSL), Inc.,* v. *The State of Colorado Department of Social Services* 1988).

Because each state dollar must be matched by at least one federal dollar, the result of what some might consider a "wink-and-nod" approach to federal oversight of state reimbursement rates is a cost savings at the federal as well as state level. But, at some critical point, lower reimbursement rates, like low enrollment rates, strongly undercut the impact of eligibility expansions, with serious implications for patient access to needed services. When reimbursement levels are too far below levels customarily paid under private plans, hospitals are forced to cross-subsidize their Medicaid patients and the newly eligible find little improvement in access to care outside the hospital. Each dollar a hospital spends to subsidize care for Medicaid patients is a dollar not available to finance care for the uninsured. For communities with large numbers of uninsured, *and* large numbers of Medicaid enrollees, low reimbursement rates can mean the loss of a community hospital. In the case of physicians and others whose participation in Medicaid is voluntary, low reimbursement rates can lower willingness to treat Medicaid patients and therefore can cause an even more direct threat to access. A public insurance policy that does not pay what the private market requires provides little purchasing power and therefore may be little better than no insurance at all.

For expanded eligibility to translate into improved access, there must be clear criteria, procedures, and incentives for scrutinizing and ensuring the adequacy of reimbursement rates. Financing eligibility expansion through reimbursement cuts is like financing economic development by printing money—it gives broadened purchasing power with one hand but removes it with the other.

Service Coverage

A final problem area for Medicaid is service coverage. Because Medicaid is a joint federal-state program, with states free to operate within general federal guidelines, state programs can and do vary considerably not only on the extent but also on the content of coverage. Federal rules on covered services mandate certain services for the categorically needy and a different list for the medically needy; with other coverage decisions left to the states' discretion. This patchwork Medicaid system results in gaps and voids in which necessary and cost-effective services are not covered.

The law also permits states to limit the amount or scope of required as well as optional services. Many states have sought to contain costs by drastically limiting the number of inpatient days that the program will cover, even when such services might be medically necessary. Alabama, for example, will cover only twelve inpatient days a year, and the situation is little better in Tennessee (fourteen days) and Mississippi (fifteen days) (Laudicina and Lipson 1988).

This system also often makes it difficult for states to implement cost-effective mechanisms for addressing the catastrophic and chronic care needs of such population groups as children or individuals with AIDS. For example, Medicaid traditionally has not paid for case-management services, or for many of the support services necessary to maintain a disabled child or a person with AIDS in the community. There have been some recent positive developments along these lines, however, and this progress could be accelerated. For example, states could be permitted, as an optional service, to allow provision of home- and community-based services to Medicaid recipients who otherwise would require institutional care. At present, states must use the more cumbersome and time-consuming waiver process to implement such programs, even though home- and community-based services have been proven to be cost effective for many groups such as individuals with AIDS, the elderly and disabled, or chronically ill children.

Implications

States have gained considerable flexibility in recent years to shape their own policies regarding eligibility, enrollment, reimbursement, and service coverage, but the combination of new federally mandated eligibility expansions and continued federal fiscal constraints creates strong pressures to finance eligibility expansions through contractions in enrollment rates, services, and especially reimbursement levels. To the extent that states succumb to such pressures, the result may be, at best, to move some of the 37 million from the uninsured to the underinsured category, thereby creating only the illusion of a solution to the direct and indirect access problem.

Private Health Insurance

While deteriorations in public programs are one cause of the growing indigent care problem, they are not the sole cause, and public program expansions cannot be the entire solution. Even if the current severe national budget constraints did not exist, America's strong and largely successful history of private employer-based health insurance coverage would show a need to shore up and protect the private coverage side of the system. While this concept is widely supported in the United States, there is far less consensus on the fundamental issue of who should pay for it. As in the case of Medicaid, moreover, it is clear that there is no cheap and easy answer to the problem: state and local initiatives that provide new mechanisms, but no new money, are likely to produce very limited change.

The workplace has long been the predominant source of health insurance in the United States. Encouraged by a federal tax structure that subsidizes health insurance and other fringe benefits by permitting employers to purchase them with pre-tax dollars, most businesses offer health insurance coverage to at least some of their workers, and most businesses with health plans make at least some arrangement for dependent coverage. The result has been extensive private coverage of workers and their families. Over 130 million of 200 million nonelderly Americans receive health care coverage, directly or indirectly, through the workplace (Chollet 1988).

Despite this strong link between insurance and work, there also is a strong, growing, paradoxical link between *non*-coverage and work. That is, while the vast majority of the insured are receiving their coverage at the workplace, the vast majority of the *uninsured* also are workers, or dependents of workers, for whom the current system somehow is not operable. Figure 16–2 shows, for example, that three quarters of the uninsured live in families with a strong, fairly consistent link to the workplace and over half live in families of full-year, full-time workers. Only 12.3 percent of the uninsured have no connection to the workplace (Chollet 1988).

While getting a job may be the most common way to obtain insurance coverage, therefore, it is not a certain route. In recent years, the link between employment and insurance has been eroding, particularly for dependents. Specifically, the data (Chollet 1988) show that three things are happening. First, employer policies are covering a declining percentage of workers. Second, other private coverage is declining, particularly in the case of children. Third, employer policies are covering fewer dependents, even in terms of absolute numbers.

At the national level, recognition of the significant erosion in private coverage has led to discussions of several proposals—most notably, the Kennedy-Waxman[4] mandated employer coverage bill—to alter incentives and legal requirements for employers. The strong presence of such proposals on the national health care agenda has clearly encouraged the formation of

---

[4]Senator Edward Kennedy (Dem., Mass.) and Congressman Henry Waxman (Dem., Calif.)

Nonelderly Population without Health Insurance By Employment Status of Family Head, 1986.

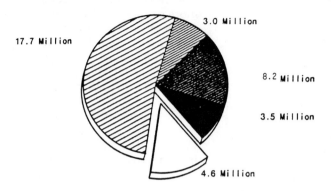

17.7 Million

3.0 Million

8.2 Million

3.5 Million

4.6 Million

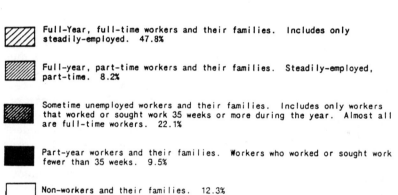

Full-Year, full-time workers and their families. Includes only steadily-employed. 47.8%

Full-year, part-time workers and their families. Steadily-employed, part-time. 8.2%

Sometime unemployed workers and their families. Includes only workers that worked or sought work 35 weeks or more during the year. Almost all are full-time workers. 22.1%

Part-year workers and their families. Workers who worked or sought work fewer than 35 weeks. 9.5%

Non-workers and their families. 12.3%

FIGURE 16–2

Source: Adapted from Chollet 1988.

task forces and study groups to develop alternative approaches, and the resulting dialogue has produced some significant evolution in the mandating proposals themselves. For example, the 1989 Kennedy-Waxman bill for the first time included a public sector expansion component, and it also included some additional incentives and protections for small and marginal businesses.

State and Local Structural Reforms

To date, however, the only concrete actions resulting from this growing national concern with private health insurance issues have taken place at the state and local level. State and local governments, in cooperation with various private sector players, are involved in a wide array of innovative and ambitious initiatives to expand private insurance coverage. The general thrust of all of these programs is to create mechanisms to enable businesses currently disadvantaged by the private health insurance system (small unincorporated firms, for example) to purchase health insurance more easily and more cheaply. These structural reforms can be grouped into four basic categories: including more people in existing groups, forming new large groups, changing the product or its delivery, and increasing product awareness (Fraser 1988; American Hospital Association 1988; Bovbjerg 1986; Wilensky 1987, 1988). As in the case of state Medicaid expansions, however, there is a very real question about the extent to which states acting alone—and, in particular, states acting alone with little new money—can counter the powerful national trends that have propelled the inexorable growth in numbers of uninsured and underinsured.

Including More People in Existing Groups

Existing large groups have a proven risk record, certain economies of scale, an established administrative apparatus, and some negotiating power with insurers and providers. One way to bring new small groups into the insurance system, therefore, can be to "piggyback" them on existing groups (Bovbjerg 1985, 1986), and sev-

eral recent initiatives have adopted this approach. In Tulsa, for example, the Health Option Plan is intended to bring together workers from small and large private plans. The core group might also consist of a public employee plan (as in West Virginia) or a public insurance program (as in Arizona).

A second, but less common way to include more people in existing groups is to improve enrollment rates for those who already belong to the group. National employer data (ICF Incorporated 1987) show that large numbers of workers who lack direct coverage from their employer are working in firms that already have an employer plan.

While some of these workers may have coverage through a spouse, many clearly are falling through the cracks, and therefore could be helped through policies designed to facilitate enrollment of workers and dependents in existing employer plans.

One federal effort of this sort is the nondiscrimination (Section 89) provision of the 1986 Tax Reform Act (P.L. 99–514), which stipulates that employee benefit policies must conform to certain federally-established formulas for equity, or else the "discriminatory excess"—the extra benefits received by one subset of employees—will be taxed. As of this writing, however, it is unclear to what extent and under what circumstances the law will result in expanded enrollment, or whether some employers might choose to achieve parity among employee groups by limiting coverage for all. The proposed formulas are generating considerable controversy and debate and several bills to postpone or rescind the legislation have been introduced.

A state approach, illustrated by legislation in New Hampshire, removes impediments to coverage of part-time employees by requiring insurers to offer all employers the option of covering part-time as well as full-time employees.

The data on uninsured workers (and, especially, worker families) within insured firms suggest, however, that real progress in closing the enrollment-eligibility gap is going to require some mechanism to make the employee share more affordable, particularly for family coverage. As discussed later, any real progress on the affordability issue is likely to require some form of targeted public subsidy.

Forming New Large Groups

A related strategy, when no handy and willing large group is available, is to form a new large group. State and local initiatives are doing this in several ways. One of the most common approaches is the grouping of employers in a multiple-employer plan. Under these arrangements, sometimes called multiple-employer trusts (METs) or multiple-employer welfare arrangements (MEWAs), two or more employers are grouped together through a central organizer or trustee, who then obtains the master insurance policy (Bovbjerg 1986; Polk 1987; Kinder 1986). In the past, these arrangements have been sponsored by labor unions, trade associations, business associations or coalitions, financial institutions, and insurers themselves. A new player with a similar arrangement is the employee leasing firm, which "hires" former small-firm employees, provides most of the common personnel functions, and then leases the employee back to the original business (ATAC 1986).

The establishment of state insurance pools provides a broader and larger grouping. Most commonly, these have taken the form of high risk pools, which focus on the small number of individuals who are medically uninsurable. But state pools can also be created to cover a broad cross-section of the population. In Washington and Oregon, such pools are being created as part of a voluntary, incentive-based mechanism, whereas in Massachusetts pooling is being done in the context of a state "pay or play" requirement, to become effective in 1992, in which firms with five or more employees either must pay a new state tax or provide health insurance for their employees.

Changing the Product

A third structural approach to lowering insurance costs is to change or deregulate the insurance product itself, to permit small firms and others newly-insured under the initiative to use some of the special exemptions, products, or delivery mechanisms available to self-insured or other large firms, for example, exemption from state mandated benefit laws, and the use of managed care options.

Increasing Product Awareness

High costs and product unavailability are not the only factors preventing employers from finding and purchasing an adequate health insurance plan. Many businesses, particularly small or emergent firms, are not aware of what products are available and how to go about selecting a product that meets their needs (National Federation of Independent Business 1985). Current initiatives to promote employer coverage are attempting to address this problem in two ways: by marketing efforts designed to promote new policies or programs, and by overall educational programs to increase product awareness and facilitate comparison shopping in the existing marketplace.

The Need for Subsidies

Each of the structural reforms described above has the potential to shave a few percentage points off of premium costs, and thereby to place small and currently-disadvantaged firms on a more equal footing with their larger and more established counterparts when it comes to locating and purchasing health insurance. Because most of the initiatives use several approaches simultaneously, the cumulative result in terms of cost savings can be significant.

Even significant cost savings may be grossly insufficient, however, given the economic resources of most uncovered workers, their families, and their employers—and given recent trends in the cost of health insurance and health care. The working uninsured face many impediments to insurance other than small group size. Uninsured firms are far more likely to be unincorporated (U.S. Small Business Administration 1987) and therefore unable to derive the full tax advantage available for the purchase of health insurance plans. The employer share of the premium is harder to come by because small businesses as a whole (and small uninsured businesses in particular) have lower levels of business assets (including cash, inventories, accounts receivable, and plants and equipment) per employee or per dollar of sales (U.S. Small Business Administration 1987). Finally, uninsured employees themselves tend to be low income—more than a third of workers lacking employer-sponsored coverage in 1986 had weekly salaries below $150 and four out of five earned less than $400 (Swartz 1989)—which means that introducing even a modest health insurance plan could represent a large percentage increase in labor costs. Low salaries also result in tight constraints on the premium share the employee can be expected to pay.

In light of average annual increases of twelve percent in health insurance premiums (Gabel, Di-Carlo, Fink and de Lissovoy 1989), moreover, a meticulously-designed program able to chip away ten percent of the cost of coverage could find such savings wiped out completely in the next mail. Given the low economic capacity of uninsured firms and the increasing costs of health care and health care coverage, initiatives that rely on structural mechanisms alone to reduce costs—that is, that allow small firms to take advantage of the same economies of scale and broad risk-sharing pools as large firms—could still miss the bulk of the working uninsured. The data clearly indicate that a sizable number of the currently uninsured would be able to pay very little toward the cost of their own coverage, much less family coverage. For some employers with many low-salaried employees, similar economic constraints may prevail. For this reason, an important strategy used in most of the current state and local initiatives is the use of private or public subsidies as a way to lower premium costs.

Providers—hospitals and, in some cases, physicians as well—are a common source of discounts in these initiatives, and some programs include insurer subsidies as well. Private donations are less common, but are included in one initiative—the Caring Program for Children (a program which insures low-income children at no cost to the family) initiated by Blue Cross of Western Pennsylvania and Pennsylvania Blue Shield, and since replicated in several other plans. While private subsidies and donations can lower premium costs somewhat, the sizable gap between the cost of coverage and available resources of currently-uncovered workers (and their employers) suggests that public subsidies will be needed.

Most private health insurance is of course already subsidized. Under federal tax law, employ-ers are able to purchase health insurance coverage with pre-tax dollars. The higher the employee's tax bracket, and the more generous the insurance plan, the greater the subsidy. For 1987, these federal supports were estimated to total $26 billion in federal income tax subsidies and $9.5 billion from social security payroll taxes (Congressional Budget Office 1986). But these subsidies obviously have been an insufficient incentive for many businesses, particularly those which have low profit levels and/or low salary structures and therefore low tax liability to begin with. For this reason, many of the state and local initiatives have provided additional public subsidies to the employer (through tax credits, subsidized premiums for former welfare recipients, and hardship funds) or, as in the state of Washington, to the employee.

The difficulty is that, given the high cost of health insurance and the low economic resources of many of the uninsured, public subsidies for private programs would need to be fairly substantial. Since much of the political appeal for private-sector approaches stems from the illusion that they can be implemented without public money, finding the funding to support these private-sector programs may be even more difficult than finding funds for Medicaid. In the face of this problem, state and local initiatives relying on public subsidies have moved very cautiously, beginning with small pilot projects. If these programs were to be done on a large-scale basis, public costs would begin to mount, and therefore these initiatives would face some of the same financial pressures already being experienced by Medicaid. If the programs are not done on a large-scale basis, however, they may provide little more than health insurance vignettes, case studies of state and local innovation which can be examined and admired while the number of uninsured continues to grow.

Conclusion

The current policy predicament is that, in the face of rapidly rising health care costs, public and private payers are desperately seeking—and, to some extent, finding—ways to contain their expenditures, though so far there has been little success in containing over-all system-wide costs. But the traditional "Robin Hood" mechanism for financing care to the uninsured—implicit cost shifts to private payers—presumes a certain level of economic irrationality or financial slippage in the system: that hospitals will be willing to care for people who do not pay, that public and private insurers and other payers will be willing to pay a little extra in order to help cover the bills of the poor uninsured, and that employees and employers will be willing to pay higher premium costs in order to help subsidize the care of workers with higher anticipated health care risks or larger families.

Increased competition and cost-consciousness in the health care environment are destroying this traditional financing system, but without creating a new mechanism to assure access and, incidentally, without solving the system-wide cost inflation problem either. Thus far, the response of most major players in the policy arena has been to search for a no-cost solution, when there clearly isn't one.

In recent years, given sizable increases in the cost of health care and health care coverage, employers have attempted to contain their own costs in a variety of ways. Some, such as the use of "second opinions" have proven to have limited effect (Congressional Research Service 1988a). But others have been quite effective, at least at the micro-level. In particular, large employers and private insurers—like Medicaid and other public payers—have been able to limit costs by transferring costs to others (increasing copayments, deductibles and employee premium shares), restricting who they will cover (denying coverage of high-risk groups or excluding coverage of preexisting conditions, for example), what they will pay for (only drugs which the Food and Drug Administration has approved for that particular use), and how much they will pay (discounted rates, avoiding any margin to cross-subsidize charity care, for example). Some of the new state and local initiatives are also adopting some of these mechanisms, and thereby reaping some of the same micro-level cost savings. The problem is that the same government sponsoring such an initiative ultimately may be picking up much of the public sector tab as well, and therefore cannot benefit to the same degree from mechanisms that limit private sector expenses by exclusion.

For example, one common device employers are using to control health insurance costs is to cut back on the share of the premium they pay for dependent coverage, with the result that a greater and greater share of the premium must be paid by the worker. A 1987 study of Service Employees International Union members, for instance, found that the employee share of the family premium commonly amounted to a third of the employee's take-home pay. Eventually, the employee share becomes so great that the employee must opt out of family coverage. The inevitable result of these factors has been a growing number of uninsured dependents of workers. Over four million children live with a parent or guardian who has employer-sponsored coverage (Chollet 1988; Gold, Kenney and Singh 1987). In fact, according to a recent study by the Congressional Research Service (1988b), most of the growth in the number of uninsured Americans since 1980 has resulted from declining employer-based coverage of children and other dependents. Ultimately, many of these uninsured dependents will generate public sector costs. While reducing dependent coverage may be a cost containment success story for the individual firm, it is a cost-generating practice from the public-sector perspective, and it clearly does not provide a model to be followed by state and local programs designed to deal with the fallout from those very "successes."

Similarly, insurers can develop a more affordable product, increase or maintain their market share, and limit their risks through medical underwriting—requiring a health examination or medical records examination and excluding from coverage those individuals or conditions with high expected health care costs. While such practices are rational, effective ways to limit the costs of insurers, employers, and individuals, the cumulative system effect (to overstate the point but slightly) is to provide insurance for those who don't need it and deny coverage for those who do.

The global problem is that, despite many years of "cost containment" initiatives, one of the few proven effective mechanisms available for an employer or insurer, or a public payer, to reduce health care costs is to stop paying for the care of others—whether those others are the poor, the sick, or even the company's own dependents.

The direction of change in the health care and insurance industry—with the increased use of experience rating, increased use and sophistication of medical underwriting, increased use of provider discounts and negotiated payments to providers, and increased emphasis on individual rather than family coverage—is to reduce the costs for one group by disassociating it from the others. Such a strategy can be effective at the firm level (at least until the firm's work force ages, or some employees become poor health risks), but it cannot work at the macro level, unless society is willing to accept, as a consequence, that some people will not receive care at all.

As discussed above, the general recognition that the access problem must be addressed is leading to very significant expansions in Medicaid eligibility, and very ambitious and innovative initiatives in private sector coverage. But failure to wrestle with the financing issue is taking away with the left hand much of what these programs are giving with the right, with the result that the cumulative impact on access may be much smaller than hoped.

More recently, increasing frustration with the twin problems of access and costs—coupled with the intense feeling on the part of all participants (government, employers, insurers, and consumers) that they are already giving more than their share—has prompted a desperate search for no-cost, quick-fix solutions, or at least solutions that move the costs to some other player. For example, the desire to address the access problem within the confines of the federal deficit clearly provided much of the impetus behind the original proposals to require employer-sponsored coverage. A more recent approach aims to solve the problem of the uninsured by making health insurance unnecessary. For example, a 1989 proposal by Congressman Brian D. Donnelley (Dem., Mass.) would have required hospitals to provide care (non-emergency as well as emergency care) to all who needed it, regardless of the patient's insurance status or ability to pay. The proposal did not, however, provide a financing mechanism.

Another, more sophisticated approach currently receiving considerable attention (See National Leadership Commission on Health Care 1989) focuses on eliminating, and capturing the current expenditures for, "unnecessary" or "ineffective" care. There is a growing recognition within the medical and policy community that practice patterns vary, that some medical care stems from liability concerns rather than medical necessity, and that up-to-date medical evidence on the utility of particular procedures is not adequately disseminated, understood, and acted upon. If expenditures for care that was not needed could be saved and spent on those who do, the theory goes, there would be more than enough to go around.

The need to restrain costs and to deliver only effective care is clearly compelling, and would be a serious matter even if no access problem existed. Faced with increasingly restrictive reimbursements from Medicare, Medicaid and private payers, providers have had strong reason to seek ways to control costs, for their own institutional well-being, as well as for the broader public good, and it is vital that they do more to increase efficiency and to ensure that care delivered is as effective as possible. Controlling costs is an important objective in its own right, and it is likely that greater efficiency could also produce some expansions in access: Reducing costs of care for Medicare and Medicaid patients would enable the public program dollar to stretch further, and decreasing costs for privately-insured patients could restrain premium costs and therefore increase the affordability of private health insurance.

To use the elimination of unnecessary or ineffective care as a financing mechanism for broadened access, however, would require a series of progressively unlikely steps: clear scientific evidence on what kinds of treatments or tests are effective in what circumstances, a somewhat likely development (Eddy and Billings 1988); mechanisms to educate the medical community and thereby change their behavior, a possible but probably lengthy and erratic process (Schroeder 1987; Kasecoff et al. 1987); and, most difficult of all, some way to assure that the money saved through increased efficiency is somehow captured and used to increase access, rather than converted to some other private or public use. For example, a corporation that presumably would have spent eight million dollars in a given year for health care, but instead only paid $7.7 million, might be most reluctant to contribute the "savings" to the cause of health care for the indigent.

Health insurance and health care clearly are expensive items—if they were cheap, everyone would have them, and this book would not need a chapter on access to care. Finding a way to control the escalating cost of health care must be a high priority for all players in the policy arena, and providers themselves have a particularly compelling public responsibility in this area. But for cost efficiencies to improve access, they must be system-wide, and there is no guarantee that even systemic improvements in efficiency will translate into improved access.

The search for ways to find true cost savings that are at the expense of neither quality of care nor the social contract, must continue. In the meantime, however, it must be recognized that covering millions of uninsured through private programs will require more than a few demonstration programs and cooperative ventures, covering them through public programs requires more than expansions in eligibility, and there are no quick-fix, no-cost solutions.

REFERENCES

American Hospital Association. 1986. *Cost and compassion: Recommendations for avoiding a crisis in care for the medically indigent.* Chicago, IL: American Hospital Association.

American Hospital Association. 1987. *Medicaid options: State opportunities and strategies for expanding eligibility.* Chicago, IL: American Hospital Association.

American Hospital Association. 1988. *Promoting health insurance in the workplace: State and local initiatives to increase private coverage.* Chicago, IL: American Hospital Association.

American Hospital Association. Forthcoming. *Financing uncompensated care: Uncompensated care pools and other provider-focused approaches.* Chicago, IL: American Hospital Association.

American Medical Association. 1988. Unpublished data from the Socioeconomic Monitoring System Survey. Chicago, IL: American Medical Association.

AMI SUB (DSL), Inc. v. The State of Colorado Department of Social Services. 1988. 698 F. Supp. 217 (D. Colo., 1988) on appeal No. 88–2482 10th Circuit.

ATAC. 1986. *Employee leasing in small versus large businesses.* Final report prepared for the Office of Advocacy. U.S. Small Business Administration.

Bovbjerg, Randall R. 1985. *Improving the lot of the Uninsured: Private and state initiatives in the individual and small group insurance markets.* Rev. Washington, D.C.: The Urban Institute.

Bovbjerg, Randall R. 1986. Insuring the uninsured through private action: Ideas and initiatives. *Inquiry* 23:403–418.

Brown, Sarah S., ed. 1988. *Prenatal care: Reaching mothers, reaching infants.* Washington, D.C.: National Academy Press.

Chollet, Deborah. 1988. *Uninsured in the United States: The nonelderly population without health insurance, 1986.* Washington, D.C.: Employee Benefit Research Institute.

Congressional Budget Office. 1986. *Reducing the deficit: Spending and revenue options.* A report to the Senate and House Committees on the Budget, Part 2. Annual Report. Washington, D.C.: Congressional Budget Office.

Congressional Research Service. 1988a. *Cost and effects of extending health insurance coverage.* Washington, D.C.: Government Printing Office.

Congressional Research Service. 1988b. *Health insurance and the uninsured: Background data and analysis.* Washington, D.C.: Government Printing Office.

Davis, Karen and Diane Rowland. 1983. Uninsured and underinsured: Inequities in health care in the United States. *Milbank Memorial Fund Quarterly* 61: 149–76.

District of Columbia Hospital Association. 1988. Prospective uninsured patient survey conducted by Lewin/ICF. Washington, D.C.: D.C. Hospital Association.

Duke University. 1986. Health care for the medically indigent: Payment and responsibility for indigent health care. April 22 presentation to the Indigent Health Care Study Commission. Raleigh, N.C.: Center for Health Policy Research and Education.

Duncan, R. Paul, Jan L. Colbert, and Jane F. Pendergast. 1986. *State University study of indigent care.* Volume 2: *The analytic report.* Gainesville, Fla.: Center for Health Policy Research, University of Florida Health Center.

Eddy, David M. and John Billings. 1988. The quality of medical evidence: Implications for quality of care. *Health Affairs* 7:19–32.

Fraser, Irene. 1988. Uninsured workers and uninsured dependents: Nine realities and thirty-two efforts to change them. Paper presented at the 1988 Annual Meeting of the American Public Health Association, Nov. 13–17. Boston.

Fraser, Irene. 1989. Medicaid: Reparing the safety net. *Michigan Hospitals* 25:23–30.

Gabel, Jon, Steven Dicarlo, Steven Fink, and Gregory de Lissovoy. 1989. *Employer-sponsored health in-*

surance in America: Preliminary results from the 1988 survey. Washington, D.C.: Health Insurance Association of America.

Gold, Rachel Benson, Asta-Maria Kenney, and Sushula Singh. 1987. Blessed events and the bottom line: Financing maternity care in the United States. New York, N.Y.: Alan Guttmacher Institute.

Gramlich, Edward M. 1987. Statement of the Acting Director, Congressional Budget Office, before the Senate Committee on Labor and Human Resources. November 4.

Hill, Ian T. 1986. Informal telephone survey of states on optional Medicaid program recipients and costs. National Governors' Association. February.

Hill, Ian. 1988. Reaching women who need prenatal care. Washington, D.C.: National Governors' Association.

Health Policy Agenda for the American People. 1988. Final report of the Ad Hoc Committee on Basic Benefits. Chicago, IL: Health Policy Agenda for the American People.

Health Policy Agenda for the American People. 1989. Including the poor: Final report of the Ad Hoc Committee on Medicaid. Chicago, IL: Health Policy Agenda for the American People.

Holahan, John F. and Joel W. Cohen. 1986. Medicaid: The trade-off between cost containment and access to care. Washington, D.C.: The Urban Institute Press.

ICF Incorporated. 1987. Health care coverage costs in small and large businesses: Final report. Prepared for Office of Advocacy, U.S. Small Business Administration.

Institute of Medicine and National Academy of Sciences. 1988. Confronting AIDS: Update 1988. Washington, D.C. National Academy Press.

Kasecoff, Jacqueline, David E. Kanouse, William H. Rogers, Lois McCloskey, Constance Monroe Dinolow and Robert H. Brook. 1987. Effects of the National Institute of Health Consensus Development Program on physician practice. Journal of the American Medical Association 258:2708–2713.

Kilbane, Kathleen and Beth Blacksin. The Demise of Free Care: The Visiting Nurse Association of Chicago. Nursing Clinics of North America 23:435–42.

Kinder, James A. 1986. Multiple employer welfare arrangements (MEWAs)—a topical discussion. Santa Ana, CA: Self-Insurance Institute of America (unpublished).

Laudicina, Susan S. and Debra J. Lipson. 1988. Medicaid and poor children: State variations in eligibility and service coverage. Alexandria, VA: National Association of Children's Hospitals and Related Institutions, Inc.

Long, Stephen H. and Jack Rodgers. 1988. Americans without health insurance: A comparison of man-

dated employment-based insurance and Medicaid expansions. Paper presented at the 1988 meeting of the American Public Health Association. Boston.

National Federation of Independent Business. 1985. Small business employee benefits. Washington, D.C.: NFIB Research and Education Foundation.

National Leadership Commission on Health Care. 1989. For the health of a nation: A shared responsibility. Ann Arbor, MI: Health Administration Press.

The National Study Group on State Medicaid Strategies. 1984. Restructuring Medicaid: An agenda for change. Washington, D.C.: The Center for the Study of Social Policy.

Polk, John. 1987. Benefit coverage: The council for smaller enterprises group health insurance programs. Facilitating Health Care Coverage for the Working Uninsured: Alternative State Strategies. Washington, D.C.: National Governors' Association.

Robert Wood Johnson Foundation. 1987. Access to care in the U.S.: Results of a 1986 survey. Princeton, N.J.: RWJ Foundation.

Rosenbaum, Sara and Dana Hughes. 1986. Financing maternity care. Paper presented at the Bush Institute Conference on Prenatal Care. May 27–28.

Rymer, Marilyn. 1984. Short-term evaluation of Medicaid: Selected issues. Baltimore: U.S. Department fo Health and Human Services, Health Care Financing Administration.

Schroeder, Steven A. 1987. Strategies for reducing medical costs by changing physicians' behavior: Efficacy and impact on quality of care. International Journal of Technology Assessment in Health Care 3:39–50.

Service Employees International Union. 1987. Access to health care: A survey of service workers (June). Washington, D.C.: Service Employees International Union.

Short, Pamela Farley, Alan Monheit, and Karen Beauregard. 1988. Uninsured Americans: A 1987 Profile. Paper presented at the 1988 meetings of the American Public Health Association. Boston.

Shuptrine, Sarah C. and Vickie C. Grant. 1988. The relationship of the reasons for denial of AFDC/Medicaid benefits to the uninsured in the U.S. Columbia, S.C.: Sarah Shuptrine and Associates.

Smith, Elmer W. 1984. Statement before the Subcommittee on Health, U.S. Senate Finance Committee. September 28.

Swartz, Katherine. 1989. The uninsured and workers without employer-group health insurance. Washington, D.C.: The Urban Institute.

Thorpe, Kenneth E., Joanna E. Siegel, and Theresa Dailey. 1989. Including the poor: The fiscal impacts of Medicaid expansion. Journal of the American Medical Association 261:1003–7.

U.S. Department of Health and Human Services. 1983. *The Medicare and Medicaid data book, 1982.* Baltimore, MD: Health Care Financing Administration.

U.S. Department of Health and Human Services. 1987. *The Medicare and Medicaid data book, 1986.* Baltimore, MD; Health Care Financing Administration.

U.S. Small Business Administration. 1987. *The state of small business: A report of the president.* Washington, D.C.: USGPO.

Wilensky, Gail. 1987. Viable strategies for dealing with the uninsured. *Health Affairs* 6:33–46.

Wilensky, Gail. 1988. Filling the gaps in health insurance: Impact on competition. *Health Affairs* 7:133–49.

West Virginia University Hospitals, Inc. v. Casey. 1988. U.S. District Court for the Middle District of Pennsylvania, No. 86–0955, November 30.

Chapter 17

Black Health Care and the American Health System:

A Political Perspective

Mitchell F. Rice

Mylon Winn

The provision and delivery of health care in the United States is not only a product of medical technology and medical science but also a product of politics and the political system. Schmandt and Wendel (1983, 213) note that health care is "abound with policy issues relating to the quantity and quality of services, the institutional structures through which they are provided, and the regulations that govern their delivery." Politics in the health delivery system involves political choices that determine priorities of medical research, the distribution of medical care and medical benefits, the supply of health professionals and the allocation of public resources to health against other societal needs.

Yet, until the 1970s, analysts in the health field gave very limited attention to the politics and policy associated with this huge industry. Further, the U.S. Department of Health and Human Services (USDHHS), the agency responsible for most of the enforcement and compliance functions in health and the administration of federal health programs, is among the largest of federal agencies. Its more than 43,000 employees serve more than 93 million beneficiaries (Rice and Jones 1987).

Moreover, even fewer analysts have explored health politics and policy as they relate to the black community. Perhaps one explanation for the paucity of research on politics and black health care is that the nature and extent of public sector involvement in the health field is difficult to describe and understand. The health care delivery system is one in which the regulated may also be the regulators, third parties rather than consumers pay for most medical care, and the financial and organizational structures of health care providers are almost mystically complex. Therefore, identifying and sorting out the role of government and other policy actors and their complex relationships becomes a difficult task. Mechanic (1986) points out the difficulty in analyzing the health care delivery system by noting that:

It is difficult to describe . . . the dimensions of an industry involving facilities, goods and services exceeding $400 billion dollars a year. The size, complexity and diversity is mind-boggling; the system of care is extraordinarily dynamic; and the high stakes intimately involve hundreds of government agencies, professional groups, business interests, consumer organizations, special interest lobbies, employees and unions, public interest groups and many others.

This chapter examines the American health care system and the black community from a political perspective. The chapter begins with a descriptive overview of the health status of the black population. It is noted that despite recent improvements in the health status of blacks, significant disparities continue to exist between blacks and whites in nearly every health status index. The next section discusses biases in the health system and argues that economic bias is the most significant problem in black health. The third section provides a review of recent government initiatives and activities aimed at improving black health. Special attention is given to offices and programs in the U.S. Department of Health and Human Services and the activities of the Congressional Black Caucus.

Federal Policy and Black Health Status: An Overview

The "Great Society" and "War on Poverty" federal programs in the mid-1960s greatly expanded the federal government's commitment and concern for improving access to health care for large numbers of America's poor and minorities. From the mid 1960s to the late 1970s more than seventy-five separate pieces of federal legislation were aimed at increasing access to health services for the economically disadvantaged (Rice and Payne 1981) including such programs as Medicaid, Medicare, Comprehensive Health Planning, Community Health Centers, as well as the recruitment and placement of minority and other health professionals in underserved communities. Federal health legislation during this period reflected an egalitarian value system which required the removal of economic barriers between health care consumers and providers.

Medicaid and Medicare are the two largest federally sponsored health insurance programs. Medicaid, enacted in 1965, is by far the nation's most expensive public program in the health care field for the poor, covering some 23 million individuals in 1986 (Treiger 1986). About 40 percent of all Medicaid enrollees are black (Schlesinger 1987). Medicaid has provided health coverage for nearly one out of every five blacks under 65 years of age and nearly half of all black children under six years of age (O'Brien, Rodgers and Baugh 1985). Medicare, enacted the same year as Medicaid, finances health care for the elderly and qualified disabled. In 1985 some 31 million individuals were covered under Medicare (USDHHS 1986a) including some ten percent of the black population (U.S. Bureau of the Census 1985; USDHHS 1984).

The Emergency Health Personnel Act of 1970, The Health Planning and Resources Development Act of 1974, and The Health Professions Assistance Act of 1976, mandated a redistribution of resources and medical personnel to favor the poor and minorities. By the 1980s these programs, along with Medicaid and Medicare, had led to marked improvement in the health of the black population (Hadley 1982). Most notable among these improvements are gains in the areas of life expectancy and infant mortality and a decline in the death rate.

As can be seen in table 17–1 black life expectancy from 1970 to 1985 increased by 5.4 years (from 64.1 years to 69.5). This increase was 1.6 years greater than that for the population as a whole during the same period (i.e., from 70.9 years to 74.7 years). While black males in 1985 continued to have the shortest life expectancy at birth, from 1970 to 1985 their life expectancy increased slightly more (5.3 years) than that of white males (3.9 years). The differential in life expectancy between white and black males declined from 8.0 years in 1970 to 6.6 years in 1985. For white and black females the differential dropped from 7.3 years in 1970 to 5.2 years in 1985.

Gains in life expectancy are indicative of lower infant mortality and lower death rates throughout life. For blacks, the infant mortality rate declined by nearly 50 percent from 1970 to 1985,

Life Expectancy at Birth, According to Race and Sex: United States, Selected Years 1970–1985.

Specified age and year	All races			White			Black		
	Both sexes	Male	Female	Both sexes	Male	Female	Both sexes	Male	Female

Remaining life expectancy in years

At birth

Specified age and year	All races			White			Black		
1970	70.9	67.1	74.8	71.7	68.0	75.6	64.1	60.0	68.3
1971	71.1	67.4	75.0	72.0	68.3	75.8	64.6	60.5	68.9
1972	71.2	67.4	75.1	72.0	68.3	75.9	64.7	60.4	69.1
1973	71.4	67.6	75.3	72.2	68.5	76.1	65.0	60.9	69.3
1974	72.0	68.2	75.9	72.8	69.0	76.7	66.0	61.7	70.3
1975	72.6	68.8	76.6	73.4	69.5	77.3	66.8	62.4	71.3
1976	72.9	69.1	76.8	73.6	69.9	77.5	67.2	62.9	71.6
1977	73.3	69.5	77.2	74.0	70.2	77.9	67.7	63.4	72.0
1978	73.5	69.6	77.3	74.1	70.4	78.0	68.1	63.7	72.4
1979	73.9	70.0	77.8	74.6	70.8	78.4	68.5	64.0	72.9
1980	73.7	70.0	77.4	74.4	70.7	78.1	68.1	63.8	72.5
1981	74.2	70.4	77.8	74.8	71.1	78.4	68.9	64.5	73.2
1982	74.5	70.9	78.1	75.1	71.5	78.7	69.4	65.1	73.7
1983	74.6	71.0	78.1	75.2	71.7	78.7	69.6	65.4	73.6
1984	74.7	71.2	78.2	75.3	71.8	78.7	69.7	65.6	73.7
1985	74.7	71.2	78.2	75.3	71.9	78.7	69.5	65.3	73.5

TABLE 17–1

SOURCE: U.S. Department of Health and Human Services, Public Health Service, Health, United States: 1987 (Washington, DC: Government Printing Office, 1987):44.

decreasing from 32.6 deaths per 1,000 live births to 18.2 per 1,000 live births (see table 17–2). The age adjusted death rates for all causes for black males decreased by 294.6 deaths from 1970 to 1985 per 100,000 population and black female age adjusted death rates for all causes decreased by 225.3 deaths per 100,000 population during the same period (see table 17–3).

However, not shown in table 1 are more recent preliminary data which indicate that the life expectancy of blacks for the first time this century has declined for two consecutive years, 1987 and 1988 (Johnson 1989, 12). While there is no empirical evidence, it seems quite clear that this condition is the cumulative effect of the Reagan Administration's restrictions, reductions and changes in health programs for the poor. Medicaid is serving a smaller proportion of those in poverty. In 1976 Medicaid covered some 65 percent of the poor. By 1984, the end of President Reagan's first term, Medicaid covered only some 38 percent of the poor (Brider 1987). With the enactment of the Omnibus Budget Reconciliation Act of 1981 (Public Law 97–35), Medicaid was reduced by some $12.8 billion mostly in federal match to the states (Rice forthcoming). In 1982 with the enactment of the Tax Equity and Fiscal Responsibilities Act (Public Law 97–248), Medicaid was reduced by another $2.2 billion through fiscal year 1985 (Rice forthcoming).

Although life expectancy and infant mortality rates and age adjusted death rates for blacks have improved considerably since 1970, health status disparities between blacks and whites continue to be the norm. In age-adjusted death rates between blacks and whites, a 50 percent difference remains (Manton, Patrick and Johnson 1987). This difference is referred to as excess deaths. If the death rates were equal, 59,000 black deaths a year would not occur (Savage, McGee and Oster 1987).[1] The black infant mortality rate is about twice the white rate (*New York Times* 1987). The incidence of low birthweight among blacks is almost two times higher than whites (Howze 1987). Blacks have more undetected diseases, higher disease and illness rates

than whites, and more chronic conditions than whites. Further, blacks in comparison to whites are more likely to (1) describe their health as fair to poor, (2) have a higher chronic limitation of activity, (3) have a larger number of restricted activity days annually, and (4) have a higher number of hospital bed days annually (USDHHS 1986a, 39). Perhaps one explanation for these differences is bias in the health system that has led to negative health consequences for blacks.

A Biased Health System

A *system* is defined as an assembly of interdependent specialized parts acting together for a common purpose or goal (Easton 1965). Accepting this definition, a health system should be one where the specialized parts act in concert for the purpose of promoting, maintaining and restoring health. However, in the United States, the present system of health care places more emphasis on *care* rather than the system and, as such, health promotion, education and prevention activities receive *secondary* consideration to treatment centered activities. One result of this focus is higher disease and illness rates in the black community that are preventable in nature through immunizations and annual physical examinations. Jesse Jackson (1988, 7) states this point in the following way:

> Our health care system is oriented toward fixing damage rather than preventing it. We spend $2,000 per person each year for health care and only $25 per person for medical research to prevent and cure illness. We pay $100,000 for intensive care for a premature baby, but we refuse to pay $800 for the prenatal that could prevent premature deaths.

The problems of health prevention in the black community are exacerbated by the lack of an adequate conceptualization of a public health strategy. Two approaches to health prevention, the proactive and reactive strategies (Jones and Rice 1987), while requiring different government re-

---

[1] Excess deaths are the difference between actual minority deaths and the number of deaths which would have been expected if the black population had the same age and sex-specific death rates as the white population.

Infant Mortality Rates*, According to Race: United States, Selected Years, 1970–1985

Number of deaths per 1,000 live births

	All races	White	Black
1970	20.0	17.8	32.6
1975	16.1	14.2	26.2
1976	15.2	13.3	25.5
1977	14.1	12.3	23.6
1978	13.8	12.0	23.1
1979	13.1	11.4	21.8
1980	12.6	11.0	21.4
1981	11.9	10.5	20.0
1982	11.5	10.1	19.6
1983	11.2	9.7	19.2
1984	10.8	9.4	18.4
1985	10.6	9.3	18.2

TABLE 17–2

SOURCE: *U.S. Department of Health and Human Services, Public Health Service, Health, United States: 1987 (Washington, DC: Government Printing Office, 1987):45.*

*Infant mortality rate is the number of deaths of infants under 1 year of age per 1,000 live births.

Death Rates for All Causes and All Ages, According to Sex and Race: United States, Selected Years 1970–1985.

	1970	1980	1981	1982	1983	1984	1985
	Number of deaths per 100,000 resident population						
All races							
All ages, age adjusted	714.3	584.8	568.2	553.5	550.5	545.9	546.1
All ages, crude	945.3	878.3	862.4	852.0	862.8	862.3	873.9
White male							
All ages, age adjusted	893.4	745.3	724.4	706.0	698.4	689.9	688.7
All ages, crude	1,086.7	983.3	965.1	951.8	957.4	951.1	960.0
Black male							
All ages, age adjusted	1,318.6	1,112.8	1,067.7	1,035.0	1,019.6	1,011.7	1,024.0
All ages, crude	1,186.6	1,034.1	991.6	960.4	963.3	958.1	976.8
White female							
All ages, age adjusted	501.7	411.1	401.4	393.3	392.7	391.3	390.6
All ages, crude	812.6	806.1	799.6	797.9	815.3	822.3	837.1
Black female							
All ages, age adjusted	814.4	631.1	599.1	581.4	590.4	585.3	589.1
All ages, crude	829.2	733.3	707.3	692.4	711.2	712.0	727.1

TABLE 17–3

SOURCE: U.S. Department of Health and Human Services, Public Health Service, Health, United States: 1987 (Washington, DC: Government Printing Office, 1987):56–57

sponses, share the same problems of implementation in the black community. Both approaches lack relevant-specific government goals and objectives (Jones and Rice 1987). Thus, it can be argued that public health prevention strategies are biased against blacks.

Further, at the heart of the United States health system is free enterprise in which an economic transaction occurs between the medical provider and the patient with a real or perceived medical problem who pays the provider to treat and/or cure the medical problem. While third party payers have complicated the transaction process, the fundamental economic relationship still holds. Economic logic dictates that the more money one has the more services one can purchase from the health system. Many blacks, however, lack the purchasing power necessary to obtain health care. A disproportionate number of blacks live in low-income households. A third of all black households have incomes below the poverty line, and almost half of all black children live in these families (Jones and Rice 1987; U.S. Congressional Budget Office 1985; Miller 1987). Moreover, an additional 40 percent of black households have incomes below 125 percent of the poverty line. Thus with nearly 75 percent of black households in or near poverty, affordable health care is out of financial reach.

Compounding this situation is the number of blacks having no medical insurance. Blacks represent about 18 percent of the total number of uninsured. Further, some 25 percent of all black children are uninsured and black children comprise some 20 percent of all uninsured children under eighteen years of age (Sulvetta and Swartz 1986).

Moreover, being employed does not guarantee medical insurance. Of the approximately 37 million uninsured individuals in the country, some two-thirds are employed (Smith 1988). About half of these individuals are employed by firms with fewer than twenty-five employees (Smith 1988). These firms are mostly in the agriculture, construction and retailing businesses and employ large numbers of blacks.

The health system operates under an assumption of patient resources. If the patient has no resources or insufficient resources, the health system responds in the following way: no services provided or not enough provided to some

individuals. Therefore, for blacks the economic emphasis in health has transformed the health system from an interdependent system (if such a system truly existed) to an independent system lacking integration that manages or cures illness at the point of exchange—a system biased against blacks. With a poverty rate for black families three times that of white households, much of the black community is unable to afford health care because of economic deprivation.

Income is one of several socioeconomic factors that affects health care. Simply put, poverty and poor health reinforce each other. As Luft (1978, 2) observes:

> People with less education [and] low paying jobs are likely to be adversely affected by a health problem. . . . Those people often begin with a greater chance of being in poverty tend to experience greater disabilities and become even more impoverished.

Clearly, the present socioeconomic conditions of blacks promote inequality in the access to health services. Jones and Rice (1987, 7) observe that "Blacks are the victims of an economic system that dictates both their ability to receive health services and the quality of their health." Thus it would seem for blacks that using the term *system* to describe the health system is misleading to the extent that the term implies organization and continuity. Rather, the health care sector is a pluralistic amalgam of many differing and varied interests, each of which is jealously protective of its share of this lucrative industry. This pluralistic arrangement works well for those individuals with financial resources. However, this arrangement has been unresponsive and insensitive to the health needs of the black community. This condition is exacerbated by the lack of input by the black community in the health policy-making process, a situation that may be associated with the tenets of a liberal, pluralistic society.

Black Health Care in a Liberal, Pluralistic Society

In 1966, the President of the American Public Health Association noted that "Clearly, in terms of health, there is a special disadvantage to being a Negro in the United States which transcends being poor" (Yerby 1966, 6). Five years later the United States Government (USDHEW 1971, 6) observed that:

> On nearly every index, we have, the poor and racial minorities fare worse than their opposites. Their lives are shorter; they have more chronic and debilitating illnesses; their infant and maternal death rates are higher; their protection, through immunization against infectious diseases is far lower. They also have far less access to health services-and this is particularly true of poor and nonwhite children, millions of whom receive little or no dental and pediatric care.

About a decade and half later the U.S. Department of Health and Human Services (1985, 1) declared that:

> Despite the unprecedented explosion in scientific knowledge and the phenomenal capacity of medicine to diagnose, treat and cure disease, Blacks have not fully benefited equally from the fruits of science or from those systems responsible for translating and using health science technology.

Health is a key indicator of a population group's well-being, and health statistics measure both progress and continuing inequities. At the heart of black health problems is the degree of governmental involvement in a liberal, pluralistic society. Liberalism as a social philosophy and pluralism in the political system dominate health care politics and health planning in the United States. A liberal, pluralistic society or community stresses the rights of various groups to have input in the public policy-making processes concerning the allocation and distribution of valued benefits, services and resources. These groups are both private and corporate, and they compete to determine the public interest. One result of competition among these groups is a bargaining process that culminates in compromise. The bargaining process becomes a far more difficult activity when valued resources approach scarcity as in the case of health resources. Blacks, in particular, are among many interest groups competing for scarce health resources.

Robert Dahl (1961), Raymond Wolfinger (1972) and Nelson Polsby (1973), leading proponents of pluralism, observe that pluralism implies that decisions result from and benefit the most influential and competitive centers of power. Accepting this observation, it is argued that pluralism has created a situation whereby the most powerful and influential have extraordinary impact on the decision/policy-making processes. Blacks as a group have had less influence and have been less competitive in policy and decision-making processes. Thus, black health inequities may be associated with the emphasis on group input in a pluralistic society. Advocacy is not seen as effective in changing the health milieu of blacks because of pluralistic assertions that the incrementalism now practiced is the only feasible way of bringing about change. Programs and proposals that threaten the basic distribution of power within the pluralist universe are viewed as radical or outside the operating standard or norm.

Further, pluralism as a political ideology has created governmental bodies that do not make effective decisions regarding health in the black community. In examining the record of federal intervention in the area of urban health, we find a lack of centralization around black health concerns. Federal health policy has been aimed at the general population and has not, for the most part, dealt with the health concerns of most of the black population. Instead of a comprehensive approach to black health problems, the pluralistic tradition has resulted in a patchwork of federal programs, policies and guidelines that have had minimal impact in the black community.

The failure of federal efforts to impact substantively on black health can be attributed to three factors: the U.S. system of federalism, the distribution of health personnel, and planning. According to Jones and Rice (1987, 9–10):

> Federalism dictates the distribution of authority for the delivery of services. . . . [T]he distribution of health professionals affects the probability of access to health services. . . . [T]he government's ability to plan dictates the ability of the system to change to meet new demands.

The federal government's expectation is that the states should be the instrument of health planning and implementation. Realistically, however, many federally financed programs are directed at local communities, resulting in the undermining of state authority. Alford (1975) has noted that neighborhood health councils were expected to assume responsibility for policy determination despite the fact that state authorities could not relinquish control in these areas.

Further, Jones and Rice (1980, 61) have argued that "local client-based associations tend to narrow health policy to a single issue preventing the exercise of authority." These local associations exert tremendous influence and may be partially responsible for the creation of an ineffective health care delivery system for blacks. Area-wide health plans produced at the local or community level tend to avoid specific programs for black residents. These plans seldom specify the physical distribution of resources to specific users (Jones and Rice 1987). Decisions concerning physical distribution, location of equipment and other resources are reserved, in most instances, for political authorities and not health planning units. In the end, however, because health planning authority is fragmented among policy bodies, political decision-making units are unable to set significant health care goals that can appease the pluralistic bases of urban health care (Clark 1978).

In the final analysis, state health planning units possess little or no control over two sources of authority—federal legislation and local implementation. Kaiser (1976) has noted that without control of these two sources of authority, state health planning units have found it difficult to develop intervention strategies and make directed change possible through health planning.

One important facet of the failure of a pluralistic government to respond to the inequities of black health care is manpower planning. Planning for adequate manpower is important for the creation of an equitable distribution of medical knowledge and resources. Without black doctors there can be no democratic way of providing incentives for a black community-based medical practice. Without an overall health manpower plan there cannot be an equitable distribution of resources. Further, while planning offers a more systematic means of providing for future situations, the failure to plan can only accentuate the problems of authority for government. Thus, it is important to examine health manpower planning to elucidate the failures of a pluralistic democracy in providing adequate health care to the black community.

Manpower Problems and Black Health Care

Approximately two-thirds of the value of health services in the United States represents labor input; somewhat less than one-sixth represents input of physical capital; and the remainder represents goods and services purchased from other industries (Sorkin 1975). The term health manpower includes not only the usual categories of physicians, dentists, and nurses but all the occupations important in the delivery of health services.

Acceptance of blacks in predominantly white medical schools has been slow in the United States. These schools have had a history of operating on a segregated basis which has resulted in segregated and overcrowded teaching institutions for blacks. The consequence of such discriminatory practices was to keep the medical profession segregated. As recently as 1985–86 blacks represented only 5.8 percent of the total enrollment in schools of allopathic medicine and as of 1983–84 comprise only 2.0 percent of the total enrollment in schools of osteopathic medicine (USDHHS 1986b, 87). Thus, racial discrimination has prevented the development of programs and opportunities for blacks in learning the skills of a physician. In contrast, licensed practical nurses and nursing aides, orderlies and attendants are overrepresented by blacks when compared to their total percentage of the population. Service work has traditionally been overrepresented by blacks while the more technical positions have been reserved for whites (Tolbert 1977; McKinney 1988).

Manpower planning requires the examination of the future market as well as the available pool of health care workers. Obviously, as the black population increases, the present level of black physicians in practice and in training will not be adequate. The federal government has played an increasing role in health manpower and development by providing the resources to solve the manpower shortage. But limitations on loan size and scholarships have significantly affected the enrollment increases among low-income minority students. Manpower planning requires the authority to allocate resources in an efficient manner in the public interest. A pluralistic government tends to bargain away this crucial source of authority rather than to assert the right to make decisions involving equity. Recent government strategies, however, have been implemented to promote equity in access to health services and improve the overall health of blacks.

Recent Government Initiatives and Black Health Inequities

In recent years several initiatives have been implemented at the federal government level to address preventive health and health status and improve overall health in the black community. The following discusses the Office of Minority Health and other programs and activities in the U.S. Department of Health and Human Services (DHHS) and the efforts of the Congressional Black Caucus (CBC) in addressing the health needs of the black population.

The Office of Secretary of DHHS

After his first few weeks as President-Elect, George Bush nominated a black as Secretary of DHHS. Dr. Louis W. Sullivan, a physician trained at Boston University's School of Medicine and President of the Morehouse School of Medicine, was confirmed by the Senate on March 1, 1989 with a 98–1 vote (Dervarics 1989, 1). His appointment was particularly praised by black medical leaders who recognize the important role of the position in black and minority health (Farrell and Wiley 1989). After nearly two months as Secretary, Dr. Sullivan demonstrated his concern for and understanding of minority health problems by calling for $42.9 million in new spending in fiscal year 1990 for scholarship and research to selected medical schools and an additional $25 million for occupational health programs (Johnson 1989). This increased funding would largely benefit minorities. The Secretary indicated that minority health care and preventative medicine would be a priority of his term in office (Johnson 1989). One of Dr. Sullivan's immediate priorities

was to strengthen the Office of Minority Health (OMH) in DHHS (Johnson 1989).

The Office of Minority Health

In 1985, DHHS released an eight volume report entitled *Report of the Secretary's Task Force on Black and Minority Health,* a very detailed and comprehensive federal examination of black and minority health status. The report documented disturbing health disparities between minorities and non-minorities and identified six major causes of death among minority populations: cardiovascular disease and stroke; cancer; homicide; suicide and unintentional injury; infant mortality; chemical dependency and diabetes (USDHHS 1985). These causes of death account for 80 percent of the excess deaths among minorities (*Federal Register* 1989, 10592).

The *Report* recommended the establishment of a federal office to focus on minority health issues. This was done with the creation of the Office of Minority Health (OMH) in December 1985 with a first year budget of three million dollars (Malone 1985). The objective of OMH is to serve as the focal point for implementing the recommendations relating to the six major causes of death enumerated in the *Report* to reduce black health disparities (OMH 1989). In 1988, OMH added AIDS as a seventh priority area because of the severity of the disease in the black and minority community (OMH 1989, 2). Of the nearly 91,000 reported cases of AIDS as of March 1989, about 27 percent are black and 53 percent of all AIDS cases among children under thirteen years of age are black cases (OMH 1989; Windom 1989). OMH is "mandated to develop policies, programs and objectives to improve the health status of minority populations" (OMH 1989, 2).

From 1985 to mid 1989, OMH initiated several programs and activities. A national information and technical assistance resource center maintains a data base of local, state, and national minority health related resources; a network of 2,000 experts from diverse public health backgrounds; and sources of complimentary and low cost services and materials (*The Nation's Health* 1989). In fiscal year 1987, OMH established and implemented a DHHS-wide minority health coordination process designed to focus the Department's attention on mechanisms and approaches to improving health disparities between minority and non minority populations (OMH 1989). This coordination effort has culminated in the formation of nine Health Issues Working Groups to examine the major disease areas affecting black and minority populations (OMH 1989). The Groups are examining cross cutting issues in the areas of health financing, health data and health professions personnel development.

OMH is also providing grant funds for coalitions of community based organizations and national organizations to promote disease reduction and to provide AIDS education and prevention. Between 1986 and early 1988, OMH awarded 26 grants under the Minority Community Health Coalition Demonstration Grant Program. In fiscal year 1988, seven grants were awarded for a sum total of $1.4 million (*Federal Register* 1989, 10593). From 1988 to early 1989 nearly 3 million dollars in grants were awarded to minority community based and national organizations for AIDS education and prevention (OMH 1989, 2). In addition to OMH, the Centers for Disease Control (Atlanta), a component of DHHS, created and filled a new position in 1988, Assistant Director of Minority Health, to focus on minority health issues.[2] A major objective of this position is to interface with minority community based organizations and develop strategies for disease prevention and health promotion.[3] The Centers for Disease Control also operates a Diabetes Control Program which has had a minority focus since 1984 (Windom 1989).

Other DHHS Programs and Activities

Other federal intervention efforts implemented to improve black health status include programs and activities in the National Institutes of Health (NIH), Health Resources and Services Administration (HRSA), and the Health Care Financing Ad-

ministration (HCFA). The National Institute of Diabetes and Digestive and Kidney in NIH sponsored a conference in September, 1988, to explore the higher rate of diabetes in blacks (Wyngaarden 1989). In 1986 the National Cancer Institute in NIH developed a Cancer Prevention Awareness Program for Blacks "to increase cancer prevention behaviors in the black population and promote life-style changes that can lower cancer risk" (Wyngaarden 1989, 200). Black colleges and universities serve as the focal points within the black community to heighten awareness about cancer risks and prevention (Windom 1989). More than 80 cancer related programs are in place that either specifically target minorities or will benefit both minorities and the general population (Windom 1989). The National Institute of Child Health and Human Development is supporting clinical research to determine those nutritional, medical and psychosocial factors contributing to the incidence of low birthweight in urban black populations (Wyngaarden 1989).

The Office of Maternal and Child Health in HRSA has awarded about 15 percent of the total Maternal and Child Health Services Block Grant Program budget allocation (some 500 million dollars annually) to special projects including some that focus on inner city minority residents and rural blacks in the South (HRSA 1989). Further, epidemiologists from the USDHHS are being placed in selected state and maternal and child health programs to improve their analytic and evaluative capability. In 1988, a $20 million perinatal care program was initiated through 206 federally supported community and migrant health centers in forty-five states (HRSA 1989). Some one-third of the clients served by the centers are black. Moreover, in collaboration with the Robert Wood Johnson Foundation, USDHHS has initiated a program under the name "Healthy Generations" to assist those states with extensive infant mortality problems (HRSA 1989).

Other programs and activities within DHHS with a focus on black and minority populations include the Administration for Children, Youth and Families. This program sponsors collaborative efforts "with local social service groups to combat the growing problem of violence and unnecessary injury in black and minority population" (Windom, 1989, p. 196). In June 1988 the Public Health Service sponsored its second an-

---

[2]Reuben Warren, D.D.S., MPH, former Dean of Meharry Medical College Dental School, is the Assistant Director of Minority health.

[3]The first author was a finalist for the position, and the objectives were articulated by the interview team during the interview process.

nual Conference on AIDS Prevention and Control. The problem of AIDS in minority communities was a special area of concern (Windom, 1989).

Congressional Black Caucus

The Congressional Black Caucus (CBC), a body of all black members of Congress, was created in 1970 to promote black interests in Congress. Former U.S. Representative Charles Diggs (Dem., Mich.) served as the first chair. Keiser (1987, 62) points out that over the years "the members of the caucus [have tended] to vote alike. . . . The group is more an independent source of initiative within the liberal coalition than it is a distinct voting bloc." The Caucus has given most attention to legislation promoting economic advancement in the black community. While the Caucus since its inception has supported health as a priority issue for Congress and the country, in recent years the health of the black community has become an important issue. In 1984, Representative Charles Rangel (Dem., N.Y.) and Representative Harold Ford (Dem., Tenn.) were part of the Ways and Means Subcommittee on Health. Representative Mickey Leland (Dem., Tex.) was on the Energy and Commerce Subcommittee on Health and Environment. Representative Louis Stokes (Dem., Ohio) was a member of the Appropriation Subcommittee on Labor, Health and Human Services.

Representative Stokes, as Chairman of the CBC Health Braintrust, one of several important issue areas of CBC[4], has stated (1988a, 14) that the CBC is "committed to supporting legislation and a Congressional budget that improves the health status and health care delivery for all Americans but particularly for [the] nation's unserved and underserved citizens." The CBC Alternative Budget for fiscal year 1988 proposed that

the federal government spend $44.11 billion for U.S. health needs, $3.27 billion more than proposed by the Reagan Administration ("The CBC Alternative" 1987). The CBC Budget objectives were (and still are) to expand access to health care for the uninsured and underinsured, improve maternal and child health care services, increase the number of minority health professionals and direct more research funding to minority health problems ("The CBC Alternative" 1987). Representative Stokes also has stated (1988b, 3) that "the health care system in America is by and large two-tiered: the affluent, who occupy one tier, receive adequate health care, and the poor, who occupy the other, do not." He further (1988a, 15) points out that:

> Health care should not be simply available for a privileged, and equal rights should be expanded to include equal health care rights as well.

In 1985, Representative Stokes, as a member of the House Appropriations Committee, was successful in attaching an amendment for an additional $10 million for two new National Institutes of Health initiatives both of which in the long term will be beneficial in improving the health status of blacks (Bowens 1985). The Stokes Amendment for fiscal year 1986 doubled the funding for research centers in the Minority Institutions Award Program and the Academic Research Enhancement Award Program.

In April, 1989, Representative Stokes called a National Black Health Summit to deal with the piecemeal and disjointed efforts of individuals and organizations in addressing black health needs (Loscocco 1989). The Summit, attended by prominent black leaders and organizations, "endorsed proposals to improve awareness of health issues and disease prevention and eliminate barriers to getting good health care" (Loscocco 1989, B1).

Conclusion

This chapter presents evidence that access to health has improved considerably for a large number of black Americans. Much of this improvement can be attributed to federal govern-

---

[4]The CBC has designated the term "Braintrust" to reflect the importance of several issue areas it has given priority including health, education, energy, aging, agriculture, civil rights, criminal justice, housing, drugs and banking and financial institutions. A black Congressional member serves as chair of each Braintrust issue area. As of September 1988, there were nineteen Braintrust issue areas. See Congressional Black Caucus, *Congressional Black Caucus Braintrusts* (mimeo) (September 16, 1988).

ment initiated health policies. Yet, on the major indicators of health status, several black/white disparities remain. Disparities are most acute for blacks who are uninsured, low income, under seventeen and over sixty-five years of age. The health care system is economically biased against these individuals. Blacks are still twice as likely to be without a regular source of care and are more likely to utilize a hospital emergency room or outpatient clinic as a primary source of care.

Poverty and powerlessness would seem to explain the health status of the black population. According to Braithwaite and Lythcott (1989, 282):

> Poverty and powerlessness create circumstances in people's lives that predispose them to the highest indexes of social dysfunction, the highest indexes of morbidity and mortality, the lowest access to primary care, and little or no access to primary preventive programs. Poverty of the spirit and resources remains the antecedent risk factor of preventable disease.

While America is a melting pot of many cultures and perspectives, most blacks are poverty stricken and in the quagmire of premature death and disability. Powerlessness is a structural problem that is embedded, reinforced and perpetuated by the fabric of social and economic institutions. Braithwaite and Lythcott (1989, 282) define powerlessness as:

> a construct of continuous interaction between the person and his/her environment. It combines an attitude of self-blame, a sense of generalized distrust, a feeling of alienation from resources of social influence, an experience of disenfranchisement and economic vulnerability, and a sense of hopelessness in the sociopolitical struggle.

The federal government response to the health status and health needs of blacks has been mixed. On the one hand, it has retreated from the regulation and financing of health services and has instead endorsed the competitive market approach as a strategy for both cost containment and promoting equity in access to health services. This role and approach will likely exacerbate existing differences between blacks and whites. Further, the changing health marketplace will have more disadvantages than advantages for blacks. Individuals who are forced to compete in a health marketplace with limited resources and bargaining power will be met with the greatest resistance.

On the other hand, the federal government has recently initiated programs and activities with a direct focus on black and minority health problems. While it is too early to assess the impact of these initiatives, it is quite clear that incrementalism and other bandages have not adequately dealt with black health issues. What is needed, as suggested by Braithwaite and Lythcott (1989, 283), on the part of both government and the health community is the development of "comprehensive and culturally sensitive approaches to address the complex and multifaceted issues of [black] health and wellness." Black congressional leaders and black community based organizations must develop a strategy that identifies health promotion priorities, inventories health resources and builds coalitions with the public and private sectors to support health interventions in the black community.

REFERENCES

Bowens, Jackie. 1985. Legislative Update. *Health care crisis: We can make a difference conference proceedings.* Washington, D.C.: District of Columbia Public Health Department, Contract #HSRA 86–113(P), Reference #457194.

Braithwaite, Ronald L. and Ngina Lythcotte. 1989. Community empowerment as a strategy for health promotion for black and other minority populations. *Journal of the American Medical Association* 261:282–283.

Brider, Patrick. 1987. Too poor to pay: The scandal of patient dumping. *American Journal of Nursing* 87:1447–1449.

Clark, Noreen M. 1978. Spanning the boundaries between agency and community: A study of health planning staff board interaction. *American Journal of Health Planning* 3:40–46.

Congressional Black Caucus. 1989. *Congressional black caucus braintrusts.* Mimeo. September 18.

Dahl, Robert C. 1961. *Who governs: Democracy and power in an American city* New Haven: Yale University Press.

Davis, Karen et al. 1987. Health care for black americans: The public sector role. *Milbank Quarterly* 65 (Supplement 1): 213–247.

Dervarics, Charles. 1989. Senate Confirms Sullivan as HHS Secretary. *Black Issues in Higher Education* 6 (1) (March 16): 1, 7.

Easton, David. 1965. *A framework for political analysis* Englewood Cliffs, N.J.: Prentice-Hall.

Farrell, Charles S. and Ed Wiley, III. 1989. Morehouse-Bush ties lead to Sullivan appointment. *Black Issues in Higher Education* 5 (21) (January 18): 1, 10.

Federal Register. 1989. 54 (48) (March 14):10592–10595.

Hadley, J. 1982. *More medical care, better health?* Washington, DC: The Urban Institute.

Health Resources and Services Administration. 1989. From the Health Resources and Services Administration. *Journal of the American Medical Association* 261:199.

HHS announces publicity campaign on minority health. 1989. *The Nation's Health* (May/June):2.

Howze, Dorothy. 1987. Closing the gap between black and white infant mortality rates: An analysis of policy options. In W. Jones, Jr. and M. F. Rice, eds. 119–139. *Health Care Issues in Black America.* New York: Greenwood Press.

Jackson, Jesse L. 1988. A prescription for America's health. *State Government News* 31 (December):6–8.

Johnson, Julie. 1989. Health chief vows minorities drive. *New York Times.* April 25, 12.

Jones, Woodrow, Jr. and Mitchell Rice. 1980. Liberalism, politics and health planning. *Journal of Health and Human Resources Administration* 3:56–66.

Jones, Woodrow, Jr. and Mitchell F. Rice. 1987. Black health care: An overview. In W. Jones, Jr. and M. F. Rice, eds. 3–20. *Health Care Issues in Black America.* New York: Greenwood Press.

Kaiser, Leland. 1976. The effective health planner. *American Journal of Health Planning.* 1:38–48.

Keiser, K. Robert. 1987. Congress and black health: Dynamics and strategies. In W. Jones, Jr. and M. F. Rice, eds. 59–77. *Health Care Issues in Black America.* New York: Greenwood Press.

Loscocco, Laurie. 1989. Stokes calls for action on blacks' health woes. *Columbus (Ohio) Dispatch,* May 5:B1.

Malone, Thomas E. 1985. Keynote address. *Health care crisis: We can make a difference, conference proceedings.* Washington, D.C.: District of Columbia Public Health Department, Contract #HSRA 86–113(P), Reference #457194.

Manton, Kenneth, Clifford H. Patrick and Katrina Johnson. 1987. Health differentials between blacks and whites: Recent trends in mortality and morbidity. *Milbank Quarterly* 65 Supplement 2: 443–461.

McKinney, Fred. 1988. Minority Employment in the Health Industry: The Effects of Restructuring. *Journal of Health and Human Resources Administration* 10:242–264.

Mechanic, David. 1986. *From Advocacy to Allocation: The Evolving American Health Care System.* New York: The Free Press.

Miller, S. M. 1987. Race in the Health of America. *Milbank Quarterly* 65(Supplement 2):500–531.

New York Times. 1987. Birth in America: A Fact Sheet, June 26.

O'Brien, M. D., J. Rodgers, and D. Baugh. 1985. *Ethnic and racial patterns in enrollment, health status, and health services utilization in the Medicaid population,* Series B, Report No. 8. Health Care Financing Administration, (September 30).

Office of Minority Health, Public Health Service, U.S. Department of Health and Human Services. 1989. *Resources persons network update* (May).

Polsby, Nelson. 1973. *Community power and political theory.* New Haven: Yale University Press.

Rice, Haynes and Larah D. Payne. 1981. Health issues for the eighties. In *The state of black America,* 119–151. New York: National Urban League.

Rice, Mitchell F. (forthcoming). Medical indigency and inner city hospital care: Patient dumping, emergency care and public policy. *Journal of Health and Social Policy.*

Rice, Mitchell F. and Woodrow Jones, Jr. 1987. Public policy compliance, enforcement and black American health: Title VI of the Civil Rights Act of 1964. In *Health care issues in black America,* W. Jones, Jr. and M. F. Rice, eds. 99–118. New York: Greenwood Press.

Savage, Daniel D., Daniel L. McGee and Gerry Oster. 1987. Reduction of hypertension—Associated heart disease and stroke among black Americans: Past experience and new perspectives on targeting resources. *Milbank Quarterly* 65 (Supplement 2): 297–321.

Schlesinger, Mark. 1987. Paying the price: Medical care, minorities and the newly competitive health care. *Milbank Quarterly* 65 (Supplement 2):270–295.

Schmandt, Henry J. and George D. Wendel. 1983. Health care in America: A political perspective. In Cities and Sickness: Health Care in Urban America, A. L. Greer and S. Greer eds., 213–244. Beverly Hills: Sage.

Smith, Lee. 1988. The Battle Over Health Insurance. *Fortune* (September 26):145–150.

Sorkin, Alan L. 1975. *Health economics: An introduction.* Lexington, MA: Lexington Books.

Stokes, Louis. 1988a. Health care: A national crisis—A national priority. *Point of View* (Congressional Black Caucus Foundation) (Special Edition):14–15.

Stokes, Louis. 1988b. The health of black America. *Health Aims* 6:3–4.

Sullivan, Louis. 1978. The education of black health professionals. *Phylon* 38:225–235.

Sulvetta, Margaret B. and Katherine Swartz. 1986. *The uninsured and uncompensated Care* Washington, DC: National Health Policy Forum.

The CBC alternative: A budget with healthy priorities. *Point of View* (Congressional Black Caucus Foundation) (Spring 1987):22.

Tolbert, George P. 1977. Meeting the health needs of minorities and the poor. *Phylon* 38:225–235.

Treiger, Karen I. 1986. Preventing patient dumping: Sharpening the COBRA's fangs. *New York University Law Review* 61:1186–1223.

U.S. Bureau of the Census. 1985. *Statistical abstract of the United States: 1986.* Washington, DC: USGPO.

U.S. Congressional Budget Office. 1985. *Reducing poverty among children.* Washington, DC: USGPO.

U.S. Department of Health, Education and Welfare. 1971. *Toward a comprehensive health policy for the 1970s: A white paper.* Washington, DC: USGPO.

U.S. Department of Health and Human Services. 1985. *Report of the secretary's task force on Black and minority health, volume I, executive summary.* Washington, DC: USGPO.

U.S. Department of Health and Human Services, Public Health Service. 1986a. *Health: United States, 1986.* Washington, DC: USGPO.

U.S. Department of Health and Human Services, Public Health Service. 1986b. *Health status of the disadvantaged: Chartbook 1986.* Washington, DC: USGPO.

Windom, Robert E. 1989. From the Assistant Secretary of Health. *Journal of the American Medical Association* 261:196.

Wolfinger, Raymond. 1972. *The politics of progress.* Englewood Cliffs, NJ: Prentice-Hall.

Wyngaarden, James B. 1989. From the national institutes of health. *Journal of the American Medical Association* 261:200.

Yerby, Alonzo. 1966. The disadvantaged and health care. *American Journal of Public Health* 56:5–9.

Chapter 18

Politics, Health and the Elderly

Inventing the Next Century— The Age of Aging[1]

William P. Brandon

The subject of the biological, social and economic needs of elderly populations, their specification by the emerging profession of gerontology and the political expression of those needs partly overlaps but is also partly distinct from the mainstream of health politics. The distinctiveness stems in large part from the fact that historically health politics in the U. S. has been focused on the provision of acute medical services, whereas aging issues resist narrow definition.

What this essay will call the "aging-support" system incorporates major subdivisions of the health care system. Thus, long-term care and Medicare are leading topics in any review of health care subjects.

Yet the aging-support system includes many social services that are not usually regarded as health considerations when one thinks about the health care of younger groups. The principal legislation in the field, the Older Americans Act of 1965, makes coordination of services a primary goal. Although the aging-support system is far from perfect in integrating social and biomedical services, there is growing recognition of the interactions among such problems as social isolation, inadequate nutrition, depression and failures of "compliance" with medical prescriptions. The emphasis placed on integration and coordination in the aging-support system contrasts with our failure even to understand how such problems of younger groups as homelessness, drug addiction, AIDS and child abuse and neglect are interconnected.

The aging-support system also illustrates how our society continually generates systems and subsystems that define new realities for us. The health care system as we now know it evolved out of a confused and heterogeneous amalgam of direct and indirect services that were available

[1]The author wishes to thank Dr. George Greenberg of the Office of the Assistant Secretary for Planning and Evaluation of the Department of Health and Human Services and Dr. Emma Quartaro of Seton Hall University for their useful comments on an earlier draft of this chapter.

in the United States a century and a half ago. The emerging aging-support system has been generated within this century. Thus, there were no nursing homes, no public pension systems aside from veteran's benefits, few private pensions and little formal retirement as recently as seventy-five years ago. New structures are arising and ideas of aging are likely to change radically in the next quarter-century. In terms of its social definition and institutional evolution, the aging-support system is roughly where the acute medical care system was a hundred years ago.

The politics of aging involves three dimensions: societal understandings, institutional structures and policy issues. After a brief general explanation of what is meant by societal understandings or meanings, I shall outline the chief institutional structures that determine policy related to the elderly. An overview of salient policy issues will follow. The essay then will explore the issue of long-term care, the most important agenda item for the elderly in the first half of the 1990s. The conclusion will compare aging policy and mainstream health policy.

Societal Understanding

Nothing in biology or in other empirical observations determines the way that we think of life or its phases. At most, physical constraints provide limits within which develop the societal understandings that give meanings and structure the details in terms of which we live out our lives. Social and political structures like Social Security, private pensions, Medicare, nursing homes and retirement communities emerge from a particular society's ways of thinking about aging and convictions regarding appropriate or desirable activities, concerns and environments for the elderly. Over time, the structures in turn become givens that guide the evolution of understandings common to the whole society, promote coherence of the values implicit in those understandings and create an impression of inevitability and legitimacy around the empirical arrangements that stem from the structures. At this level of analysis it is difficult to disentangle "subjective" from "objective" realities, because one reinforces the other and changes reverberate

across these artificial distinctions (Winch 1958, 1970; Brandon 1982).

Several brief examples will help to clarify the thesis that how we think of aging—and hence its reality—is a social creation (Estes 1983). Perhaps the clearest example is the understanding of retirement as a natural phase of life. In North America and England during much of the nineteenth century, while the nature of work undertaken by elderly people might change as their physical powers waned, the idea of crossing a line in time or chronological age in which one stopped productive work altogether was not widely accepted (Quadagno 1984, 422–424, 436). Formal retirement depended upon the availability of pension schemes. Private pensions could become common only with the concentration of capital and profit produced by large-scale industrial enterprises. Industrialization reduced the heterogeneity of work that had allowed responsibilities in agriculture or traditional hand-manufacturing to be altered to accommodate failing physical strength, eyesight or mental ability (Kreps 1971, 40, 44). As late as 1940, when Social Security began paying benefits, about 40 percent of those sixty-five and over were "retired." By 1984 about 90 percent were "retired" (U.S. Bureau of the Census 1942, 1986).[2]

Another example of the relation between social meanings and institutional structures is the nursing home, a physical dwelling associated with a way of life. It is easy to forget that the Kerr-Mills Act of 1960 and Medicaid (1965) virtually created the nursing home industry in this country (Brasfield 1987). In contrast, some social welfare states like Sweden and the United Kingdom strive to keep elderly persons living in their own homes by providing home-care and other services and by de-emphasizing skilled nursing facilities (Zappolo and Sundstrom 1989; Johnson 1989; Jazwiecki and Schwab 1989). Consequently, individuals in those societies may not experience the same feelings of guilt or failure or run the risks of financial ruin that often attend

---

[2]These statistics are based on the assumption that data about labor force activity for those 65 and over can be used to infer retirement patterns. Respondents, mostly women, who reported in the 1940 survey that they were "engaged in home housework" were considered to be retired. This interpretation is necessary to be consistent with the 1940 data. Males 65 and over had a retirement rate of 16 percent in 1940.

decisions in the United States regarding the entry of an elderly person in long-term care institutions.

The "plasticity" that makes it possible for different societies to evolve different ways for the elderly to live is also illustrated by the formation of powerful groups in this country that articulate the political interests of the elderly. The U.S. began its universal social health insurance program, Medicare[3], by covering the elderly who receive Social Security. In contrast, other industrial nations began government health coverage for workers and expanded it to the rest of society. During the fifteen years of struggle to pass Medicare, proponents had to conceptualize retirees as a group who were uniquely needy, at least in regard to obtaining and paying for health care (Marmor 1973).[4] This campaign eventually established the legitimacy of demands that society be responsible for providing health care for the elderly. As we shall see in the section dealing with social structures, the effort to enact Medicare generated or strengthened many of the interest groups that institutionalize a view of politics based on age cohorts.

Because the parameters of health insurance were fixed by its initial circumstances, expansions of Medicare have mainly involved providing better protection for current beneficiaries rather than extending coverage to *additional* population groups. Even groups and institutions like the Gray Panthers and the Villers Foundation, which favor universal entitlement and explicitly reject the struggle of one age group against others, probably reinforce our society's tendency to organize aging-support issues around age-defined cohorts. Although the Gray Panthers and the Villers Foundation eschew " ageist" principles (Kuhn 1988; Gray Panthers 1987, 13; Villers Foundation 1986), the fact that those who respond to their call for "empowerment" are preponderantly over sixty or retirees suggests that in reality these organizations function by mobilizing subgroups of older Americans who otherwise might not become active on issues of aging-support. In contrast, the elderly in other industrial nations are not so organized as political or social pressure groups focused narrowly on aging-support issues. Rather, their elderly are commonly incorporated into broad-based and socially active labor and political structures.

The fact of social plasticity makes us at least collectively responsible for the condition of the elderly in our society. This consideration is especially important in regard to the future of aging in America. Pointing out that baby-boomers have focused attention on, and often altered social values when they were young, Betty Friedan (1983) asks why we should expect them to fall passively into accepted twentieth century patterns when they become old in the next century. The elderly will be far more numerous after 2015 than at any other time in U.S. history. Some research suggests that they may be healthier (Fries 1980, 1983; Manton 1982). As the first generation without *any* experience of the depression and as the beneficiaries of private pensions and Social Security that increases with the cost of living, they will be the most affluent cohort of elderly.

In his seminal *Centuries of Childhood,* the French historian Philippe Aries (1962, 22) wrote:

> It is as if, to every period of history, there corresponded a privileged age and a particular division of human life: 'youth' is the privileged age of the seventeenth century, childhood of the nineteenth, adolescence of the twentieth.
>
> The variations from one century to another bear witness to the naive interpretation which public opinion has given, in each and every period, of its demographic structure, when it could not always form an objective idea of it.

Is it far-fetched to ask whether the twenty-first century will be the century of old age and whether our generation will be the one that is privileged simultaneously to explore and to invent a new human experience?

---

[3]Social insurance, which is contrasted with means-tested welfare programs, involves universal entitlement of some easily recognized group.

[4]The image of the elderly as poor and frail, if not actually sick, remains the predominant image of the aged in America. Even professionals dealing with the elderly commonly intone the phrase "the elderly living on fixed incomes," even though the indexing of Social Security to the cost of living made the elderly the largest class of Americans who enjoy protection against the ravages of inflation for a significant proportion of their incomes.

Increasingly, however, advocates of the elderly want to change the stereotype of the aged as victims deserving of social help. Instead, diversity among the elderly is emphasized. At issue is whether the general population regards victims as autonomous individuals deserving of dignity and respect rather than pity and paternalism however charitable.

Institutional Structures

Much of what government does that affects the elderly is conducted by parts of the government that are not organized specifically to deal with the needs of the elderly. In these arenas advocates of the aging clash, bargain, or cooperate with other groups representing a multitude of interests in society. It is here, for example, that aging interest groups encounter the significant substantive lobbying efforts of the American Medical Association, hospital interests, employers concerned about the costs of retirement benefits, and unions. Over the long term the relative power of the elderly in relation to these other interests will depend on the ability of the elderly to mobilize and to work together.

Yet an aging-support policy system has recently been created. In part, the system's components that are entirely dedicated to elderly issues serve largely symbolic purposes; in part, they constitute administrative routines that are capable of reaching the elderly. The government structures established in Congress to respond to the needs of the elderly are a creation of the 1960s and early 1970s. The first Commissioner of Aging was not appointed until 1965. Interest groups representing the elderly were relatively weak as late as the first half of the 1970s (Pratt 1976). By 1980, however, voices were beginning to be raised expressing concern that the elderly might become an organized political force of staggering proportions (Samuelson 1978, 1987b; Ossofsky 1978).

The chief institutional features of the political landscape can usefully be divided into three categories: government entities, interest groups and private service institutions. Government entities, the public sector, includes government agencies like the Administration on Aging, Congressional committees and subcommittees, and programs. Programs like the Social Security program involve bureaucratic structures—the Social Security Administration—which administer the program and promote debate about related issues. For example, when Medicare was passed in 1965 after a fifteen year struggle, the Social Security Administration provided considerable information supporting the need for government-financed medical care for the elderly. As activi-

ties, programs are also the focus of political disagreements and controversy.

Interest groups, which are usually constituted as voluntary, not-for-profit corporations, are institutions that try to influence public entities. Like private institutions they also often provide significant services to their members. For many years the largest and therefore potentially the most powerful interest group—the American Association of Retired Persons (AARP)—served the information and insurance needs of a growing membership but was not very active in influencing federal or state government. It did not even work actively for Medicare in 1965 (Pratt 1976, 90-91).

Finally, private institutions are those not-for-profit non-governmental or for-profit institutions that provide services to the elderly. They range from nursing homes and home health agencies and adult day care centers to more informal social groups that are composed mainly of the elderly. Many of the interactions between private institutions and government involve government efforts to regulate the private sector. Consequently, private institutions commonly form interest groups designed to protect their own interests.

The pragmatic distinctions among governmental entities, interest groups and private institutions are useful in ordering the discussion that follows, but should not be pressed too far. Private institutions often attempt to influence government actions and interest groups receive significant revenue from the sale of services. Government entities are far from shy about trying to influence other government institutions or interest groups. Like AARP, some institutional structures may change over time in ways that require reclassification.

Government Entities

In the executive branch responsibility for government programs to aid the elderly is diffuse. Using 1978 data, Carol Estes counted at least eighty different federal programs benefitting the elderly directly or indirectly through "cash assistance, in-kind transfers or direct provision of goods and services" (Estes 1983, 77–82). These programs are scattered among six cabinet departments and seven independent agencies. Tax, regulatory or employment policies would add to the number of programs benefiting the elderly.

In 1978 the outspoken advocate for the elderly, Representative Claude Pepper (Dem., Fla), who chaired the House Select Committee on the Aging, and a correspondent for the *National Journal* disputed both the number and the value of programs that could be regarded as benefitting the elderly (Samuelson 1978, and 1978b; Ossofsky 1978). Their debate vividly demonstrates the difficulty even in defining what programs belong to the aging-support system. It also focused on the question whether the elderly receive a disproportionate share of the GNP in relation to their numbers or average economic status.

The confusion in determining the extent of Federal aid to the elderly arises in part from the fact that the federal government is largely organized by function rather than according to beneficiaries or "clientele" groups.[5] Income security and health programs are examples of functional organization. Thus, the Social Security Administration handles old age, survivor and disability insurance (OASDI) and the Supplemental Security Income program (SSI), which is a national means-tested program for low-income elderly, blind and the totally disabled. The Health Care Financing Administration (HCFA) is responsible for Medicare, which is an entitlement of the disabled on Social Security and renal dialysis patients in addition to the eligible elderly, and for Medicaid, the means-tested federal-state program to provide health care to qualifying poor persons without regard to age.

The Administration on Aging, which was established under the Older Americans Act of 1965 (PL 89–73), is more important as a symbol of national commitment than for its power as measured in money or staff. It is the apex of a diffuse, decentralized network that directs money to local government, specialized area aging agencies and states where allocation decisions are made among a list of approved types of activities. The Older Americans Act and its amendments can be considered as a prototypical New Federalism

program in which the federal government provides funds in broadly defined "block grants" which allow area agencies and state government to decide what programs to fund. Although permitted to deliver services themselves, they were primarily intended to promote and coordinate the services delivered by private institutions and other government entities, and their funding has never been sufficiently generous for them to become major providers of service.

Whereas the many programs under the Older Americans Act were decentralized from the early 1970s and federal control was relaxed even further under President Reagan's New Federalism, Congress largely frustrated the efforts of David Stockman, former Director of the Office of Management and Budget, to consolidate public health programs into block grants or to cap federal expenditures for Medicare and Medicaid. While successful in prohibiting changes in basic programmatic structures, liberals in Congress like Henry Waxman (Dem., Calif.), chair of the House Commerce Subcommittee on Health and Environment, had to accept sharp cuts in annual operating budgets for health during the Reagan years (Sorian 1989). Programs under the Older Americans Act did not fare any better.

The relevant Congressional committees also illustrate the distinction between government entities that demonstrate symbolic concern and those with substantive responsibility for programs. The House Committee on Ways and Means and its Health Subcommittee under Chairman Fortney (Pete) Stark (Dem., Calif.), and the Senate Finance Committee must approve any changes in Medicare. This prerogative results from the fact that the payroll deduction for Medicare is a tax and therefore is subject to the tax committees. Substantive health policies, such as those embodied in The Public Health Service Act and Medicaid, fall under the jurisdiction of the House Committee on Energy and Commerce and its Subcommittee on Health and Environment. In recent years, however, an accommodation has been reached to share jurisdiction over health matters between Commerce's Subcommittee on Health and the Environment and the Health Subcommittee of Ways and Means.

In the Senate issues that are generally addressed by Energy and Commerce in the House go to Labor and Human Resources, where Sena-

---

[5]The Departments of Agriculture, Commerce, Labor and the newly-created Department of Veterans' Affairs constitute exceptions to the generalization that federal programs are organized with reference to function rather then client group.

tor Edward Kennedy (Dem., Mass.) and David Durenberger (Rep., Minn.) play important roles. The bulk of *health* issues will be decided by these two committees and the two tax committees in each chamber; non-health matters of interest to the elderly are assigned to the appropriate Senate committee according to the nature of the program.

There are two important committees that deal exclusively with matters related to the elderly, but they are not responsible for initiating legislation. The House Select Committee on Aging and the Senate Special Committee on Aging have great freedom to investigate issues regarding the elderly and to hold oversight hearings. The late Claude Pepper built the House Select Committee into a particularly powerful source of information and advocacy.

Interest Groups

The Administration, Congress and organized groups representing interested parties largely determine federal policies relating to the aged. As late as 1969 Theodore Lowi could characterize the elderly as "unorganized and apathetic" and therefore powerless in the struggle to achieve Medicare (Lowi 1969, 64).

No one would describe the elderly in these terms in the 1980s in light of their importance in successfully opposing Administration proposals to cut Social Security benefits early in the Reagan presidency, in influencing the great Social Security compromise of 1983, and in the bargaining that led to the expansion of Medicare in 1988 to cover catastrophic health expenses.

There are four mass-membership organizations whose primary focus is the interests of the elderly—the American Association of Retired Persons/National Retired Teachers Association (AARP/NRTA, the National Association of Retired Federal Employees (NARFE), the National Council of Senior Citizens (NCSC), and the Gray Panthers. Only AARP and NARFE existed before 1960.

American Association of Retired Persons (AARP)

AARP, the largest of the organizations with 30 million members in 1988 (table 18-1), was founded as a retired teachers' association in 1947 and prospered from the sale of life and health insurance to the elderly. It only began vigorously to try to exercise political influence in 1970 over the issue of control of the 1971 White House Conference on Aging (Pratt 1976, 145–53).

National Association of Retired Federal Employees (NARFE)

NARFE began in 1921 with the initiation of the federal employee pension system; at the beginning of 1989 it had almost 500,000 members (Dennis Harrington, personal communication) (table 18-1). It helps members deal with their individual problems relating to federal benefits—case work—and monitors legislative action affecting members' interests. NARFE does not invest a great deal of energy on matters relating to broader issues of aging that are not directly related to the self-interest of its membership. For example, its major objective during bargaining leading up to the Social Security compromise of 1983 was to avoid the inclusion of federal workers in Social Security (Light 1985, 82–3).

National Council of Senior Citizens (NCSC)

The NCSC began as Senior Citizens for Kennedy in 1960 under union aegis (table 18-1). With additional aid from the Democratic National Committee the organization began to grow by developing local senior citizens clubs across the country. NCSC focused almost entirely on Medicare until that legislation was enacted (Pratt 1976, 88–89). It still focuses on income security and health issues. Its unity of purpose, grassroots foundations in about 4000 active local clubs, access to AFL-CIO lobbying resources and experience of coalition building made it a potent force in the debates about Social Security in the early 1980s. These advantages, according to Light (1985, 75–78), offset the difference in NCSC's 4 million members and AARP's 14 million in determining the relative effectiveness of the two most important senior citizens organizations on this important issue.

Organizational Characteristics of Selected Major Elderly-Focused Interest Groups

Interest Group[a]	Year Founded	Membership Mid 70s	Membership 88–89	Full-time Employees (Late 1988)	1987 Revenue (Millions)
AARP/NRTA	1947	9,000,000	30,000,000	1200	235.9
Gray Panthers	1970	N.A.	60,000[c] 10,000[d]	6[f]	0.7
GSA	1945	2000	6800	N.A.	1.8
NARFE	1921	182,000	500,000	90[g]	2.0
NCOA	1950	1900[b]	6500[e]	110	36.6
NCPSSM	1982	N.R.	5,000,000	55	30.0
NCSC	1961	3,000,000	N.A.	150–200	57.3[i]
Villers Foundations	1981	N.R.	N.R.	22[h]	2.0[i]

[a] N.R. = not relevant, N.A. = not available.
[b] In addition, 5,000 *Senior Citizen Centers* belonged to NCOA.
[c] At large members.
[d] In local networks.
[e] Center membership is not available.
[f] An additional 7 are part-time.
[g] At national headquarters
[h] Data from the *1983–1984–1985 Report*; dollar figure is the total value equal of grants awarded in 1985.
[i] Fiscal year July 1, 1987–June 30, 1988.

TABLE 18–1

SOURCES: *Personal communications from Robert DeFillippo (AARP), Jean Hopper (Gray Panthers), Linda Harootyan (GSA), Denis Harrington (NARFE), Sandra Adams (NCOA), Jack McDavitt (NCPSSM). Published materials: NCSC. Progress report: January 1989. Washington, D.C.: NCSC 1989; The Villers Foundation,* Report 1983, 1984, 1985.

Gray Panthers

The Gray Panthers, which were first organized in 1970, has a broad social justice agenda that transcends issues benefiting only the elderly (table 18–1). It also describes itself as an intergenerational group. In a signed editorial in its official newspaper *Network,* charismatic founder Maggie Kuhn (1988) proposed that the Gray Panthers should concentrate on organizing college campuses and urged local networks to have members of diverse ages. Yet despite this aspiration, the Gray Panthers are clearly focused on the task of consciousness raising, empowering and organizing of the elderly. The organization has 60,000 at-large members and 10,000 who are active in local grass-roots networks; the national budget is about $700,000 (Gray Panthers n.d.; Frances Humphreys, pers. com.) (table 18–1). Its imaginative lobbying and protest activities and network membership magnify its effectiveness beyond its numbers. However, its leadership is well aware of the fact that the Gray Panthers must enter into coalitions with larger organizations.

The political orientations of these organizations reflect their origins. NARFE aggressively pursues the narrow self-interest of its membership without regard to political orientation. Retirees from the professions who often held conservative views made up the bulk of AARP membership in its early years. The organization, which is now middle-of-the road, still seems reluctant to risk offending members, many of whom are more attracted by the services and information that it offers than by its ideological commitment. In contrast, the NCSC reflects the mainstream liberal outlook of the large proportion of its members who are former union members and of its leadership, which is predominantly composed of retired labor leaders. The Gray Panthers champion both the causes and methods of the 1960s. Thus its newspaper agitates for racial equality, anti-ageism, peace and universal health care through a national health service (or "socialized medicine").

In addition to the elderly mass-membership groups, two other organizations merit mention: the National Council on Aging (NCOA) and the American Gerontological Society, the major professional organization.

National Council On the Aging (NCOA)

The NCOA, which was founded in 1950, describes itself as "the nation's leading resources center in the field of aging" (NCOA n.d.); its organizational and individual members are involved in all facets of the aging network. It engages in advocacy on national and state levels and also tests programs. For example, NCOA takes credit for developing "Meals on Wheels" into a national program. Its extensive programs require it to have a large annual budget, which in both 1986 and 1987 amounted to about 37 million dollars (NCOA, 1988, xviii) (table 18–1). Many senior centers are affiliated with NCOA and provide some of its membership, but professionals and organizations that provide services to the elderly constitute much of its constituency.

Gerontological Society of America (GSA)

The GSA was founded in 1945 "to promote the scientific study of aging, to encourage exchanges among researchers and practitioners . . . and to foster the use of gerontological research in forming public policy" (Gerontological Society 1987). It engages in research projects and "education" to inform government officials and interest groups about gerontological issues (Gerontological Society 1987, 1, 2). In some respects, then, it resembles an organization like the American Public Health Association (APHA), but its lobbying and advocacy efforts are not yet as large as APHA's. One measure of the increasing importance of gerontology and aging-support issues is the tripling of its membership from about 2000 members in the mid-1970s (Pratt 1976, 87) to about 6800 at the beginning of 1989 (Linda Harootyan, pers. com.) (table 18–1).

This section has developed several themes. The emergence of an increasingly distinct aging-support system began with the development of government civil service pensions and social security and became increasingly differentiated from other medical and social service programs during the fifteen year campaign that followed the decision in 1951 to pursue social health insurance only for the elderly (Marmor 1973, 13–15). Nonetheless, federal agencies and committees charged with the most important substantive decision-making generally combine responsibility for aging-support issues with other domestic policy issues. Different executive and legislative entities—the Administration on Aging, the House Select Committee on Aging and the Senate Special Committee—embody the important symbolic dimension which aging issues now demand (Edelman 1964). The interest groups that focus on the elderly have become increasingly strong in the last twenty years. They span a wide range of political outlooks and use diverse methods.

As the numbers of elderly grow, such writers as Phillip Longman (1987) fear that they will become politically invincible. (See also Feldstein 1988, 199–204.) The elderly vote in much greater percentages than any other age group. Yet gerontologist Robert H. Binstock (1989) argues that the very diversity of the elderly serves to keep them from forming an effective voting block: "A person who celebrates an older birthday does not suddenly change a lifetime of political attachment, self- and group identities and specific economic and social interests."

It is now time to examine how such important aging issues as income security, catastrophic illness insurance and long-term care are addressed through the interaction of government structures, interest groups and private institutions.

Three Policy Issues

Sometimes political elites and the average voter fail to discern the same broad fundamental issues, but in the arena of aging policy they currently identify the same issues. Interviews of Washington insiders conducted by the author in 1988 revealed that the three leading areas of political concern around aging issues are health care, long-term care and income security.[6] A Gallup poll of voters of all ages in June 1988, showed that "health care, retirement and long-

term care" were the most important family policy issues in the presidential campaign (American Association of Retired Persons 1988).[7] Although the Washington insiders and ordinary voters agree in a generic ranking of the issues, the politics of agenda-building (Cobb and Elder 1972) suggests that elites rather than the grass roots will largely provide the substantive definition of specific issues. Thus, the task of this section is to discuss briefly income security, which constitutes the context of discussions about the politics of aging, to outline some of the chief political and policy issues connected with providing and financing acute health care for the elderly—particularly catastrophic coverage—and to focus in more detail on long-term care.

Income Security

The major income transfer program benefitting the elderly and the cornerstone of retirement income is Social Security. It is the single most important government program in keeping large numbers of citizens out of poverty (Pear 1988; U.S. Bureau of the Census 1988). Since 1972, Social Security has been indexed so that it rises with increases in the cost of living. Even in the 1980s the poverty rate among the elderly declined while poverty in the general population increased.[8]

The imbalance in the Social Security Trust Funds during the 1970s and early 1980s was a significant threat to the financial security of the elderly. One of the major achievements of the 1980s was the eleventh-hour cooperation be-

---

[6]The author interviewed staff employed by the Congressional Research Service of the Library of Congress, a Republican Senator who is active on health issues, the majority side of the House Ways and Means Committee, the Executive Office of the President, AARP, and the Villers Foundation. The author greatly appreciates the cooperation shown him by his informants.

[7]Voters of all ages show considerable concern about issues affecting the elderly, but the elderly do not demonstrate a corresponding concern for issues that transcend the interest of their age cohort. The four issues about which more than 60 percent of all respondents said they were "very concerned" were health care costs, retirement income, the cost of federal taxes and long-term care. The AARP/Gallup survey shows that the elderly focus on "their" issues. Respondents sixty-five and over did not register a 60 percent "very concerned" about any other family issue, nor did 60 percent of them agree that federal taxes were a problem (American Association of Retired Persons 1988).

[8]The poverty rate of the elderly declined to 12.4 percent in 1987 from 15.3 percent in 1980, while the poverty rate of the general population increased to 13.6 percent in 1987 from 13 percent in 1980 (Martin Tolchin quoted in Iglehart 1989, 334).

tween Congress, the President and major private interests that resulted in returning Social Security to a sound financial basis.

The process by which that agreement was reached is important. It involved establishing the National Commission on Social Security Reform (which was also known as the Greenspan Commission after its chairman Alan Greenspan). This bipartisan commission and others like it served during the Reagan Administration as a way for the outspoken conservative President to ease away from his seemingly implacable public opposition to the Democratic Congress without angering supporters on the political right. On an issue as controversial as Social Security, the myth of a sacred compromise resulting from secret negotiations that needed to be enacted as a package to succeed also served to protect members of Congress from Social Security beneficiaries upset about the postponement of a cost-of-living-allowance (COLA), from federal employees and retirees who were angered about including new civil servants in Social Security; and from other disgruntled interests (Light 1985, 198–203). Although the U. S. National Commission on Social Security Reform (1983) did useful work, it was behind-the-scenes negotiations between David Stockman and former Social Security Commissioner Robert Ball that produced the compromise (Light 1985; Moynihan 1988).

The outcome proved to be successful. Before the package passed the House (282–148) and the Senate (88–11), Social Security reserves were declining rapidly. The compromise, which accelerated scheduled tax increases in the short-term and reduced benefits (which principally have long-term effects), coupled with the end of the economic recession of 1982–83 will make Social Security financially sound well into the next century.[9] The one remaining danger is that the federal government will be tempted to use burgeoning Social Security surpluses to reduce the deficit or for other purposes.

Acute Health Care

In contrast to the effective action on Social Security, the Medicare Part A Trust Fund remains in potential financial peril. Part A of Medicare, which covers inpatient hospital care and other related care of about 30 million persons sixty-five and over and 3 million younger disabled persons, depends on contributions from payroll taxes. In the mid-1980s it appeared that the Trust Fund would be in deficit by the early 1990s. However, a generally healthy economy with decreasing unemployment and efforts to contain Medicare costs including the Prospective Payment System (PPS) keep extending the projected date when the Trust Fund will go into deficit.[10] Under the most likely assumptions about income and costs, the *1988 Annual Report* of the Medicare Trustees projects that the Medicare Trust Fund will be "completely exhausted shortly after the turn of the century" (Federal Hospital Insurance Trust Fund Board of Trustees 1988, 2, 42, 85, 92; Russell and Manning 1989; Sloan, Morrisey and Valvona 1988).

In the early 1990s, however, political attention is likely to be focused on Medicare Part B, which pays for physicians services, outpatient hospital services and other medical expenses of both those aged sixty-five and over and of those who are long- term disabled. From 1983 to 1987 Part B expenditures doubled, a growth rate that was "40 percent faster than the economy as a whole" (Federal Supplementary Medical Insurance Trust Fund Board of Trustees 1988, 2, 38). Congress established the Physician Payment Review Commission to recommend sweeping changes in physician payment and directed the Health Care Financing Administration to fund a study of the resource-based relative value scale by Dr. William Hsiao at Harvard University (Hsiao et al. 1988; Hsiao et al. 1988b). The Resulting changes

---

[9]The 1988 Report of the Social Security Board of Trustees calculates that under the most likely intermediate assumptions (IIB) the combined Trust Funds will accumulate staggering reserves up until 2015 and will decline until the assets and current income are less than benefits in 2048 (Federal OASI and DI Trust Fund Board of Trustees 1988, 1, 141–2). Obviously, sixty years provides plenty of time to take timely action to avoid deficits.

[10]PPS, which was introduced in 1983, pays hospitals set fees for types of cases determined by the Diagnosis-Related Group (DRG) under which a case falls. (There is still some modification to allow for hospital-specific characteristics.) This "prospective" system replaced cost-based retrospective reimbursement. Hospitals therefore know in advance how much they will receive for a given case. If they can reduce the costs of treating a patient—for example, by discharging the patient earlier than is the average for patients in the DRG—then the hospital can keep the savings that it generates.

in part B enacted in 1989 are likely to be as important for physician reimbursement as the implementation of PPS for hospital payment in the early 1980s (Sorian 1989b).

In light of increasing Medicare costs, threatening Trust Fund bankruptcy and an intractable overall federal deficit, it is logical to ask why would President Reagan propose to enhance Medicare coverage by adding catastrophic protection. In particular, why would a Republican administration, which vociferously opposed the expansion of federal "entitlement" programs like Medicare, propose a significant addition? Moreover, anyone with Washington experience could have predicted that Congress would likely accept the general proposal but make it more generous. In fact, Congress changed the Administration bill by reducing the amount that individuals would have to pay before qualifying for catastrophic provisions, added outpatient prescription coverage, and altered the proposed financing to make it progressive. (Funding was "progressive" because the more affluent elderly, i.e., the 40 percent with the highest incomes, would partially subsidize average and low income elderly by paying more of the program costs.) Even the timing was unusual: new legislative initiatives are not common in the waning years of the second term of an administration.

Part of the explanation for passage of this legislation is that for the first time the full cost of an entitlement program for the elderly would be paid by the beneficiaries rather than current workers or taxpayers. Thus, those who supported the bill could, in the jargon of the time, claim that it was "budget neutral." Because relatively few beneficiaries would have bills that are large enough to trigger benefits for catastrophic costs, the bill's price was fairly cheap. It was estimated that the entire costs for the five year phase-in period (1989–93) would only amount to 30.8 billion (Iglehart 1989, 330).

Although the government structures and interest groups described earlier participated actively in efforts to pass or defeat the catastrophic bill, the politics of its initiation is an interesting lesson in the role of individuals and chance in political developments. Dr. Otis Bowen was appointed as Reagan's last Secretary of Health and Human Resources at the end of 1985. He brought at least two qualifications to the job. As a former governor of Indiana he had independent political standing. The other advantage was that he had recently completed work as chair of a Federal advisory committee studying Medicare that had explored the possibility of extending Medicare to cover financially catastrophic medical events. Thus, he came to Washington with an issue already selected and knowledge of some HHS civil servants who would help him accomplish his objective (Pear 1987). At about the same time, a reporter caught President Reagan unprepared when she asked what could be done about the plight of the ill elderly at one of his rare news conferences. The President's answer promised some sort of action. Shortly thereafter, brief mention in the State of the Union message for 1986 also indicated that some action on catastrophic medical costs would ensue. Dr. Bowen and the HHS civil servants exploited this invitation by producing massive studies on the nature of the problem and what to do about it (U.S. DHHS 1986; U.S. DHHS, Office of the Assistant Secretary for Planning and Evaluation n.d.; U.S. DHHS, Technical Work Group on Private Financing of Long-Term Care for the Elderly 1986). The elderly interest groups began to regard an extension of Medicare acute care to cover acute catastrophic illness costs as the only possible expansion of the program. Reluctantly AARP accepted beneficiary financing.

Dr. Bowen encountered some of his toughest battles in getting White House permission to present an administration bill. The media attention received by his Department's efforts and the public positions of the President provided Dr. Bowen with the leverage he needed to defeat the negative voices of such White House staff as James C. Miller, Director of the Office of Management and Budget, and such personal friends of Reagan as Attorney General Edwin Meese. The political need to counter an impression that the Administration opposed programs for the elderly was also undoubtedly an important consideration (Pear 1987; Iglehart 1989; Rovner 1988b; Congressional Quarterly Almanac 1988).

Interest group lobbying both for and against the bill was most evident during the Congressional deliberations. AARP was instrumental in securing the support of the then newly-selected Democratic Speaker James Wright (Dem., Tex), who needed a chance to show his commitment to liberal "Democratic" causes. He joined liberals like Stark, Waxman and Pepper, who wished to use the administration's initiative to achieve a significant expansion of Medicare coverage. The drug benefit was selected as the new program element to be added to Medicare, although Congressman Pepper tried to use the bill as a vehicle for the expansion of long-term home care. Active support for the measure was also provided by NCSC (Iglehart 1989; Rovner 1988b; Congressional Quarterly Almanac 1988).

Once the proposal had survived its White House opponents perhaps the strongest opposition came from commercial health insurers, especially Mutual of Omaha, and the brand-name pharmaceutical companies and their trade association. The insurers wished to avoid losing any business in selling supplementary Medicare policies (the so-called "Medigap" policies) and the name-brand drug producers feared that the new drug benefit would bring increased government regulation. The drug companies were so opposed to the bill that they carried the battle outside of Washington by trying to convince elderly citizens that the drug benefit was not in their best interest. Going outside of the Washington beltway to grass-roots America was a risky lobbying tactic, which may actually have hurt the Pharmaceutical Manufacturers Association. It irritated some legislators, threatened AARP, and even failed to win the support of several major drug manufacturers (Iglehart 1989; Rovner 1988b; Congressional Quarterly Almanac 1988).

Despite the advantages to Medicare patients of enhanced catastrophic coverage, the bill once enacted engendered major criticism on several counts. First, the new catastrophic coverage would pay only the fees that Medicare deemed appropriate. Because many physicians set fees higher than the Medicare fee schedule (or "balance bill" patients), many patients qualifying for catastrophic coverage still faced significant out-of-pocket payments.

Second, the Catastrophic Coverage Act did little about the most common catastrophe among the aged—the need for extensive nursing home care. Critics regarded the legislation as, at best, clearing the decks for the struggle to provide genuine security to the nation's elderly (Brandon 1989; Rovner 1988 and 1988b).

A third and more politically telling criticism

came from a segment of the elderly themselves. The immediate effect of the passage of the Act was to anger many of the more affluent elderly, who would have to pay up to a maximum of $800 ($1600 for a couple) in income-related premiums in 1989.[11] They complained that they had been singled out for a discriminatory tax increase. What was called an "income-related premium" looked remarkably like a tax: it was compulsory for those sixty-five and over and most Medicare beneficiaries would have paid it with their income taxes. Flat premiums that all beneficiaries must pay (such as the $4 per month that all beneficiaries would have to pay for Catastrophic and the Medicare Part B premium) are more acceptable to upper-income elderly, for they look like the "user fees" that became widespread substitutes for increased tax rates in the 1980s.

The significance of the issue is far reaching. Even financial participation in the form of fixed premiums is uncommon in aging support programs.[12] In Medicare, only Part B, which is voluntary insurance, requires the elderly to contribute anything. Because federal general revenues pay three-quarters of the costs, Supplemental Medical Insurance is financially so attractive that it has become almost universal. All other Social Security and medical programs are financed by taxing workers, employers or in the case of Medicaid, the general public.

The attack on the payment scheme was initiated by grass-roots opposition that sprang up in a number of states. It probably began in Nevada where it was led by a sixty-four year-old retired airline pilot. The National Committee to Preserve Social Security and Medicare (NCPSSM), a dissident organization headed by James Roosevelt which claims 5 million members, capitalized on the issue (table 18). NCPSSM was joined by NARFE. In response, AARP embarked on an en-

[11]The maximum annual income-related premium was to rise to $1,050 in 1993. Only 10 percent of beneficiaries have the taxable incomes of $45,000 (or $90,000 married, filing jointly) that would have required them to pay the maximum in 1993. Sixty percent would have paid nothing more than the monthly $4 increase in Part B premiums that are withheld from Social Security benefit checks (Firshein 1989; Rovner 1988).

[12]An exception to the generalization is the provision of the Social Security compromise of 1983 that began taxing half of Social Security benefits as income for those with incomes above $25,000 (or $32,000 married, filing jointly). The income tax, of course, is a progressive tax.

ergetic campaign to explain the advantages of the new legislation to its members. Some in Congress admitted that they had failed to explain the legislation and its financing adequately and belatedly began trying to educate the public (Firshein 1989; Iglehart 1989). The *New York Times* (1989) entered the dispute with an editorial entitled "Fair is Fair for Medicare" that observed:

> It's understandable that people accustomed to subsidized health care will complain when they must pay something for new benefits. But that's no reason for the rest of us, now paying heavy payroll taxes to support the subsidy, to be misled.

The affluent elderly and their supporters, however, were successful in getting Congress to repeal the Catastrophic Coverage Act less than a year after it took effect. But in doing so, they paradoxically may have made further expansion of Medicare almost impossible. For increases in payroll tax rates and the base salary on which they are levied are likely to generate resistance. Thus, any expansion of Medicare, whether for catastrophic or long-term care, will require beneficiaries to pay a large proportion of the bill, and, if they are unwilling to do so, such expansion is highly unlikely.

Long-Term Care

The most vexing health problem for the elderly is long-term care. There are many dimensions to this problem:

1. The numbers of elderly will rise dramatically in the next century to about 22 percent of the population (or 66 million people 65 and over (Berke 1989).
2. Increasing longevity means that there will be more of the "old-old" who generate the greatest need for long-term care.
3. Individuals find that direct financing or insurance against future long-term care needs is the most difficult health finance problem.
4. There is a chronic shortage of available long-term care services in most parts of the country.
5. Long-term care commonly requires both so-

cial services and health care, which have traditionally been separated in the U.S. to the detriment of each and the frustration of those assigned to coordinate them.

The problems of long-term care are increasingly becoming political issues.

The Anatomy of Long-Term Care Problems

The politicization of long-term care is resulting in an overly narrow focus on finance. Many of the underlying problems faced by patients and their families are not fundamentally financing issues, but instead are questions regarding the organization and delivery of care. The consequence of the disjunction between private problems and public issues is that the political resolutions of public issues, when finally generated, are likely to leave many citizens dissatisfied. Some of the problems of organizing and delivering long-term care are even likely to be exacerbated by attempts to force misguided solutions that are determined by the alignment of political forces.

In today's climate the responsible public servant begins by comparing institutional costs with the cost of those home expenses that it is reasonable to consider reimbursing. The problem has become operationalized by asking whether institutional care (for example in nursing facilities) or home- or community-based long-term care is likely to save more money. The conventional wisdom used to be that it is cheaper to care for all but the most impaired patients in their homes. However, a number of careful studies using control groups, often along with random assignment and multi- variate statistical techniques, show the counter-intuitive conclusion that the home- and community-based care provided in such studies does not save money that would otherwise have been spent for institutional care (Weissert, Cready, and Pawelak 1988; Rivlin and Wiener 1988, 190–202).

Quiet concern has also been raised about the possibility that providing long-term home care will inadvertently *monetize* home care; that is that paid care will slowly drive out unpaid care. Paying for services that family and friends have been supplying outside of market arrangements inevitably leads to increasing dependence on paid care and rising public and private costs.

Moreover, as Titmus' classic *Gift Relationship* (1971) suggests, quality may be lower when services are bought and sold rather than freely given. Although Riven and Wiener (1988, 197, 202) find an increase in paid service associated with a small decrease in unpaid voluntary caregiving, they discount its significance.

The non-political delivery question that patients and their families want someone to ask is whether a patient's health status, quality of life, or subjective satisfaction is typically greater when home- or community-based care permits patients to remain at home. Evidence in thirty-one studies suggest that mortality is little affected and indices of physical functioning registered mixed results but nothing startling. The most positive findings in favor of home- and community- based care were in the broad category of psychosocial outcomes. Within this category, however, studies did register a decline in the functioning of informal social supports, which may be the result of introducing paid services in the home. "Increased life satisfaction appears to be a relatively consistent benefit of community care. Caregivers and patients who use community care are more satisfied" (Weissert, Cready, and Pawelak 1988, 347–366). This observation leads health care researchers to question whether saving money ought to be the *sine qua non* for offering support for home- and community-based services (Weissert, Cready, and Pawelak 1988, 367; Rivlin and Wiener 1988, 198–9).

Gerontologists and health services researchers who focus on the delivery of services to the elderly must deal with a vast number of unsolved problems and unanswered questions. For example, there are problems faced by mentally and physically impaired elderly living alone, such as the possibility of accidents or fire, the likelihood of social isolation, and difficulties in assuring nutritious and palatable nourishment. These problems must be balanced against the loss of self-esteem or even clinical depression that may result from the loss of independence due to long-term institutionalization, very real problems with the quality of care—including nutrition—in nursing homes and intermediate care facilities, etc. Such decisions have to be made for each case in light of personal characteristics and the availability—or, too often, the lack of availability—of

home and community services in a specific patient's community.

This broad-scaled characterization of the kinds of problems facing service providers suggests the countless issues that face professionals in the aging-support system. Because this chapter is an essay on the *politics* of aging, it can only nod at the kinds of problems that are difficult to translate adequately into the political discourse currently used to settle society's public business.

The common ground on which the problem definitions discerned by health workers and the formulation of public issues should focus is the organization and delivery of care. Both the concerned caregiver and the public servant want to give the elderly citizen what he or she wants so long as its bad effects including high costs are minimized. Although costs must be considered, they should not be the only criterion.

The reality, however, is that so long as budget problems are the principal focus in Washington and the state capitals, it will be difficult for politicians to define long-term care needs as more than problems in health care finance. Some grandstanding or symbolic gestures may obscure this fact, but the underlying focus on the financial definition seems unchangeable. Thus, it is necessary to conclude this section by examining the options that face the federal government as it comes under increasing pressure to take some action to increase its financing of long-term care.

Three Options for Long-Term Care

There are three broad options for financing long-term care services.[13] While each comes with implications for the organization of care and therefore for the delivery of services, our discussion will be restricted chiefly to the financial implications of each alternative.

Medicaid as National Nursing Home Insurance. Continuing the current system in which Medicaid pays for more than 40 percent of the cost of nursing home care is always possible. Since relatively few elderly qualify as "poor" by official income criteria, most of those for whom government ultimately pays have exhausted their private re-

---

[13]This section draws on Brandon 1989.

sources—called "spending down"—before receiving Medicaid assistance. Although the Catastrophic Protection Act had sought to ease some of the rules that forced "spousal impoverishment" (Iglehart 1989; Rovner 1988), elderly individuals and couples who live independent and economically productive lives still often have to turn to means-tested welfare to pay for long-term care in their final years. Medicaid, which was initially regarded as serving the large group of mothers and children receiving Aid to Families with Dependent Children (AFDC), has developed into a perverse kind of national nursing home health insurance program that covers elderly Americans after they pay a gigantic and variable deductible amounting to their life savings.

There are some steps that could be taken to ameliorate the current system. An obvious development is to liberalize the qualifications necessary for the elderly to qualify for Medicaid (Rivlin and Wiener 1988, 203–9). Another suggestion is the Reverse Annuity Mortgage (RAM), a form of home equity conversion that allows an elderly homeowner to tap the heretofore non-liquid assets represented by the family home. Under this arrangement banks or other financial institutions pay monthly fixed amounts to elderly residents in return for ownership of the real estate when the aged person dies. The best evidence is that making available assets that are currently non-liquid can help some individuals cope with long-term care costs, but does not constitute a systematic solution (Rivlin and Wiener 1988, 123–145).

Pauperization caused entirely by the bad luck of needing extended long-term care seems cruel and unnecessary. This belief, the fact that long-term care is the most common financial catastrophe encountered by the elderly, and the focus on long-term care by AARP and the Villers Foundation during the 1988 Presidential primaries has caused long-term care to join the problem of controlling physician payments at the top of the nation's health agenda. Long-term care is relatively rare: only 5 percent of those sixty-five and over are in nursing homes at any one time. Yet it is so expensive at an average of about $25,000 a year that few retirees have enough liquid resources to pay for extended periods of long-term care. This distribution of risks (relatively low) and

costs (high) are the sort that invite the development of insurance to guard against the financial consequences of malign events.

Private Long-Term Care Insurance. Private insurance is now sold to protect individuals against the financial consequences of long-term care. Despite much publicity about the growth of a private market for long-term care insurance and enthusiastic encouragement from the Reagan administration, there are good reasons why only about 425,000 policies were in force in April, 1987 (U.S., DHHS, Task Force on Long-Term Health Care Policies 1987, 72–74). Unless one begins to pay for insurance well before retirement, when the possibility of needing expensive long-term care becomes apparent, premiums are too expensive for the individual to purchase. Private insurance companies are also not eager to promise service benefits or indemnity benefits that are indexed for inflation, because the future incidence and costs of long-term care defy accurate prediction. Private insurance companies, of course, are required to have reserves set aside against future claims.

Under the most optimistic assumptions about adequate supply and full information, Rivlin and Wiener (1988, 73–78) estimate that between 25 percent and 64 percent of the population in the critical years 2016 to 2020 will be able to afford private long- term care insurance. The range in percentages depends on the quality of the insurance product, which in turn determines its price. Those policies that were affordable to as many as half of the population offered no more than one year of nursing home coverage or required purchase early in the insured's working career.

Social Insurance. Social insurance would provide a way to avoid the problems of predicting future demand and costs and determining adequate reserve requirements. Social Security and Medicare Part A are examples of social insurance. Compulsory public long-term care insurance would avoid the problem of adverse selection, because everyone within a given group would have to participate. The difficulty of calculating reserves and predicting future costs and demand do not arise, because social insurance can use each year's income to pay obligations as they arise. Federal taxing power guarantees that government promises will be kept.

Both social insurance and private insurance might lead to an expansion of demand and price increases. Even public comprehensive coverage of long-term institutional care at its current costs would strain the federal government. Although nursing home costs are *less* than 10 per cent of national health expenditures, this amounts to almost 40 billion dollars per year. At the time of this writing legislative proposals on nursing home care were being developed by Senator George Mitchell (Dem., Maine) Senator Kennedy and retired Social Security Commissioner Robert Ball. Each claimed his legislation would cost about $18 billion in 1988 dollars. Yet none of the proposals—expensive as they were—were comprehensive. Mitchell proposed to cover care after individuals or their insurance had paid for the first two years. Kennedy wanted to cover the first half-year of nursing home care with a publicly financed program and then pool taxes and beneficiary premiums to cover the costs of longer stays. Ball agreed with Kennedy's focus on the early months of nursing home care. He believed that the government should try to preserve those patients' assets because a significant proportion of them would recover sufficiently to return to their homes. He also proposed covering longer stays for those with a spouse living in the community on the grounds that avoiding "spousal impoverishment" is appropriate public policy. In contrast, he believes that protecting the assets of single individuals faced with the need for extended long-term care is an interest of those who will inherit the assets rather than a public priority (Kosterlitz 1988).

Informed opinion suggests that there is an understanding in Congress about acceptable federal revenue sources that could be used to finance coverage of long-term care. One idea that is popular in Congress is to remove the maximum on the tax base for Medicare or Social Security (currently set at $45,000). If the cap were removed, the extra revenue from affluent workers could be used to pay for long-term care. Increasing the estate tax, which is very low, and the perennially favorite "sin taxes" on cigarettes and liquor are identifiable additional revenue sources (Kosterlitz 1988). The elderly who will benefit from any new protection can also expect to contribute.

Coming Choices and Lessons from the Past

The principal message of this chapter is that the experience of aging in America for the indefinite future is going to be determined by choices made in the next few years. Some sophistication is required to understand how these important choices are likely to be made. The history of the acute medical care system suggests that many will be implicit or even inadvertent, rather than the outcome of formal decision-making processes. Such societal choices are no less the measure of a civilization than its explicit decisions. (Oakeshott 1962, 123 et seq.)

This essay has emphasized the relatively recent emergence of a definable aging-support system providing income, social services (including transportation) and health care. In keeping with the political focus of this book, the chapter provided considerable detail about the relevant public structures and those private interests that have developed to support and influence them.

Yet much of the future aging-support system is likely to remain in the private sector, as the long-term care system has an even higher ratio of proprietary institutions to nonprofit and public institutions than the hospital system (Donabedian, et al. 1986, 230, 278–79).

However, neither the private role in financing long-term care nor the mix of nursing homes, home-based or community-based delivery modes are yet definitively fixed. As Medicaid financing of nursing home care becomes less acceptable to increasingly affluent elderly and as the demand for, and availability of, home care increases, pressure will increase for changes in funding. At issue are fundamental choices that will affect the structure of living, dying and illness in the next century. Also implicit in the decision to finance long-term care through either public or putatively private means is a choice involving the ideal of one-class of care for all and the potential for separate levels of care for the affluent and for those who have to pauperize themselves before receiving government-funded care.

Three Lessons

The mixed public-private nature of the acute health care system in the U.S. may well be replicated in the aging-support system that is emerging. The evolution of the health care system provides three useful lessons for the choices that must be made about the aging support in the next decade or two.

- Although Medicare and Medicaid have provided massive amounts of funding for acute health care, the original legislation contained a self-denying ordinance which promised that nothing in the Act would affect the practice of medicine.

The self-denying clauses of Titles XVIII and XIX contradict the substance of the Act. It is impossible to infuse large amounts of new revenues into a system without affecting practices. The announced intent not to interfere with established private arrangements merely encouraged providers to use the new resources to intensify the trends toward high technology, hospital-based specialty care that were already in vogue. Faced with what by the standards of the late 1960s were unacceptable cost increases, the federal government soon began to impose regulations that were designed to control costs.

Two considerations make such massive infusions of money and subsequent cost-containment regulation unsatisfactory. Because regulation is a reaction to developments in the private sector, it is inevitably one step behind the evolution of the system. Both interventions are typically financial in nature or ultimate intent and therefore do not usually deal directly with the problems and bottlenecks of the organization and delivery of health services.

Focusing on financial arrangements while attempting to deny the need for rational reform and expansion of the organization of services would be a disaster for the aging-support system. Any significant new federal action to cover long-term care is essentially a promise of access to covered services. Yet long-term care is less established and less uniform than the hospitals and other services that made up the acute medical care system in 1965. While area aging agencies do some planning for social services, few proactive community planning systems insure that an appropriate mix of long-term care services is available in communities where they are needed (Ford and Burns 1987). Such rational planning is

necessary to make long-term care services readily available.

- Medicare gave a large role as government paymasters to private insurance carriers and Blue Cross-Blue Shield plans (which were incorporated as not-for-profits).

At least three consequences of incorporating private insurance companies into government reimbursement schemes should be noted. The role of Blue Cross and other private carriers in Medicare facilitates efforts to market their private "Medigap" supplementary policies. Local and regional variation in Medicare operational definitions and procedures resulting from the participation of numerous private carriers and fiscal intermediaries has hindered the development of uniformity in what is supposed to be a national program. In addition, use of local insurance data as the basis for calculating Medicare reimbursement for physicians' services has frozen in place a system with wide and often inequitable geographical variation in what Medicare pays doctors. This "usual, customary and reasonable" reimbursement (UCR) has been widely blamed for discouraging physicians from entering primary care specialties and from practicing in rural or economically underdeveloped areas of the country.

At present the insurance companies do not have a large stake in the aging-support system (aside from life insurance). The Medicare experience suggests that the best way to achieve a national system that would reorganize the delivery of long-term care is to enter the field before the insurance companies develop a major stake in providing or reimbursing services for the elderly. Providing social insurance for long-term care would require a planned, comprehensive system with checks and balances to assure both cost-control and quality of care. Paradoxically, such a system will be easier to build in the near future than during the crisis years of the early twenty-first century, when the demographic facts will make it too expensive.

- Programs to establish neighborhood health centers and HMOs constitute two notable federal attempts to change the way medicine is practiced in the U.S.

In at least these two instances the federal government was "proactive" rather than reactive. The neighborhood health center movement attempted to institutionalize the ideology of comprehensive health services during Johnson's War on Poverty in the 1960s and early 1970s (Brandon 1977; Sardell 1988). The second effort occurred when Congress and the Executive agreed to promote health maintenance organizations to encourage efficiency and equity in health care delivery and to reap savings (Brown 1983; Brandon 1980). Both programs had to be sold as panaceas in order to secure sufficient support. Although not achieving all of their ambitious goals, these programs are noteworthy examples that show that the federal government can foster alternative modes of medical practice.

Positive organizational change cannot be motivated entirely by fiscal considerations (although cost-containment was an important consideration in the federal support for HMOs). The federal government in the 1960s was not constrained by a mammoth budget deficit. Financial concerns at that time were often expressed in terms of total health care costs rather than the current narrow focus on government's *portion* of the bill. Cost-shifting involving private payers was a much greater government concern in the 1960s and 1970s than in the 1980s.

The current narrow focus on balancing the federal budget is incompatible with any systematic enlargement of the government's responsibility for the aging-support system. Services cannot be significantly expanded and access increased without increasing expenditures. Thus, the availability of resources for the aging-support system ultimately depends on the performance of the economy and societal decisions about where to spend any additional resources.

This overview of the acute medical care system and its implications for the aging-support system suggest the continuing validity of Saward's law that "if form follows function, function follows funding." When the late Ernest Saward enunciated his half-facetious "law," government was still able to direct significant amounts of money to projects to effect ends that it chose. It had the confidence necessary to plan and implement government programs with a view to improving the organization and delivery of services. Cost-shifting and other provider responses prove that

function still follows funding when government devotes its energies to reducing the cost of its purchases of services from the private sector.

These "lessons" and their application to issues of the elderly are fairly obvious, but they bear emphasizing. Major changes in resources change programs. One may think in advance about these changes—a practice that used to be dignified by the name "planning." Alternatively, one may let events happen and feign surprises. It will be easier to promote planned change before great vested interests like insurance companies achieve a position that enables them to force government to share power with them. Finally, we should not lose our nerve and commitment to act. Government has acted effectively in the past, despite considerable recent propaganda to the contrary. Whether we will be in a position to make major improvements in aging support depends on the ability of the U.S. economy to continue creating abundant wealth. If there is "discretionary" national income, however, we may choose to spend it on worthy causes like children or education rather than investing it in even more security for the elderly.

Thus, the future of at least the long-term care portion of the aging-support system may be decided in part by the economic future of the country. If we are to develop a rational, comprehensive, government-funded and -monitored system which does not permit two classes of care or facilities, we must develop some way to see around the budget deficit blinders that currently preclude significant innovation in domestic public policy. The sort of aging-support system that we establish is a societal choice for which we must collectively be at least partially responsible.

REFERENCES

Aaron, Henry J. and William B. Schwartz. 1984. *The painful prescription: Rationing hospital care.* Washington, DC: The Brookings Institution.

American Association of Retired Persons. 1988. The AARP/Gallup survey of family policy issues: Summary of findings. July, photo copy (n.p.).

Aries, Philippe. 1962. *Centuries of childhood: A social history of family life,* trans. Robert Baldick. New York: Alfred A. Knopf.

Berke, Richard L. 1989. Census predicts population

drop in next century: 300 million peak For U.S. *New York Times,* February 1: A1, A18.

Binstock, Robert H. 1989. The phantom old-age vote. *New York Times,* January 2:23.

Brandon, William. 1977. Politics, administration and conflict in neighborhood health centers. *Journal of Health Politics, Policy and Law* 2:79–99.

Brandon, William P. 1982. 'Fact' and 'value' in the thought of Peter Winch: Linguistic analysis broaches metaphysical questions. *Political Theory* 10:215–244.

Brandon, William P. 1989. Cut off at the impasse without real catastrophic health insurance: Three approaches to financing long-term care. *Policy Studies Review* 8.

Brandon, William P., Emma K. Lee and Mark J. Segal. 1980. Testing the anti-regulatory arguments of the market reformers: New data on the HMO-HSA relationship. *Journal of Health and Human Resources Administration* 2:391–428.

Brasfield, James M. 1987. The management of invisible Policies: Medicaid and long term care. Paper presented at the meeting of the Southwestern Social Science Association. Dallas TX. March 18–21.

Brown, Lawrence D. 1983. *Politics and health care organization: HMOs as federal policy.* Washington, DC: The Brookings Institution.

Cobb, Roger W. and Charles D. Elder. 1972. *Participation in American politics: The dynamics of agenda-building.* Boston: Allyn and Bacon.

Congressional Quarterly Almanac. 1988. Congress passes catastrophic-costs measure. *Congressional Quarterly Almanac: 100th Congress 1st Session— 1987.* Washington, DC: Congressional Quarterly Inc.

Donabedian, Avedis, *et al.* 1986. *Medical care chartbook,* 8th ed. Ann Arbor, MI: Health Administration Press.

Edelman, Murray. 1964. *The symbolic uses of politics.* Urbana, IL: University of Illinois.

Estes, Carroll L. 1983. *The aging enterprise: A critical examination of social policies and services for the aged.* San Francisco: Jossey-Bass.

Federal Hospital Insurance Trust Fund Board of Trustees. 1988. *The 1988 Annual Report,* H. R. Doc. 100–193, 100th Cong., 2d Sess. Washington, DC: USGPO.

Federal Old-Age and Survivors Insurance and Disability Insurance Trust Fund Board of Trustees. 1988. *The 1988 annual report.* H. R. Doc. 100–192, 100th Cong., 2d sess. Washington, DC: USGPO.

Federal Supplementary Medical Insurance Trust Fund Board of Trustees. 1988. *The 1988 annual report.* H. R. Doc. 100–194, 100th Cong., 2d sess. Washington, DC: USGPO.

Feldstein, Paul J. 1988. *The politics of health legislation:*

An economic perspective Ann Arbor, MI: Health Administration Press.

Friedan, Betty. 1983. Paper presented to the Hastings Center-Harvard Medical School Project on Ethics and the Care of the Aging, Harvard Medical School, Boston, May 25–26.

Fries, James F. 1980. Aging, natural death, and the compression of morbidity. *New England Journal of Medicine* 303:130–5.

Fries, James F. 1983. The compression of morbidity. *Milbank Memorial Fund Quarterly* 61:397–419.

Firshein, Janet. 1989. Congress confronts catastrophic fallout. *Medicine and Health Perspectives* 43 (January 9).

Ford, Doris and Mark Burns. 1987. The politics of domain consensus: application to long-term care. *Journal of Health and Human Resources Administration* 9:423–447.

Gerontological Society of America. 1987. To meet the Challenge of Aging: Annual Report 1987. Washington, DC: Gerontological Society of America.

Gray Panthers. 1987. *Disability task force newsletter: Age & youth in action* 3 (March).

Gray Panthers. n.d. Gray Panthers fact sheet. Photocopy.

Hsiao, William C., et al. 1988. Estimating physicians' work for a resource-based relative-value scale. *New England Journal of Medicine* 319:835–841.

Hsiao, William C., et al. 1988. Resource-based relative values: An overview *Journal of the American Medical Association* 260:2347–2353.

Iglehart, John K. 1989. Medicare's new benefits: 'Catastrophic' health insurance. *New England Journal of Medicine* 320:329–336.

Jazwiecki, Tom and Teresa Schwab. 1989. Conclusion. In *Caring for an aging world: International models for Long-term care, financing, and delivery,* edited by Teresa Schwab, 366–76. New York: McGraw-Hill.

Johnson, Malcolm. 1989. Long-term care for the elderly in England In *Caring for an aging world: International models for long-term care, financing, and delivery,* edited by Teresa Schwab New York: McGraw-Hill. 162–192.

Kosterlitz, Julie. 1988. The coming crisis. *National Journal* (August 6):2029–2032.

Kreps, Juanita M. 1971. *Lifetime allocation of work and income: Essays in the Economics of aging.* Durham, NC: Duke University Press.

Kuhn, Maggie. 1988. Editorial. *Network* 17 (November-December):13.

Light, Paul. 1985. *Artful work: The politics of social security reform.* New York: Random House.

Longman, Phillip. 1987. *Born to pay: The new politics of aging in America.* Boston: Houghton Mifflin.

Lowi, Theodore J. 1969. *The end of liberalism: Ideology,*

policy, and the crisis of public authority. New York: W. W. Norton.

Manton, Kenneth G. 1982. Changing concepts of morbidity and mortality in the elderly population. *Milbank Memorial Fund Quarterly* 60:183–244.

Marmor, Theodore R. 1973. *Politics of Medicare.* Chicago: Aldine.

Moynihan, Daniel P. 1988. Conspirators, trillions, limos in the night. *New York Times,* May 23, A19.

Murphy, Michelle M. 1988. Elderly lobby group continues to thrive . . . but image on Capitol Hill still tarnished. *Congressional Quarterly Weekly Report* 46 (March 26):778–9.

National Committee to Preserve Social Security and Medicare, n.d. What is the National Committee. Washington, DC: NCPSSM.

National Council on the Aging, Inc. 1988. NCOA at work: Annual report 1987. Washington, DC: NCOA.

National Council on the Aging, Inc. n.d. NCOA: Helping you improve the lives of older Americans. Washington, DC: NCOA.

New York Times. 1989. Fair is fair for Medicare. March 31, A34.

Oakeshott, Michael. 1962. Political education In *Rationalism in Politics,* 110–136. London: Methuen.

Ossofsky, Jack. 1978. Correspondence. *National Journal* 18 (March 11):408–9.

Pear, Robert. 1987. Working Profile: Thomas R. Burke: The man behind the medicare expansion plan. *New York Times,* February 18.

Pear, Robert. 1988. Social Security said to bridge gap in income. *New York Times,* December 28: A1, A20.

Pratt, Henry J. 1976. *The gray lobby.* Chicago: University of Chicago Press.

Quadagno, Jill S. 1984. From Poor Laws to Pensions: The Evolution of Economic Support for the Aged in England and America. *Milbank Memorial Fund Quarterly* 62 (Summer):417 446.

Rivlin, Alice M. and Joshua M. Wiener. 1988. *Caring for the disabled elderly: Who will pay?* Washington, DC: The Brookings Institution.

Rovner, Julie. 1988. Catastrophic-costs measure ready for final hill approval. *Congressional Quarterly Weekly Report* 46 (June 4):1494–5.

Rovner, Julie. 1988b. 'Pepper Bill' pits politics against process. *Congressional Quarterly Weekly Report* 46 (June 4): 1491–3.

Russell, Louise B. and Carrie Lynn Manning. 1989. The effect of prospective payment on Medicare expenditures. *The New England Journal of Medicine* 320:439–444.

Samuelson, Robert J. 1978. Another look at those figures on the aged. *National Journal* 18 (March 11):399.

Samuelson, Robert J. 1978b. Busting the U.S. budget—The costs of an aging America. *National Journal* 18 (February):256–60.

Sardell, Alice. 1988. *The U.S. experiment in social medicine The community health center program, 1965–1986.* Pittsburgh, PA: University of Pittsburgh Press.

Sloan, Frank A., Michael A. Morrisey and Joseph Valvona. 1988. Effects of the Medicare prospective payment system on hospital cost containment: An early appraisal. *Milbank Quarterly* 66:191–220.

Sorian, Richard. 1989. A Reagan retrospective. *Medicine and Health Perspectives* 43 (January 16).

Sorian, Richard. 1989b. "Physician payment reform: On the brink," *Medicine and Health Perspectives* 43 (March 27).

Sorian, Richard, ed. 1989c. Six states eye mandatory insurance. *Medicine and Health* 43 (March 27):2.

Titmus, Richard M. 1971. *The gift relationship: From human blood to social policy.* New York: Pantheon Books.

U.S., Bureau of the Census. 1942. *Statistical abstract of the United States 1941.* Sixty-third number. Washington, DC: USGPO.

U.S., Bureau of the Census. 1986. *Economic characteristics of households in the United States: Fourth quarter 1984.* Current Population Reports, Series P-70, No. 6, Household Economic Studies. Washington, DC: USGPO

U.S., Bureau of the Census. 1988. *Measuring the effect of benefits and taxes on income and poverty: 1986.* Current Population Reports, Series P-60, No. 164-RD-1, Washington, DC: USGPO

U.S., Department of Health and Human Services. 1986. *Catastrophic illness expenses: Report to the president.* Washington, DC: DHHS, November.

U.S., Department of Health and Human Services, Office of the Assistant Secretary for Planning and Evaluation. N.d. *Insuring catastrophic illness for the general population.* (n.p.: DHHS).

U.S. Technical Work Group on Private Financing of Long-Term Care for the Elderly. 1986. *Report to the secretary on private financing of long-term care for the elderly.* Draft (n.p.: November).

U.S. National Commission on Social Security Reform. 1983. *Final report.* Washington, DC: USGPO.

U.S., DHHS, Task Force on Long-Term Health Care Policies. 1987. *Report to Congress and the secretary,* HCFA Pub. No. 87–02170 Washington, DC: USGPO.

Villers Foundation. 1986. *The Villers Foundation: Report 1983–1984–1985.* (n.p.).

Winch, Peter. 1958. *The idea of a social science and its relation to philosophy.* London: Routledge & Kegan Paul.

Winch, Peter. 1970. Understanding a primitive society.

In *Rationality,* edited by Bryan R. Wilson, 78–111. New York: Harper and Row.

Weissert, William G., C. Matthews Cready, and James E. Pawelak. 1988. The past and future of home- and community-based long-term care. *Milbank Quarterly* 66:309–388.

Zappolo, Aurora A. and Gerdt Sundstrom. 1989. Long-term care for the elderly in sweden. In *Caring for an aging world: International models for long-term care, financing, and delivery,* edited by Teresa Schwab, 22–57. New York: McGraw-Hill.

Chapter 19

The Politics of Public Health:

The Dilemma of a Public Profession[1]

Camilla Stivers

A man may be a walking dictionary, living encyclopedia, bacteria wizard, or virtue personified,
and yet not intelligent as to government.
William H. Allen
Efficient Democracy (1906)

The mission of public health as seen by public
health professionals is to prevent disease and
promote health on a community-wide basis. Like
most professionals, public health professionals
believe that practice should be grounded in science. Knowledge about causes of disease, methods of transmission, preventive techniques, and
the administration of community-wide programs
forms the core of public health expertise, and in
the eyes of its members justifies the profession's
claims to autonomy and legitimacy. Public
health professionals see their skill and dedication
as the key to assuring conditions for the health of
entire populations, and argue that society should
accord them the authority to practice as they
think best. Yet, as a public profession, public
health is confronted with the necessity for political responsiveness. Practice must serve not only
scientific and professional concerns but values
that result from political bargaining and compromise with a range of constituencies, among
whom elected officials are paramount.

Public health as practiced in state and local
health departments in the United States[2] is accorded low status among actors in the policy process and is politically weak. This essay will suggest, based on contemporary and historical
evidence, that the political plight of the profession of public health can be traced to its failure

---

[1]Although the viewpoint of this chapter departs considerably
from that expressed in the Institute of Medicine report, I would
like to thank the members of the IOM's Committee on the
Future of Public Health, who taught me much, and especially
the committee chair, Richard Remington, who critiqued an earlier draft of this chapter from a perspective it could not have
done without.

[2]This essay focuses on the state and local level where "classic"
public health originated and is still practiced.

to come to terms with the public nature of its practice and to find an effective way of joining knowledge with power in the service of the public good.

Contemporary Public Health Practice

Unlike most other professions, the self-definition of public health is not consistent with its operational definition, that is the actual activities carried on by state and local health departments. Theoretically, the mission of public health can be expanded to encompass a vast range of concerns. From the profession's perspective, almost any aspect of living can be related to the health of society and thus appropriately be considered a potential public health matter. For example, decent jobs and adequate housing contribute to people's good health. This more expansive interpretation of the public health purview is reflected in C. E. A. Winslow's widely quoted definition of the field:

> Public health is the science and the art of (1) preventing disease, (2) prolonging life, and (3) promoting physical health and efficiency through organized community efforts for (a) the sanitation of the environment, (b) the control of communicable infections, (c) the education of the individual in personal hygiene, (d) the organization of medical and nursing services for the early diagnosis and preventive treatment of disease, and (e) the development of the social machinery to ensure everyone a standard of living adequate for the maintenance of health, so organizing these benefits as to enable every citizen to realize his birthright of health and longevity (Hanlon 1969, 4).

In actual practice, however, the responsibilities of state and local health departments are in tension with the profession's self-image. Several incongruities can be observed. First, no health department's activities encompass the broad scope of the Winslow definition. In addition, there is great heterogeneity of duties and functions among the various state and local entities responsible for public health. Thus, there appears to be no consistent societal response to the profession's overall claim to authority. Another ten-

sion is reflected in the fact that many health departments, particularly on the local level, have been assigned the responsibility for providing direct medical care to individuals (i.e., the uninsured and many Medicaid patients who have been turned away by private providers). As we have seen above, public health claims the right to *organize* medical care services but not to provide them directly, a duty that in practice diverts resources away from prevention activities. Finally, many if not most of the people actually doing the work of public health in agencies are not public health professionals by training, a situation at odds with the classic claim of every profession, that outsiders have no right to do its work. Let us now consider each of these tensions in a bit more detail, based on findings from a 1988 study by the Institute of Medicine (IOM) in which the author served as associate study director.[3]

What State and Local Health Departments Do

Since the earliest days of the Republic, even before the Constitution, states have had the responsibility of protecting the health and welfare of their citizens (the "police power"). Local governments on the other hand come into being as a result of state action. Consequently, states are the central authorities in the nation's public health system. State health departments vary greatly in their organization and scope of responsibilities. Some can be found within human service "super agencies" while others are independent. Some act as the chief environmental, mental health, and/or Medicaid agency for their states, but in each case about two-thirds of the state health departments do not have this respon-

---

[3]As its final report states, the IOM study of public health "was undertaken to address a growing perception among the Institute of Medicine membership and others concerned with the health of the public that this nation has lost sight of its public health goals and has allowed the system of public health activities to fall into disarray" (Institute of Medicine 1988 1). During the two-year study, interviews were conducted with more than 350 people from inside and outside state and local health departments in six states, and data were reviewed on the organization, staffing, and financing of state and local health in the United States as a whole and on the scope and severity of fourteen of the nation's major public health problems.

sibility. Nearly all states collect and analyze vital statistics, do epidemiological studies and laboratory analyses, screen the population for various diseases, and do some health-related research. Nearly all engage in some type of health education activity. Most state health departments engage in inspection and quality assurance activities such as food and milk control, health facility licensing, and environmental protection, particularly with respect to public and individual water supplies and sewage disposal systems. Nearly all are involved in maternal and child health, prenatal and family planning services, immunizations, chronic diseases and dental services. Nevertheless, although it is possible to list functions performed by "nearly all" or "most" state health departments, few generalizations can be made about how deeply or in what manner (e.g., data collection, research, policy planning, or direct service provision) these agencies are involved in any particular activity, or which health problems they address.

Even more diversity exists at the local level. In some states, local health departments are operated directly by the state health department itself. In most states, however, local health departments are under the jurisdiction of a general-purpose unit of local government, usually a county but sometimes a city or town. Because of great differences among localities in their population size and revenue base, local health departments range from agencies larger in size and scope than some state health departments to bare-bones operations with one- or two-member staffs. In many sparsely populated areas, there is no local health department—perhaps a circuit-riding nurse or sanitarian from the state visits these areas occasionally, but often nothing at all exists in the way of public health activity, and there is no public official specifically responsible for public health.

Given this great variation in size, it is not surprising that the functions performed by local health departments are even less consistent than those of the states. Most local health agencies are involved in environmental inspections, in health education, and in control of venereal disease and tuberculosis. In contrast to states, however, a great many local health departments provide personal health services, particularly to those who would otherwise not be able to afford

such services. The IOM study found that having to serve as "provider of last resort" constitutes a difficult duty for local health agencies. Because the need of individuals for medical care is so immediate and compelling, agency resources are inevitably drawn away from population-wide disease prevention and health promotion activities (Institute of Medicine 1988, 97–98, 109).

The IOM study concluded that the diversity of organizational arrangements and responsibilities reflected in state and local health agencies suggests that there is no clear organizational focus for state and local public health in the United States, and little agreement among its units of government about what "public health" means operationally. The study uncovered numerous examples of gaps and confusions in the public health system that reflect this lack of focus (Institute of Medicine 1988, 125). For example, in one community poor women were presenting themselves at the hospital emergency room in labor, never having seen a physician during their entire pregnancy (Institute of Medicine 1988, 117). In another case, neither local nor state officials knew who among them had the authority to act in case a toxic materials spill threatened the local water supply (Institute of Medicine 1988, 123).

The difficulty of arriving at an operational definition of public health is further complicated by the fact that a great many public health agency personnel have no specific training in public health. The public health profession itself frankly acknowledges, even prides itself on, its multi-disciplinary nature, including within the fold not only physicians, nurses, and sanitarians, but industrial hygienists, statisticians, community health educators, and others. But the tie that binds these different perspectives together, according to the profession, that is, training in a distinctive body of knowledge centering around the "mother science" epidemiology (Institute of Medicine 1988, 40), is not widespread among existing state and local agency staffs. For example, only about one-third of local health department directors have a master's degree in public health, and most public health nurses have little formal public health training beyond what they may have received in nursing school.

In practice, contemporary public health in the United States is both narrower in scope of authority and more diffuse in actual responsibility than the profession's vision of itself. Public health agencies are faced with a complex array of tasks. In addition to long-standing concerns such as protection of the water supply, maternal and child health, vital statistics, and health education, new challenges such as AIDS, toxic waste control, and care of the indigent patient have been added to the menu of health department responsibilities.

The IOM study concluded that, despite obvious expertise, dedication, hard work, and some success on the part of many professionals, on the whole public health agencies are ill-equipped to cope with the functions they perform, let alone fulfill the broader vision of the profession. The study traced the current difficulties of public health to fragmented authority, antiquated laws, frequently inadequate fiscal resources, and lack of public understanding and support.

Problems with Contemporary Public Health Practice

Fragmented authority for carrying out public health functions began in the 1960s as the leadership role in protecting the environment was gradually removed from public health departments and lodged in newly-created departments of environmental services or ecology. This development appears to have been a response to the proliferation of environmental programs and permit requirements that took place as environmental hazards worsened. In a climate of growing concern over pollution, the traditional "health department model" for handling environmental problems "appeared increasingly outdated" (Rabe 1986, 31). In the same way, Medicaid and other War on Poverty programs went to other public agencies, or, in the latter case, bypassed government entirely in favor of non-profit community organizations. Such fragmentation concerns public health professionals not only because of growing confusion about who has the power to act to solve health problems, but also because they fear neglect—due to lack of knowledge—of the health dimensions of issues removed from their control. In addition organizational separation usually brings with it duplicative and uncoordinated program planning.

Separate data systems in different agencies, it is believed, also hinder the kind of broad assessment and surveillance on which effective action depends.

Moreover, public understanding of the public health mission has suffered as a result of the organizational disarray (Institute of Medicine 1988) of contemporary U.S. public health. Subsuming health departments under umbrella human service agencies has made it difficult to emphasize the society-wide benefits realized from public health action, as distinguished from the help provided to individual—usually poor—clients by human service programs. Public health has come to be seen, by legislators and the general public alike, as a welfare program. In addition, the tendency to remove environmental health and other responsibilities from health departments has led to a generalized "conventional wisdom" that public health agencies are incapable of solving complex, important problems.

Another difficulty with public health practice today is the fact that state public health laws are in many cases seriously outmoded. Many state statutes delineating public health authority and responsibility date from the first few decades of this century—some even earlier. In addition, as Gostin (1986) argues, the statutory powers provided are too restrictive and offer too few due process guarantees to deal with new diseases such as AIDS, where outdated measures like full isolation and quarantine are inappropriate and the conflict between individual freedom and community safety is extreme. Overly restrictive laws become politically unfeasible, according to Gostin, leaving public health administrators with too much unfettered administrative discretion.

Public health agencies face yet another difficulty in the form of inadequate funding, although the same could probably be said for most governmental activity today. Public health professionals argue that the fiscal problems of health departments are particularly acute, because they have had to take on much broader responsibilities in recent years, such as the care of indigent patients and dealing with AIDS. At the same time, federal support for state and local public health has declined markedly, as the federal government has cut public health-related block grants. The size of state and local public health budgets barely held steady during the 1980s, reflecting, of course, a reduction in spending power when inflation is taken into account. The effect of these trends has been exacerbated in particular states and localities where recovery from the steep recession in the early 1980s was slow to materialize, and in the country at large by the growing needs of an aging population, outdated and ill-maintained water and sewer systems, and the generalized persistent rise in health care costs, which continues to outpace inflation.

Perhaps the most striking of all the difficulties facing public health today is a lack of public knowledge and support. State and local health departments not only have no apparent constituency, a serious handicap in a political system where organized interest groups play a key role in policy decisions, but in addition the general public has little knowledge of what health departments actually do. The IOM study found during a series of site visits that while many people who are not trained or employed in public health generally understand and favor the public health mission, they have little awareness of specific activities or programs carried on by public health agencies in their communities and the benefits they produce. When asked, respondents could furnish definitions of public health such as, "It's things that benefit everybody . . . Promoting health on a general level . . . What the private sector can't or won't do"; but when queried about what the local or state health department does specifically, most were able to make only vague suggestions, such as, "They take care of poor people . . . You can go there to get a shot . . . Don't they inspect restaurants?" (Institute of Medicine 1988, 37, 41).

The Political Dilemma of Public Health

The legal, organizational, fiscal and constituency problems of public health are largely rooted, it is argued here, in the profession's view of politics as a contaminant of rational, scientific and expert decision-making and implementation. While there are individual exceptions, as a group public health professionals, taking a dim view of politics, have failed to develop the level and kind of political skills necessary in order to get laws updated, structures improved, resources

expanded and a constituency mobilized. Before considering the extent to which professionalism *per se* may lie at the heart of the public health perspective on politics, however, let us look for a moment at the political dilemma of public health in states and localities across the United States. Evidence of this dilemma, excerpted from but reflective of over 350 unpublished interviews conducted by the IOM study group, is found both in what those who interact with state and local health departments have to say about them and their staffs as well as in what public health people themselves say about their political situations.

To take the external perspective first, many legislators, private health care providers, appointed officials, and members of the general public interviewed by the IOM study team view public health departments and their personnel as timid, passive, and out of the policy mainstream. As one respondent put it, "The health department has never done anything. . . . Public health people are just survivors." Another commented, "I never saw the state health department assess problems and develop a strategy. . . . They take a Band-Aid approach." Still another put it this way, "Public health is infantile politically, not strong, not vocal." As might be expected in an era in which candidates for executive office routinely run on anti-government platforms, public health agencies also come in for their share of "bureaucrat bashing." The IOM interviewers heard that public health practitioners are "consummate bureaucrats, saving their own jobs." Another noted, "It's a bottomless pit . . . a ponderous bureaucracy . . . no one leader can change it." Perhaps most troubling to the study group were comments to the effect that "Politicos don't turn to the health department for advice." Even favorable assessments tended to take the form of damning with faint praise, as in: "They're doing the best they can with what they have" (Institute of Medicine 1988, unpublished interview data).

Public health people, for their part, are inclined to the view that politics are outside their realm, or at best a necessary evil. For example, one state health official commented, "We state it like it is; we don't mess with problems that don't have solutions." Another put it, "The professionals should make the decisions and then take the heat." Those interviewed were apparently well aware that their views have little effect on policy decisions. "The state doesn't recognize public health concerns unless there's a public outcry. The department develops statistics, but statistics don't make people act." And again, "We get frustrated when the public and the legislature don't listen. The staff says, 'What's the use? Nobody really cares about public health' " (Institute of Medicine 1988, unpublished interview data).

The results of the IOM study interviews paint a picture in which those who interact with and observe public health staffs view them as paper-shufflers and time servers, enmeshed in red tape, out of touch with reality, politically naive and ineffective; while agency personnel themselves mourn the fact that nobody pays any attention to their expertise and bemoan the presence of politics in the policy process.

Professionalism and Politics

Having offered an assessment of the current policy status of public health and suggested that the current "disarray" in which the IOM report finds the nation's public health system is fundamentally political rather than simply a matter of inadequate funds or poor organization, this essay must now make its central argument, namely that the political problems of public health are related to the profession's failure to come to terms with what it means to be a public sector professional.

Professionalism in the Public Sector

The problematic nature of public sector professionalism can be understood by reflecting on the classic features of the professional role and the extent to which these are in tension with public service. The sociological literature defines a profession as paid, full-time work, requiring formal education that imparts a systematic body of knowledge and a set of practical skills to be practiced in the work setting. Professionals are also characterized by an ethic of service to clients; by the use of expert judgment not reducible to a set of formalizable rules; and by the claim to auton-

omy on the basis of expertise: that is, professional knowledge and its application in practice are so specialized, so esoteric, that no outsider is qualified to say whether or not a member of the profession is competent (Freidson 1984; Bledstein 1976; Vollmer and Mills 1966).

The socialization process in most professions ensures that members acquire a sense of mission that shapes both theory and practice. Convinced of the worth of their calling, i.e., that their work contributes to the welfare of the community, professionals see themselves as uniquely dedicated to serving in the area over which they claim knowledge (Meigh 1966; Greenwood 1966). Even more than commitment, however, professionals ground their legitimacy claims in objective expertise, in the science they apply in practice, which they see as unbiased by partisan interests and therefore as by its nature in the public interest.

Professionalism practiced in the public sector raises difficulties on at least two counts. Professionals who are employees of any organization, including public agencies, are faced with the necessity of sacrificing some of the autonomy they claim. This is because their work forms only a part of the set of capacities necessary to achieve organizational goals, meaning that organizational professionals must regulate their work to fit broader frameworks and must sometimes respond to organizational fiat instead of professional standards (Scott 1966).

The more complex problem stems from the *public* nature of public sector professionalism. (Mosher 1982; Bell 1985). Professionals in public service must not only possess specialized skills and fit them to agency purposes, they must also take into account the governmental context in which they work. In the case of the United States, our system of representative democracy imposes a necessary constraint on the exercise of professional judgment in the public sector. The "objective" authority of expertise is only a part of the process of deciding what to do. Executive agencies, including public health departments, must join with other constituencies in the bargaining and negotiation that characterize the policy process. Public sector professionals cannot reasonably expect other policy actors to treat professional judgments as neutral while all other interests are seen as biased. Bell (1985, 87) makes the point as follows:

> By conceptualizing the positions of [interest] groups as essentially alien to the merits . . . [professionals] treat those positions, in effect, as important in proportion to the power of those who take them.

Instead, Bell argues, professionals should begin with the assumption that interest groups do not work their will simply on the basis of sheer power, but by arguing in terms of principles that are widely accepted in society (e.g., the public interest). As Bell suggests, by acknowledging that these principles have validity and by critically assessing interest group positions, public professionals could help make policy argument more principled. Such a stance, however, would mean according a less privileged place to professional claims of objectivity.

Public Health Professionals and Politics

Since the translation of public health knowledge into action takes place within the context of public service, effective public health practice brings with it the peculiar set of constraints suggested above, restrictions that other health professions—for example, private-practice medicine, the profession *par excellence*—do not face. The IOM study findings suggest that while some public health professionals are politically astute and effective, in general the profession gives relatively little attention to the gap that exists in the public sector between knowing what is the case and deciding what to do about it. Public health professionals place great faith in the ability of statistical and epidemiological studies to diagnose problems. To the professional eye, the ambiguities in problematic situations are only a result of inadequate data. Given "good" data, the correct, professional solution becomes obvious, while the interpretations of politicians and other interests are seen as biased. Thus, public health professionals are able to view politics as a contaminant of what would otherwise be rational and objective, that is, professional decisions instead of seeing the characteristics of the policy process—pulling and hauling, constituency building, persuasion—as essential to democratic government.

Public health personnel tend to see themselves as engaged in a lonely struggle to promote public goods such as infectious disease control that have no organized advocates. Sincerely believing that their values and aims are consistent with, even identical with, the public interest, they lose sight of the fact that public decision-making entails bargaining, negotiation and compromise: convincing others rather than merely furnishing what the profession feels is incontrovertible proof.

Taking the legitimacy of the public health knowledge base for granted, the profession has a limited understanding of the issue of public accountability. Public sector professionals have the obligation to hold themselves demonstrably and tangibly accountable to the public, both directly and through elected representatives. This answerability in practice is what helps to ensure that decisions of public-sector professionals are responsive to the widest possible definition of the public interest rather than exclusively professional norms. As Mosher (1982, 212) notes:

> Any effort to remove an area of governmental activity from general political responsibility—to protect it from politics—is, *per se*, a threat to administrative morality since it encourages the administrator to approach his problems narrowly, to minimize or neglect or ignore the general interest.

There is some evidence from the historical record that the gap between public health knowledge and effective political practice was not always as wide as it now appears. Indeed, contrary to the frequent call among present-day public health professionals for a purer mode of practice like that of earlier days, history suggests that public health has never been "above" politics. Although organized public health came out of a reform era that abhorred political pollution as much as the environmental variety, some of the early successes of public health can be traced to political circumstances and to leaders who were able and pragmatic political strategists. In the concluding section of this chapter, we will explore how such an understanding of the history of public health might offer guidance for the present and future.

Political Lessons from Public Health History

Three aspects of the history of public health offer evidence that public health has never been completely apolitical and that, indeed, important public health measures in specific locations and at specific moments in history owe their success at least partially to favorable political circumstances and the political skill of key individuals. For one thing, the history of public health reveals that public health knowledge has always had political dimensions and implications. Like all knowledge, public health reflects a set of intellectual and value assumptions that can be seen reflected in what is said to be known and how it is applied to problems. Another important aspect of the history of public health is its development as part of the much broader Progressive reform movement in the latter half of the nineteenth and early twentieth centuries: a movement, as we will see, that presented itself as non-partisan but which had deeply political roots. A third source of understanding lies in the actions of public health leaders who were successful in instituting health and safety measures because they understood politics and knew how to play it. Following a review of these three perspectives on the history of public health politics, we will conclude with a brief reflection on the relationship over time between the profession of public health and private-practice medicine, in order to suggest how long-standing tension between the two has shaped the profession of public health and its self-understanding, a self-image which in turn has led to the profession's current political handicaps.

The Politics of Public Health Knowledge

Despite the public health profession's treatment of scientific knowledge, derived particularly from epidemiology and biostatistics, as objective and unbiased, a review of public health history suggests that it has never been safe to regard public health knowledge as self-evidently neutral: instead, this knowledge has had political dimensions since the earliest period in U.S. history.

A case in point is the yellow fever epidemic along the eastern seaboard from 1793 to 1795, which brought the first organized local boards of health into being in order to deal with the threat (Duffy 1978). At the time, no one knew what caused yellow fever. There was a host of conflicting theories about causes, prevention, and cures. Medical science was divided as to whether the source of the illness was environmental, the result of poor sanitation or unhealthy climate, or whether it was transmitted from person to person. In Philadelphia, conflicting theories divided along political lines: Federalist physicians largely subscribed to the notion that the disease was being brought into the city by refugees from an uprising in Haiti, while Republican doctors generally believed the source of the fever to be environmental (Pernick 1978). Such an alignment did not develop at random. The environmental theory lent itself to broad-scale actions to improve domestic sanitation, an approach that was consistent with the Republicans' decentralized approach to government. The contagion theory on the other hand required immediate governmental action such as quarantines or barring refugees from disembarking in port, measures better suited to the Federalist acceptance of strong central government. A bitter argument developed between proponents of these two points of view, a dispute that was eventually settled by political compromise—both kinds of measures were instituted—an outcome that, considering the primitive state of medical knowledge at the time, served the public interest by making concerted action possible (Pernick 1978; Schwartz 1977).

Another example of the political dimension of public health knowledge is the effect the discovery of bacteria had on the field. In its early days, public health was defined in terms of its aim to prevent disease and keep whole populations healthy, rather than by any specific body of theory and methodology. Conventional wisdom seesawed back and forth between environmental approaches and those based on theories of contagion. There was strong opinion to the effect that disease represented moral failing on the part of the affected individual, and cleanliness and godliness were indeed linked in the minds of many public health physicians. But the diffuse and uncertain character of the knowledge base meant that the question of qualification for public health action was apt to be settled more by personal commitment than by knowledge. The early membership of the American Public Health Association included persons of good will with practical goals but little formal health training. Since there were no right answers on disease control, there was also no possibility of exclusive expertise (Rosenkrantz 1974).

Once the bacterial origin of many diseases became accepted, however, the bacteriology laboratory came to symbolize a newly scientific public health, drawing attention away from exclusively environmental action such as street cleaning and housing reform, and beginning the development of standardized methods requiring trained experts for successful implementation (Fee 1987; Rosenkrantz 1974). Since bacteria theory seemed to suggest that preventing disease had little to do with changing behavior, the question of responsibility for prevention shifted from susceptible individuals themselves to experts who claimed specific skills (Rosenkrantz 1972).

The shift from environmental to germ theory was not total, however. Dirty environments contribute to bacteria growth; therefore, basic sanitation could still support disease control. In addition, there was a period when public health physicians remained unsure about how best to apply the findings of bacteriology in practice, as in the purification of milk. The range of possible action on both environmental and bacteriological fronts ensured that medical disputes would be drawn into the political arena. Leavitt's (1982) account of the Milwaukee milk war illustrates this point. Medical opinion divided over which was the best strategy for protecting public health, that is, simply certifying milk, thus not altering the nutritional quality of raw milk; sterilizing to destroy all germs; pasteurization, which left some bacteria; or tuberculin testing of cows. As Leavitt (1982, 245) observes, "Because of the lack of professional cohesion, medicine alone rarely solved a public health problem." Political solutions were necessary because political unanimity was impossible.

The history of public health, then, shows that the knowledge base has been in a continuing process of development and change, as a result of shifting views about the causes of disease and methods of prevention; that assertions about the nature of public health "science" were more or less congruent with particular political philosophies; and that contention about science inevitably politicized the decision-making process. A final illustration may drive the point home. As Fee (1987) and others have shown, germ theory set in motion a dynamic that raised the profile of the medical aspect of public health in contrast to elements grounded in sanitary engineering, and thus inexorably moved public health into conflict with private-practice medicine. In the 1930s, a particularly vivid debate developed within the American Public Health Association, between progressives who wanted public health and medical care unified in a single health system and conservatives who favored keeping the definition of public health within its traditional prevention-oriented boundaries. Fee (1987, 228) points out that this debate reflected a broader division in political thinking about the New Deal. Progressives looked to the federal government for public health legislation, while conservatives wanted to keep the focus of government activity at the state and local level. A bifurcated health system meant, and means today, failure to integrate prevention and cure, public health and private medicine. This dichotomy had and still has its roots in definitions of knowledge.

The Politics of Reform

Although public health action in the United States dates back to the nation's early days, professionalization and the creation of a discipline arose as a part of the reform movement that dominated the latter years of the nineteenth century and persisted into the twentieth. Progressive reformers presented themselves and their positions on issues as non-partisan. Beginning ostensibly with the aim of "throwing the rascals out," that is, getting rid of machine patronage, politics, and corruption, the movement nevertheless had a substantive agenda that served the interests of upper- and upper-middle class persons:

regaining control of city governments taken over by immigrant groups (Hays 1964; Schiesl 1977). Couched in terms of "efficient and expert" government, professionalism in public service was also a strategy of "the better sort" for displacing those occupying patronage jobs with people of their own kind. As Hays (1964) argues, the class dimensions of Progressive reform are displayed not in its rhetoric but in practice: almost half the reformers were professional men (few professionals of the time were women), and crucial support for the movement came from upper class business and professional leaders.

Fear of immigrants and their strange ways had already blended with reform idealism in the early public health movement. In Massachusetts, the famous Shattuck Report of 1850[4] on sanitation and public health stated that the living conditions of the immigrants threatened society as a whole, and argued that good health was associated with clean living. The Shattuck Report advocated professional, full-time "sanitarians" and called for professorships of sanitation in American colleges (Bledstein 1976). A similar impetus lay behind reform efforts in New York City in the 1860s, where physicians, spurred by a cholera epidemic, performed a sanitary survey of the city in cooperation with the newly formed Council on Hygiene and Public Health. The Council used the report to embarrass Tammany Hall, the city's noted political machine, and secure passage of a Metropolitan Board of Health bill by the state legislature. The metropolitan scope of the board would, of course, threaten the Tammany municipal power base (Duffy 1968; Schwartz 1977).

As the reform movement moved into full swing in the late nineteenth century, public health leaders, who were mainly upper-class physicians, turned their attention to health officers then serving in city and state health departments. These were largely patronage jobs. Few of the physicians had any specialized training, and they were promoted or removed from office on the basis of their alliances with political leaders. Since the medical profession of the time had little power of its own, many physicians had looked upon a public health appointment as a way up the career ladder (Fee 1987; Rosenkrantz 1974). By the 1890s, however, the discovery of bacteria began to move public health into a new, scientific era, while at the same time the medical profession began to organize and professionalize itself. Public health leaders, who were also physicians, set about a similar professionalization effort.

As Fee (1987) suggests, the professionalization of public health was a deliberate strategy aimed at removing public health from direct political control, defining the necessary knowledge base for public health practice, and determining the requisite training for the new profession. The strategy was successful. With the founding of schools of public health, potential health officers received training in the "medical model" of public health rooted in the germ theory of disease, with sanitary engineering relegated to a secondary role in the curriculum.

Thus reform efforts in public health, while they assuredly improved the qualifications of city and state health officers, also served upper-class and medical interests, imbuing public health with a professionalism modeled after entrepreneurial private medicine, a development that over time became increasingly problematic both for society and for the strength of the profession itself.

The Politics of Public Health Leadership

Although the norm of leadership in public health today generally preserves the aspects of nonpartisanship and expert objectivity it took on as the profession developed during the reform era, several important moments in the history of public health suggest that the success of efforts to protect the health of the public depended on whether public health leadership was able to create or take advantage of favorable political conditions. An early example is reflected in Rosenkrantz's (1974) history of the Massachusetts Board of Health, particularly during its "golden years" spanning the turn of the century. She ar-

[4]The Shattuck Report is a landmark event in the history of public health. Lemuel Shattuck, a Massachusetts bookseller and statistician, collected vital statistics on the Massachusetts population which pointed up differences in death and illness rates in different localities. Shattuck argued that these differences could be attributed to the foulness of the air in dirty urban neighborhoods and to the immoral life-style of (heavily immigrant) urban populations. His report called for government to step in where the failure of individuals to take responsibility for cleanliness threatened entire populations.

gues that, while a good bit of the Board's authority and prestige in this period can be traced to the competence and commitment of the professional men associated with it, political conditions also made an important difference. Republicans dominated elective office during the period, and the Board's active role as a regulatory agency was consistent with Republican expectations:

> Civic responsibility to protect the "public interest" from ignorance, irresponsibility, or selfishness . . . had long been assumed by successive generations of enlightened Republicans . . . [who] had never yielded . . . substantial power to immigrant groups or their children, although such new citizens made up more than half the state's population by 1900. Yet Massachusetts workers . . . were protected from . . . unsanitary factory conditions to a degree unknown in other industrial states (Rosenkrantz 1974, 135).

Thus the Board's success in regulating worksites lay partly in the fact that such efforts were consistent with the interests and values of partisan politicians.

The career of Hermann Biggs, health officer of New York City in the early twentieth century, illustrates the difference one person can make when political acumen is combined with scientific knowledge. The issue involved the reporting of tuberculosis cases by private physicians. Public health officials believed the disease to be contagious, and compulsory reporting was viewed as a necessary measure to prevent its spread. Physicians on the other hand looked on reporting as an infringement on patients' rights and a threat to their own livelihoods.

Biggs and his colleagues faced a difficult situation. Too much physician enmity would not only stall the public health measure, it would also bring the state legislature down on New York City's Tammany-controlled government. By using his political skills to define issues, however, Biggs worked out compromises that eventually brought the physicians around. Biggs framed the issue of reporting in terms of the general welfare rather than as a benefit to the poor (who were most of the TB cases); offered departmental patronage to some physicians; was flexible about phasing in enforcement measures; provided active services to patients so that physicians could

not develop lay support for their resistance; and soft-pedaled other controversial issues at the time. By these measures Biggs was able to implement TB reporting successfully over a period of several years (Fox 1978). Leavitt (1982) chronicles similar political competence on the part of certain public health leaders in Milwaukee during the reform era.

A more contemporary example of the importance of political skill in public health leaders is suggested in FitzGerald's (1986) account of the efforts of Mervyn Silverman, health officer of San Francisco, to close gay bathhouses in the hope of retarding the spread of AIDS in that city. FitzGerald shows that, although Silverman received a great deal of negative press over his apparent foot-dragging on the bathhouse closures, and eventually lost his job because the criticism he received became a political liability to elected officials, in reality Silverman's actions were a deliberate strategy to win the confidence of the gay community before taking action. That community's suspicion of the city government was extreme, and Silverman realized that a hard line would simply strengthen their resistance. He proceeded with a staged education campaign, the formation of advisory groups with gay and non-gay members, and a great deal of networking and negotiation. His strategy worked. Eventually he was able to close the baths without noticeable protest from the gay community.

Other similar examples of political astuteness on the part of contemporary public health leaders can undoubtedly be found. The profession continues, however, to give much greater weight to scientific expertise than to political effectiveness in the ideal model of public health leadership.

Public Health and Private Medicine

The historical evidence has suggested that the boundary between the disciplines of public health and private medicine has never been mutually acceptable and tension-free. We have seen that through the mid-nineteenth century, the value of involvement in public health action by upper-class physician-leaders lay more in commitment than expertise, while the ordinary physician frequently regarded a paid public health position as a means of acquiring status in an age when medicine still struggled for generalized societal esteem. With the discovery of the role of bacteria in disease, however, the relative position of the two disciplines began to shift. Physician unease at the effect sanitary action was having on disease rates was exacerbated as germ theory began to display its potential to generate even more effective disease control measures. As physicians took steps around the turn of the century to raise their profession's status in the eyes of society, the field of public health became a strategic target. This struggle took the form of staking claims over domains of professional knowledge and practice.

Rosenkrantz (1974) argues that the unsolved question of differential susceptibility to disease provided the grounds for medicine's assertion of unique expertise. Neither the old-style sanitation campaigns (e.g., cleaning up the water supply) nor the newer measures emerging from bacteriological research solved the mystery of why some people fell ill and others in apparently identical circumstances did not. Individual vulnerability and fear of disease and death could not be assuaged by community-wide action, but required the private physician's promise of expert judgment and personal attention. As a result, over time medicine laid successful claim to exclusive efficacy in matters where the link between cause and cure was less than assured and where knowledge of the individual patient was therefore seen as an important guide to therapeutic action. The public health professional's domain became restricted to intervention where standardized, straightforward approaches would bring results. Public health could not guarantee the fates of individuals, but it could promise significant action from a community-wide perspective.

Not being able to promise to save individuals, only the community-at-large, the professional practice of public health became separated from people, and public health activity, when viewed in contrast to the "miracles" performed by the medical profession, acquired an anonymity that precluded the kind of support that grateful clients can afford professionals who provide personal care. Faced with a *de facto* interprofessional rivalry over the terrain of health knowledge and practice, public health found itself at a

disadvantage, lacking the natural practice links with individual clients which supported the status claims of physicians. Struggling in the turf battle with private-practice medicine, public health professionals attempted to make a virtue of apparent necessity, asserting a self-definition they were, in a sense, being handed by default. Interprofessional rivalry aside, there is little inherent logic in the current assignment of tasks between public health agencies and private physicians. The line between prevention and cure does not correspond neatly to the division between community-based and individual services. Physician-entrepreneurs routinely innoculate patients and thus prevent the spread of disease in the community, while health departments in many localities provide acute medical care to poor persons: evidence that the division of labor between public health and private medicine is rooted in politics rather than in clearly distinguishable domains of professional knowledge.

Conclusions

As the Institute of Medicine study findings imply, the political power of public health, particularly when contrasted to private medicine, is inadequate to develop the support needed to deal with the public health challenges of the present and future. This essay has attempted to make the case that clear organizational focus, increased fiscal resources and other needs of public health will be difficult to marshal as long as public health professionals continue to attempt to insulate practice from the political process. While society depends on public health action grounded in scientific knowledge, the governmental framework in which public health is practiced requires that science be transformed into policy, a process that depends inherently on professional skill in making a political case for expert recommendations. Even purportedly neutral knowledge, history suggests, has political dimensions, because whatever strategies are recommended as "the best way" will inevitably serve some interests and undermine others. This suggests the need for public health professionals to be able to turn their right answers into the good reasons that will win support for their proposals. As the epigraph at the head of this chapter suggests, public sector professionals need a broader form of expertise than do their counterparts in the private sector: they must be "intelligent as to government."

The IOM report cites the dedication and skill of hard-working public health professionals across the country and calls on the nation to begin the process of restoring public health capacity to deal effectively with community health problems, which has eroded in recent years. But as the Progressive reform movement a century ago demonstrates, the call for reform is never, and is never received as, simply a nonpartisan effort to build technical skills and organizational structures. Change in the public sector is inherently political. The politics of public health will not get better until public health professionals get better at politics.

REFERENCES

Bell, Robert. 1985. Professional values and organizational decision making. *Administration and Society* 17:21–60.

Bledstein, Burton. 1976. *The culture of professionalism: The middle class and the development of higher education in America.* New York: Norton.

Duffy, John. 1968. *The history of public health in New York City 1625–1866.* New York: Russell Sage.

Duffy, John. 1978. Social impact of disease in the late 19th century. In *Sickness and health in America: Readings in the history of medicine and public health,* edited by Judith Walzer Leavitt and Ronald L. Numbers, 395–402. Madison, WI: University of Wisconsin Press.

Fee, Elizabeth. 1987. *Disease and discovery: A history of the Johns Hopkins School of Hygiene and Public Health 1916–1939.* Baltimore and London: The Johns Hopkins University Press.

FitzGerald, Frances. 1986. A reporter at large: The Castro—II. *New Yorker* (July 28):44–63.

Fox, Daniel. 1978. Social policy and city politics: Tuberculosis reporting in New York, 1889–1900. In *Sickness and health in America: Readings in the history of medicine and public health,* edited by Judith Walzer Leavitt and Ronald L. Numbers, 415–432. Madison, WI: University of Wisconsin Press.

Freidson, Eliot. 1984. Are professions necessary? In *The authority of experts: Studies in history and the-*

ory, edited by Thomas L. Haskell, 3–27. Bloomington, IN: Indiana University Press.

Gostin, Larry. 1986. The future of communicable disease control: Toward a new concept in public health law. *The Milbank Quarterly* 64 (Supp.): 79–96.

Greenwood, Ernest. 1966. The elements of professionlization. In *professionalization,* edited by Howard M. Vollmer and Donald L. Mills, 9–18. Englewood Cliffs, NJ: Prentice-Hall.

Hanlon, John J. 1969. *Principles of public health administration.* St. Louis: Mosby.

Hays, Samuel P. 1964. The politics of reform in municipal government. *Pacific Northwest Quarterly* 55:157–169.

Institute of Medicine. 1988. *The future of public health.* Washington: National Academy Press.

Leavitt, Judith Walzer. 1982. *The healthiest city: Milwaukee and the politics of health reform.* Princeton, NJ: Princeton University Press.

Meigh, Edward. 1966. Associational goals—business management. In *Professionalization,* edited by Howard M. Vollmer and Donald L. Mills, 162–168. Englewood Cliffs, NJ: Prentice-Hall.

Mosher, Frederick. 1982. *Democracy and the public service.* 2d ed. New York: Oxford.

Pernick, Martin S. 1978. Politics, parties and pestilence: Epidemic yellow fever in philadelphia and the rise of the first party system. In *Sickness and health in America: Readings in the history of medicine and public health,* edited by Judith Walzer Leavitt and Ronald L. Numbers, 241–256. Madison, WI: University of Wisconsin Press.

Rabe, Barry G. 1986. *Fragmentation and integration in state environmental management.* Washington: Conservation Foundation.

Rosenkrantz, Barbara G. 1974. Cart before horse: Theory, practice and professional image in American public health, 1870–1920. *Journal of the History of Medicine* 29:55–73.

Rosenkrantz, Barbara G. 1972. *Public health and the state: Changing views in Massachusetts, 1842–1936.* Cambridge, MA: Harvard University Press.

Schiesl, Martin J. 1977. *The politics of efficiency: Municipal administration and reform in America 1800–1920.* Berkeley, CA: University of California Press.

Schwartz, Joshua Ira. 1977. *Public health: Case studies on the origins of government responsibilities for health services in the United States.* Ithaca, NY: Environmental Health Planning Training Program, Department of City and Regional Planning, Cornell University.

Scott, Ronald Bodley. 1966. Occupational images and norms—Medicine. In *Professionalization,* edited by Howard L. Vollmer and Donald L. Mills, 114–119. Englewood Cliffs, NJ: Prentice-Hall.

Vollmer, Howard L. and Donald L. Mills, eds. 1966. *Professionalization*. Englewood Cliffs, NJ: Prentice-Hall.

Chapter 20

The New Politics of AIDS

Leonard S. Robins
Charles H. Backstrom[1]

Introduction

The discovery of an unusual pattern of diseases among male homosexuals—gays—was reported in June, 1981 (Centers for Disease Control 1981). By the end of the 1980s, Acquired Immune Deficiency Syndrome (AIDS)[2] was one of the most widely known and feared diseases in the United States. Because at least one million people are estimated to carry the AIDS virus (Heywood and Curran 1988), the 1990s will see massive increases in the numbers of people who will need care for the disease, and who will die from it. Even discovery of an effective vaccine or great reduction in all the various types of behaviors that spread the disease—both highly doubtful in the short run—will not eliminate AIDS as a major health problem at least through the last decade of the Twentieth Century.

An intense debate has ensued over what should be the appropriate public policy response to this epidemic. Because AIDS is a gruesome disease that may invariably be terminal,[3] because its virus carriers can transmit the disease without themselves showing symptoms, and because it primarily affects socially disdained groups of people, the disease is a special blend of sex, drugs, and death suffused with value dimensions that make health policy formation regarding it intensely political.

In an earlier article (Backstrom and Robins 1989) we established a conceptual framework for

[1]The authors wish to thank William Hathaway, James Karpiac, and Patrick Lenihan for their comments on earlier drafts of this chapter.

[2]For purposes of this article we will refer to the Human Immunodeficiency virus (HIV) that produces AIDS as the AIDS virus. We will also refer to the diseases that appear because of the breakdown of the immune system as AIDS, and follow the Centers for Disease Control (CDC).

[3]We are not here concerned as to whether the AIDS virus inevitably leads to death or whether AIDS inevitably leads to death, because the very high percentages of both of those occurrences dictate the same public policy responses.

analyzing the political aspects of policy issues faced in dealing with AIDS in the United States (see Table 20–1). Here we deal with the five major goals of AIDS policy outlined there, but in a different way. This chapter takes up each policy goal in turn, beginning with the thrust of early writings on the subject. Next, present realities are contrasted with this "conventional wisdom." Then present policy issues are explained, with specific attention given to the political dimensions of various controversies. The chapter concludes by indicating how the overall shape of the American polity and society and its health care delivery system have affected AIDS policy, and, conversely, how experience with AIDS is likely to affect the American polity and society and its health care delivery system.

One final preliminary point. Public policy choices concerning AIDS cannot (or perhaps more appropriately should not) be based merely on abstract values. Rather, effective decision-making will have to recognize that medical science and technologies concerning AIDS are rapidly evolving, and the resulting changes require adjustments in policy response. This point will be illustrated frequently in the analysis.

Comprehending the Extent of AIDS

Nearly all the authors studying the initial indifference to AIDS emphasize the long delay in getting the Reagan Administration to recognize its seriousness and significance. This is usually attributed to hostility to those initially primarily at risk—gays (Shilts 1987).

While there is still considerable dispute about the scope and magnitude of the epidemic, *all* public policy makers now consider AIDS a very serious health issue demanding major governmental endeavors. Not a single member of Congress, to the best of our knowledge, has argued that biomedical funding for AIDS research should be dramatically cut "because only gays and drug users get the disease."

The major debate today regarding the extent of AIDS is over the chances that AIDS will break out extensively into the general heterosexual population. Public health officials have to be very careful about the impressions they give as they

try to lead the discussion on this issue. They must steer a careful course between downplaying the threat of AIDS and overdramatizing it. The present and probable future magnitude of AIDS presses them toward emphasizing the threat in order that their programs receive sufficient attention and funding to deal effectively with it. Yet overdramatizing the threat could incite panic that would produce policies that are simultaneously both harsh and counterproductive.

The current consensus is that AIDS in the next few years is likely to be largely confined to gays, bisexuals, IV-drug users, and the sexual partners of bisexuals and IV-drug users—that is, that AIDS will not become widely distributed in the rest of the population. Nonetheless, stressing the magnitude of the AIDS threat constitutes good public health policy. First, understatement, in contrast, diminishes the perceived seriousness of the threat, delays behavior change, and thereby might even contribute to a breakout into the low-risk population. Second, despite today's reduced fear, if substantial numbers of people were ever to suspect that health professionals had underestimated the danger, loud calls would be heard demanding much more repressive measures than most health professionals would propose even under very pessimistic scenarios. Thus, by presenting data in an overly optimistic way, the results might ultimately be an overreaction rather than the serious but sober consideration health professionals hope for.

The most notable current trend in the spread of AIDS is the relative shift in those acquiring the AIDS virus away from gays and to intravenous (IV)-drug users. Thus, because of the greater prevalence of IV-drug users among the "underclass," and although there are numerous African-American and Hispanic gays and white IV-drug users, the disease is increasingly becoming one of people of color. The special growth of AIDS among African-Americans is contributing to, but, it must be emphasized, is only one cause of, the worsening status of African-American health in the United States. In 1987 and 1988 African-American mortality in absolute and not just relative terms *increased* in the United States (Rice and Winn, ch. 17 in this volume). Clearly, the problem of AIDS in minority communities will not be solved in isolation from solutions to their overall health and socioeconomic problems.

Selected Political Aspects of Aids Policy

A. Goals of AIDS Policy	B. Policy Decisions Required	C. Political Aspects of Decisions	D. Recommended Political Strategies
1. Comprehending the seriousness of AIDS as a health problem.	Developing the appropriate level of policy; response to it.	Downplaying the potential threat fails to generate sufficient support for strong action; overdramatizing the threat leads to hysteria and ineffective, draconian action.	When there is legitimate uncertainty, err on the side of emphasizing risks.
2. Research on prevention and treatments.	a. Determining roles of various types of research in overall program against AIDS. b. Whether to speed drug approval.	a. Temptation to see problems solely as biomedical. b. Strong pressures for fast approval.	a. Emphasize no magic bullet. b. Accelerate general FDA reform.
3. Finding those who have been exposed.	a. Deciding whether to test. b. Voluntary or compulsory testing. c. Getting high-risk people located and tested.	a. Strong consensus in U.S. on testing. b. Public health v. individual rights. c. Fear of social and economic discrimination.	a. Support appropriate testing. b. Argue cost-effectiveness. c. Shift case for antidiscrimination from ideological to results-oriented criteria.
4. Prevention of spread.	a. Establishing the degree of personal restriction. b. Insuring availability of counseling. c. Choosing the appropriate type of education. d. Assuring use of clean needles.	a. Superficial attractiveness of counterproductive overregulation. b. Giving benefits to unpopular groups. c. Appearance of condoning unpopular behavior. d. Abetting illegal behavior by providing clean needles.	a. Stress individual responsibility backed up by civil commitment for wanton behavior and criminal penalties for assault. b. Target counseling at high-risk people; education for low-risk. c. Use voluntary groups for explicit messages. d. Consider local political culture.
5. Care of victims.	a. Limiting denial of insurance. b. Obtaining accessible, cost-effective, and quality care.	a. Resistance by private insurers to absorbing costs of AIDS. b. Bias toward "high-tech" health care.	a. Emphasize role of insurance availability for AIDS control. b. Reform of national health system.

TABLE 20–1

Research Toward Biomedical Prevention and Treatment

After an initially slow start that drew much criticism from AIDS activists, funding for biomedical research grew dramatically from $3.4 million in 1982 to $603 million in 1988 (Smith 1989), boosting the National Institute of Allergies and Infectious Diseases from a small division into one of the largest within the National Institutes of Health (NIH). Perhaps even more important, a much higher proportion of grant requests for AIDS research was being funded than for other diseases.

This increase should not, in retrospect, have been surprising. Research funding is politically the easiest public policy on AIDS to achieve, for two reasons. First, the American public overestimates the ability to solve social and medical problems quickly by research leading to a technological "fix." Second, funding biomedical research to relieve human suffering is above ideology; it is the one form of action on which the political left (Senator Edward Kennedy, Dem., Mass.) and right (Senator Jesse Helms, Rep., N.C.) can agree (Rovner 1987).

The current challenge to increased funding of biomedical research on AIDS comes not primarily from those who downgrade the seriousness of AIDS, but rather from those who feel that the explosion in funding for research on AIDS has resulted in an unfair deemphasis of research on diseases they feel are more important.

This "war of the diseases" may truly be a case of fighting the wrong enemy. Several rather obvious statements about possible effects of large expenditures on AIDS research can be made: that an unwillingness by the national government to raise taxes means more use of tough comparative cost-benefit analyses of programs; that, other things being equal, closely-related programs (cancer) are more likely to be cut than unrelated programs (defense); and that research scientists in the late 1980s somewhat shifted their attention to AIDS as the "hot" new subject. But against these assertions it can be said, first, that much biomedical research is basic in nature and has general applicability to many diseases. The knowledge gained from the study of the immune system—a key element in AIDS research—

is, for example, likely to have real benefits for the treatment and possible cure of many other diseases. Second, the argument that AIDS research funding takes money away from cancer or other biomedical research implies a fixed-sum allotment for biomedical research, that is, a zero-sum game. No empirical evidence has been presented for this assertion. While it is true that the Reagan Administration tried to fund biomedical research on AIDS out of existing funds for other NIH research, Congress successfully resisted this strategy and funded AIDS research with "new money."

What does seem likely is that the recent wide dissemination of information on the high level of biomedical research spending on AIDS compared to that for other major diseases (Winkenweider, Kessler, and Stolec 1989) will provide effective ammunition necessary for those who wish to cap spending for biomedical research on AIDS, that is, not cut spending, but end the explosive increase in funds provided for this purpose. This would in any event have been inevitable in the next few years—massive budget expansions for even the most worthwhile endeavor cannot continue indefinitely.

Another pressing biomedical research public policy issue is the time it takes the Food and Drug Administration (FDA) to approve drugs for treating AIDS and its symptomatic diseases. One of the main early complaints of AIDS activists was that the FDA has been a "bottleneck" in getting effective drugs from the laboratory to the patient.

In recent years, however, the political pressures brought by persons with AIDS (PWAs) and their supporters have caused the FDA to drastically shorten and simplify the process required to gain FDA approval of drugs that might alleviate the symptomatic diseases produced by AIDS (Spector 1989). It must be further pointed out that FDA overcaution is not unique to AIDS. Indeed it really is not the product of bureaucratic torpitude, but rather results from a Congressional mandate in the Kefauver/Harris 1962 Amendments to the Pure Food and Drug Act, which were triggered by the thalidomide scare and the resulting feeling that extraordinary care should be taken before approving new drugs (Harris 1964).

The dispute about AIDS drugs is thus only another in a series of long-running attacks on the FDA's procedures for introducing new drugs. Experts have long contended that negative health consequences due to excessive delays in introducing new drugs exceed the health benefits of delaying their introduction to safeguard against unanticipated negative side effects, or from using drugs that turn out to be ineffective (Fuchs 1974). Up to now, public pressure for faster FDA approval for AIDS drugs has had a slight spillover in improving and simplifying procedures for approval of drugs for other health problems. Certainly it would be preferable to focus on general reform of FDA procedures rather than to keep making exceptions for AIDS drugs, but one cannot expect AIDS advocates to take a long-term perspective on this question.

No one should anticipate an AIDS vaccine or medication for a full cure in the short run. But remarkably rapid progress has been made by developing predictors for the onset of AIDS symptoms (T-helper cell counts), prophylaxis to stave off the principal opportunistic disease characteristic of AIDS (pentamidine spray against pneumocystis pneumonia), and drugs to delay the progress of the disease to total disability and death (AZT). Trials are underway to identify predictors of the onset of the disease and to inhibit early replication of the AIDS virus (Rhame and Maki 1989).

In the long run, science is likely to be much more successful in preventing and treating AIDS, but drugs will never completely eliminate AIDS. Experience has shown that declining cases reduce fear, awareness, and employment of vaccines and curative drugs. In addition, as with syphilis and gonorrhea, drug-resistant strains appear. A truly "magic bullet" for AIDS is unlikely (Brandt 1988).

Finding Those Who Have Been Exposed

It might seem obvious that the attempt to control AIDS should be based on public health methods traditionally used for other infectious diseases: surveillance of the disease's spread, testing those who are at high risk of contracting the disease, reporting to public health officials the names of people with the disease, and tracing and treating their contacts. But AIDS differs from other infectious diseases in several notable respects. First, symptoms are long delayed, requiring getting people to test who don't feel or look sick. Second, those primarily at risk of acquiring the disease are engaging in behavior that is either technically illegal, or at least morally frowned upon by large majorities of the public. Third, those having AIDS or even the AIDS virus often report being subject to discrimination resulting in loss of jobs and housing. Finally, whereas diseases such as gonorrhea can be cured with penicillin, there is no known cure for AIDS at the present time.

Gay activists, given their understandable fears of harassment by government agents and discrimination in civil society, were initially suspicious of all AIDS testing programs. Now most—though not all—gay spokesman are supportive of voluntary and anonymous testing, but typically oppose mandatory testing, mandatory reporting to public health authorities of those who test positive for the AIDS virus, and programs of government contact tracing—"partner notification" (Bayer 1989). Initially, the impetus for the change was on the growing realization of the serious threat that AIDS presented to gays, but now the primary reason is the aforementioned development of drugs to prevent or at least delay the onset of some of the typically fatal opportunistic diseases associated with AIDS. Before these drugs there was no obvious positive medical benefit to offer to induce someone to undergo AIDS testing despite possible negative social consequences.

Nevertheless, gay spokesman continue to strongly insist that unless confidentiality and anti-discrimination ordinances are enacted, preventive public health programs such as testing are doomed to failure, because at-risk populations will not cooperate in activities that have the by-product of placing them at still greater risk of economic and social discrimination.

Analytically, the debate over testing is usually framed in terms of *widespread, mandatory* testing. These two points, however, while related, are not interchangeable. One has to do with *compulsion,* the other with *scope.*

The political dimension of this question is that as long as the issue of massive mandatory testing is conceptualized as one of public health versus the right to privacy, the movement for massive mandatory testing will remain strong and have frequent, albeit not universal, success. AIDS is the classic kind of public health issue for which politicians and the public are willing to override civil liberties. What must instead be emphasized is the *impracticality* of mandatory mass testing.

One can oppose mandatory testing of very large groups solely on the basis of cost-effectiveness. Ultimately this was successfully done in Illinois and Louisiana, where laws requiring AIDS tests before issuance of marriage licenses were repealed. In Illinois, the incentive to repeal came from the showing that these tests cost over $200,000 for each case of AIDS virus found and deprived counties bordering on Indiana and Wisconsin of approximately 20 percent of their expected marriage license fees (Pierson and Egler 1989).

Moreover, massive testing is likely to overburden present high-quality laboratories and lead to the use of marginal facilities which will be created to handle the increased demand. This will inevitably result in many people being diagnosed as having the AIDS virus who in fact do not ("false positives"), causing them undue hardship in the period their status remains uncorrected.

Mandatory testing is also unwise for the two main groups at highest risk for AIDS—gays and IV drug users. While it would certainly be desirable if members of these groups were tested, making it compulsory would be highly unproductive. Members of these groups already have strong incentives to be "invisible"; attempting to force them to test (no one has offered a practical proposal on how this could be done anyway) would only hurt the battle against AIDS by driving them away from the health care system.

Mandatory testing, however, does not necessarily involve large groups. One might well consider mandatory testing for certain especially endangered and relatively easy-to-regulate populations, such as prisoners and convicted prostitutes, although even with these there are complications.

The vital current challenges are how to increase the rate of voluntary testing among those likely to be carrying or acquiring the AIDS virus and how to increase reporting and partner notification of those testing positive without discouraging people from being tested. While nobody knows the exact number of persons with the AIDS virus, everybody agrees that the vast majority of people—over 80 percent—with the virus and those at high-risk of getting it have not been tested (Presidential Commission on the Human Immunodeficiency Virus Epidemic 1988).

Medical personnel who have been exposed to the blood of a patient typically want to know as quickly as possible whether they have received the AIDS virus (Rhame 1989). Why do gays and IV-drug users and their advocates seem to have a different attitude? One cannot know for sure, but there is clearly one major difference—the perception among high-risk groups that they will suffer dire social and economic discrimination if they have the virus. This includes job loss, social discrimination, ostracism from family, loss of health insurance, even criminal charges; indeed, the threat is felt to be present just for having the test, even if it turns out to be negative.

An obvious response is to enact laws that forbid discrimination against those having the AIDS virus or AIDS, or encourage interpretations of existing laws forbidding discrimination against the disabled to include those who have the AIDS virus or AIDS. Expanding anti-discrimination statutes is never easy politically, and has proved especially difficult when it involves homosexuals and drug users, but the desperate need to control AIDS presents an opportunity to shift the case for such laws from one about the desirability of protecting a discriminated-against group to the argument that essential disease control mechanisms cannot work without first lowering discrimination.

Recognizing the unlikelihood of complete fairness and tolerance, however, absolute privacy of information about being tested and test results must be assured. Yet if high-risk persons do volunteer for testing, and test positive, failure to report results and notify partners is a disservice to society. This juxtaposition of seemingly inconsistent aims can be resolved by gaining greater understanding and acceptance of the distinction that public health officials make between *anonymity* and *confidentiality*. Anonymity for those testing positive means that only they know they have it. Confidentiality means that those they don't want to know they have it don't in fact find out. While reporting a positive test to a health department sacrifices anonymity, a person with the AIDS virus obviously needs to be referred to a physician, and should be advised to seek the support of friends and other available services that will eventually be needed, which also is impossible with anonymity. Thus, true anonymity is not desirable.

But quite in contrast is confidentiality. One's employers, workmates, and personal service vendors are typically not in danger and have no need to know one's AIDS-virus status. Thus complete professionalism and legal protections to assure confidentiality are required. The highly successful record of public health agencies in maintaining confidentiality must be stressed, thereby diminishing the exaggerated fears, especially of gays, of breaches of professional responsibility in this regard. Other *medical* providers have been less fastidious about confidentiality, and to close this gap, tighter legal requirements and penalties may well need to be devised.

Overcoming resistance to testing and reporting is only the first task of public health authorities. Their traditional techniques also require tracing the sexual or needle-sharing contacts of those testing positive for AIDS. This adds a new dimensions of privacy invasion—telling others and trying to get them to test. The perceived threat of this is often greater than of getting oneself tested.

To avoid these disincentives to testing, some alternative test sites have stressed anonymity to the point of sacrificing all reporting and contact tracing. Yet the case for the traditional public health approach is now clearly stronger than it would have been even as late as the mid-1980s, because the previously mentioned new drug therapies mean that partner notification has moved beyond being an important element of health education to becoming an important possible medical benefit to those being notified.

One possible way out of serious conflict between advocates of anonymous testing and mandatory reporting is for public health departments to persuade, and if necessary pressure, health providers and counselors to go beyond technical delivery of services and advocate to their patients the benefits of cooperating with the health department in reporting and partner notification. Increased reporting and contact tracing obviously benefits the public's health, but will also

ultimately benefit patients psychologically by enabling them to take a major step in helping to fight AIDS. Conversely, if clinicians downplay the benefits of reporting and partner notification, patients are unlikely to cooperate, and if pushed by attempts at mandatory reporting, are likely to frustrate the whole effort by giving false names.

One pair of AIDS researchers/clinicians, despairing of achieving satisfactory levels of testing through any of these means, advocate universal (but voluntary) testing of anyone coming in contact with health providers—such as at every physical examination—believing this will remove the stigma and fear of testing because it will then be routine (Rhame and Maki 1989). But it is doubtful that the benefits would justify the major expenditures for physicians' costly time and for the tests and laboratory work required. The tens of millions of additional AIDS tests would also magnify the strain on laboratories and the number of people enduring the consequences of false positive test results.

A policy question that will likely soon emerge is *how* people should be tested. A new, at-home test kit for AIDS is available as a potential possible alternative method for testing, which, it is widely agreed, has substantial reliability and lower cost than on-site testing. It also provides anonymity both in fact and appearance.

These features might be particularly helpful to the drive for increased testing, but there are good reasons for the FDA to have not yet approved home testing kits. Not only are reporting and notification lost, but even more critical, all authorities believe the severe psychological shock upon receiving proof that one has the AIDS virus can best be dealt with by personal counseling (Institute of Medicine 1988).

The determinative question is, therefore, whether at-home testing would primarily be used by those who would or would not otherwise get tested. If its primary effect is *increased testing of the untested,* it would seem to be a good idea. If, however, it primarily shifts present testing from the clinic or physician's office to the home, the judgment on home testing should be based on whether savings in costs outweigh the loss of counseling, as well as one's beliefs about the "right" to have as an option an alternative that public health professionals regard as inferior.

Prevention of Spread

Despite the concentration of public health officials on testing/reporting/tracing, the implication that their absence is the core of the AIDS problem is a major oversimplification. Testing, reporting, and tracing by themselves do not prevent the spread of the AIDS virus. And, as has been mentioned, there is currently no drug that can be given to those who test positive for AIDS that will make them non-communicable, nor a vaccine that can be given to still negative partners that will prevent them from getting the AIDS virus. Only modification of risky behavior can prevent people from spreading or acquiring the AIDS virus.

AIDS activists were greatly apprehensive that fear of AIDS—coupled with hatred for gays—would lead to repressive physical restrictions on those having, or being at high risk of getting, the virus, in the name of preventing the spread of the disease. They strongly oppose such proposals as quarantine in themselves, but they also warn that such extreme proposals or even milder restrictions are counterproductive in that they will decrease cooperation by high-risk groups.

Public health authorities also oppose most proposals for restriction, for such measures typically are both unfairly harsh and punitive and unlikely to be effective in this, the most individualistic society in the world. Successful opposition to these proposals, however, lies in understanding the reasons for their appeal, and responding to them in a manner that reduces that appeal.

The operative political reality is, as was true in the debate over mandatory testing, that as long as the issue is conceptualized as one of public health versus the right to privacy, the movement for repressive restrictions will remain strong. Proposals for restriction are politically attractive to elected officials, because enacting them gives the appearance that public officials are being decisive in time of crisis. The battle probably will be lost unless the *impracticality* of most of the proposed restrictions is somehow made the central issue.

Support for quarantine, for example, arises because of a false analogy of AIDS to other diseases, such as tuberculosis or typhoid. Quarantine could be argued for a disease like tuberculosis, which can be spread by the presence of an infected person in the same room, although it should be noted that history suggests that quarantine in itself is often not a successful policy even for such diseases (Musto 1986). Likewise, occupational restrictions can legitimately be sought for a disease like typhoid, where an infected person should not handle food. Neither of these situations is true of AIDS because AIDS is not spread through casual contacts.

Some who do not advocate quarantine have nonetheless proposed defining certain acts as crimes. One of these would be intentionally spreading AIDS. Another would be wanton promiscuity by a known AIDS carrier. A third could be the transmission of the disease even without prior knowledge of one's virus status.

The task for health professionals is to emphasize that these are differing problems requiring different solutions. In fact, there is probably no need for new law on the intentional spreading of AIDS, since assault is likely to be covered by present statutes. In the case of non-compliance by an AIDS carrier who has been warned to stop his/her behavior, civil commitment procedures, carefully hedged by due process, could be used. Criminalizing consensual behavior that risks transmission of AIDS when neither partner believes they have it, is in truth only a modernized call for new and tougher sodomy laws. Public health authorities typically vigorously resist these sometimes politically popular proposals for criminalizing AIDS because they believe a punitive stance would seriously weaken the fight against AIDS by lessening cooperation in both testing, reporting, and notification, and in programs of health education and behavior modification that are most essential to combat the disease.

But opposing even the mildest non-criminal restrictions on wanton behavior could boomerang. Not only can a strong case be made for taking action against those intentionally and knowingly spreading AIDS, but even more important, unless action is taken against the few that might deliberately spread the disease, the public may well mistakenly demand more intrusive legislation to curb sodomy in the belief that public health officials are not doing enough to stop the spread of AIDS. Carefully describing the egregious degree of behavior that is sought to be curbed, and tailoring reasonable and productive restrictions, should both make thoughtful policy choices more probable and avoid serious chilling of cooperation on the part of the vast majority of affected people who do not wish to harm others.

Voluntary programs of health education and behavior modification to prevent the spread of AIDS are currently the most important steps that can be taken in the fight against AIDS. Unfortunately, actually stopping the spread of AIDS requires behavior changes of the most personal nature. Adjusting sexual activities and methods of drug use are extremely difficult, and scientific knowledge about how this can be accomplished is limited.

Yet change is not impossible. As a result of AIDS, gays in recent years have greatly, though far from totally, reduced their risky behavior, demonstrating that change is possible in even such an elemental function as sexual behavior. This has been especially true for those who test positive for the AIDS virus, contrary to the impression people reading about Patient Zero (Shilts 1987) might have. Those who test negative also reduce their risk, though many fewer do so (Coates, Morin, and McKusick 1987).

Significant permanent behavior change is likely to require substantial counseling. But counseling is very expensive, because it usually involves face-to-face contact with a professional, one-to-one, or at most in small groups. Moreover, the amount of counseling available is limited by the supply of trained personnel.

Needle-sharing drug users present special problems in the control of AIDS. Already engaged in self-destructive behavior, they are the least amenable high-risk group to educational and counseling programs. Yet evidence indicates that even they are changing somewhat the manner in which they use needles as a result of their fear of AIDS (Green and Miller 1987).

Some public health officials favor reducing the risk of AIDS transmission among IV-drug users by programs to provide free needles, for example through needle exchange—requiring that a used needle be turned in before a clean one is handed out. All available empirical evidence (admittedly limited) shows that needle provision not only reduces AIDS, but it also leads drug addicts to be more likely to apply for treatment programs (Lambert 1988). The reason seems to be that

such programs give addicts an increasing feeling that they can alter or modify their way of life and also a feeling of increased trust (or lessening of distrust) in the promise of public authorities that they want to *help* addicts overcome their addiction and not just *punish* them for their addiction.

These programs are highly controversial, because they appear to abet drug use. It is significant that in the United States these programs are typically occurring in states such as New York, Oregon, and Washington that have liberal political cultures. Some state and local health professionals who favor free needle exchange do not advocate it because they fear it would not be worth the cost of possible political backlash that would imperil possibly more beneficial programs.

Perhaps the most productive action that could currently be taken in preventing AIDS is expansion of drug-treatment programs to handle the large numbers of abusers awaiting assistance (Presidential Commission on the Human Immunodeficiency Virus Epidemic 1988). It is distressing to note that the implementors of the war on drugs in the Bush Administration seem to have used the valid insight that the ultimate solution is reduction in the demand for drugs as a basis for increasing the resources for punishing rather than treating drug addicts (Barrett 1989).

Concentrating on prevention of the spread of AIDS by persons presently known to have the virus has often obscured an even more fundamental aspect of stopping the epidemic—getting people who do not have the virus to accept the responsibility for their own continued safety. This requires new directions in education and counseling, and a new urgency for it. Persuading heterosexuals who do not perceive themselves at risk and teenagers who typically think they are invulnerable are hefty challenges.

Some state are responding by requiring local schools to institute an AIDS curriculum, often beginning in early grades. But this runs into long-standing and well-organized opposition to any kind of public sex education. The most common fear of the opponents is that discussion of sexual behaviors appears to condone or even advocate them. Worries are increased because most authorities believe anti-AIDS messages must be explicit enough to force people to identify their own behaviors as risky and to visualize themselves enjoying new practices (Brandt 1988).

Unfortunately, pointing out that United States teenage girls have both the highest abortion and out-of-wedlock birth rate in the Western world, while not having any higher rate of sexual intercourse (Kantrowitz, Hager, et al. 1987) has not seemed to be able to convince the opponents of effective sex education of its necessity. Still, the fear of AIDS provides a further persuasive argument for those who believe in the necessity of effective sex education, and the fact that there is new money for AIDS education indirectly provides a boost for all sex education (Kenney, Guardado, and Brown 1989).

Two final points: first, education by public authorities is less persuasive than if done by private groups, especially by peers (Green and Miller 1987). Thus, subsidizing voluntary groups to carry out AIDS education is likely to be more efficient and also may help blunt, though not totally divert, the opposition of groups who object to having public officials involved with sex education. Second, standardized educational materials are probably not sufficient to reach minorities. Messages will be more effective when tailored and delivered by people who understand specific cultural constraints and opportunities.

Care of Patients

AIDS activists were very critical of the initial response of the health care delivery system to the problem of caring for PWAs. They bitterly noted that those few physicians and institutions who were willing to treat AIDS patients were viewed as second-class citizens by the medical community. Again, they attributed this reaction to general homophobia among both providers and funders (Shilts 1987).

AIDS activists also condemned the loss of health insurance for those who test positive for the AIDS virus as being both unjust and a barrier to testing and seeking medical care. They also complained about the acute-care emphasis of much of the treatment for AIDS, with many arguing that alternatives to hospital-based care would simultaneously both improve quality and decrease cost. Nevertheless, things have improved somewhat in recent years.

First, an increasing percentage of care for PWAs is now community-based. The San Francisco model is increasingly recognized as the ideal to be striven for, and not only in caring for PWAs. Second, though no insurance company can be forced to issue policies to persons with pre-existing conditions, such as testing positive for the AIDS virus, at least a few states forbid insurance companies from excluding persons who are thought to be at high risk of getting AIDS from coverage through establishing overly broad exclusions based on occupations stereotyped as attracting gays (Hatch 1989). Finally, associates of medical personnel and health institutions have reiterated the professional duty of providers to care for everyone—including AIDS patients (Goldsmith 1987). This makes the role of state regulators in enforcing non-discrimination—for example against nursing homes who do not want to take AIDS patients—less politically controversial, because the government is acting against individuals and institutions who are not meeting professional norms.

Projecting the total cost of handling the care for PWAs is not simple. Clearly, costs will increase dramatically in coming years, because, as previously noted, the number of those already carrying the AIDS virus who develop the opportunistic diseases that signal AIDS will dramatically increase.

A more theoretically interesting question for purposes of policy analysis however is whether—adjusted for inflation—costs *per case* for those with AIDS will increase or decrease in coming years. One scholar (Hellinger 1988) argues that these costs will decrease because AIDS is increasingly being treated on an outpatient, community-based model rather than in inpatient hospital facilities. It is important to note, however, that this author (for good methodological reasons) did not include in his study those who had the AIDS virus but did not have the disease. Moreover, his analysis, as he himself emphasized, did not consider the cost effects of treatment that might extend the length of life for people with AIDS. Therefore, if improved drug therapies are discovered and distributed that delay the progression of the virus, of actual AIDS, and/or of death, one quite possible unpleasant side effect will be to increase the cost of caring for each person with the virus or AIDS.

Long experience with "intermediate health

care technologies"—those that ameliorate but do not solve the health problem—suggests that they typically tend to be "add-ons" rather than "replacements for" other means of dealing with a patient and that they hence typically ultimately increase costs (Evans 1984). If AIDS, as many health professionals are now asserting, is becoming a "chronic" disease, then experience with the costs of chronic diseases should provide a sober warning to anyone who thinks the problems of controlling costs for AIDS will be easily solved.

Nonetheless, it is possible that more familiarity with treating AIDS patients will both increase quality and result in cost savings that will overpower the cost increasing effects of drugs that help, but do not cure. It is even more necessary to emphasize that the benefits from the new drugs that will undoubtedly be developed for people with AIDS will probably be worth well more than their costs. This is true because the AIDS drugs already developed are prolonging the time in which individuals can lead a high quality of life and be economically productive members of society rather than merely keeping people very sick longer (Simpson 1989). If, however, newly-to-be-discovered drugs to fight AIDS delay death but not debilitating illness, then their cost-benefit balance would be much more problematic.

Another health care issue that may arise for PWAs is their eligibility for Medicare. AIDS patients are eligible, like others considered disabled, for Medicare after they have been diagnosed as having the disease for two years. While some of the elderly have grumbled about payments from "their" program going to AIDS patients, until now this has not been a serious issue, simply because the vast majority of people with AIDS died before they became eligible for Medicare. But this will be less and less true in coming years. In addition to the war of the diseases, then, the predominantly young AIDS patients could become unwilling participants in a war of the generations.

AIDS in General Perspective

AIDS is an obviously extremely grave disease, but it is still only one disease. We wish, therefore, to conclude by examining AIDS, even if by necessity somewhat speculatively, in the overall context of the American political and social system generally and its health care delivery system in particular. Our aim will be to answer two questions, each of which has three parts: how have the American political and social systems and its health care delivery system shaped how we have dealt with AIDS, and how has AIDS affected our overall political and social systems and health care delivery system?

How Has the American Political System Affected AIDS

In what respects, if any, has AIDS policy developed differently from what would have been predicted given the structure and operation of the American political system?

Perhaps the easiest way to present our views on this question is by contrasting them in part with those of Sandra Panem (1988) on how the United States government should have been organized to fight AIDS at the outset and how it should be organized to fight future health emergencies (Robins and Backstrom 1989).

In brief, Panem argues that the United States' effort against AIDS has not been coordinated; there has been no overall strategy regarding research, testing, tracking, or education, nor any overall plan for organizing and financing health care delivery to those suffering from AIDS.

Panem recommends reorganization under a "czar" of many federal agencies to bring about the necessary coordination to handle AIDS and any future emergencies. This would be intended to end the bureaucratic infighting among several National Institutes of Health (NIH), the Centers for Disease Control (CDC), the Health Care Financing Administration (HCFA), Health Services and Resources Administration (HSRA), the Alcohol, Drug Abuse and Mental Health Administration (ADAMHA), Food and Drug Administration (FDA), National Science Foundation (NSF), Veterans Administration (VA), and Department of Defense (DOD). An undersecretary in the Department of Health and Human Services for health emergencies is seen as the answer to solve the coordination problems. This prescription can be challenged on the grounds that single-agency (or czar) control might possibly sacrifice healthy multiple experimentation and competition in attacking AIDS. Would the decisions of an emergency manager necessarily be better than those that have been made up to now?

Panem also advocates a pre-appropriated emergency fund, with great executive flexibility as to how it could be used. This would bypass the slow bargaining of the federal budget process, escape Gramm-Rudman-Hollings reductions, and soften the impact of health emergencies on local governments where they hit first. Yet even if Congress could be persuaded to tolerate a large fund lying around in a period of perpetual budget deficits, disputes would still arise as to whether a disease should be called an emergency, with attendant lobbying and political intervention. An enduring recrimination about AIDS is, after all, that it was not seen by appropriate federal agencies to be an emergency for some years. Moreover, at what point would a disease cease to qualify as an emergency?

Panem also wants to sort out clearly the responsibilities of federal, state, and local governments, essentially bringing the latter under federal direction during health emergencies. But calling for national government dominance in dealing with AIDS ignores the very real gains in competence that are evident among the states (Lipson, ch. 9 in this volume). In fact it has been argued that there has been a relative lack of federal involvement in AIDS policy and a relatively vigorous state response (Lipson, ch. 9 in this volume). It should be noted, however, that federal expenditure on AIDS are much greater, and they are likely to increase further when AIDS patients in proportionately greater numbers begin to qualify for Medicare. Moreover, at the local level it is surprising how much San Francisco and New York City have done with relatively little help from their respective state governments, though the fact that these cities have many resources and are politically liberal should perhaps have made this more expected. Nonetheless, the point that AIDS *policy* has been largely state-based rather than "made in Washington" is largely true, and thus is in broad consonance with the American political system.

In summary, the localistic, incremental nature of AIDS policymaking is very much shaped by the general contours of the American political system. This is not to say that bold action is impossible, but given the *gradual* realization of the seriousness of the AIDS problem, in part caused by the initial inability of most gay activists to grasp the full implications of AIDS, this should not have been expected. Moreover, even bold action is likely to occur "American style," that is, with major roles assigned to state and local governments and the private sector. Advocates for effective AIDS policy who ignore the American political system's "way of doing business" put their entire effort in jeopardy.

How Has American Society Affected AIDS

American values have also greatly shaped the American response to AIDS. While a majority of Americans as measured by public opinion polls seem in the abstract to believe Americans have a right to guaranteed health care and economic security, those same polls show strong resistance to the increased taxes necessary to effectuate such rights (Rochefort, ch. 13 in this volume). It should not be surprising, therefore, that the onset of AIDS has often meant the loss of employment and the attendant loss of health insurance, the combination leading to impoverishment.

Americans in their role as private individuals have been warm and generous in their willingness to help those with AIDS more than perhaps could have been expected given their biases. In their roles as public citizens and taxpayers, however, Americans have maintained their expected conservatism. Here also, therefore, things have been pretty much as might have been predicted.

More positively, the American emphasis on individual freedom and willingness to tolerate diversity has resulted, until now, in an avoidance of the governmental repression against those with AIDS and gays in general that many greatly feared. The imposition of quarantine has become the policy of Castro's Cuba, not that of the United States (Bayer 1988).

Let us conclude this section with a conjecture. How would United States policy toward AIDS have differed if it had been a disease primarily of white heterosexuals? First, we believe it certainly would have been taken seriously earlier and more intensely by government at all levels and society as a whole. Second, while funding for biomedical research, would, we believe, have accelerated even faster than it did, it is unlikely that spending would *now* be at a considerably higher level than it is. Third, the pressures on the FDA would, we believe, have been even greater and therefore would probably have resulted in an even faster changing of its standards for drug approval, though again things might not be much different *now*.

While some of the policy problems in dealing with AIDS would have been greatly reduced if it had been a white, middle-class disease, some of the problems that did occur might in fact have been exacerbated. In particular, a strong argument can even be made that if AIDS were a disease that struck randomly, pressures for restriction might have even been greater, for as long as AIDS was perceived as largely a disease of gays and drug users, there was less panic among the general public.

On balance, of course, early public policy decisions would have been better if AIDS were a disease the majority of the public could perceive getting. But explaining AIDS policy—especially *now*—as almost solely a function of attitudes toward those most likely to get it would be a serious error.

How Has the Health System Affected AIDS?

AIDS policy has been greatly affected by the general characteristics of the nation's overall health care system.

First, the problem of obtaining insurance and paying for health care for PWAs is only too real, but this problem is not uniquely AIDS-specific. Individual employers and health insurers are increasingly seeking to screen applicants for drug use, alcoholism, and other diseases—not just AIDS. Moreover, there is a growing trend of employers either offering no insurance at all, or requiring increasing cost-sharing from their employees (Fraser, ch. 16 in this volume).

Second, although the French were at least equally responsible for the discovery of AIDS (Shilts 1987), most of the major biomedical research on AIDS has been done in the United

States, and it is likely that if a vaccine and cure are found for AIDS, they will be found here. There is nothing unusual in this, for the United States is far and away the world's leader in biomedical research, probably doing more than the rest of the world combined.

Finally, given the weakness of public health in the United States (Stivers, ch. 19 in this volume), the relative success so far experienced by public health professionals in influencing the debate over AIDS is pleasantly surprising. Whether in the "hard" public health of testing, reporting and tracing, or the "soft" public health of opposition to restrictions like quarantine and emphasis on voluntary action for behavioral change, public health professionals have emerged as the group with the most influence in public policymaking on AIDS.

How Has AIDS Affected the Political System?

The reverse side of the question of how AIDS policy has been shaped by the general socio-political and health policy environment is how AIDS has affected American politics, society, and its health system. Without implying that AIDS has produced revolutionary effects, its overall impact can be fairly characterized as substantial.

Politically, the main impact of AIDS has probably been on the politics of the gay community. Prior to AIDS, its goals were first to "get government off the back of gays" and then to seek non-discrimination laws. After AIDS, the goals of gay groups inevitably became more complex. They continued, of course, to seek non-discrimination laws, in particular against those with AIDS and more generally for all gays and lesbians. They now, however, are also pressing for massive new funding for biomedical research, more lenient FDA approval of anti-AIDS drugs, and generous governmental funding for health care and social services for PWAs.

In terms of general political affiliation, the gay perception of a highly inadequate—to say the least—response to AIDS of many members of the Reagan Administration led, along with the growing influence of the religious right in the Republican party, to gays giving more support to the Democratic party. This has not been a total net gain for the Democrats. While they gained increased support from one constituency, they lost votes among those who dislike homosexuals. Moreover, this further reinforced the image of the Democratic party as being comprised of "special interests"—gays, feminists, African-Americans, unionists, and others—who make it unable to speak for the country as a whole. Operationally, while increased gay support probably usually helps elect Democrats to Congress and to state and local offices, it also probably makes it harder for the Democrats when they try for the presidency. The reason for this seems to be a public acceptance of Congress and the state legislatures as appropriate places for the brokering of interests, but the President is viewed as someone who should be above the control of special interests.

How Has AIDS Affected Society?

Perhaps the most widely heralded contention about the effect of AIDS upon American culture is that it has brought the sexual revolution to an end. Among gays, sexual behavior had, of necessity, to change dramatically, and, as previously noted, by and large it has (Coates, Morin, and McKusick 1987). Moreover, attempts at philosophically justifying anonymous sex as exemplifying a new and better "gay lifestyle" have largely ceased (Beauchamp 1989). Whether these changes will be permanent is, of course, uncertain.

The effects on the heterosexual population of the fear of AIDS are, however, much more uncertain. The swinging lifestyle and the singles bar are less glorified than in the past, but there are several reasons for believing that the degree of overall change in heterosexual behavior is likely to be less than many have hoped. For instance, as has already been noted, American teenagers do not have more sex than those in Western Europe, but the absence of sex education about and accessibility to contraceptives means they— white as well as African-American—have both more abortions and more births (Kantrowitz, Hager, et al. 1987). There is, unfortunately, no reason to assume this will soon change. Similarly, men and women are delaying marriage,

hoping first to complete their education or training and then successfully embark on their careers. Moreover, while the divorce rate slightly declined in the late 1980s, the United States still has by far the highest percentage of divorces in the world (Kantrowitz, Wingert, et al. 1987). Thus, urging sexual abstinence is not likely to be very effective.

The argument here is not that changing values about sex are unimportant. Rather it is that widespread sex outside of marriage is inevitably here to stay. Even the fear of AIDS cannot overcome this existential fact. The issue, then, is not whether AIDS will cause the end of the sexual revolution; it will not if this means no sex. The hope is, however, that it will cause an increase in more responsible sexual behavior.

An additional important effect of AIDS on American society that should be noted is that people in developed countries can no longer believe they are secure from plagues or epidemics. Comprehending and coping with AIDS itself presses the general public to the limits of its understanding and tolerance. Whether we will have learned enough from battling AIDS to handle further threats with some equanimity, or whether the difficulty of this struggle will cause people to react with heavy-handed, even cruel self-protective measures to the inevitable next crisis (McNeill 1976) remains an open question that hopefully will not have to be answered soon.

Another and more controversial effect of AIDS on society is its effect on societal attitudes and actions toward gays. To imply a single, unidirectional effect would be inaccurate, for AIDS has both simultaneously increased hostility to gays and increased respect for them as human beings.

The negative effects are more direct and visible. First, an increased number of gays are reporting isolated acts of violence directed against them because of their sexual orientation (Barron 1989). This, obviously, may merely be in large part a function of more gays than previously either being willing to report such acts to the police or being more open about their sexual orientation and thus presenting more potential targets for homophobes.

Less easily empirically quantifiable, but no less real, has been a growing understanding and acceptance of gays as a visible and more integral part of the larger community. This has risen as more and more people are personally touched by relatives and friends who suffer and die from AIDS. It is true that one author complained of sympathy for gays arising only when they are sick (Rist 1989), but given previous responses to those having epidemic diseases or sexually-transmitted diseases, this is a strange complaint indeed.

Whether this positive sentiment can soon overcome anti-gay hostility sufficiently to engender requisite support for passage in many jurisdictions of anti-discrimination laws to protect gays is doubtful. National opinion polls show a growing unwillingness of the public to legalize homosexual relations between consenting adults. In fairness, these same polls do show continued backing for prohibiting discrimination in employment against homosexuals (Gallup 1988).

What has been most lacking is for leaders at the highest level to make open symbolic gestures of support for those affected by AIDS and to broadly endorse the recommendations of the President's Commission on AIDS (President's Commission on the Human Immunodeficiency Virus Epidemic 1988). These omissions show that AIDS has not fundamentally improved the acceptance of gays as full members of society.

Finally, a noteworthy social effect of AIDS has been a shift in the values of gays toward greater emphasis on becoming a caring community (Altman 1986). This raises their own feelings of worth and capacity and thereby is likely ultimately to increase their ability to effect social change.

How Has AIDS Affected the Health System?

Finally, what effects has AIDS had on the health care delivery system? First, as has been previously noted, public health professionals have been more successful so far in dealing with AIDS than many observers of that profession might have anticipated. More basically, although certainly nothing they sought, the AIDS epidemic has increased the morale of public health professionals because, after being eclipsed when antibiotics had tamed earlier epidemics and concern turned to chronic diseases like heart, can-

cer, and stroke, they once again are in the forefront of health concerns.

AIDS has also affected public health professionals by forcing them to generally reconsider their legal powers. It turns out that alarmists' calls for new laws for controlling the behavior of those testing positive for the AIDS virus are largely unnecessary because laws already on the books, typically dating back to the Nineteenth Century, give public health nearly dictatorial power (Gostin 1986). It is only now, as public health professionals typically oppose restrictive new AIDS legislation because they think it would be counter-productive, that they are reexamining the old laws and quietly telling appropriate legislators that such laws should be repealed, modified to conform to modern concepts of fair procedure, or allowed to remain on the books as dead letters.

A second major issue concerns whether and how FDA procedures for approval and distribution of drugs for AIDS will result in overall general changes in the manner in which the FDA approves drugs. This seems likely for two main reasons. First, this process was already occurring to some extent. Second, the leadership of FDA should find it easier to bureaucratically justify changes for AIDS drugs in the context of generally overhauling FDA procedures. Subsequent events will confirm or refute this hypothesis.

A third major issue is whether AIDS will trigger fundamental revisions in the system for paying for health care in the United States. One of the major improvements that could occur would be if the health care system were reformed through enactment of national health insurance. Regrettably, the health care system has up to now successfully resisted this direction, and in and of itself AIDS seems insufficient to produce such a major change.

Finally, AIDS care is likely to change as the disease primarily shifts from predominantly white gays to African-American and Hispanic IV-drug users. On the average the latter have fewer resources for obtaining private care, and collectively they have no major community support networks. Hence, the models of effective and economical non-institutional care provided for AIDS patients—especially brilliantly in San Francisco—may be unsuccessfully applied to the new populations having AIDS and cynically cited as a rationale for cost containment. More positively, these models will be remembered and emulated as role models for other communities and for other diseases.

In summary, AIDS has affected as well as been affected by its broader environment, though not always as people have expected or thought. What is clear is that the effects of AIDS are subtle and deep. Health policy analysts must inevitably focus on the direct health effects of the disease, the number of cases, priorities in biomedical research, the modalities of testing, the effectiveness of education, and the costs of care. The observer of general policymaking and social trends will, however, both find much to learn from AIDS and have much to contribute to our understanding of how AIDS has affected our polity and society.

REFERENCES

Altman, Dennis. 1986. *AIDS In the mind of america.* Garden City, NY: Anchor Press.

Backstrom, Charles and Leonard Robins. 1989. The political elements in policymaking on AIDS. *New England Journal of Human Services* 9,2:13–19.

Barrett, Paul. 1989. Drug czar Bennett favors jailing dealers, users over treatment, education in national effort. *Wall Street Journal,* July 21:A16.

Barron, James. 1989. Homosexuals see 2 Decades of gains, but fear setbacks. *New York Times,* June 25:1:1.

Bayer, Ronald. 1988. Presentation at annual convention of the American Public Health Association, Boston, November.

Bayer, Ronald 1989. *Private acts, social consequences: AIDS and the politics of public health.* New York: Free Press.

Beauchamp, Dan E. 1989. *The health of the republic: Epidemics, medicine, and moralism as challenges to democracy.* Philadelphia: Temple University Press.

Brandt, Allan. 1988. AIDS in historical perspective: Four lessons from the history of sexually transmitted diseases. *American Journal of Public Health.* 78:367–371.

Centers for Disease Control. 1981. Pneumocystis pneumonia—Los Angeles. *Morbidity and Mortality Weekly Report* 30:250–252.

Coates, Thomas, Stephen Morin, and Leon McKusick. 1987. Behavioral consequences of AIDS antibody testing among gay men *Journal of the American Medical Association* 254,14:1889.

Evans, Robert G. 1984.*Strained mercy: The economics of health care in Canada.* Toronto: Butterworths.

Fuchs, Victor. 1974. *Who shall live?* New York: Basic Books.

Gallup, George Jr. 1988. *The Gallup Poll: Public opinion 1987.* Wilmington, DE: Scholarly Resources.

Goldsmith, Marsha, 1987. AMA house of delegates adopts comprehensive measures on AIDS. *Journal of the American Medical Association* 258,4:425–426.

Gostin, Larry. 1986. The future of communicable disease control: Toward a new concept in public health law. *Milbank Quarterly* 64,1:79–96.

Green, John and David Miller. 1987. The psychosocial impact of AIDS and human immunodeficiency virus. In *Current topics in AIDS,* edited by M. S. Gottlieb, D. J. Jeffries, D. Mildvan, A. J. Pinching, T. C. Quinn, and R. A. Weiss, 287–302. Chichester, UK: Wiley.

Harris, Richard. 1964. *The real voice.* New York: Macmillan.

Hatch, Michael, 1989. Personal interview with Commissioner of Commerce, State of Minnesota. July 12.

Hellinger, Fred J. 1988. National forecasts of the medical care costs of AIDS: 1988–1992. *Inquiry* 25:469–484.

Heyward, William L. and James W. Curran. 1988. The epidemiology of AIDS in the U.S. *Scientific American* 259,4:72–81.

Institute of Medicine, National Academy of Sciences. 1988. *Confronting AIDS: Update 1988.* Washington, DC: National Academy Press.

Kantrowitz, Barbara, Mary Hager, Pat Wingert, Ginny Carroll, George Raine, Monroe Anderson, Deborah Witherspoon, Janet Huck, and Shawn Doherty. 1987. Kids and contraceptives. *Newsweek* 109, 10 February 16):54–58.

Kantrowitz, Barbara, Pat Wingert, Leanne Gordon, Renee Michael, Deborah Witherspoon, Eric Calonius, David Gonzalez, and Bill Turque. 1987. How to stay married. *Newsweek,* 110,1 (February 16):52–57.

Kenney, Asta, Sandra Guardado, and Lisanne Brown. 1989. Sex education and AIDS education in the schools: What states and large school districts are doing. *Family Planning Perspectives* 21,2:56–64.

Lambert, Bruce. 1988. The free-needle program is under way and under fire. *New York Times*(November 13):4:6.

McNeill William. 1976. *Plaques and people.* Garden City, NY: Anchor Press.

Musto, David. 1986. Quarantine and the problem of AIDS. *Milbank Quarterly* 64,1:97–117.

Panem, Sandra. 1988. *The AIDS bureaucracy: Why society failed to meed the AIDS crisis and how we might improve our response.* Cambridge, MA: Harvard University Press.

Pierson, Rick and Daniel Egler. 1989. Repeal of AIDS testing passes. *Chicago Tribune* June 12:1:1.

Presidential Commission on the Human Immunodeficiency Virus Epidemic. 1988. *Report*. Washington, DC: USGPO.

Rhame, Frank, M.D. 1989. Personal interview with Director of Infection Control. University of Minnesota Hospital and Clinic. June 21.

Rhame, Frank and Dennis G. Maki. 1989. The case for wider use of testing for HIV infection. *New England Journal of Medicine* 320:1248–1254.

Rist, Darrell Y. 1989. The Deadly Costs of An Obsession: AIDS as Apocalypse. *Nation* 248,6:181–200.

Robins, Leonard and Charles Backstrom. 1989. Book review of Sandra Panem, the AIDS bureaucracy: Why society failed to meet the AIDS crisis and how we might improve our response. *Journal of Health Politics, Policy, and Law* 14:428–431.

Rovner, Julie. 1987. Congress is stalemated over AIDS epidemic. *Congressional Quarterly Weekly Report* 45:2486–2988.

Simpson, Margaret, M.D. 1989. Personal interview with Director of Sexually Transmitted Diseases. Hennepin County (MN) Medical Center. July 7.

Shilts, Randy. 1987. *And the band played on: Politics, people, and the AIDS epidemic*. New York: St. Martins.

Smith, Pamela. 1989. *Federal funding for AIDS research and prevention*. Washington, DC: Congressional Research Service.

Spector, Michael. 1989. A revolution in how drugs are tested. *Star Tribune* July 6:14A.

Winkenwerder, William, Austin R. Kessler, and Rhonda M. Stalec. 1989. Federal spending for illness caused by the human immunodeficiency virus. *New England Journal of Medicine,* 320:1598–1603.

Epilogue

Health Politics and Policy in the 1990s

Leonard S. Robins

Readers of this book seeking to synthesize the meaning of its various chapters must inevitably come to the judgment that in the United States in the 1980s health politics and policy revolved around the issues of health care cost containment and adequate access to health care, with cost containment dominating the agenda. It is possible to arrive at three conclusions concerning these issues:

First, the problem of rising health care costs (as measured by the rate of increase of the share of the gross national product devoted to health care) was as bad at the end of the decade as at the beginning; the problem of inadequate health insurance coverage was worse.

Second, by the end of the decade, political and business elites had become fully aware of the need for dealing with these problems, which caused them to be ranked high on the political agenda.

Third, in the 1980s the United States took serious and important actions to control health care costs. (Indeed, as shown in Chapter 16, some of the measures taken to control health care costs were important contributors to the growing number of people in the United States without any or sufficient health insurance.) While a multitude of previous specific actions—detailed in Chapter 6—were taken in the 1970s to control costs, these are now widely acknowledged, and indeed were perceived by many at the time, as being generally weak and minor. Yet despite the decision to pay hospitals for Medicare patients on the basis of Diagnostic Related Groups (DRGs), the growing involvement of business in efforts to control health care costs, the proliferation of Health Maintenance Organizations (HMOs), Preferred Provider Organizations (PPOs), and other managed care arrangements, health care costs have continued to escalate.

The clear failure to solve the cost problem and the increasing access problem have created a sense of frustration among politicians, business leaders, policy analysts, and in the health care community as a whole. In the 1970s, blame could be placed on an inadequate perception of the magnitude of the problems and timid, half-hearted, and generally weak public and private responses to them. Neither of these is any longer true.

The current conventional wisdom is, therefore, profoundly pessimistic about both the status quo and the possibility and prospects for significant and effective reform. Nevertheless, there are important potential developments in health politics, forthcoming developments in health policy, and potential and forthcoming developments in American politics and policy as a whole that should help the United States deal with its health care cost problem and improve its overall health care system. They are the subject of this epilogue.

Potential Developments in Health Politics

There are two potential developments in health politics which could have tremendous impact on health policy in the 1990s. They involve possible changes in the policy views of the American Medical Association and in the strategy of the business community.

The American Medical Association

Beset by ever-tighter external regulation on the practice of medicine, fearful of being sued for malpractice, and embarrassed by the growing number of uninsured and rising medical care costs, the American physician is a troubled professional. The response of the American Medical Association (AMA) has been to resist oversight of the profession by both government and insurers, push for malpractice reforms that decrease malpractice insurance costs to physicians, fight for bringing all of the poor under a more generous and remunerative Medicaid program (thereby *increasing* costs), and oppose structural reforms that would limit physician incomes. In short, the AMA has been doing just about what one would expect.

Yet medical associations in other countries

have frequently not adopted the same policies. They all act in the same way in the sense that their primary goal is the self-interest of their membership, but other associations perceive that self-interest differently. Specifically, many of them have come to accept the argument made in Chapter 14 that health care cost containment is the necessary precondition for clinical freedom, and consequently have not vigorously opposed effective health care cost containment policies.

Is it likely that the AMA will come around to this approach? Probably not. Still, growing physician dissatisfaction with the status quo should not be underestimated, and physician openness to new thinking is growing. Moreover, the AMA's policy positions have over the years been quite reflective of the views of its members. While any organization finds it difficult to change direction, if the membership indicates it desires a different course, the organization is likely to respond.

Finally, as demonstrated in Chapter 12, the power and influence of the AMA as a force for change would be even greater than as a force that primarily serves to defend the status quo. Currently, both the public and the Congress essentially view the AMA as the trade union of physicians. They admire their own physician—not the AMA. Currently, the AMA relies on professional authority and political pressure for its influence and power. Its power and influence would be greatly strengthened if it could also rely on moral authority.

The Business Community

The business community's interest in health care cost containment is, of course, primarily the result of the seemingly inexorable rise in health care costs. It was heightened by the general slowdown of economic growth in the 1970s and the rise of corporate debt in the 1980s, which led firms to be more cost conscious.

Initially the business community approached the challenge in a "can-do" manner, confident that by moving from being just a bill-payer to becoming an active participant in managing care it would wring the waste out of the system. This more active business role in managing health benefits has improved efficiency and restrained costs. Unfortunately, it has not reduced the rate of health care cost increases. As a result business has become increasingly pessimistic about its ability to control health care costs.

More recently, business has sought to have employees pay a higher share of their own health care costs as a means of controlling the costs to business. One advantage cited for this approach is that it will cut overall health care costs because the consumers of health care will be more careful shoppers when they have to pay more for what they use. This is theoretically possible, though Chapter 15 demonstrates the serous weaknesses in this approach. It is a certainty, of course, that if employees pay a higher percentage of health care costs, business expenditures will be relatively less.

But cost sharing has met strong and bitter resistance from employees. It has become very clear that extensive health benefits are not primarily caused by the tax advantages fringe benefits enjoy over wages, but rather are due to their being very popular and highly desired by employees. The proposed curtailment of health benefits is therefore often a good way to provoke a strike.

The ultimate in cost sharing is, of course, 100 percent patient responsibility, that is, no health insurance. The increase in the uninsured shows that some employers are great believers in this "solution." Since most employers accept the validity of health insurance, however, and since there is major employee resistance to cutting benefits, there are clear limits to cost sharing from both the perspective of the employer as well as the employee.

It might seem obvious that growing employer doubts about their capacity to control health care costs coupled with a general belief in health insurance would lead to a greater acceptance of an increased role for government in providing health insurance and controlling costs. But business retains its general hostility to government regulation of business and the welfare state. While the majority in business continue to oppose national health insurance, however, some are reexamining the question and many are less hostile to it. Like the medical community, the business community is potentially in flux regarding its approach to health politics and policy.

Future Developments in Health Policy

The discussion of future developments in health policy need not be as speculative as the previous discussion of potential developments in health politics. This is because there were a number of major initiatives in health policy taken in late 1989 and early 1990. This section will examine the likely long-term consequences of three of the most important of these initiatives. Specifically, we will consider the possible long-term policy impacts of legislation mandating that physician reimbursement under Medicare be based on a resource-based relative value scale, Oregon's proposal for controlling Medicaid spending, and the Supreme Court's decision to give states more circumstances under which they can limit a woman's right to an abortion.

Resource-Based Relative Value Scale (RBRVS)

In the last days of the 1989 session, Congress changed the way in which Medicare Part B reimburses physicians. Upon implementation, reimbursement would no longer be primarily on a usual, customary, and reasonable fee for services basis. Instead, physicians would be reimbursed on the basis of the relative value of the resources expended in patient treatment.

The intended result was to increase the rewards for preventive and primary care procedures (primarily performed by those in family practice and internal medicine) and decrease payments for severe, acute care procedures (often performed by surgeons). The AMA and most of organized medicine (though not the surgeons) ultimately supported this change on the principle of equity among its members.

The leading advocates of this change were primarily driven by the felt need to redistribute income among physicians. They were also, however, interested in two other objectives. First, they believed that increasing the rewards for preventive and primary care relative to acute care would divert health resources from acute care and into preventive and primary care. This, they argued, would simultaneously increase access to health care, improve health outcomes, and help control health care costs over time.

Second, at least some of the supporters hoped that the more centralized and prospective process of determining fees inherent in an RBRVS would also more directly help control health care costs. These supporters hoped that an RBRVS would do for physician reimbursement what the DRG method of reimbursement did for hospital reimbursement.

Whether these results will in fact occur is, of course, problematic. Moreover, opponents have real doubts—both empirical and theoretical—about RBRVS. Empirically, they worry that increasing fees to family physicians and internists and decreasing fees to surgeons will ultimately lead to *increased* health care costs, for surgeons will inevitably seek and may well find new ways to make up for the presumed loss of income they are supposed to incur. Theoretically, opponents point out that pricing under usual and customary fees was at least quasi-market based, and that RBRVS has all the problems inherent in central government "command" pricing. In this regard, the problems inherent in updating the RBRVS are likely to be particularly fearsome.

Although RBRVS may not have been the best way to break an unsatisfactory status quo on the method of physician reimbursement, it did break it. Specific flaws of RBRVS can be fixed as they become apparent over the years.

An indirect political effect of RBRVS might be to change the political balance of power within the physician community away from surgeons and toward internal medicine and family practitioners. If this were to occur, it would weaken the most conservative element of organized medicine—the group most opposed to national health insurance. This would not, of course, convert the AMA into a liberal organization, but it would be another reason for the AMA to be more receptive to new ways of thinking.

Finally, it is necessary to reemphasize the point made in Chapter 3 that an RBRVS is, despite the continued rhetoric promoting competition and markets, yet another major new regulatory initiative.

The Oregon Approach to Controlling Medical Spending

A state's spending on Medicaid is a function of four variables:

(1) the percentage of the population and the services covered by Medicaid as a result of federal regulations,

(2) the additional percentage of the population a state decides shall be eligible for Medicaid,

(3) the additional services a state decides shall be eligible for Medicaid, and

(4) the compensation the state provides for various services.

Thus, a state with a large percentage of its population eligible for Medicaid as a result of federal mandate may be heavily spending on Medicaid even though it has not extended eligibility for services beyond the minimum federal requirements. Conversely, a state that has expanded both the population and services eligible for Medicaid may nonetheless be spending relatively little on Medicaid if it is stringent in its compensation for those services or if it has a small population eligible for Medicaid under federal mandate. Therefore, by varying eligibility, services covered, or compensation, states have considerable discretion and control over their Medicaid expenditures.

The State of Oregon's Medicaid burden is not unduly heavy. Though in 1987 it was thirtieth among the states in population, it was thirty-fourth in the amount it spent on Medicaid and thirty-second in the number of persons receiving Medicaid (Bureau of the Census, 1989: 19 and 362). Nonetheless, in 1989 Oregon decided that the cost increases inherent in its desire to increase the percentage of the population covered by Medicaid had to be balanced by cost reductions elsewhere.

The truly unique aspect of Oregon's decision was that it did not follow the usual cost containment approaches of freezing reimbursement rates or restricting coverage of "non-essential" services like eyeglasses, dental care, and podiatric care. Instead, in 1990 Oregon developed an elaborate formula for comparatively evaluating the costs and benefits of specific services, with the intention of discontinuing coverage for services that did poorly according to the formula. Its exact details aside, two unique features of the formula need to be stressed: First, in addition to objective facts like cost and longevity, the formula includes the subjective factor of "quality of well-being;" Second, under the formula preventive and primary care services typically receive high scores, while acute care services—sometimes including life-saving operations—frequently receive low scores.

How might this system work? Its proponents hope that it will result in an expansion in the percentage of those who are eligible for Medicaid (the "medically needy", provide a more beneficial benefits package, and do so without raising costs by eliminating coverage for high-cost, low-benefit procedures. They also hope that Oregon will follow its stated intention of using the formula for selecting the mandated benefits that employers must provide their employees under state law by no later than 1995.

While both of these goals are possible, considerable skepticism is in order. The plan may not, in practice, reduce costs, because if Oregon expands eligibility and decides on the procedures not to cover, medical practitioners may well find a way to do them anyway. Additionally, Oregon will have a larger constituency demanding increased services for those eligible for Medicaid. (Those who believe the Reagan cuts in eligibility and benefits should be more fully reversed will not, of course, object.)

More theoretically, whatever the merit of the Oregon plan for controlling Medicaid spending, it has serious flaws as the basis for employer-based health insurance. The working population operationally sees health insurance primarily as a program of *financial protection.* It is always most interested and willing to pay for insurance that covers expensive hospitalizations. Conversely, the public frequently opts for lower cost insurance at the expense of limited preventive and primary care coverage and deductibles, even though health experts warn that this frequently results in the type of benefits package least beneficial for health. Avoiding this dilemma is one of the most important arguments for national health insurance. In this specific context, however, the outcome is likely to be pressure by both employers and employees that will result in a rejection of the formula as the basis for the services to be covered under mandated employer coverage.

If one shuns the exaggerated importance for good or ill ascribed to the Oregon plan by its supporters and opponents and simply asks whether it is likely to result in more efficient Medicaid spending, the answer is probably yes.

The fundamental debate over Oregon's plan, however, is political. It seems to imply that the only means of controlling health care costs is through rationing, and as noted in Chapter 15, proponents of the status quo in the United States health system desire to frame the debate this way.

Throughout this discussion, however, the Oregon plan has been described as a program for allocating Medicaid spending rather than rationing health care. The reason is that Oregon is *not* rationing health care. Rationing is dealing with shortage by allocating a limited supply on the basis of equality or need. In Oregon, except for certain rural areas, there is no general shortage of health care services. Indeed, there is a relative shortage of the services for which the plan would increase demand (preventive and primary care) and a relative surplus of the services for which the plan would decrease demand (surgery). Moreover, the plan does not apply equally; it applies only to the poorest Oregonians. It is, of course, frequently true that the poor in the United States are the test market for bold new health care delivery experiments. In this case, being on the cutting edge is clearly a mixed blessing.

The New Politics of Abortion

Having an abortion requires that, at a minimum, a woman consider the following issues:

(1) whether or not she wants to have a baby,
(2) the relative safety of having a baby as opposed to the risks of having an abortion,
(3) the relative cost of having a baby as opposed to that of having an abortion, and
(4) possible legal penalties associated with having an abortion as opposed to those associated with having a baby.

In China, the government encourages women in a variety of official and unofficial ways to have abortions if they have had one child and that child is still alive. The government of the United States has never encouraged abortion, and throughout most of the Twentieth century prior to 1973, most of the states—the level of government that had primary policy responsibility for this issue—made abortions illegal except under certain limited (sometimes very limited) circumstances.

In 1973 in *Roe v. Wade* the Supreme Court radically changed this. It made all abortions legal in the first trimester of pregnancy, severely limited the right of the states to restrict abortions in the second trimester, and granted considerable discretion to states only in the last trimester. Since the vast majority of abortions occur in the first trimester, the Supreme Court essentially created a full right to an abortion.

As a consequence of the *Roe* decision those opposed to abortion rights had to limit themselves to actions designed to induce women to want to have the babies and the modification or reversal of *Roe*. If, for example, public hospitals are legally forbidden to perform abortions and physicians and hospitals are successfully pressured to not perform abortions, then a woman desiring one might reconsider because she feared the health consequences of a poorly performed abortion. Similarly, while abortions are much cheaper than pregnancies, if Medicaid refuses to pay for them, they are more expensive to the woman and she may therefore decide to have the baby.

Between 1973 and 1989 the pro-life movement was generally politically stronger than the pro-choice movement. An increasing number of limitations on abortion were enacted, though they never were strong enough to limit the vast majority of abortions.

The reason for this greater strength of the pro-life movement was not its greater overall appeal to the public. While opinion polls gave a somewhat different picture of public opinion depending on how questions were asked (a problem discussed in the context of national health insurance in Chapter 13), the majority of the public clearly wanted to keep abortions legal in most of the circumstances under which they occur. Instead, the key to the strength of the pro-life movement was the greater *intensity* of feeling on the part of the pro-life supporters in contrast to those who were pro-choice.

In its last decision of the 1988–89 term, the Supreme Court in *Webster v. Reproductive Health Services* limited the scope of *Roe* and gave the states greater discretion in limiting abortions.

While the Court seemed to suggest that further limitations, if not the actual reversal of *Roe,* were forthcoming, the consequences were not quite what the pro-lifers had hoped for. Admittedly some states, most notably Pennsylvania, curbed abortion rights. In many more states, however, the pro-choice movement won both major electoral and legislative victories. It appears that the rights created by *Roe* have largely been institutionalized in our society, regardless of what future Supreme Court rulings may do to further limit or eliminate the U.S. Constitutional restraints on state action.

Politically, what accounts for this? First, the dilution of *Roe* by *Webster* has energized the pro-choice movement. Ordinarily, political disappointment leads to political apathy. In this case, however, it appears that *Roe* itself produced pro-choice apathy because the right of abortion appeared to be fully protected by the Court. The realization that this was no longer true brought an intensity to the pro-choice movement that essentially matched that of the pro-lifers.

Second, since 1973 millions of women have had safe, legal, and inexpensive abortions. Public opinion polls have repeatedly shown these women to be the strongest supporters of abortion rights in the United States. Whether the liberalized abortion rights granted under *Roe* would have been supported by the American people in 1973 is uncertain. In the decades of the 1970s and 1980s, however, an important constituency, albeit one that frequently does not want to identify itself, has developed in support of abortion rights.

Finally, even though most of the pro-choice leadership is politically liberal and most of the pro-life leadership is politically conservative, the recent success of the pro-choice movement has revolved around its ability to tap anti-big government sentiment. Public opinion polls typically show general support for abortion rights, but many circumstances under which people would be willing to limit the right to an abortion. But when people are asked whether they believe *government* should make the decision instead of a woman and her physician, they overwhelmingly say no.

Antipathy to *Roe*—a liberal pro-choice decision—helped build the political strength of pro-lifers and indirectly helped the conservative movement and President Ronald Reagan dominate politics and policy in the late 1970s and 1980s. *Webster*—a conservative pro-life decision—has helped build the political strength of pro-choicers and may indirectly help liberals in the political and policy struggles of the 1990s.

Health Politics and Policy in Broader Perspective

Just as the politics of abortion has had an impact on the overall politics of the United States, so overall political and policy developments in the United States have major impacts on health policy and politics. This last section will therefore concentrate on two overall developments that are likely to have a major, albeit indirect, effect on health politics and policy in the 1990s: the increased politicization of the disabled and the end of the Cold War.

Increased Politicization of the Disabled

In 1990, Congress passed the Americans With Disabilities Act. It was, by general consensus, the most important piece of civil rights legislation since the historic 1964 Civil Rights Act. By extending to the disabled the protection already given to victims of racial and sexual discrimination, over forty million Americans have received new protection against discrimination.

The political struggle for the Act strengthened the political power and influence of the disabled in two ways: First, it gave the disabled a basis for greater *political unity,* making them less likely to conceptualize themselves just as blind or deaf or mobility-impaired (Noah, 1990); Second, winning this legislative battle convinced the disabled that they could be successful in the political process, thereby inevitably stimulating additional increased *political activity* by them.

One of the most important goals of the supporters of the Disabilities Act was to increase the participation of the disabled in the mainstream of society. Probably their most fervent wish was that ending discrimination in employment would not only help the currently employed disabled, but would also encourage more of the disabled to seek and obtain employment.

If this occurs, the disabled have to overcome yet another obstacle. Becoming employed will remove their Medicaid or Medicare eligibility. Obtaining health insurance through their employer will be very difficult as employers—especially the majority who self-insure—make ever greater efforts to deny employer-based coverage to those with pre-existing conditions. Conversely, requiring the disabled to buy private health insurance will be such a burden that most of them will lose the economic benefits of employment. The unfortunate result is likely to be that many will in fact opt to stay on Medicaid or Medicare.

Representatives of the disabled are fully aware of this scenario. They are consequently strong supporters of a variety of additional efforts to provide insurance coverage for the uninsured. Ideally, from their perspective, the United States would enact national health insurance (Noah, 1990), for this would be the optimum in "mainstreaming."

It is doubtful whether the new political influence of the disabled will be sufficient to bring about national health insurance. It is quite likely, however, that the increased political influence of the disabled will be an important and useful force for engendering change in the United States health care system.

The End of the Cold War

While the crackdown on the democratization movement in China in the spring of 1989 made it bitterly clear that political liberalization in communist countries is at least temporarily reversible, the breaking of the communist stranglehold in Eastern Europe can, nonetheless, be said to mark the beginning of the post-Cold War period. What are some of the likely consequences for United States politics and policy generally and health politics and policy in particular?

First, Presidents Reagan and Bush will get credit for these events. While Democrats may say they did not cause them, the developments occurred during their terms in the White House. Since Presidents are usually blamed for the bad, whether a result of Presidential policies or not, it is only fair they receive credit for the good. If this were the only force operating, it would be even harder for a Democrat to win the Presidency than it has been recently.

In the long run, however, it is by no means clear that the Republicans will generally benefit from the end of the Cold War. Public opinion polls consistently show the Republicans are very strongly favored over the Democrats on foreign and defense policy, but the parties are much more evenly matched on domestic affairs, with Republicans somewhat favored on overall handling of the economy, and Democrats clearly favored on health, education, the environment, and other specific issues. If foreign and defense policy issues become less important to voters, the Democrats will benefit.

Despite the limits of presidential influence on health politics and policy described in Chapter 5, a Democrat in the White House—especially a liberal Democrat in the Kennedy-Johnson tradition—would have a major direct impact on health politics and policy by promoting increased coverage and global budgeting. Perhaps equally importantly, a liberal Democratic president would have a powerful indirect effect on health via increased national government support for such things as parental leave, early child care, and sheltering the homeless.

Moreover, even if the political balance of power in the United States between the political parties remains unchanged, the end of the Cold War is likely to have major consequences for health policy. First, even if most of the "peace dividend" goes to reduce the federal deficit, some will be left for new domestic policy initiatives, including health policy initiatives. Second, a major reorientation will occur from an emphasis on the strength of the military to the strength of the economy as the key to national security. The dissatisfaction with the increasing drain the poorly working health sector is currently placing on our nation's economic competitiveness will then add another political force for change.

In conclusion, the objective evidence from the health sector provides ample grounds for pessimism about the possibility of successful major structural change in the health care system of the United States. The 1990s, however, give every indication of being a decade of concern for

groups not in the mainstream of our society and the first decade since the 1930s in which the United States and its political leadership are not understandingly preoccupied by war or the threat of war or the need to avoid war via maintaining the strongest military force in the world. It is not unreasonable to hope and expect that in giving increased emphasis to domestic renewal we will somehow find a way to significantly, if not radically, change and improve our health care system.

REFERENCES

Bureau of the Census. 1989. *Statistical Abstract of the United States,* Washington, D.C.: U.S. Department of Commerce.

Noah, Timothy. 1990. "Legislation Will Give Disabled People Greater Leverage to Gain Access to Jobs," *Wall Street Journal,* May 23, B:1.

Appendix

Chronology and Capsule Highlights of the Major Historical and Political Milestones in the Evolutionary Involvement of Government in Health and Health Care in the United States

Theodor J. Litman

1730 American seamen (then British subjects) taxed to pay for hospital care.

1760 New York City adopts licensure requirement for physicians to practice medicine.

1772 New Jersey legislature adopts an act to regulate medical practice requiring that all persons wishing to practice medicine be examined and approved by any two judges of the Supreme Court. This act serves as a colonial prototype of later state boards of medical examiners.

1780 Virginia taxes seamen for hospital care.

1798 The Fifth Congress passes act to tax seamen for health care and establishes the U.S. Marine Hospital Service to provide medical care for sick and disabled seamen—in essence, the first prepaid medical care program in the United States.

1809 The Commonwealth of Massachusetts adopts the nation's first compulsory vaccination (small pox) law.

1846 In response to a call from the New York State Medical Society, a preliminary meeting of delegates from medical societies and colleges from throughout the United States is held at New York University to explore the establishment of a national physicians' organization (a forerunner of the American Medical Association— AMA).

1847 The American Medical Association is established. Under its charter, representation is to be comprised of delegates from state, county, and local medical societies, institutions, and medical colleges in a fixed numerical ratio.

1854 Congress passes a bill providing for federal financing of the indigent insane, signifying the first federal action dealing with public welfare. The measure, however, is vetoed by President Pierce on the grounds that the federal government should not be involved in any welfare program.

1855 The first state board of health is established in Louisiana. (Freedman 1951).

1872 The American Public Health Association (APHA) is founded.

1878 National Quarantine Act is passed.

1891 The National Confederation of State Medical Examining and Licensing Boards is founded.

1899 The classic legal recognition for the practice of state aid to church-related welfare institutions such as hospitals is given by the U.S. Supreme Court in the Case of *Bradfield v. Roberts* 175 US 299 (1899).

1902 The Public Health Service is reorganized and renamed the Public Health and Marine Hospital Service.

1904 A uniform curriculum, recommended to all faculties, is adopted by the National Confederation of State Medical Examining and Licensing Boards.

1905 The U.S. Supreme Court upholds the constitutionality of Massachusetts Compulsory Vaccination Law [*Jacobson v. Commonwealth of Massachusetts* 197 US 11 (1905)].

1906 The first bill to establish a national children's bureau is introduced.

1906 PL 59–384, the Pure Food and Drug or "Wiley" Act is passed prohibiting the transport of adulterated and misbranded foods and drugs in interstate commerce.

1909 President Theodore Roosevelt calls together a conference (later to be known as the first White House Conference on Children) of some 200 professional and lay leaders interested in the care of dependent children.

1910 The Flexner Report, commissioned by the Carnegie Foundation, condemns the current state of medical education in the United States and proposes major reforms that are to transform medical education from a guild apprenticeship model to a university-hospital-based enterprise modeled after that of the Johns Hopkins University.

1912 On a vote of 54 to 20 with 17 not voting in the Senate and 177 to 17 with 190 not voting in the House, a bill calling for the establishment of a children's bureau is passed and approved by President Taft.

1912 Social insurance, including health insurance, is endorsed in the platform of the Progressive party and espoused by its candidate, Theodore Roosevelt.

1912 The Public Health and Marine Hospital Service is renamed the U.S. Public Health Service.

1913 The American College of Surgeons (ACS)

is formed to further a more structured examination of surgical practice in the United States.

1916—
1920 Several state commissions study a standard bill for health insurance and conclude that it is neither needed nor wanted. State interest then wanes.

1916 Samuel Gompers, one of organized labor's early patriarchs, reaffirms his opposition to any form of government-sponsored compulsory health insurance as infringing upon labor's right to bargain.

1917 Congress passes amendment to War Risk Insurance Act to provide medical benefits to veterans with service-connected disabilities.

1917 The AMA's house of delegates passes resolution stating principles to be followed in government health insurance plans.

1918 First federal grants to states for public health services.

1920 The AMA's house of delegates reverses its position, declaring its unequivocal opposition to compulsory health insurance.

1920 Congress passes the first Vocational Rehabilitation Act. Passage rests less on humanitarian than utilitarian terms; that is, it would put people on the productive tax rolls.

1921 Congress enacts (PL67–97) the first Maternity and Infancy Act (Sheppard-Towner) which provided grants to states to develop health services for mothers and children. The act is a prototype for federal grants-in-aid to the states.

1924 Congress passes World War Veteran's Act providing more liberal hospital benefits to all war veterans.

1924 A bill to remove a prohibition against contraceptives and information on contraception fails to win congressional approval.

1929 The first Blue Cross plan in the United States is established at Baylor University in Dallas, Texas.

1929 Assailed and opposed in Congress as "drawn chiefly from the radical, socialistic, behavioristic philosophy of Germany and Russia" and denounced by the AMA as an "imported socialistic scheme," the Sheppard-Towner Act is allowed to lapse.

1930 The National Institute of Health (NIH) is created as the administrative home for the medical research of the Public Health Service (PHS).

1932 The report of the Committee on the Cost of Medical Care (CCMC) is published calling for the organization of the U.S. medical services on a group practice, pre-payment basis. Despite the preeminence of its compilers and extensive documentation, the report is rejected out of hand by the AMA as socialistic and inimical to the best interests of the people of the United States.

1933 Enactment of the Federal Emergency Relief Act affords the first federal financing of medical care for the aged as funds are made available to states through the Federal Emergency Relief Administration (FERA) to pay medical expenses for people receiving relief. However, in most states, only emergency medical and dental care are provided for.

1935 On January 17 President Franklin D. Roosevelt sends to Congress the report of the President's Committee on Economic Security, which is to form the basis of the Social Security Act (PL 74–271) (SSA) passed later that year. The report endorses the principle of compulsory national health insurance (NHI) but makes no specific program recommendations. In his accompanying message, the president states that he is not planning to recommend adoption of "so-called health insurance at this time," His decision not to recommend national health insurance reportedly is based, in part, on the fear that opposition to it would endanger passage of the entire Social Security Act, and, in part, on the belief that the nation's medical facilities were inadequate to sustain such a program and needed to be beefed up first through public health facility grants and other similar efforts.

1935 July 15 the first government health insurance bill is introduced in the Congress—the Epstein Bill sponsored by Senator Capper.

1935 Congress passes and the president signs (August 14) the Social Security Act (PL

74–271), which includes provisions for grants-in-aid to states for maternal and child care, aid to crippled children, aid to the blind, the aged, and other health-impaired people.

1935 The first National Health Survey is conducted.

1936 Congress authorizes federal regulation of industrial safety in companies doing business with the government through passage of the Walsh-Healy Act (PL 74–846).

1937 The first categorical institute, the National Cancer Institute, is established under the National Cancer Institute Act (PL 75–244).

1938 The National Health Conference calls for expansion of public health services, provision of medical services to people at the lowest income levels at public expense, and medical insurance at the state level for the rest of the population.

1938 The LaFollette-Bulwinkle Act (venereal disease—VD control) (PL 75–540) provides grants-in-aid to states and other authorities to investigate and control VD.

1938 The federal Food, Drug and Cosmetic Act (PL 75–717) extends federal authority to act against adulterated and misbranded food, drugs, and cosmetic products, banning new drugs until approved by the federal Food and Drug Administration (FDA).

1939 Senator Robert Wagner (Dem., N.Y.) introduces a bill based on recommendations of the 1938 National Health Conference calling for federally subsidized state medical care compensation. No action is taken, however.

1939 The Public Health Service is transferred from the Treasury Department to the new Federal Security Agency by the Reorganization Act of 1939 (PL 76–19).

1939 The AMA, the District of Columbia Medical Society, and the Harris, Texas, Medical Society are indicted for violation of the Sherman Antitrust Case over their efforts to restrict physicians in prepaid group practice from practicing medicine.

1940 After a lengthy trial, the AMA and the District of Columbia Medical Society are found guilty of restraint of trade in their battle against prepaid medicine. Despite their legal reversal, organized medicine is

successful in getting legislation passed at the state level prohibiting the corporate practice of medicine. Many such restrictions remain in existence today and limit the growth and development of health maintenance organizations (HMOs).

1941 The Nurse Training Act (PL 77–146) gives schools of nursing support to increase their enrollments and help strengthen their facilities.

1941 The Physicians Forum, a liberal-based physician's organization, is formed by dissident members of the New York County Medical Society to work for the adoption of compulsory health insurance.

1942 Rhode Island becomes the first state to pass a health insurance law.

1942 A *Fortune* magazine poll reports that 75 percent of the public favors national health insurance.

1943 The first Wagner (Sen. Robert, Dem., N.Y.), Murray (Sen. James E., Dem., Montana), Dingell (Rep. John D., Sr., Dem., Mich.) Bill (S1161, HR2861) calling for sweeping revisions and broadening of the Social Security Act including a compulsory national health system for people of all ages, financed through a payroll tax, is introduced in the Senate and the House. No action is taken on the measure, however, by the seventy-eighth Congress. Opponents call the bill "the most virulent scheme ever to be conjured out of the mind of man" and depict a revised version to mean "the end of freedom for all classes of Americans."

1944 President Roosevelt, in his January 11 State of the Union Message, outlines an Economic Bill of Rights, which includes "the right to adequate care and the opportunity to achieve and enjoy good health." Although interpreted by many to imply that the president favored a national health insurance system, no subsequent recommendations of any such enabling legislation to Congress is forthcoming.

1944 The APHA adopts a set of principles on comprehensive health care for all people in the United States financed through social insurance supported by general taxation or by general taxation alone.

1944 All public health service authorities are consolidated into a single statute (42 U.S. Code) under the Public Health Service Act (PL 78–410).

1945 Wagner, Murray, and Dingell reintroduce the same broad bill that they had sponsored in 1943.

1945 November 19, President Harry S. Truman sends a message on health legislation to Congress calling for comprehensive, pre-paid, medical insurance for all people of all ages, to be financed through a 4 percent rise in the Social Security Old Age and Survivors Insurance Tax. His proposal is quickly introduced in the Senate and House by Senators Wagner and Murray and Representative Dingell. The bill, however, languishes in Congress and no action is taken.

1946 The National Mental Health Act (PL 79–487) authorizes major federal support for mental health research, diagnosis, prevention and treatment, establishes state grants-in-aid for mental health, and changes the PHS Division of Mental Health to the National Institute of Mental Health.

1946 Recognizing a shortage in health care services and the antiquated status of the nation's hospital facilities, Congress enacts the Hospital Survey and Construction Act (PL 79–725) (Hill-Burton) providing for national direct support for the development of community hospitals, ostensibly rural facilities, and for the first time attempts to mandate, at least, rudimentary standards for construction and the insistence on regional planning. At the same time, however, the act carries a hidden time bomb that only comes to light 30 some years later, that is, a requirement that recipients provide a "reasonable volume of services to those unable to pay"—a free care obligation—and make their facilities "available to all persons residing in their service areas"—a community service obligation.

1946 The Communicable Disease Center is established in Atlanta, Georgia, and the Census Bureau's Division of Vital Statistics is transferred to the Public Health Service as the National Office of Vital Statistics.

1946 California passes a compulsory health insurance act.

1948 National Health Act (PL 80–655) establishes the National Heart Institute, pluralizing NIH.

1949 Flushed with success after upset victories in the 1948 presidential and congressional elections that found the Democratic party in control of both houses of Congress plus the White House, President Truman again calls for compulsory national health insurance in his January 5 State of the Union Message.

1949 Hearings on bills embodying the proposals sponsored by Senators Murray and Wagner (S1679) and Representative Dingell and others (HR43121) produces bitter controversy and heavy lobbying on both sides of the issue.

1949 The AMA sets up $3.5 million war chest and mobilizes a massive campaign to defeat what they consider to be socialized medicine and a threat to the free practice of medicine in the United States, using the talents of the California public relations firm of Whitaker and Baxter for a fee of $100,000 and assessing each physician $25 to support their efforts. No congressional action in either house is taken.

1950 The president repeats his earlier request for compulsory national health insurance, but again no congressional action is forthcoming. Instead, Congress moves to help the states provide medical care for welfare recipients supported by the four federal-state public assistance programs for the indigent, that is, Old Age Assistance (OAA), Aid to Dependent Children (ADC), Aid to the Blind (AB), and Aid to the Permanently and Totally Disabled (APTD). Amendments to the Social Security Act provide for federal sharing with the states in vendor payments, that is, payments to providers as well as the direct payments of living expenses to recipients.

1950 PL 81–507 establishes the National Science Foundation as an autonomous entity and strengthens the concept of federal support for university-based research in physical, medical, and social sciences.

1951 Durham-Humphrey amendments (PL 8–2–

215) establishes category of prescription drugs requiring labeling and medical supervision.

1952 The Joint Commission on Accreditation of Hospitals (JCAH) is established.

1952 A bill (S3001, HR 7484–85) is introduced in Congress by Senator Murray and Representatives Dingell and Celler (Emanuel D., Dem., N.Y.) calling for the payment of hospitalization costs for retired people and their dependents or survivors under the Social Security Old-Age and Survivors Insurance (OASI) System. No action is taken, however.

1953 The Federal Security Agency (FSA) is transformed into the Department of Health Education and Welfare (DHEW) and elevated to cabinet status.

1954 The Hill-Burton Act amended (PL 83–482, Medical Facilities Survey and Construction Act) to expand the scope of the program to include nursing homes, rehabilitation facilities, chronic disease hospitals, and diagnostic or treatment centers.

1954 Responsibility for maintenance and operation of Indian Health facilities is placed in PHS rather than Bureau of Indian Affairs (PL 83–568).

1955 The U.S. major trade unions—the American Federation of Labor (AFL) and Congress of Industrial Organization (CIO)—merge (AFL-CIO) and set health insurance for the aged as a top priority.

1955 The American Hospital Association's Board of Trustees passes a resolution recommending federal subsidies to the states to begin voluntary health insurance programs for older people, and the concept is approved by the association's house of delegates.

1955 PL 84–377 Polio Vaccination Assistance Act provides assistance to state vaccination programs.

1956 The Social Security Act is further amended to permit separate federal matching funds for medical care payments on an individual basis in addition to cash assistance.

1956 The Dependents Medical Care Act (PL 84–569) sets up CHAMPUS program of primarily inpatient medical care for military dependents.

1956 PL 84–911, the Health Amendments Act of 1956, constitutes the first federal legislation addressed specifically to the question of health manpower, authorizing traineeships for public health personnel and advanced training for professional nurses.

1956 The National Health Survey Act (PL 84–652) provides for a continuing survey and special sickness and disability studies of the U.S. population.

1956 PL 84–941 transfers responsibility for the Library of Medicine to the Public Health Service.

1957 The Forand (Rep. Aime J., Dem., R.I.) Bill (HR9467) calling for an increase in the Social Security OASI payroll tax to provide for up to 120 days of combined hospital and nursing home care as well as necessary surgery for aged OASI beneficiaries is introduced. Although no action is taken by the Congress, the Forand bill begins to draw increasing public interest and debate. Both the American Hospital Association (AHA) and American Nurses Association (ANA) endorse the bill.

1958 The AMA sets up the joint council to improve the health care of the aged comprised of the AMA, AHA, the American Dental Association (ADA), and the American Nursing Home Association, which concludes that the health care of the aged does not need improvement. Not represented in the council is the ANA, which in 1957 had supported in principle the Forand bill.

1958 PL 85–929, the Food Additive Amendment to the Food, Drug and Cosmetics Act, requires premarketing clearance for new food additives, establishes a generally recognized as safe (GRAS) category, and prohibits under the so-called Delaney clause, the approval of any additive "found to induce cancer in man or animal."

1958 The Small Business Administration is authorized to provide loans to nursing homes through the Small Business Act and the Small Business Investment Act.

1958 A program of formula grants to Schools of Public Health is established (PL 85–544).

1959 The House Ways and Means Committee holds hearings on Forand's reintroduced bill, but no action is taken.

1959 Blue Cross negotiates contract with Civil Service Commission to provide health insurance coverage for federal employees under PL 86–352, Federal Employees Health Benefits Act. Contract serves as a foot-in-the-door and a prototype for Blue Cross' later involvement in Medicare-Medicaid.

1960 The Forand bill becomes a major political issue, supported on one hand by organized labor and liberal Democrats and opposed on the other by the AMA, most Republicans including President Eisenhower, most business and insurance groups, and political conservatives.

1960 March 31, the House Ways and Means Committee on a 17 (Dem. 7, Rep. 10) to 8 (Dem. 8, Rep. 0) vote to table the Forand bill. Voting in favor of killing the bill are Committee Chairman Wilber D. Mills (Dem., Ark.) and six other southern representatives.

1960 May 4, in testimony before the Ways and Means Committee, the Eisenhower administration unveils its own "Medicare" program, which it proposes will help the needy aged meet the costs of catastrophic illness without using the compulsory national health insurance feature proposed under the Forand bill. Under the administration's plan, federal matching grants would be offered to the states to help them pay for a varied list of specified medical, hospital, and nursing costs for elderly persons with incomes of $2,500 a year or less ($3,800 for a couple). Individuals would have the option of receiving cash payments to help them purchase private commercial health insurance.

1960 August, Congress passes the Kerr (Sen. Robert S., Dem., Okla.)—Mills (Rep. Wilbur D.) Bill (PL 86–778—Title XVI of the Social Security Act) providing additional federal matching funds to the states for vendor payments under the Old Age Assistance Act as well as federal matching funds for the medically needy aged, creating a new public assistance category—Medical Assistance for the Aged (MAA). The significance of the MAA program (Bernard and Feingold 1970) lay in (1) its recognition of medical indigence, (2) its introduction of open funding by the federal government, and (3) the introduction of some minimal standard to the substance and administration of public assistance medical care.

1961 White House Conference on Aging is held and the issue of medical care to the elderly is debated.

1961 The King-Anderson bill, embodying President Kennedy's proposal to provide health insurance for the elderly through the social security system is introduced in both houses of Congress by Senator Anderson (Clinton, Dem., N. Mex.) and Representative King (Cecil, Dem., Calif.) [Note: As a senator, the president had earlier sponsored a Senate version of the Forand bill (S 2915)]. Although normally an administration's legislative initiatives are sponsored by the highest ranking member of the president's party on the committee with jurisdiction over it, since both Senate Finance Committee chairman Harry F. Byrd (Dem., Va.) and Ways and Means chairman Mills were opposed to the president's proposal, the bill carried the sponsorship of Congressman King and Senator Anderson. The latter had earlier proposed a revised version of the Forand-Kennedy bill in the Senate Finance Committee in 1960 but it was rejected. Hearings on the proposed legislation are held by the Ways and Means Committee but no action is taken.

1962 The AMA sets up AMPAC, a political action committee analogous to the AFL-CIO's COPE to fight the Kennedy proposal for medical care for the aged.

1962 PL 87–692, Health Services for Agricultural Migratory Workers Act authorizes federal aid to clinics serving migratory agricultural workers and their families.

1962 PL 87–781, Kefauver-Harris drug amendments require improved manufacturing practices, better reporting, assurances of efficacy, as well as safety and strengthened regulation of the drug industry.

1962 January 3, the AHA drops its opposition to federal funding averring that the source of funding is of secondary importance and federal assistance a necessity.

1962 Continued inaction by the House Ways and Means Committee leads Senator Anderson to offer a revised version of the administration's medical care for the aged proposal as an amendment on the floor of the Senate, to the Public Welfare Amendment (HR10606) that already had been passed by the House. The Anderson amendment, cosponsored by five Republicans, headed by Senator Jacob K. Javits (Rep., N.Y.), proposes a one-quarter of one percent increase on the OASDI payroll tax on each employer and employee and three-eights of one percent on the self-employed, as well as a rise to $5,200 in the wage base for the tax, with additional revenues to be earmarked to pay for all or most of the costs of a long list of hospital (90 days inpatient care), nursing home (180 days, skilled care), and diagnostic services for people 65 years of age and older eligible for OASDI old age benefits, as well as certain other people not otherwise eligible for OASDI benefits.

1962 July 17, In a dramatic roll call vote, Senate Republicans and Southern Democrats unite to kill the Anderson amendment on a 52 (Dem. 21, Rep. 31) to 48 (Dem. 43, Rep. 5) vote.

1963 Health Professions Educational Assistance Act (PL 88–129) provides construction money for health professions schools, funds tied to increase enrollment requirements to assist with the school's operating expenses, plus loans and scholarship programs. It authorizes support to medical schools for the first time and establishes the presence of the federal government in health-related educational institutions.

1963 The Blue Cross Association of America under the leadership of its president, Walter McNerney, issues report in support of government financing of medical care for the aged, noting the problem the high cost of

health care poses for the elderly, the hospitals, and the third-party carriers as well.

1963 PL 88–156, Maternal and Child Health and Mental Retardation Planning Amendments, initiate program of comprehensive maternity, infant care and mental retardation prevention.

1963 PL88–164, Community Mental Health Centers Construction Act seeks to bring comprehensive mental health services to patients in their own communities and further deinstitutionalization.

1963 PL 88–206, Clean Air Act, authorizes direct grants to state and local governments for air pollution control. Establishes federal enforcement in interstate air pollution.

1963 The AMA raises several million dollars to fight Medicare.

1964 PL 88–525 authorizes the food stamp program for low-income people to purchase nutritious foods for a balanced diet.

1964 PL 88–581, Nurse Training Act, provides special federal effort for training professional nursing personnel.

1964 The Hill-Burton act amended to set aside monies for the modernization and replacement of health care facilities.

1965 Congress amends the Social Security Act (PL 89–97) providing for medical care for the elderly (Medicare—Title 18) and grants to the states for medical assistance to the poor (Medicaid—Title 19), on a vote of 307 to 116 in the House and 70 to 24 in the Senate, and President Lyndon B. Johnson signs it into law on July 30. The act also extends social security coverage to physicians.

1965 The conservative Association of American Physicians and Surgeons urges its 16,500 members not to cooperate with the program. The AMA, on the other hand, cautions against a physician's boycott. The legislative defeat leads to the forced retirement of Dr. Morris Fishbein, former editor of the *Journal of the American Medical Association* (1924–1949) and the long-time, erstwhile spokesman of organized medicine as executive secretary of the AMA. He is replaced by Dr. Frank Blasingame who later is summarily dismissed in 1968.

1965 PL 89–239 amends the Public Health Service Act and establishes a nationwide network of Regional Medical Programs (RMPs) for heart disease, cancer, and stroke. The legislation is an outgrowth of the President's Commission on Heart Disease, Cancer and Stroke headed by Dr. Michael DeBakey.

1965 PL 89–272, Clean Air Act Amendments, provide for federal regulation of Motor Vehicle Exhaust (Title I) and establishes program of federal research and grants-in-aid in solid waste disposal (Title II).

1965 PL 89–290, Health Professions Educational Assistance Amendments, provide scholarships, loans, and construction aid to schools of medicine, osteopathy, and dentistry. Introduces provision of 50 percent forgiveness of loans for service in personnel shortage areas.

1965 Congress authorizes a program of Special Project Grants for health of school and preschool children under Title V of the Social Security Act Amendments (PL 89–97), including the delivery of compulsory health services to low-income children. Out of this legislation comes the Children and Youth (C and Y) projects and clinics administered through the Maternal and Child Health Service (Lewis et al. 1976).

1965 PL 89–73, The Older Americans Act, establishes an Administration on Aging within DHEW headed by a commissioner of aging appointed by the president. It declares 10 objectives for older people, which are the joint responsibility of federal, state, and local governments.

1965 PL 89–92, The Federal Cigarette Labeling and Advertising Act, requires that all cigarette packages or containers offered for sale in the United States must bear the warning statement: "Caution: Cigarette Smoking May be Hazardous to your Health." The new law preempts the field of cigarette labeling, precluding any federal, state, or local authority in the area.

1966 An amendment (PL 89–749) to the Office of Economic Opportunity (OED) legislation formalizes the Comprehensive Health Services Program, including the provision for the establishment of neighborhood health centers.

1966 PL 89–749, The Comprehensive Health Planning Act, is passed to promote comprehensive planning for health services, personnel, and facilities in federal-state-local partnership.

1966 PL 89–614 broadens eligibility to CHAMPUS and extends benefits beyond inpatient care.

1966 PL 89–642, Child Nutrition Act, establishes federal program of research and support for child nutrition, including authorization for school breakfast program.

1966 PL 89–751, Allied Health Professions Personnel Act, provides initial effort to support the training of allied health workers.

1967 Amendment to the Social Security Act (PL 90–248) seeks to raise the quality of care provided in nursing homes, establishing a number of conditions of nursing home participation under Medicare and Medicaid. Creats a new class of facility—the intermediate care facility. Establishes educational requirements for long-term care facility administrators (Kennedy amendment). The latter constitutes the first time that educational requirements for licensure are mandated by legislative fiat at the federal level.

1968 PL 90–407, amends the National Science Foundation to include major support of applied research in the sciences.

1968 PL 90–490, Health Manpower Act, authorizes formula institutional grants for training all health professionals and adds pharmacy and veterinary medicine to the professions covered.

1968 The Social Security Act is amended to strengthen the nursing home enforcement activities of the individual states. No federal matching funds may be paid to any nursing home that does not fully meet state requirements for licensure. States are also required, as part of their medical assistance program for skilled nursing home care, to evaluate each patient's needs prior to admission, followed by regular and periodic inspections of the care being given to medical assistance patients in nursing homes.

1969   PL 91–173, Federal Coal Mine Health and Safety Act, provides for protection of the health and safety of coal miners.

1969   PL 91–190, National Environmental Policy Act, creates the Council on Environmental Quality to advise the president on environmental matters; requires preparation of environmental impact statements before major federal actions.

1969   In an effort to slow the rise in Medicaid costs, the secretary of DHEW issues regulations setting an upper limit (75th percentile of customary charges) on fees to be paid to individual practitioners.

1970   PL 91–222, Public Health Cigarette Smoking Act, bans cigarette advertising from radio and television.

1970   The Communicable Disease Center is renamed the Center for Disease Control (CDC), and its functions are broadened under PL 91–464 to address other preventable conditions in addition to infectious disease.

1970   PL 91–596, Occupational Safety and Health Act (OSHA), provides federal program of standard setting and enforcement to assure safe and healthful conditions in the workplace.

1970   PL 91–616 establishes National Institute of Alcohol Abuse and Alcoholism and provides comprehensive aid program to states and localities.

1970   PL 91–623, Emergency Health Personnel Act, provides for assistance to health manpower shortage areas through the establishment of the National Health Service Corps.

1971   In his February health message to Congress, President Nixon introduces the notion of health maintenance organizations (HMOs) as the cornerstone of his administration's national health insurance proposal.

1971   The health industry is singled out for special stringent controls under the Economic Stabilization Act (and are the last segment of the economy to be relieved of such controls 3 years later).

1971   PL 92–157, Comprehensive Health Manpower Training Act, covering programs for students in medicine, osteopathy, dentistry, veterinary medicine, optometry, pharmacy, and podiatry replaces institutional formula grants with capitation grants. Provides for schools to receive a fixed sum of money for each student in return for agreeing to increase its enrollment by a specified percentage. Adds interest subsidies and loan guarantees to outright grants for construction (the sole previous financing mechanism under earlier programs) as the federal government assumes an active role in the funding of primary care. The act is the most comprehensive piece of health manpower legislation to date. A shift from support to control is evident (Losteller and Chapman 1979).

1972   PL 92–303 amends the Federal Coal Mine Health and Safety Act, providing benefits and other assistance for coals miners suffering from black lung disease.

1972   PL 92–426 establishes a Uniformed Services University of the Health Sciences and an Armed Forces Health Professions Scholarship Program.

1972   PL 92–433, The National School Lunch and Child Nutrition Amendments, adds funds to support nutritious diets for pregnant and lactating women and for infants and children (the WIC program).

1972   PL 92–541 authorizes the Veterans Administration (VA) to help establish eight state medical schools and provides grant support to existing medical schools.

1972   PL 92–573, Consumer Product Safety Act, creates Consumer Product Safety Commission and transfers enforcement of hazardous substances, flammable fabrics, poison prevention packaging acts to the commissions.

1972   PL 92–585, Emergency Health Personnel Act Amendments of 1972, establishes Public Health and National Health Services Corps scholarships.

1972   PL 92–603, amendments of the Social Security Act. Establishes, over the bitter opposition of organized medicine, Professional Standards Review Organizations (PSROs) to monitor the need and quality of care rendered to recipients of federal health programs. Extends health insurance benefits to the disabled and end-stage renal disease patients.

1972 PL 93–154, Emergency Medical Services Systems Act, provides aid to states and localities to establish coordinated cost-effective Emergency Medical Service (EMS) Systems.

1972 Blue Cross at McNerney's urging and in response to public pressure concerning conflict of interest, severs formal ties with AHA.

1973 PL 93–227 Health Maintenance Organization Act, provides assistance for the establishment and expansion of HMOs. Authorizes $375 million over a 5-year period for grants, loans, and loan guarantees for feasibility studies, development studies, and initial operations for new and existing HMOs.

1973 Congress passes the Older Americans Act that shifts the Administration on Aging from HEW's Social and Rehabilitation section to the Office of the Secretary, establishes the National Clearinghouse for Information on Aging, creates the Federal Council on Aging, and authorizes funds for the establishment of gerontology centers and grants for training and research in the field of aging.

1973 The National Institute of Occupational Safety and Health (NIOSH) is incorporated into the Center for Disease Control.

1973 Supreme Court (Roe vs. Wade, 410 U.S. 113, 93 S. Ct. 705) declares laws outlawing abortion unconstitutional.

1974 PL 93–247, Child Abuse Prevention and Treatment Act, creates a National Center on Child Abuse and Neglect, authorizes research and demonstration grants to states and other private and public agencies.

1974 PL 93–296, Research in Aging Act, establishes National Institute on Aging within the National Institutes of Health (NIH).

1974 PL 93–523, Safe Drinking Water Act, requires the Environmental Protection Agency to set national drinking water standards and aid states and localities in their enforcement.

1974 Moss (Sen. Frank, Dem., Utah) Senate Subcommittee on Nursing Homes issues extensive report detailing abuses in the nursing home industry.

1975 PL 93–641, The National Health Planning and Resources Development Act, sets up national designation of local health systems areas and authorizes major federal reorganization of health planning programs. Establishes a national certificate of need (CON) program.

1975 Rhode Island enacts first state catastrophic health insurance program.

1976 PL 94–484, Health Professions Educational Assistance Act, requires medical schools to have 50 percent of their graduates nationally entering primary residencies by 1980. Continues capitation payments but no longer requires enrollment increases as a condition for funding. Mandates that recipient schools reserve positions in their classes for U.S. students studying at foreign medical schools as a condition for receiving federal financial support. The latter provision is heatedly opposed by the U.S. medical schools as an unwarranted infringement on their right to determine admissions. Northwestern, Indiana, and Yale universities announce that they will not comply even if it should mean loss of federal funding.

1976 Medicare and Medicaid are transferred from the Social Security Administration and Social and Rehabilitation Service (SRS) and combined into a new agency, the Health Care Financing Administration (HCFA).

1976 Over the strenuous opposition of the hospital industry, Congress tightens up the immigration rules amending the Immigration and Nationality Act (Sections 101 and 212) to restrict the entry of alien physicians into the United States and imposes stringent constraints on the licensure of foreign medical graduates including the requirement of passage of the VISA and/or FLEX exam, declaring that "there is no longer an insufficient number of physicians and surgeons in the United States" and that "there is no further need for affording preference to alien physicians and surgeons in admission to the United States."

1977 PL 95–210, Rural Health Clinics Act, extends Medicare and Medicaid coverage to new health practitioners in rural clinics.

1977   The Carter administration proposes placing a cap (9 percent) on increases in hospital revenues to be reimbursed by federal programs by limiting what they can spend. The industry counters by proposing its own voluntary program deemed Voluntary Effort (VE).

1977   PL 95–215, Health Professions Education Amendments. Bowing to medical school pressure. Congress repeals the requirement that medical schools, as a condition of receiving capitation funds, must reserve an adequate number of positions in their classes for United States citizen foreign medical students (USFMS).

1978   The DHEW secretary, Joseph Califano, issues controversial bed supply guidelines to control excess hospital bed capacity in the United States. Rural and western sections of the country take strong exception, seeing the proposal as a further intrusion of the federal government on what they consider to be a local or state matter.

1980   The Department of Education is split off as a separate department from DHEW and the remainder is renamed the Department of Health and Human Services (DHHS).

1980   Medicare and Medicaid amendments of the Omnibus Reconciliation Act of 1980 (PL 96–499) results in significant changes in both programs, including simplification of methods for state reimbursement of nursing homes, increased funding for state Medicaid fraud-control units, changes in utilization review requirements, coverage of nurse-midwife services, reimbursement under both programs for hospital swing beds, and a measure for state enrollment in Medicare part B.

1980   The Center for Disease Control is reorganized and renamed Centers for Disease Control.

1981   President Reagan proposes the consolidation of 26 categorical health programs into two large block grants. Instead, Congress responds by creating four health block grants: preventive health (combining eight programs: home health, rodent control, water fluoridation, health education, risk reduction, health incentive grants, emergency medical services, rape crisis cen-

ters, and hypertension), health services, primary care, and maternal and child health care, authorizing all for 3 years or until the end of fiscal year (FY) 1984. (The Omnibus Budget Reconciliation Act of 1981, (PL 97–35). Several other programs originally targeted for block grants, that is, family planning, childhood immunization, VD research and treatment, migrant health center, tuberculosis, primary care research and demonstrations, retain their categorical status, and a new adolescent family life program is authorized.

1981   Capitation grants to schools of medicine, osteopathy, dentistry, veterinary medicine, optometry, podiatry, pharmacy, and nursing are eliminated.

1981   The provision for free medical care for merchant seamen is eliminated as of October 1, 1981, with existing public health hospitals slated for closure by end of fiscal year 1982.

1982   President Reagan proposes in a single bold stroke to create a "new federalism" transferring responsibility of many human services to the states.

1982   Office of Management and Budget considers proposals to trim the cost of Medicare by requiring the elderly to demonstrate need as a condition of receiving benefits. The introduction of a means test is acknowledged to constitute a significant change in the program, making Medicare less of an insurance program and more of an income assistance one.

1982   Congress passes the Tax Equity and Fiscal Responsibility Act (TEFRA) authorizing Medicare reimbursement for hospice services.

1982   The State of Arizona implements a new and experimental Medicaid Program known as the Arizona Health Care Cost Containment System (AHCCS). Its predominant feature is its reliance on competitive bidding to establish a complete acute care delivery system for its indigent population and to set capitated reimbursement rates for participating providers.

1982   The Health Resources and Services Administration is established through the merger of the Health Resources Administration and the Health Services Administration.

1982   Congress seeks to encourage and facilitate the development and approval of drugs for rare diseases and conditions by passage of the PL 97–414, the Orphan Drug Act.

1982   Congress passes PL 97–248, the Tax Equity and Fiscal Responsibility Act (TEFRA), which seeks to control costs by placing limits on total hospital costs per discharge adjusted to reflect each hospital's case mix. Places a ceiling on the annual rate of increase in total costs per discharge while providing a token incentive payment for hospitals that operate below the established limits. Also authorizes Medicare payments for hospice services but includes a "sunset provision" which allows the benefit to expire in 1986.

1982   Congress declines to kill PSROs (Professional Standards Review Organizations), transforming them into PROs (Peer Review Organizations) instead.

1983   Congress establishes a new Medicare hospital prospective payment (reimbursement) system based on the use of diagnostic related groups (DRGs) as part of the 1983 Amendments to the Social Security Act (PL98–21), signed into law June, 1983.

1983   On September 1, the Health Care Finance Administration ushers in a new era of Medicare hospital reimbursement with the publication of regulations implementing the DRG-based prospective payment system.

1984   Congress imposes a temporary (15 month) freeze on physician fees under Medicare as part of the Deficit Reduction Act (DEFRA) and adds the Child Health Assurance Program to Medicaid.

1984   Amendments to the Child Abuse Prevention and Treatment Act (PL 98–457) involving the states and Infant Care Review Committees in medical decisions about the treatment of handicapped newborns are passed.

1985   The Balanced Budget and Emergency Deficit Control Act, (H.J. Res. 372, PL 99–177) otherwise known as Gramm-Rudman, Hollings, mandates that if projected deficits exceed predetermined targets, federal spending is to be reduced according to a prescribed formula.

1985   The Reagan Administration seeks and Congress rejects placement of a cap on the exclusion of the amount contributed by employer to a worker's health benefit plan from the employee's taxable income.

1985   As part of the Consolidated Omnibus Budget Reconciliation Act of 1985 (COBRA), hospice care is made a permanent part of the Medicare Program. Payment rates under the program are raised and the states are given the ability to provide hospice services under the Medicaid Program. In addition, employers are required to continue health insurance for employees and their dependents who otherwise would lose their eligibility because of reduced work hours or termination of employment. Coverage is also extended to survivors and separated or divorced spouses of workers. Continuation of employer contributions, however, is not required.

1986   The Secretary of Health and Human Services, Otis Bowen, submits recommendations to the President calling for the expansion of federal health programs to provide coverage for catastrophic care.

1986   Congress enacts two omnibus budget bills: COBRA, the Consolidated Omnibus Budget Reconciliation Act and SOBRA, the Sixth Omnibus Budget Reconciliation Act. Both seek to clean up Medicare's prospective payment system for hospitals and gradually close some of the more gaping holes in Medicaid.
PL 99–272, PL 99–509. (Medicare), inner city hospitals serving a "disproportionate" share of poor patients are given a Medicare payment boost of as much as 15 percent. Payments for graduate medical education (GME) however, are scaled back, with direct GME support of residents and interns limited to five years of postgraduate work. Attempts to end support for foreign medical graduates fails, but passage of a tough new qualification test is required.
New penalties are imposed on hospitals that transfer (dump) poor patients to public and other facilities. Medicare hospice

benefit is made permanent, and restrictions are imposed on the growth of the Part A deductible. Physician fees are frozen for nearly three years and placed under federal controls beginning in 1987.

PL 99–278, PL 99–509 (Medicaid). Administration proposal to put the lid on federal Medicaid funding is rejected twice. Under COBRA, Medicaid coverage is mandated for pregnant women in two-parent families with an unemployed bread-winner. SOBRA, on the other hand, encourages coverage for pregnant women in families with incomes below the poverty line.

1986 Omnibus Health Act (PL 99–660). States are allowed to offer coverage to all pregnant women, infants up to one year of age, and, on a phased-in basis, children up to five years of age with incomes up to the federal poverty line.

1986 In a twelfth hour package of health bills, Congress provides for a federal vaccine injury compensation system (National Childhood Vaccine Injury Act) that would bypass the courts, limiting out-of-court awards to income losses plus $250,000 for pain and suffering or death; affords members of peer review committees protection from most damage suits filed by physicians who they discipline; mandates (Health Care Quality Improvement Act) creation of a national physician malpractice and discipline data bank to which physicians and hospitals are required to report information on licensure actions and malpractice claims paid; repeals PL 93–641, the 1974 National Health Planning and Resource Development Act, effective January 1, 1987, throwing responsibility for Certificate of Need programs to the states.

1987 Passage of the Omnibus Budget Reconciliation Act (PL 100–203) provides a number of significant changes in the Medicaid Program including additional options for children and pregnant women. Requires states to extend coverage to children up to age six with an option of allowing for coverage up to age eight. Encourages the provision of Medicaid clinic services to the homeless at shelters, soup kitchens and other such locations.

Also substantially amends and adds to the Medicaid nursing home law by eliminating the old law's distinction between skilled nursing facilities (SNFs) and intermediate care facilities (ICFs) and repeals its requirement that states pay less for ICF than SNF services. Requires that facilities maintain or enhance the quality of life of each resident and operate a quality assurance program, conduct and periodically update a standardized assessment of each resident's functional capacity; mandates that by October 1st, 1990, nursing homes serving Medicaid patients provide 24 hour nursing including at least one registered nurse on duty eight hours a day, seven days a week plus one licensed nurse on duty 24 hours per day seven days per week, plus employment of at least one full-time social worker in facilities of more than 120 beds. Nurse's aids are required to have at least 75 hours of pre-service training. While states may wave these requirements, each must have in effect by July 1, a preadmission screening program for all mentally ill or mentally retarded individuals to determine the appropriateness of placement in an SNF or ICF as well as review all mentally ill or mentally retarded nursing home residents to determine whether continued placement is appropriate.

In addition, OBRA '87 authorizes states to provide home and community based care to persons age 65 and over who otherwise would likely require care in a skilled nursing or intermediate care facility without prior treatment in such facilities. Finally, the act calls for the Secretary of Health and Human Services to establish federal qualifications for nursing home administrators.

1987 The National Health Service Corps (NHSC) Program (PL 100–177) is re-authorized and amended. Under a new loan repayment program, students who have completed their training or are in their final year may have up to $20,000 ($25,000 if Native Americans) of their educational and related loans repaid by the federal government in return for providing services to designated needy areas. The law also authorizes payment to states for loan repayment programs in which the state is responsible for 25 percent of program costs. Repayment for students who default on their scholarships since obligation is set at three times the amount of the scholarship, plus interest.

1987 The era of federal involvement in local regulation of health care capital spending ends as HHS terminates Section 1122 Capital review agreements with 16 states and the Virgin Islands. Begun in 1972, the program was the oldest federal effort at capital regulation and provided a separate capital review system operated by the states with some help from HHS. Coupled with the repeal of the 1974 National Health Planning and Resource Development Act in 1986, the Reagan Administration appears to have succeeded in its goal of dismantling the federal health planning apparatus.

1987 Following passage of the House's own version in late July, the Senate on an 86–11 vote, October 27, virtually assures ultimate enactment of a catastrophic insurance measure. The two bills (HR 2470; S. 1127), remarkably similar in scope, attempt to limit out-of-pocket expenditures by the elderly for Medicare-covered services. Both offer expanded coverage of short-term nursing home and home health care; both seek to finance the new benefits by taxing the upper-income elderly while charging the rest of the nation's 32 million beneficiaries relatively minor amounts. In addition, over the opposition of both the prescription drug industry and the Reagan administration, both provide for the first time, coverage of prescription drugs.

1987 Following an eleven year court battle, the AMA, America College of Surgeons and American College of Radiologists are found guilty of anti-trust and conspiracy in their efforts to restrain the practice of chiropractic medicine.

1987 Congress replaces the National Health Service Corps Scholarship Program with a loan repayment plan to keep medical students from defaulting on their government loans.

1987 Senator Edward Kennedy (Dem., Mass.) introduces legislation that would require employers to provide a minimum package of health benefits to any worker employed 17.5 hours or more a week and extends such coverage to spouses and dependents. Proposal draws support from some members of the automobile industry, but most corporations and small businesses, as well as the Reagan administration, oppose it.

1987 Oregon becomes the first state in the Union to limit organ transplants to kidneys and corneas under its Medicaid program. The decision arises after the state legislature opts for expanding its prenatal care program at the expense of providing additional funds for organ transplants. In so doing, the legislature makes explicit their preference, within the constraints of limited public resources, for investing in preventive services that can benefit many, rather than spend large sums for high tech procedures that would benefit only a few.

1987 The Reagan administration is accused of attempting to exert political control over government funded health services research. In testimony before a congressional committee, the former director of the National Center for Health Services Research tells of efforts by the Administration to stifle research that is not in agreement with its political aims, including recommending the creation of research agenda boards made up of political appointees to screen all research projects.

1987 The Surgeon General's annual report on smoking asserts for the first time that inhalation of cigarette smoke by non-smokers (passive smoking) is a cause of disease, including lung cancer. The report calls for the establishment of smoke-free work sites.

1988 Enactment of PL 100–360, the Catastrophic Health bill marks the largest expansion of the Medicare program in twenty-three years. Benefits which include outpatient drugs and a cap on enrollee co-payment costs for covered services are to be phased in over a four year period and financed entirely by enrollee premiums, with 37 percent of the costs to be covered by a fixed monthly premium, and the remainder by an income-related, supplemental premium—an income surtax to be paid by less than half (40 percent) of the enrollees.

1988 In the largest mailing on health ever done in the United States, some 45 million pieces, the Department of Health and Human Services sends out informational materials on the dangers of AIDS and methods of prevention to every residential address in the country.

1988 The Institute of Medicine issues its report on the status of public health in the U.S. While finding much to commend in the nation's public health efforts, the twenty-six member committee notes an even longer list of "problems," including citizen ignorance of what public health protection does for them, the difficulty public health officials have in communicating the urgency of prevention and other efforts to the public and its elected representatives, and the disorganization within and lack of coordination among agencies that carry out public health activities.

＊1988 The Department of Health and Human Services publishes rules that family planning clinics which receive federal funds may not do anything to assist women to obtain an abortion or increase the availability or accessibility of abortion for family planning purposes. The action is immediately challenged in the courts by Planned Parenthood, the American Public Health Association, the National Family Planning and Reproductive Health Association and other advocacy groups.

1988 Massachusetts enacts the first law in the nation to mandate competitive, universal health insurance coverage of an entire state's population.

1988 In a unanimous decision, the Supreme Court (*West v. Atkins*) confirms the right of prisoners to adequate health care in prisons and makes it clear that the constitutional mandate to provide such care is the same whether given by a full-time state employee or is contracted out.

1988 After initial controversy and delay, the Presidential Commission on the Human

Immune Deficiency Virus epidemic (AIDS) issues its final report to President Reagan. Emphasizing that in general the nation's response has been seriously deficient, the report proposes nearly 500 recommendations including a call for a national law barring discrimination against persons with AIDS, AIDS-related complex and those infected with the AIDS virus; a federal law penalizing improper diclosure of HIV-antibody test results; increased federal and state funds for drug abuse treatment; expedited consideration of AIDS budget requests from the Public Health Service; expanded access to voluntary HIV testing; and new efforts to provide less expensive noninstitutional care to AIDS patients.

1989 For the first time the federal government (Health Care Financing Administration) releases information on the quality of the nation's more than 15,000 nursing homes.

1989 Senate Finance Committee splits its health subcommittee into two in order to ease its workload. Responsibility for Medicaid and making health insurance coverage available to the nation's uninsured is to be handled by the subcommittee on Health and Families and the Uninsured, and oversight of Medicare budget issues and the search for ways to cover the cost of long term nursing home care is to rest with the subcommittee on Medicare and long term care.

1989 As part of the Omnibus Budget Reconciliation Act of 1989 (PL. 101–239) Congress calls for the establishment of the Agency for Health Care Policy and Research (AHPR) to succeed the National Center for Health Services Research and Health Care Technology Assessment (NCHSR). The purpose of the new agency is to enhance the quality, application and efficiency of Health Care Services and improve access to services.

1989 In response to intense pressure (over 5 million cards, letters, petitions and telegrams) from Senior Citizen groups and individuals (primarily upper and middle income elderly), upset over its funding provisions which would require many of them to pay an income tax surtax, the House votes 360 to 66 to repeal and the Senate, 73 to 26 to sharply cut back on the 1988 Catastrophic Coverage Act. Efforts by the Senate to save several features of the Act (i.e., unlimited inpatient hospital coverage, thirty-eight days of home health care per spell of illness, eighty hours a year of respite care, unlimited hospice care, $50 in coverage toward mammography screening for elderly and disabled women, as well as some Medicaid protection for low income elderly and poor pregnant women and infants) in the Conference Committee fail and the law, passed just sixteen months earlier, is repealed. As a result of the Congressional action, Medicare's previous Part A deductible and co-payment requirements as well the requirement of a three day hospital stay in order to be eligible for skilled nursing home care are revived.

1989   In its continuing effort to try to hold down costs, Congress adopts as part of its Medicare physician reforms, included under the FY (Fiscal Year) 90 budget legislation, a new volume performance standard (VPS) and directs the Department of Health and Human Services to establish a Medicare relative value scale (RVS) fee schedule, with a five year phase in.

REFERENCES

Becker, Dorothy D. and Ruth R. Johnson. 1980. *Chronology health professions legislation, 1956–1979.* DHHS Publication No. (HRA) 80–69, Bureau of Health Professions, Washington D.C.: USGPO.

Berliner, Howard S. 1973. The origins of health insurance for the aged. *International Journal of Health Services* 3, (3):465–474.

Bernard, Sydney E. and Eugene Feingold. 1970. The impact of Medicaid. *Wisconsin Law Review* 1970 (2):726–755.

Blendon, Robert *et al.*, eds. 1976. *Baselines for setting health goals and standards.* Papers on the National Health Guidelines. DHEW Publication No. (HRA) 76–640, Washington D.C.: USGPO.

Brown, Lawrence D. 1986. Introduction to a decade of transitions. *Journal of Health Politics, Policy and Law* 11(4): 569–583.

Chapman, Carleton B. and John M. Talmadge. 1970. Historical and political background of federal health care legislation, health care: Part I. *Law and Contemporary Problems* 35: Spring, 334–347.

Chapman, Carleton B. and John M. Talmadge. 1971. The evolution of the right to health concept in the United States. *The Pharos*, 34, (1): 30–51.

Congressional Quarterly. 1963. Medical care for the aged. *Congressional Quarterly special report.* Washington D.C.: Congressional Quarterly Service, Inc., August 15–17.

Corning, Peter A. 1969. *The evolution of Medicare . . . from idea to law.* Office of Research and Statistics, Social Security Administration, Department of Health, Education and Welfare. Research Report No. 29. Washington D.C.: USGPO.

Feingold, Eugene. 1966. *Medicare: Policy and politics.* San Francisco, CA.: Chandler Publishing Co.

Fishbein, Morris. 1947. *A history of the American Medical Association.* Philadelphia: W.B. Saunders Co.

Freedman, Ben. 1951. The Louisiana State Board of Health *American Journal of Public Health* 41:Fall, 1279–1285.

Freund, Deborah A. and Edward Neuschler. 1986. Overview of Medicaid capitation and case management initiatives. *Health Care Financing Review* Annual Supplement:21.

Gardner, John W., Wilbur J. Cohen and Ralph K. Huitt. 1965. *1965: Year of legislative achievements in health, education and welfare,* Office of the Secretary, DHEW, Washington, D.C.: USGPO.

Langwell, Kathryn M. and James P. Hadley. 1986. Capitation and the Medicare program: History, issues and evidence. *Health Care Financing Review,* 1986 Annual Supplement: 9–20.

Lewis, Charles E., Rashi Fein and David Mechanic. 1976. *A right to health.* New York: John Wiley and Sons.

Losteller, John O. and John E. Chapman. 1979. The participation of the United States Government in providing financial support for medical education. *Health Policy and Education:* 27–65.

Pegels, C. Carl. 1981. *Health care of the elderly.* Germantown, MD., Aspen Systems Corporation: 10, 14.

Wilson, Florence A. and Duncan Newhauser, eds. 1985. *Health services in the United States.* Cambridge, MA.: Ballinger Publishing Co., 2nd edition.

Bibliography

General Reference Guides To Congress, Legislation, and Governmental Affairs

Current Government Documents

▓ Theodor J. Litman ▓

Bills and Resolutions. One free copy of all legislation is printed daily after it is introduced and is available from one's member of Congress. One free copy of a bill, committee report, conference report, or public law may be obtained by sending a request along with a self-addressed mailing label to either Senate Document Room SH-B 04 or House Document Room H-226, U.S. Capitol, Washington, D. C., 20510.

Congressional Directory. Issued annually. Contains brief biographical sketches of each member of Congress, complete rosters of standing and special committees assignments by members, as well as maps of all congressional districts. Also lists major executives of all government agencies and members of the diplomatic corps. Available from the Superintendent of Documents, Government Printing Office (GPO).

The Congressional Record. Published in its present form since 1973. A verbatim transcript, subject to revision by members of Congress, of the proceedings and floor debates of the U.S. Senate and House of Representatives, including extension of remarks and materials inserted at the request of members of Congress. Bound sets consist of 15–20 parts per year, including separate index and, since 1947, *Daily Digest* volumes. A *Daily Digest* is included at the back of each issue. Single copies may be obtained by sending 75¢ to the Congressional Record Office, H-112, U.S. Capitol, Washington, D.C., 20515.

Committee Reports. When each piece of legislation goes to the floor, it is accompanied by a report that generally analyzes the bill, describes its purposes, and states the view of the committee members as to the desirability of its enactment. Available from the publications clerk of the appropriate committee.

Digest of Public General Bills. Cumulative compilation providing a brief description of each public bill introduced during the session.

Published approximately five times per year. Indexed by subject matter. Available from the Government Printing Office (GPO).

Federal Register. Published 5 days each week. Contains notices of proposed rule making as well as proposed regulations and changes and all legal documents of the executive branch. Available from the Government Printing Office (GPO).

Focus On. Published six times a year; each issue presents a thorough analysis of a single topic of major interest to state health policymakers and providers. Prepared by leading health care policy researchers and writers, the reports present the latest thinking on the topic and describe current policy and practice.

Forum. Bimonthly publication. Official magazine of the Health Care Financing Administration (HCFA). Covers all aspects of health care financing as well as HCFA programs and activities. Available from the Government Printing Office (GPO).

General Accounting Office Reports. Issued on an irregular basis by the General Accounting Office (GAO), the investigative and program auditing arm of Congress, pursuant to a special request by a congressional committee. Single copies may be obtained free of charge by writing the U.S. General Accounting Office, Document Handling and Information Services Facility, P.O. Box 6015, Gaithersburg, MD 20760. A free monthly listing of reports with summaries may be obtained by writing the General Accounting Office, 441 G. Street N.W., Washington, D.C. 20548.

Health Care Financing Review. Quarterly publication of the Health Care Financing Administration's Office of Research, Demonstrations and Statistics. Presents statistics on Medicare, Medicaid, national health expenditures, and related subjects, as well as reports on agency-supplied research. Demonstration and evaluation projects. Available from ORDS, HCFA, Room 1-E-9 Meadows Bldg., 6340 Security Blvd., Baltimore, MD 21235.

Index to U.S. Government Periodicals. Published quarterly. Index to articles appearing in periodicals produced by over 100 federal departments and agencies.

Intergovernmental Health Policy Project (IHPP).

2100 Pennsylvania Avenue, N.W., Suite 616, Washington, D.C., 20037. Devoted exclusively to research on health and health-related law and programs in the 50 states, and funded principally by contracts from the Health Care Financing Administration and the U.S. Public Health Service; IHPP is based at George Washington University. Publications include:

Issue Briefs. Published 20–25 times per year by the National Health Policy Forum, each brief provides a comprehensive examination of a current or emerging issue of principal concern to federal health policy makers including: a complete overview of the policy issue, its legislative history, the current state of debate, summaries of relevant studies, and descriptions of publications pertinent to the discussion.

Monthly Catalog of U.S. Government Publications. Monthly publication with annual cumulative index. Lists every document published by the federal government that is made available to the public, including House and Senate documents, hearings, and reports, as well as those of federal departments and agencies. Available from the Government Printing Office. (GPO).

Perspective. Published three to five times a year. HCFA's how-to publication for Medicaid and Medicare carriers, Medicare carriers and intermediaries, state, and local agencies. Articles address program techniques, procedures, and operations' management. Available from Health Care Financing Administration (HCFA).

Rules of the House and Senate. Published separately for the House and Senate at least once each Congress. Provides a useful reference on jurisdiction of committees, procedures in handling of legislation, precedents, etc.

Social Security Bulletin. Official monthly publication of the Social Security Administration. Offers feature articles, regular reports, notes, statistics, and analyses of public and private expenditures for hospital care and physicians services. Provides review of private health insurance and Medicare and Medicaid experience. Available from the Government Printing Office.

State Health Notes. Published ten times a year, it

provides up-to-date information on significant health policy trends and innovations occurring in the states, including analysis of significant federal and state health legislation and regulations; descriptions and reviews of major public health programs; highlights of innovative state programs; summaries of congressional activity in the health arena; as well as important findings and recommendations from the latest health policy research carried out by the states.

U. S. Code. There are 14 volumes and supplements. Published every 6 years, with annual supplements until the next publication. Compiled by subject under 50 titles. Includes all the general and permanent laws of the United States. Available from the Government Printing Office (GPO).

U.S. Government Manual. Issued annually. Official handbook of the federal government. Describes purposes and programs of most government agencies, including listings of top personnel. Contains brief references to the statuatory authority for federal programs by department or agency as well as organization charts and statements of purpose of various administrative units in the executive branch and the names and titles of principal administrative officers.

U. S. Statutes at Large. Official edition of federal laws arranged numerically in order of enactment. Includes subject and name index, list of bills enacted into law, guide to legislative history of bills enacted, and tables of laws affected. Usually consists of one of more volumes for each legislative session.

Commercial Publications

Almanac of American Politics. Contains biographies, group ratings, committee assignments, voting records, and lobby interests of members of Congress as well as political, demographic, and economic make-up of each member's state or district. Published by E.P. Dutton, 2 Park Avenue, New York, New York, 10016.

Congress and the Nation. Volume I (1945–1964), Volume II (1965–1968). Congressional Quarterly. A 3,100-page two-volume set. Documents all major legislative actions and national political campaigns from 1945 to 1968. Published by Congressional Quarterly, Inc.

Congress and Health: An Introduction to the Legislative Process and its Key Participants. Provides description of how a bill becomes a law. Gives practical information on how to determine the current status of a bill. Lists committees and subcommittees having significant impact on health legislation, including a brief description of their jurisdictions as well as names, photographs, and phone numbers of the six most important health subcommittees and the names of their staff members who handle health issues.

Commerce Clearing House Congressional Index. Weekly looseleaf publication. Lists, indexes, summarizes, and reports progress of bills and resolutions in Congress. Pending measures are indexed by number, subject, author, and headline term. Voting records of members of Congress on each bill and status tables of action taken on each bill in the House and Senate are given. Published by Commerce Clearing House, 4025 W. Peterson Avenue, Chicago, Illinois, 60646.

Congressional Information Service/Index to Publications of the U.S. Congress (CIS). Private commercial reference work. Abstracts and indexes all congressional committee hearings and all House and Senate reports, documents, and special publications. Available from Congressional Information Service, 4520 East-West Highway, Washington, D.C., 20014.

Congressional Quarterly's Guide to the Congress of the United States. A 1,000-page volume documenting the origins, development and operations of the U.S. Congress. Explains how Congress works, including its powers, pressures on it, and prospects for change.

Congressional Quarterly Weekly Report (CQ). Weekly report, published since 1945, of major congressional actions in the House and Senate. Contains all roll call votes taken in each chamber plus weekly political roundups. Includes rosters, updated committee and subcommittee assignments, presidential texts, and so on.

Congressional Quarterly Almanac. Published each spring since 1945. Presents a thorough review of the legislative and political activity of each session of Congress, as well as a summary of the terms of the U.S. Supreme Court.

Congressional Staff Aides for Health Legislation. Directory of the names, addresses, and phone numbers of senators and representatives and their staff aides assigned responsibility for health matters.

Congressional Staff Directory. Published annually. Contains staffs, lists of employees of members and committees. Available from Congressional Staff Directory, 300 New Jersey Ave. S.E., Washington, D.C.

Health Legislation and Regulation. Published weekly (50 issues). Originally, a publication of McGraw Hill, it is now distributed by Faulkner and Gray, Inc. Noted for its detailed briefings and ongoing analyses of Congressional health care developments, it provides detailed reports on the federal health budget, insurance coverage and interviews with Congressional health leaders. Includes comprehensive summaries of major health legislation and regulations as well as updates on new bills in Congress. Faulkner and Gray's Healthcare Information Center, 4401 Connecticut Avenue N.W., Box 12, Washington, D.C., 20008–2379.

Medicine and Health. A weekly (50 issues a year) newsletter, originally published by McGraw Hill and now distributed by Faulkner and Gray, Inc. Provides brief coverage of health care developments in Congress, HHS, the White House, the Executive branch, as well as reports on health care providers, associations and insurers including the current status and probable fate of health bills on Capitol Hill. A special four page section called "Perspectives" offers a provocative analysis of a different topic each week. Faulkner and Gray's Healthcare Information Center, 4401 Connecticut Avenue N.W., Box 12, Washington, D.C., 20008-2379.

National Health Council's Relations Handbooks: 1740 Broadway, New York, New York, 10019.

National Health Directory. Published annually. Directory of more than 6,000 key health and medical officials within Congress, including health legislative aides, federal agencies, state governments, federal regional offices, and congressional districts. Complete list of members of the six major congressional committees on health; current titles, addresses and phone numbers of health decision makers in offices of the governor, state agencies, and state legislators. Available from Science and Health Communications Group, Inc., 1740 N. Street. N.W., Washington, D.C., 20036.

National Journal Report. Weekly periodical reviews congressional activities, lobbying, campaign and policy issues. Includes chart of roll call votes. Spotlights federal officials and election campaign reports and analyzes executive action. Especially informative is the discussion on health policy issues by John Iglehart.

Private Health Organizations' Government Relations Directory. Lists major private health organizations and groups with major interest in health policy as well as names and phone numbers of their staffs assigned to lobby in Washington, D.C.

Washington Health Record. A weekly publication (50 issues) originally published by McGraw-Hill and now distributed by Faulkner and Gray, Inc. Lists presidential proclamations, federal regulations and notices, legislative activities including committee and floor actions on House and Senate bills. Faulkner and Gray's Healthcare Information Center, 4401 Connecticut Avenue N.W., Box 12, Washington, D.C., 20008–2379.

Other Sources

American Medical News. Weekly tabloid-size newspaper published by the AMA. Distributed free to association members as part of their dues and offered on subscription basis to others. Covers policy positions and activities of organized medicine at both the national and state level as well as governmental actions of interest to the medical profession.

Drug Research Reports (The Blue Sheet). A weekly

newsletter published by a commercial firm, providing special coverage of government activities in the drug, medical, and allied research fields. Reports on congressional committee hearings and health bills and reviews congressional and executive branch actions in the area of health and health care.

Hospitals. Semimonthly journal of the American Hospital Association. Particular attention is directed to two sections: "News at Deadline" and "Washington Briefs," located at the beginning and end of each issue, which focus on policy developments and government actions affecting the hospital industry.

Medical Care Review. Quarterly. Originally published by the School of Public Health at the University of Michigan and now published under the auspices of the Health Administration Press. Includes items from several of the nation's leading newspapers, for example, the *New York Times,* the *Washington Post,* the *Wall Street Journal,* and the *Christian Science Monitor,* as well as abstracts of new releases from the Department of Health and Human Services, the *Congressional Record,* and the major health care journals.

The Nation's Health. Tabloid-size newspaper of the American Public Health Association. Contains reports of current status of state and federal actions in the field of health and health care and comments on government activities as they relate to the public's health.

Warren, David G., "Current Resources for Health Law Research," Journal of Health Politics, Policy and Law, Vol. 11, Spring 1986, pp. 137–161.

The Politics of Health and Health Care

Begun, James W. and Ronald C. Lippincott. "A Case Study in the Politics of Free-Market Health Care." *Journal of Health Politics, Policy and Law* Vol. 7 (Fall 1982): 667–687.

Bellin, Lowell E. "The Intellectual Decline of the Health Care Left." *Medical Care* Vol. 18 (September 1980): 960–968.

Bergman, Abraham B. *The 'Discovery' of Sudden Infant Death Syndrome: Lessons in the Practice of Political Medicine.* Seattle, Washington: University of Washington Press, 1988.

Brown, J. H. U. and Southwest Research Consortium. *The Politics of Health Care.* Cambridge: Ballinger Publishing Co., 1978.

Cater Douglass and Philip R. Lee, eds. *Politics of Health.* New York: Medcom Press, 1972.

Edelman, Murray. "The Political Language of the Helping Professions." *Politics and Society* Vol. 4, No. 3 (1974): 295–310.

Facchinetti, Neil J. and W. Michael Dickson. "Access to Generic Drugs in the 1950's: The Politics of a Social Problem." *American Journal of Public Health* Vol. 72 (May 1982): 468–475.

Falcone, David. "The Challenge of Comparative Health Policy for Political Science." *Journal of Health Politics, Policy and Law* Vol. 1 (Summer 1976): 196–213.

Fox, Daniel M. *Health Policies, Health Politics: The British and American Experience, 1911–1965.* Princeton: Princeton University Press, 1986.

Fox, Daniel M. and Robert Crawford. "Health Politics in the United States." In Howard E. Freeman, Sol Levine and Leo G. Reeder, eds., *Handbook of Medical Sociology.* New York: The Free Press, 1979, 3d ed.: 392–411.

Goldsmith, Seth B. "Political Party Platform Planks: A Mechanism for Participation and Prediction?." *American Journal of Public Health* Vol. 63 (July 1973): 594–601.

Hodgson, Godfrey. "The Politics of Health Care: What is it Costing You?" *The Atlantic* Vol. 232 (October 1973): 95–61.

Hodgson, Godfrey, "The Politics of Health Care: What is it Costing You?" In David Kotelchuck, ed., *Prognosis Negative, Crisis in the Health System.* New York: Vintage Books, 1976:304–316.

Kaufman, Herbert. "The Political Ingredient of Public Health Services: A Neglected Area of Research." *Milbank Memorial Fund Quarterly* Vol. 44, pt.1 (October 1966): 13–34.

Krause, Elliott. "Health and the Politics of Technology." *Inquiry* Vol. 8 (September 1971):51–59.

Lee, Philip R. and A.E. Benjamin. "Health Policy and the Politics of Health Care." In Stephen J. Williams and Paul R. Torrens, ed., *Intro-*

duction to Health Services. New York: John Wiley and Sons, 1988, 3d ed. 457–479.

Lepawsky, Albert. "Medical Science and Political Science." Journal of Medical Education Vol. 42 (October 1967):905–917.

Lewis, Irving J. "Science and Health Care—The Political Problem." New England Journal of Medicine Vol. 281. (October 16, 1969): 888–896.

Lewis, Oscar. "Medicine and Politics in a Mexican Village." In Benjamin D. Paul, ed., Health, Culture, and Community. New York: Russell Sage Foundation, 1955:403–434.

Margolis, Richard J. "Where Does it Hurt: America's Medical Crisis and the Politics of Health Reform." The New Leader Vol. 57 (April 15 1974): 3–35.

Marmor, Theodore R., Amy Bridges and Wayne L. Hoffman. "Comparative Politics and Health Policies: Notes on Benefits, Costs, Limits." In Douglas E. Ashford, ed., Comparing Public Policies: New Concepts and Methods Vol. 4. Beverly Hills: Sage Publications (1978): 59–80.

Marmor, Theodore R. and Andrew B. Dunham. "Political Science and Health." In Thomas Choi and Jay Greenberg, eds., From Social Science Approaches to Health Services Research. Ann Arbor: Health Administration Press, 1982:55–80.

Marmor, Theodore R. and Andrew Dunham. "Political Science and Health Services Administration." In Theodore R. Marmor Political Analysis and American Medical Care. New York: Cambridge University Press, 1983:3–44.

Marmor, Theodore R., Donald A. Withman and Thomas C. Heagy. "Politics, Public Policy and Medical Inflation." In Michael Zubkoff, ed., Health: A Victim or Cause of Inflation. New York: Prodist, 1976: 299–316.

McKinlay, John B., ed. "Politics and Law in Health Care Policy." A Selection of Articles from the Milbank Memorial Fund Quarterly. New York: Prodist, 1973.

McKinlay, John B., ed. Politics and Health Care. A Milbank Reader, No. 6. Cambridge: MIT Press, 1981.

Mechanic, David. Politics, Medicine and Social Science. New York: John Wiley & Sons 1974.

Mendeloff, John, Politics and Bioethical Commissions. "Muddling Through" and the "Slippery Slope." Journal of Health Politics, Policy and Law Vol. 10 (Spring 1985):81–92.

Middleton, William J. "Politics of Liberating the Health System." The Black Scholar Vol. 5 (May 1974):16–25.

Millman, Michael L. "Politics and the Expanding Physician Supply." Unpublished doctoral dissertation, Columbia University, 1977, Microfilm No. 77–24, 110.

National League for Nursing. People, Power, Politics for Health Care. New York: National League for Nursing, 1976.

Navarro, Vicente. "Social Class, Political Power and the State: Their Implications in Medicine—Parts 1 and 2." Journal of Health Politics, Policy and Law Vol. 1 (Fall 1976): 256–284.

Powell, John E. Medicine and Politics: 1975 and After. Turnbridge Wells, England: Pitman Medical, 1976.

Record, Jane Cassels. "Medical Politics and Medical Prices: The Relation Between Who Decides and How Much it Costs." In Kenneth M. Friedman and Stuart H. Rakoff, eds., Toward a National Health Policy: Public Policy and the Control of Health Care Costs. Cambridge: Lexington Books, 1977.

Riska, Elainne and James A. Taylor. "Consumer Attitudes Toward Health Policy and knowledge About Health Legislation." Journal of Health Politics, Policy and Law Vol. 3 (Spring 1978):112–123.

Silver, George A. "Medical Politics, Health Policy, Party Health Platforms, Promise and Performance." International Journal of Health Services Vol. 6, No. 2 (1976):331–343.

Swanson, Bert E. "The Politics of Health." In Howard E. Freeman, Sol Levine and Leo G. Reeder, eds., Handbook of Medical Sociology. Englewood Cliffs, N.J.: Prentice-Hall, 1972, 2d ed.:435–455.

Taylor, Peter. The Smoke Ring: Tobacco, Money and Multinational Politics. New York: Pantheon Books, 1984.

Weaver, Jerry L. "Health Care Costs as a Political Issue: Comparative Responses of Chicanos and Anglos." Social Science Quarterly Vol. 53 (March 1973):846–854.

Weller, G. R. "From 'Pressure Group Politics' to 'Medical-Industrial Complex': The Development of Approaches to the Politics of Health." *Journal of Health Politics, Policy and Law* Vol. 1 (Winter 1977):444–470.

Wildavsky, Aaron. "Doing Better and Feeling Worse: The Political Pathology of Health Policy." *Daedalus* Vol. 106 (Winter 1977):105–123.

Zola, Irving K. "In the Name of Health and Illness: On Some Socio- Political Consequences of Medical Influence." *Social Science and Medicine* Vol. 9 (February 1975): 83–87.

Abortion

Karson, Stephen M. *Abortion: Politics, Morality, and the Constitution: A Critical Study of Row vs. Wade and Doe vs. Bolton and a Basis for Change.* Latham, M.D.: University Press of America, 1984.

Paige, Constance and Elisa B. Karnofsky. "The Antiabortion Movement and Baby Jane Doe." *Journal of Health Politics, Policy and Law* Vol. 11 (Summer 1986):255–270.

Roemer, Ruth. "Abortion Law Reform and Repeal: Legislative and Judicial Developments." *American Journal of Public Health* Vol. 61 (March 1971):500–509.

Schneider, Carl E. and Maris A. Vinovskis. *The Law and Politics of Abortion.* Lexington, MA.: Lexington Books, 1980.

Steinhoff, Patricia G. and Milton Diamond. *Abortion Politics: The Hawaii Experience.* Honolulu: University of Hawaii Press, 1977.

AIDS

Bayer, Ronald. *Private Acts, Social Consequences. AIDS and the Politics of Public Health.* New York: The Free Press, 1988.

Buchanan, Robert J. "State Medicaid Coverage of AZT and AIDS-Related Policies." *American Journal of Public Health* Vol. 78 (April 1988): 432–436.

Griggs, John, ed. *AIDS: Public Policy Dimensions.* New York: United Hospital Fund of New York, 1987.

Hellinger, Fred J. "National Forecasts of the Medical Care Costs of AIDS: 1988–1992." *Inquiry* Vol. 25 (Winter 1988):469–484.

Hummel, Robert F., William F. Leavy, Michael Rampolla, and Sherry Chorost, eds. *AIDS: Impact on Public Policy. An International Forum: Policy, Politics, and AIDS.* New York: Plenum Publishing, 1988.

Judson, Franklyn N. and Thomas M. Vernon, Jr. "The Impact of AIDS on State and Local Health Departments: Issues and a Few Answers." *American Journal of Public Health* Vol. 78 (April 1988):387–393.

Krieger, Nancy. "AIDS Funding: Competing Needs and the Politics of Priorities." *International Journal of Health Services* Vol. 18, No. 4 (1988):521–542.

Krieger, Nancy and Joyce C. Lashoff. "AIDS; Policy Analysis and the Electorate: The Role of Schools of Public Health." *American Journal of Public Health* Vol. 78 (April 1988): 411–417.

Lee, Philip R. and Peter S. Arno. "The Federal Response to the AIDS Epidemic." *Health Policy* Vol. 6, No. 3 (1986):259–267.

Panem, Sandra. *The AIDS Bureaucracy (Why Society Failed to Meet the AIDS Crises and How We Might Improve Our Response).* Cambridge: Harvard University Press, 1988.

Rabin, Judith A. "The AIDS Epidemic and Gay Bathhouses: A Constitutional Analysis." *Journal of Health Politics, Policy and Law* Vol. 10 (Winter 1986):729–748.

Richland, Jordan H. "Role of State Health Agencies in Responding to AIDS." *Public Health Reports* Vol. 103 (May–June 1988): 267–272.

Rowe, Mona and Caitlin C. Ryan. *AIDS: A Public Health Challenge, State Issues, Policies and Programs.* Washington, D.C.: Intergovernmental Health Policy Project, George Washington University, October 1987.

Rowe, Mona and Caitlin C. Ryan. "Comparing State-Only Expenditures for AIDS." *American Journal of Public Health* Vol. 78 (April 1988):424–431.

Shilts, Randy. *And The Band Played On: Politics, People and the AIDS Epidemic.* New York: St. Martins Press, 1987.

Singer, Eleanor, Theresa F. Rogers and Mary Concoran. "The Polls—A Report: AIDS."

Public Opinion Quarterly Vol. 51 (Winter 1987): 580–595.

Cancer

Eisenberg, Lucy. "The Politics of Cancer." *Harpers* Vol. 243 (November 1971):100–105.

Epstein, Samuel S. *Politics of Cancer.* San Francisco: Sierra Club Books, 1978.

Hixson, Joseph. *The Patchwork Mouse, Politics and Intrigue in the Campaign to Conquer Cancer.* Garden City, N.Y.: Anchor Press/Doubleday and Co., 1976.

Lally, John J. "Social Determinants of Differential Allocation of Resources to Disease Research: A Comparative Analysis of Crib Death and Cancer Research." *Journal of Health and Social Behavior* Vol. 18 (June 1977):125–138.

Levine, Adeline G. *Love Canal, Politics and People.* Lexington, MA.: Lexington Books, 1982.

Markle, Gerald E. and James C. Peterson, eds. *Politics, Science and Cancer: The Laetrile Phenomenon.* Boulder, CO.: Westview Press, 1980.

Rettig, Richard A. *Cancer Crusade: The Story of the National Cancer Act of 1971.* Princeton, N.J.: Princeton University Press, 1977.

Strickland, Stephen P. *Politics, Science and Dread Disease: A Short History of United States Medical Research Policy.* Cambridge: Harvard University Press, 1972.

Whelan, Ellen Haas. "Government: Hindrance or Help in the Cancer War?" In Bernard H. Siegan, ed., *Government, Regulation and the Economy.* Lexington, MA.: Lexington Books, 1980.

Competition-Regulation

Altman, Drew. "The Politics of Health Care Regulation: The Case of the National Health Planning and Resources Development Act." *Journal of Health Politics, Policy and Law* Vol. 2 (Winter 1978):560–580.

Ashby, John L., Jr. "The Impact of Hospital Regulatory Programs on Per Capita Costs, Utilization and Capital Investment." *Inquiry* Vol. 21 (Spring 1984):45–59.

Avellone, Joseph C. and Francis D. Moore. "The Federal Trade Commission Enters a New Arena: Health Services." *New England Journal of Medicine* Vol. 299 (August 31, 1978):478–483.

Barth, Peter S. "The Tragedy of Black Lung: Federal Compensation for Occupational Disease." Kalamazoo, Ml.: Upjohn Institute for Employment Research, 1987.

Battistella, Roger M. and Thomas P. Weil. "Pro-competitive Health Policy: Benefits and Perils." *Frontiers of Health Services Management* Vol. 2 (May 1986):3–27.

Bauer, Morris L. "Regulating Physician Supply: The Evolution of British Columbia's Bill 41." *Journal of Health Politics, Policy and Law* Vol. 13 (Spring 1988):1–26.

Bice, Thomas W. "The Politics of Health Care Regulation." in Theodor J. Litman and Leonard Robins, eds., *Health Politics and Policy.* New York: John Wiley and Sons, 1984:274–289.

Chesney, James D. "The Politics of Regulation: An Assessment of Winners and Losers." *Inquiry* Vol. 19 (Fall 1982) 235–245.

Christoffel, Tom and Katherine K. Christoffel. "The Consumer Product Safety Commission's Opposition to Consumer Product Safety: Lessons for Public Health Advocates." *American Journal of Public Health* Vol. 79 (March 1989):336–339.

Cohen, Harris S. "Regulating Politics and American Medicine." *American Behavioral Scientist* Vol. 19, No. 1 (1975):122–136.

Curran, William, Richard Steele and Ellen Ober. "Government Intervention on Increase," *Hospitals* Vol. 49 (May 16, 1975):57–61.

Day, Patricia and Rudolf Klein. "The Regulation of Nursing Homes: A Comparative Perspective." *Milbank Memorial Fund Quarterly* Vol. 65, No. 3 (1987):303–347.

Dranove, David and Kenneth Kone. "Do States' Rate Setting Regulations Really Lower Hospital Expenses?" *Journal of Health Economics* Vol. 4 (June 1985):159–165.

Eby, C.A. and Donald R. Cohodes. "What Do We Know About Rate Setting?" *Journal of Health Politics, Policy and Law* Vol. 10 (Summer 1985):299–327.

Feldstein, Paul J. "The Emergence of Market Competition in the U.S. Health Care System. Its Courses, Likely Structure and Implications." *Health Policy* Vol. 6, No. 1 (1986):1–20.

Finkler, Merton D. "State Rate Setting Revisited." *Health Affairs* Vol. 6 (Winter 1987):82–89.

Fuchs, Victor R. "The 'Competition Revolution' in Health Care." *Health Affairs* Vol. 7 (Summer 1988):5–24.

Gaumer, Gary L. "Regulating Health Professionals: A Review of the Empirical Literature." *Milbank Memorial Fund Quarterly* Vol. 62 (Summer 1984): 380–416.

Grabowski, Henry G. *Drug Regulation and Innovation,* Evaluative Studies No. 28, Washington, D.C.: American Enterprise Institute for Public Policy Research, 1976.

Greenberg, Warren. *Competition in the Health Care Sector: Ten Years Later.* Durham, N.C.: Duke University Press, 1988.

Joskow, Paul. *Controlling Hospital Costs: The Role of Government Regulation.* Cambridge, MA.: MIT Press, 1984.

Kavaler, Florence, Howard R. Kelman, and Alan P. Brownstein. "Regulating Health Care. Prospects for the Future." *Journal of Public Health Policy* Vol. 1 (September 1980):230–240.

Kennedy, Donald. "Health, Science, and Regulation: The Politics of Prevention." *Health Affairs* Vol. 2 (Fall 1983): 39–51.

Krause, Elliott A. "The Political Context of Health Service Regulation." *International Journal of Health Services* Vol. 5, No. 4 (1975):593–608.

Levin, Arthur. *Regulating Health Care. The Struggle for Control.* New York: Academy of Political Science, 1981.

Levine, Adeline G. *Love Canal: Science, Politics, and People.* Lexington, MA.: Lexington Books, 1982.

Luft, Harold S. "Competition and Regulation." *Medical Care* Vol. 23 (May 1985):383–400.

MacSheoin, Thomas. "The Dismantling of U.S. Health and Safety Regulations Under the First Reagan Administration: A Bibliography." *International Journal of Health Services* Vol. 15, No. 4 (1985):585–608.

McCaffrey, David P. *OSHA and the Politics of Health Regulation.* New York: Plenum Publishing Corp., 1982.

McCall, Nelda, Thomas Rice and Arden Hall. "The Effect of State Regulations on the Quality and Sale of Insurance Policies to Medicare Beneficiaries." *Journal of Health Politics, Policy and Law* Vol. 12 (Spring 1987) 53–76.

Melhaldo, Evan M. "Competition Versus Regulation in American Health Policy." in Evan M. Melhaldo, Walter Feinberg and Harold W. Swartz, eds., *Money, Power and Health Care.* Ann Arbor, MI, Health Administration Press, 1988:15–102.

Mendeloff, John M. *Regulation Safety. An Economic and Political Analysis of Occupational Safety and Health Policy.* Cambridge: MIT Press, 1979.

Mendeloff, John M. *The Dilemma of Toxic Substance Regulation: How Overregulation Causes Underregulation.* Cambridge, MA: MIT Press, 1988.

Merrill, Jeffrey and Catherine McLaughlin. "Competition Versus Regulation: Some Empirical Evidence." *Journal of Health Politics, Policy and Law* Vol. 10 (Winter 1986):613–623.

Meyer, Jack A., ed. *Incentives Versus Controls in Health Policy.* Washington, D.C.: American Enterprise Institute for Public Policy Research, 1987.

Morford, Thomas G. "Nursing Home Regulation: History and Expectations." *Health Care Financing Review* 1988 Supplement (December 1988):129–132.

Morrisey, Michael A., Frank A. Sloan and Samuel A. Mitchell. "State Rate Setting: An Analysis of Some Unresolved Issues." *Health Affairs* Vol. 2 (Summer 1983):36–47.

Mosher, James F. and Lawrence M. Wallack. "Government Regulation of Alcohol Advertising: Protecting Industry Profits Versus Promoting the Public Health." *Journal of Public Health Policy* Vol. 2 (December 1981):333–353.

Pauly, Mark V. "Is Medical Care Different? Old Questions, New Answers." *Journal of Health Politics, Policy and Law* Vol. 13 (Summer 1988):227–238.

Rice, Donald. "Government Regulation of the Hospital Industry in Colorado." *Journal of Public Health Policy* Vol. 2 (March 1981):58–69.

Rolph, Elizabeth S., Paul B. Ginsburg and Susan D. Hosek. "The Regulation of Preferred Provider Arrangements." *Health Affairs* Vol. 6 (Fall 1987):32–45.

Schramm, Carl J. "Revisiting the Competition/Regulation Debate in Health Care Cost Containment." *Inquiry* Vol. 23 (Fall 1986):236–242.

Schramm, Carl J., Steven C. Renn and Brian Biles. "Controlling Hospital Cost Inflation: New Perspectives on State Rate Setting." *Health Affairs* Vol. 5 (Fall 1986):22–33.

Schwartz, Teresa M. "Protecting Consumer Health and Safety: The Need for Coordinated Regulation Among Federal Agencies." *George Washington Law Review* Vol. 43 (May 1975):1031–1076.

Sloan, Frank A. "Rate Regulation as a Strategy for Hospital Cost Control: Evidence from the Last Decade." *Milbank Memorial Fund Quarterly* Vol. 61 (Spring 1983):195–221.

Smith, Barbara E. *Digging Our Own Graves: Coal Miners and the Struggle Over Black Lung Disease.* Philadelphia: Temple University Press, 1987.

Spitz, Bruce and John Abramson. "Competition, Capitation and Case Management. Barriers to Strategic Reform." *Milbank Memorial Fund Quarterly* Vol. 65, No. 3 (1987):348–370.

Thomas, Constance. "CON Changes Taper Off." *State Health Notes,* No. 67. Washington, D.C.: Intergovernmental Health Policy Projects, George Washington University, October 1986.

Cost Containment

Abel-Smith, Brian. *Cost Containment in Health Care: A Study of Twelve European Countries 1977–1983,* occasional papers on Social Administration, No. 73. Bedford, England: London Square Press, Brookfield Publishing Company, 1984.

Birch, Stephen. "DRGs U.K. Style: A Comparison of U.K. and U.S. Policies for Hospital Cost Containment and Their Implications for Health Status." *Health Policy* Vol. 10, No. 2 (1988):143–154.

Christianson, Jon B. and Kenneth R. Smith. *Current Strategies for Containing Health Care Expenditures.* Bridgeport, CT.: Robert B. Luce, Inc., 1985.

Christianson, Jon B. and Diane G. Hillman. *Health Care for the Indigent and Competitive Contracts: The Arizona Experiment.* Ann Arbor, MI.: Health Administration Press, 1986.

Christianson, Jon B., Diane G. Hillman and Kenneth R. Smith. "The Arizona Experiment: Competitive Biding for Indigent Medical Care." *Health Affairs* Vol. 2, No. 3 (1983):88–103.

Davis, Karen, Gerard F. Anderson, Steven C. Renn, Diane Rowland, Carl J. Schramm, and Earl Steinberg. "Is Cost Containment Working?" *Health Affairs* Vol. 4 (Fall 1985): 81–94.

Evans, Robert G. "Finding the Levers, Finding the Courage: Lessons for Cost Containment in North America." *Journal of Health Politics, Policy and Law* Vol. 11, No. 4 (1986):585–615.

Fraser, Irene. "Medicare Reimbursement for Hospice Care: Ethical and Policy Implications of Cost-Containment Strategies." *Journal of Health Politics, Policy and Law* Vol. 10 (Fall 1985):565–578.

Fuchs, Victor. "Has Cost Containment Gone Too Far?" *Milbank Memorial Fund Quarterly* Vol. 64, No. 3 (1986): 479–488.

Lave, Judith R. "Cost Containment Policies in Long-Term Care." *Inquiry* Vol. 22 (Spring 1985):7–23.

McCall, Nelda, Douglas Henton, Susan Haber, et al. "Evaluation of Arizona Health Care Cost Containment System., 1984–85." *Health Care Financing Review* Vol. 9 (Winter 1987):79–90.

McCarthy, Carol M. "DRGs—Five Years Later." *New England Journal of Medicine* Vol. 318 (June 23, 1988):1683–1686.

McCue, Jack D., ed. *The Medical Cost-Containment Crisis: Fears, Opinions, and Facts.* Melrose Park, IL.: Health Administration Press, 1989.

Mechanic, David. "Cost Containment and the Quality of Medical Care: Rationing Strategies in an Era of Constrained Resources." *Milbank Memorial Fund Quarterly* Vol. 63 (Summer 1985):453–475.

Menges, Joel. "From Health Services Research to Federal Law: The Case of DRGs." In Marion Ein Lewin, ed., *From Research into Policy. Improving the Link for Health Services.* Washington, D.C.: American Enterprise Institute for Public Policy Research, 1986:20–23.

Rosko, Michael D. and Robert W. Broyles. "The Impact of the New Jersey All-Payer DRG System." *Inquiry* Vol. 23 (Spring 1986):67–75.

Sapolsky, Harvey M. "Prospective Payment in Perspective." *Journal of Health Politics, Policy and Law* Vol. 11, No. 4 (1986):633–645.

Schramm, Carl J. "State Hospital Cost Containment: An Analysis of Legislative Initiatives." *Indiana Law Review* Vol. 19, No. 4 (1986):919–954.

Schramm, Carl J. and Jon Gabel. "Prospective Payment—Some Retrospective Observations." *New England Journal of Medicine* Vol. 318 (June 23, 1988):1681–1682.

Sheingold, Steven H. "Unintended Results of Medicare's National Prospective Payment Rates." *Health Affairs* Vol. 5 (Winter 1986):5–21.

Disability and Rehabilitation

Berkowitz, Edward D. "Rehabilitation: The Federal Government's Response to Disability, 1935–1954." Unpublished doctoral dissertation, Northwestern University, 1976. Also, New York: Arno Press, 1980.

Brandt, Allan M. "Polio, Politics, Publicity and Duplicity: Ethical Aspects in the Development of the Salk Vaccine." *International Journal of Health Services* Vol. 8, No. 2 (1978): 257–270.

Howards, Irving, Henry P. Brehm and Saad Z. Nagi. *Disability: From Social Problem to Federal Program.* New York: Praeger Publishers, 1980.

Krause, Elliott A. "The Political Sociology of Rehabilitation." In Gary L. Albrecht, ed., *The Sociology of Physical Disability and Rehabilitation.* Pittsburgh, PA.: University of Pittsburgh Press, 1976: 201–222.

Morris, Robert, ed. *Allocating Health Resources for the Aged and Disabled. Technology versus Politics.* Lexington, MA.: Lexington Books, 1981.

Rivlin, Alice M. and Joshua M. Wiener. *Caring for the Disabled Elderly: Who Will Pay?* Washington, D.C.: The Brookings Institution, 1988.

Scotch, Richard K. *From Good Will to Civil Rights: Transforming Federal Disability Policy.* Philadelphia: Temple University Press, 1984.

Spingarn, Natalie Davis. *Heartbeat: The Politics of Health Research.* Washington, D. C.: Robert B. Luce, 1976.

Stone, Deborah. *The Disabled State.* Philadelphia: Temple University Press, 1984.

Drugs

Blank, Charles H. "Delaney Clause: Technical Naivete and Scientific Advocacy in the Formulation of Public Health Policies." *California Law Review* Vol. 62 (July-September 1974): 1084–1120.

Campbell, Rita Ricardo. *Drug Lag; Federal Government Decision Making,* Hoover Institution Studies No. 55. Stanford, CA.: Hoover Institution Press, 1976.

Greenberg, Daniel S. "Report of the President's Biomedical Panel and the Old Days at the FDA." *New England Journal of Medicine* Vol. 294 (May 27, 1976): 1245–1246.

Landau, Richard L., ed. *Regulating New Drugs,* Chicago, IL.: University of Chicago, Center for Policy Study, 1973.

Peltzman, Sam. *Regulation of Pharmaceutical Innovation: The 1962 Amendments,* Research Evaluative Studies No. 15. Washington, D.C.: American Enterprise Institute for Public Policy Research, 1974.

Rock, Paul E., ed. *Drugs and Politics.* New Brunswick, N.J.: Transaction Books, 1977.

Schroeder, Richard C. *The Politics of Drugs: Marijuana to Mainlining.* Washington, D.C.: Congressional Quarterly, 1975.

Silverman, Milton and Philip R. Lee. *Pills, Profits and Politics.* Berkeley, CA.: University of California Press, 1974.

Steslicke, William E. *Doctors in Politics: The Political Life of the Japan Medical Association.* New York: Praeger Publishers, 1973.

Wardell, William M. and Louis Lasagna. *Regula-*

tion and Drug Development. Washington, D.C.: The American Enterprise Institute for Public Policy Research, 1975.

Health Care Finance (see also Medicare and Medicaid; National Health Insurance)

Anderson, Gerard F. "National Medical Care Spending." *Health Affairs* Vol. 4 (Fall 1985): 100–107 and Vol. 5 (Fall 1986): 123–130.

Anderson, Gerard F. "Payment Reform in the United States." *Health Policy* Vol. 6, No. 4 (1986): 321–328.

Eastaugh, Steven R. *Financing Health Care: Economic Efficiency and Equity.* Dover, MA.: Auburn House Publishing Co., 1987.

Enthoven, Alain. "Managed Competition in Health Care and the Unfinished Agenda." *Health Care Finance Review* (1988 Supplement): 105–119.

Enthoven, Alain. "Managed Competition of Alternative Delivery Systems." *Journal of Health Politics, Policy and Law* Vol. 13 (Summer 1988): 305–322.

Feldman, Roger. "Health Care. The Tyranny of the Budget." In David Boaz, ed., *Assessing the Reagan Years.* Washington, D.C.: CATO Institute, 1988.

Fuchs, Victor. "Has Cost Containment Gone Too Far?" *Milbank Memorial Fund Quarterly* Vol. 64, No. 3 (1986): 479–488.

Ginsburg, Paul B. "Physician Payment Policy in the 101st Congress." *Health Affairs* Vol. 8 (Spring 1989): 5–20.

Glaser, William A. "Juggling Multiple Payers: American Problems and Foreign Solutions." *Inquiry* Vol. 21 (Summer 1984): 178–188.

Glaser, William A. *Paying the Hospital: The Organizational Dynamics and Effects of Differing Financial Arrangements.* San Francisco, CA.: Jossey-Bass, 1987.

Langwell, Kathryn and Lyle M. Nelson. "Physician Payment Systems: A Review of History, Alternatives and Evidence." *Medical Care Review* Vol. 43 (Spring 1986): 5–58.

Levit, Katharine and Mark S. Freeland. "National Medical Care Spending: Datawatch." *Health Affairs* Vol. 7 (Winter 1988): 124–136.

McMenamin, Peter. "Medicare Part B: Rising As-signment Rates, Rising Costs." *Inquiry* Vol. 24 (Winter 1987): 344–356.

Ron, Aviva. "Sharing in the Financing of Health Care: Government, Insurance and the Patient." *Health Policy* Vol. 6, No. 1 (1986): 87–101.

Schieber, George J. and Jean-Pierre Poullier. "International Health Care Spending. Datawatch." *Health Affairs* Vol. 5 (Fall 1986): 111–122.

Schramm, Carl J., Steven C. Renn and Brian Biles. "Cost Inflation: New Perspectives on State Rate Setting." *Health Affairs* Vol. 5 (Fall 1986): 22–33.

Somers, Anne R. "Financing Long-Term Care for the Elderly: Institutions, Incentives, Issues." In Institute of Medicine. National Research Council. *America's Aging Health in an Older Society.* Washington, D.C., Institute of Medicine, National Academy Press, 1985: 182–233.

Health Insurance and the Uninsured

Black, Jeanne T. "The Employed Uninsured and the Role of Public Policy." *Inquiry* Vol. 23 (Summer 1986): 209–212.

Bovbjerg, Randall R. and William G. Kopit. "Coverage and Care for the Medically Indigent: Public and Private Options." *Indiana Law Review* Vol. 19, No. 4 (1986): 857–917.

Bowler, M. Kenneth. "Changing Politics of Federal Health Insurance Programs." *PS* Vol. 20 (Spring 1987): 202–211.

Butler, Patricia A. *Too Poor to be Sick. Access to Medical Care for the Uninsured.* Washington, D.C.: American Public Health Association, 1989.

Cohodes, Donald R. "America: The Home of the Free, the Land of the Uninsured." *Inquiry* Vol. 23 (Fall 1986): 227–235.

Davis, Karen and Diane Rowland. "Uninsured and Underserved: Inequities in Health Care in the United States." *Milbank Memorial Fund Quarterly* Vol. 61 (Spring 1983): 149–176.

Enthoven, Alain. "A New Proposal to Reform the Tax Threat of Health Insurance." *Health Affairs* Vol. 3 (Spring 1984) 21–39.

Evans, Robert G. "Public Health Insurance—The

Collective Purchase of Individual Care." *Health Policy* Vol. 7, No. 115 (1987): 115–134.

Feder, Judith, Jack Hadley and Ross Mullner. "Falling Through the Cracks: Poverty, Insurance Coverage, and Hospital Care for the Poor, 1980 and 1982." *Milbank Memorial Fund Quarterly* Vol. 62 (Fall 1984): 544–566.

Fein, Rashi. *Medical Care, Medical Costs: The Search for a Health Insurance Policy.* Cambridge: Harvard University Press, 1986.

Fox, Daniel M. and Daniel C. Schaffer. "Tax Policy as Social Policy: Cafeteria Plans, 1978–1985." *Journal of Health Politics, Policy and Law* Vol. 12 (Winter 1987): 609–664.

Freedman, Benjamin and Francoise Baylis. "Purpose and Function in Government-Funded Health Coverage." *Journal of Health Politics, Policy and Law* Vol. 12 (Spring 1987): 97–112.

Holmes, Martin. "Tax Policy and the Demand for Health Insurance." *Journal of Health Economics* Vol. 3 (December 1984): 203–221.

Long, Stephen H. "Public Versus Employment-Related Health Insurance: Experience and Implications for Black and Non-black Americans." *Milbank Memorial Fund Quarterly* Vol. 65, Supplement 1 (1987): 200–212.

McCall, Nelda. *Medigroup—Study of Comparative Effectiveness of Various State Regulations.* Menlo Park, CA: SRI International, 1983.

McCall, Nelda, Thomas Rice and Arden Hall. "The Effect of State Regulations on the Quality and Sale of Insurance Policies to Medicare Beneficiaries." *Journal of Health Politics, Policy and Law* Vol. 12 (Spring 1987): 53–76.

Monheit, Alan C., Michael M. Hagan, Marc L. Berk and Gail R. Wilensky. "Health Insurance for the Unemployed: Is Federal Legislation Needed?" *Health Affairs* Vol. 3 (Spring 1984): 101–111.

Monheit, Alan C., Michael M. Hagan, Marc L. Berk and Pamela J. Farley. "The Employed Uninsured and the Role of Public Policy." *Inquiry* Vol. 22 (Winter 1985): 348–364.

Mulstein, Suzanne. "The Uninsured and the Financing of Uncompensated Care: Scope, Costs, and Policy Options." *Inquiry* Vol. 21 (Fall 1984): 214–229.

Regula, Ralph. "National Policy and the Medi-

cally Uninsured." *Inquiry* Vol. 24 (Spring 1987): 48–56.

Reinhardt, Uwe E. "Health Insurance for the Nation's Poor." *Health Affairs* Vol. 6 (Spring 1987): 101–112.

Rice, Thomas and Jon Gabel. "Protecting the Elderly Against High Health Care Costs." *Health Affairs* Vol. 5 (Fall 1986): 5–21.

Thorpe, Kenneth E. "Uncompensated Care Pools and Care to the Uninsured: Lessons from the New York Prospective Hospital Reimbursement Methodology." *Inquiry* Vol. 25 (Fall 1988): 354–363.

Wilensky, Gail R. "Viable Strategies for Dealing with the Uninsured." *Health Affairs* Vol. 6 (Spring 1987): 33–46.

Wilensky, Gail R., Pamela J. Farley, and Amy K. Taylor. "Variations in Health Insurance Coverage: Benefits versus Premiums." *Milbank Memorial Fund Quarterly* Vol. 62 (Winter 1984): 53–81.

Health Maintenance Organizations

Bauman, Patricia. "The Formulation and Evolution of the Health Maintenance Organization Policy, 1970–1973." *Social Science and Medicine* Vol. 10 (March–April 1976): 129–142.

Brown, Lawrence D. *Politics and Health Care Organization: HMO's as Federal Policy,* Washington D.C.: The Brookings Institution, 1983.

Falkson, Joseph L. *HMO's and the Politics of Health System Reform.* Chicago: American Hospital Association and Robert J. Brady Co., 1980.

Moran, Donald W. "HMO's, Competition and the Politics of Minimum Benefits." *Milbank Memorial Fund Quarterly/Health and Society* Vol. 59, No. 2 (Spring 1981): 190–208.

Schlesinger, Mark. "On the Limits of Expanding Health Care Reform: Chronic Care in Prepaid Settings." *Milbank Memorial Fund Quarterly* Vol. 64, No. 2 (1986): 189–215.

Health Planning (also see Competition-Regulation)

Altman, Drew. "The Politics of Health Care Regulation: The Case of the National Health Planning and Resources Development Act." *Journal of Health Politics, Policy, and Law* Vol. 2 (Winter 1978): 560–580.

Altman, Drew and Harvey M. Sapolsky, "Writing the Regulations for Health," *Policy Sciences.* Vol. 7 Dec 1976, 417–438.

Binstock Robert H. "Effective Planning Through Political Influence." *American Journal of Public Health* Vol. 59 (May 1969): 808–813.

Brown, Lawrence D. *The Political Structure of the Federal Planning Program.* Washington, D.C.: The Brookings Institution, 1982.

Brown, Lawrence D. "Common Sense Meets Implementation: Certificate of Need Regulation in the States." *Journal of Health Politics, Policy and Law* Vol. 8 (Fall 1983): 480–494.

Conant, Ralph W. "The Politics of Health Planning." Hospital Progress Vol. 50 (January 1969): 51–56.

Desario, Jack. "Demise of Health Planning in the United States: The Politics of Incremental Health Policy Formation." *Journal of Health Politics, Policy and Law* Vol. 3 (June 1982): 164–177.

Dowell, Michael A. "Hill Burton: The Unfulfilled Promise." *Journal of Health Politics, Policy and Law* Vol. 12 (Spring 1987): 153–175.

Feingold, Eugene. "The Changing Political Character of Health Planning." *American Journal of Public Health* Vol. 59 (May 1969): 803–807."

Hyman, Herbert H., ed. *The Politics of Health Care: Nine Case Studies of Innovative Planning in New York City.* New York: Praeger Publishers, 1973.

Ingman, Stanley R. "Politics of Health Planning." Unpublished doctoral dissertation, University of Pittsburgh, 1971, Microfilm No. 71–23, 656.

James, A. Everette, Jr., et al., "Certificate-of-Need in and Antitrust Context" (research note): *Journal of Health Politics, Policy and Law* Vol 8 (Summer 1983): 314–315.

Kaufman, Herbert et al. "The Politics of Health Planning." *American Journal of Public Health* Vol. 59 (May 1969): 795–813 [(1) Herbert Kaufman: Introduction, 795–796; (2) Basil J.F. Mott: The Myth of Planning Without Politics, 797–803; (3) Eugene Feingold: The Changing Character of Health Planning 803–

807; (4) Robert H. Binstock: Effective Planning Political Influence, 808–813.

Klarman, Herbert E. "National Policies and Local Planning for Health Services." *Milbank Memorial Fund Quarterly/Health and Society* Vol. 54 (Winter 1976): 1–28.

Levin, A. L. "Health Planning and the U. S. Government." *International Journal of Health Services* Vol. 2, No. 3 (1972): 367–376.

Mick, Stephen S. and John D. Thompson. "Public Attitudes Towards Health Planning Under the Health Systems Agreement." *Journal of Health Politics, Policy and Law* Vol. 8 (Winter 1984): 782–800.

Mott, Basil J.F. "The Myth of Planning Without Politics." *American Journal of Public Health* Vol. 59 (May 1969): 797–803.

Mott, Basil J. F. " Politics and International Planning," *Social Science and Medicine* Vol. 8 (May 1974) 271–274.

Mueller, Keith J. "Federal Programs Do Expire: The Case of Health Planning. *Public Administration Review* Vol. 48 (May–June 1988): 719–725.

Rodwin, Victor G. *The Health Planning Predicament: France, Quebec, England, and the United States.* Berkeley, CA: University of California Press, 1984.

Rohrer, James E. "The Political Development of the Hill-Burton Program: A Case Study in Distributive Policy." *Journal of Health Politics, Policy and Law* (Spring 1987): 137–152.

Rothstein, P. *The Closing of St. Francis Hospital: A Case Study in the Politics of Health Planning.* New York: Health Policy Advisory Center of the Institute for Policy Studies, 1968.

Seder, Richard H. "Planning and Politics in the Allocation of Health Resources." *American Journal of Public Health* Vol. 63 (September 1973): 774–777.

Sloan, Frank A., James F. Blumstein and James M. Perrin, eds. *Cost, Quality and Access in Health Care: New Roles for Health Planning in a Competitive Environment.* San Francisco: Jossey-Bass Publishers, 1988.

Warde, James J. "The Role of Local Government in Health Planning." *Journal of Health Politics, Policy and Law* Vol. 1 (Winter, 1977): 387–390.

Health Policy (Also See Rationing)

Axinn, June and Mack J. Stern. "Age and Dependency: Children and the Aged in American Social Policy." *Milbank Memorial Fund Quarterly* Vol. 63 (Fall 1985): 648–670.

Bailey, Mary Ann, "Rationing" and "American Health Policy." *Journal of Health Politics, Policy and Law* Vol. 9 (Fall 1984): 489–501.

Battistella, Roger M. and Robert J. Buchanan. "National Health Policy: Efficiency—Equity Syncretism." *Social Justice Review* Vol. 1, No. 3 (1987): 329–360.

Bauman, Patricia. "The Formulation and Evolution of the Health Maintenance Organization Policy, 1970–1973." *Social Science and Medicine* Vol. 10 (March–April 1976): 129–142.

Bayer, Ronald and Jonathan D. Moreno. "Health Promotion: Ethical and Social Dilemmas of Government Policy." *Health Affairs* Vol. 5 (Summer 1986): 72–85.

Beauchamp, Dan E. *Health of the Republic: Epidemics, Medicine, and the Moralism as Challenges to Democracy.* Philadelphia: Temple University Press, 1988.

Blendon, Robert J., Carl J. Schramm, Thomas W. Maloney and David E. Rogers. "An Era of Stress for Health Institutions: The 1980's." *Journal of the American Medical Association,* Vol. 245, May 8, (1981), pp. 1843–1845.

Blumstein, James F. and Michael Zubkoff, "Public Choice and Health: Problems, Politics and Perspectives on Formulating National Health Policy," *Journal of Health Politics, Policy and Law,* Vol. 4, Fall 1979, pp. 382–413.

Bowler, M. Kenneth, "Changing Politics of Federal Health Insurance Programs," *PS,* Vol. 20, Spring 1987, pp. 202–211.

Brown, Jonathan B. and Richard B. Saltman, "Health Capital Policy in the United States: A Strategic Perspective," *Inquiry,* Vol. 22, Summer 1985, pp. 122–131.

Brown, Lawrence D. "The Formulation of Federal Health Care Policy." *Bulletin of the New York Academy of Medicine* Vol. 54 (January 1978): 45–58.

Brown, Lawrence D. *The Scope and Limits of Equality as a Normative Guide to Federal Health Care Policy.* Washington, D.C.: The Brookings Institution, 1979, General Series Reprint, No. 350.

Brown, Lawrence D. "Introduction to a Decade of Transition." *Journal of Health Politics, Policy and Law* Vol. 11, No. 4 (1986): 569–583.

Brown, Lawrence D. *Health Policy in Transition: A Decade of Health Politics, Policy and Law,* Durham, N.C.: Duke University Press, 1987.

Brown, Lawrence D., *Health Policy in the United States: Issues and Options, Occasional Paper Number Four,* New York: Ford Foundation, 1988.

Dallek, Geraldine. "Frozen in Ice. Federal Health Policy During the Reagan Years." *Health/ PAC Bulletin* (Summer 1988): 4–14.

Davis, Karen. "Reagan Administration Health Policy." *Journal of Public Health Policy* Vol. 2 (December 1981): 321–332.

deKervasdóue, Jean, John R. Kimberly and Victor G. Rodwin, eds. *The End of an Illusion: The Future of Health Policy in Western Industrialized Nations.* Berkeley: University of California Press, 1985.

DeSario, Jack P. "Health Issues and Policy Options." *PS,* Vol. 20 (Spring 1987): 226–231.

Dobson, Allen and Ronald Bialek. "Shaping Public Policy from the Prospective of a Data Builder." *Health Care Financing Review,* Vol. 6 (Summer 1985): 117–134.

Doty, Pamela. "Family Care of the Elderly: The Role of Public Policy." *Milbank Memorial Fund Quarterly* Vol. 64, No. 1 (1986): pp. 34–75.

Dunham, Andrew B. and Theodore Marmor. "Federal Policy in Health: Recent Trends and Different Perspectives." In Theodore J. Lowi and Alan Stone, eds., *Nationalizing Government: Public Policies in America.* Beverly Hills, CA.: Sage Publications, 1978.

Etheridge, Lynn. "An Aging Society and the Federal Deficit." *Milbank Memorial Fund Quarterly* Vol. 62 (Fall 1984): 521–543.

Falcone, David. "The Challenge of Comparative Health Policy for Political Science." *Journal of Health Politics, Policy and Law* Vol. 1 (Summer 1976): 196–213.

Fein, Rashi. "Social and Economic Attitudes Shaping American Health Policy." *Milbank Memorial Fund Quarterly/Health and Society,* Vol. 58 (Summer 1980): 349–385. Also in John B. McKinlay, ed., *Issues in Health Care Policy.* Cambridge: MIT Press, 1981: 29–65.

Fein, Rashi. *Medical Care, Medical Costs: The*

Search for a Health Insurance Policy. Cambridge, MA.: Harvard University Press, 1986.

Fox, Daniel M. "The Consequences of Consensus: American Health Policy in the Twentieth Century." Milbank Memorial Fund Quarterly Vol. 64, No. 1 (1986): 76–99.

Fox, Daniel M. Health Policies, Health Politics: The British and American Experience, 1911–1965. Princeton: Princeton University Press, 1986.

Fuchs, Beth C. and John F. Hoadley. "Reflections from Inside the Beltway: How Congress and the President Grapple with Health Policy." PS Vol. 20 (Spring 1987): 212–220.

Ginzberg, Eli. "The Future Supply of Physicians: From Pluralism to Policy." Health Affairs Vol. 1 (Fall 1982): 6–19.

Ginzberg, Eli. "The Monetization of Medical Care." New England Journal of Medicine Vol. 310 (May 3, 1984): 1162–1165.

Ginzberg, Eli and Miriam Ostow. The Coming Physician Surplus. In Search of a Public Policy. Savage, MD.: Rowman and Littlefield Publishers, Inc., 1985.

Goggin, Malcolm L. Policy Design and the Politics of Implementation: The Case of Child Health Care in the American States. Knoxville, TN.: University of Tennessee Press, 1987.

Havighurst, Clark C. Health Care Law and Policy. Readings, Notes and Questions. Westbury, New York: Foundation Press, 1988.

Ibrahim, Michel A. Epidemiology and Health Policy. Rockville, MD.: Aspen Systems Corp., 1985.

Ingraham, Norman R. "Formulation of Public Policy in Medical Care: Dynamics of Community Action at Local Level." American Journal of Public Health Vol. 51 (August 1961): 1144–1151.

Kars- Marshall, Cri, Yvonne W. Spronk-Boon and Marjan C. Pollemans. "National Health Interview Surveys for Health Care Policy." Social Science and Medicine Vol. 26, No. 2 (1988): 223–233.

Klein, Rudolf. "Economic Versus Political Models in Health Care Policy." In John B. McKinlay, ed., Issues in Health Care Policy, Cambridge: MIT Press, 1981: 66–79. Also in "Models of Man and Models of Policy: Reflections on Exit, Voice and Loyalty Ten Years Later." Milbank Memorial Fund Quarterly/

Health and Society Vol. 58 (Summer 1980): 416–429.

Kronenfeld, Jennie Jacobs and Marcia Lynn Whicker. U.S. National Health Policy: An Analysis of the Federal Role. New York: Praeger Publishers, 1984.

Leader, Shelah and Marilyn Moon, eds. Changing America's Health Care System: Proposals for Legislative Action. Washington, D.C.: American Association of Retired Persons, Public Policy Institute, 1988.

Lee, Philip R. and A.E. Benjamin. "Health Policy and the Politics of Health Care." In Stephen J. Williams and Paul R. Torrens, eds., Introduction to Health Services, New York: John Wiley and Sons, 1988, 3d ed.: 457–479.

Lewin, Marion Ein, ed. The Health Policy Agenda: Some Critical Questions. Washington, D.C.: American Enterprise Institute, 1985.

Lewin, Marion Ein, ed. From Research into Policy. Improving the Link for Health Services. Washington, D.C.: American Enterprise Institute for Public Policy Research, 1986.

Light, Paul. Artful Work: The Politics of Social Security Reform. New York: Random House, 1985.

Marmor, Theodore R. "American Medical Policy and the 'Crisis' of the Welfare State: A Comparative Perspective." Journal of Health Politics, Policy and Law Vol. 11, No. 4 (1986): 617–631.

Marmor, Theodore R. and James A. Morone. "The Health Programs of the Kennedy Johnson Years: An Overview." In Theodore R. Marmor's Political Analysis and American Medical Care. New York: Cambridge University Press, 1983: 131–154.

Marmor, Theodore R., Amy Bridges and Wayne L. Hoffman. "Comparative Politics and Health Policies: Notes on Benefits, Costs and Limits." In Douglas E. Ashford, ed., Comparing Public Policies: New Concepts and Methods. Beverly Hills, CA.: Sage Publications, 1978, Vol. 4: 59–80.

Marmor, Theodore R. and Jon B. Christianson. Health Care Policy. A Political Economy Approach. Beverly Hills, CA.: Sage Publications, 1982.

Marmor, Theodore R. Donald A. Withman and Thomas C. Heagy, "Politics, Public Policy and Medical Inflation." In Michael Zubkoff, ed., *Health: A Victim or Cause of Inflation.* New York: Prodist, 1976: 299–316.

McLachlan, Gordon and Alan Maynard, eds. *The Public/Private Mix for Health.* London: Nuffield Provincial Hospitals Trust, 1982.

McKinlay, John B., ed. *Issues in Health Care Policy.* A Milbank Reader, Cambridge: MIT Press, 1981.

Mechanic, David. "Some Dilemmas in Health Care Policy." *Milbank Memorial Fund Quarterly/Health and Society,* Vol. 59 (Winter 1981). Also in John B. McKinlay, ed., *Issues in Health Care Policy.* Cambridge: MIT Press, Winter 1981,: 80–94.

Mechanic, David. *From Advocacy to Allocation: The Evolving American Health Care System.* New York: The Free Press, 1986.

Melhaldo, Evan M., Walter Feinberg and Harold W. Swartz, eds. *Money, Power and Health Care.* Ann Arbor, MI.: Health Administration Press, 1988.

Meyer, Jack A. *Incentives Versus Controls in Health Policy: Broadening the Debate.* Washington, D.C.: American Enterprise Institute, 1985.

Meyer, Jack A. and Marion Ein Lewin, eds. *Chart up the Future of Health Care: Policy, Politics and Public Health.* Washington, D.C.: American Enterprise Institute for Public Policy Research, 1987.

Mick, Stephen S. "Contradictory Policies for Foreign Medical Graduates." *Health Affairs* Vol. 6 (Fall 1987): 5–18.

Mitchell, Faith and Claire Brindis. "Adolescent Pregnancy: The Responsibilities of Policy Makers." *Health Services Research* Vol. 22 (August 1987): 399–437.

Morris, Jonas. *Searching for a Cure: National Health Policy.* Berkeley: Morgan Publishing Co., 1986.

Navarro, Vicente. "Federal Health Policies in the United States: An Alternative Explanation."- *Milbank Memorial Fund Quarterly* Vol. 65, No. 1 (1987): 81–110.

Raffel, Marshall W. and Norma K. Raffel. *Perspectives on Health Policy: Australia, New Zealand, United States.* New York: John Wiley and Sons, 1987.

Rhoads, Steven E., ed. *Valuing Life: Public Policy Dilemmas.* Boulder, Colo.: Westview Press, 1980.

Riska, Elainne and James A. Taylor. "Consumer Attitudes Toward Health Policy and Knowledge About Health Legislation." *Journal of Health Politics, Policy and Law* Vol. 6, No. 2 (1976): 331–343.

Rochefort, David A. *American Social Welfare Policy: Dynamics of Formulation and Change.* Boulder, CO.: Westview Press, 1986.

Roemer, Ruth. "The Right to Health Care—Gains and Gaps," *American Journal of Public Health* Vol. 78 (March 1988): 241–247.

Sass, Hans-Martin and Robert U. Massey, eds. *Health Care Systems, Moral Conflicts in European and American Public Policies.* Higham, MA.: Kluwer Academic Publishing Co., 1988.

Silver, George A. "Ordering Social Objectives: National Health Service and National Health Insurance as Policy Options in Organizing the Medical Care System." *Yale Journal of Biology and Medicine* Vol. 5 (1978): 177–184.

Sorian, Richard. *The Bitter Pill: Tough Choices in America's Health Policy.* Washington, D.C.: McGraw-Hill, 1988.

Starr, Paul. "Medical Care and the Pursuit of Equality in America." In "President's Commission for the Study of Ethical Problems in Medical and Biomedical Behavior Research." *Securing Access to Health Care* Vol. 2. Washington, D.C.: United States Government Printing Office, 1983: 3–49.

Stone, Deborah A. *Policy Paradox and Political Reason.* Glenview, IL.: Scott, Foresman and Co., 1988.

Straetz, Ralph A. and Marvin Lieberman. "Health Policy Studies by Political Scientists." *Policy Studies Journal* Vol. 3 (Winter 1974): 195–200.

Straetz, Ralph A., Marvin Lieberman and Alice Sardell. *Critical Issues and Health Policy.* Lexington, MA.: Lexington Books, 1981.

Torrens, Paul R. "Historical Evolution and Overview of Health Services in the United States." In Stephen J. Williams and Paul R. Torrens, eds., *Introduction to Health Services.* New York: John Wiley and Sons, 1988, 3d ed.: 3–32.

VanEtten, Geert and Frans Rutten. "The Social Sciences in Health Policy and Practice." *Social Science and Medicine* Vol. 22, No. 11 (1986): 1187–1194.

Waters, William J. and John T. Tierney. "Hard Lessons Learned." *New England Journal of Medicine* Vol. 311 (November 8, 1984) 1251–52.

Weeks, Lewis E. and Howard J. Berman. *Shapers of American Health Care Policy: An Oral History.* Ann Arbor, MI.: Health Administration Press, 1985.

Hospitals

Derzon, Robert A. "The Politics of Municipal Hospitals." In Douglass Cater and Philip R. Lee, eds., *Politics of Health.* New York: Medcom Press, 1972.

Feder, Judith and Bruce Spitz. "The Politics of Hospital Payment." *Journal of Health Politics, Policy and Law* Vol. 4 (Fall 1979): 435–463.

Jaeger, Boi Jon. "Government and Hospitals: A Perspective on Health Politics." *Hospital Administration* Vol. 17 (Winter 1972): 39–50.

Joskow, Paul L. *Controlling Hospital Costs. The Role of Government Regulation.* Cambridge: MIT Press, 1981.

Lindsay. Cotton M. *Veterans Administration Hospitals: An Economic Analysis of Government Enterprise.* Washington, D.C.: American Enterprise Institute for Public Policy Research, 1975.

Raphaelson, Arnold H. and Charles P. Hall, Jr. "Politics and Economics of Hospital Cost Containment." *Journal of Health Politics, Policy and Law* Vol. 3 (Spring 1978): 87–11.

Rosner, David. "Gaining Control: Reform Reimbursement and Politics in New York's Community Hospitals, 1890–1915." *American Journal of Public Health* Vol. 70 (May 1980): 533–542.

Long Term Care

Avorn, Jerry. "Benefits and Cost Analysis in Geriatric Care. Turning Age Discrimination into Health Policy." *New England Journal of Medicine* Vol. 310 (May 17, 1984): 1294–1301.

Axinn, June and Mark J. Stern. "Age and Dependency: Children and the Aged in American Social Policy." *Milbank Memorial Fund Quarterly* Vol. 63 (Fall 1985): 648–670.

Barfield, Claude. "New Federalism and Long Term Care of the Elderly." Update, *Health Affairs* Vol. 2 (Spring 1983): 113–125.

Binney, Elizabeth A. and Carroll L. Estes. "The Retreat of the State and its Transfer of Responsibility: The Intergenerational War." *International Journal of Health Services* Vol. 18, No. 1 (1988): 83–96.

Brecher, Charles and James Knickman. "A Reconsideration of Long Term Care Policy." *Journal of Health Politics, Policy and Law* Vol. 10 (Summer 1985): 245–274.

Burke, Thomas R. "Long Term Care: The Public Role and Private Initiative." *Health Care Financing Review,* 1988 Supplement (December 1988): 1–5.

Culyer, A.J. and Stephen Birch. "Caring for the Elderly: A European Perspective on Today and Tomorrow." *Journal of Health Politics, Policy and Law* Vol. 10 (Fall 1985): 469–488.

Doty, Pamela. "Long Term Care in International Perspective." *Health Care Financing Review,* 1988 Supplement (December 1988): 145–155.

Estes, Carroll L. "Social Security: The Social Construction of a Crisis." *Milbank Memorial Fund Quarterly* Vol. 61 (Summer 1983): 445–461.

Estes, Carroll L. "Long Term Care and Public Policy in an Era of Austerity." *Journal of Public Health Policy* Vol. 6 (December 1985): 464–475.

Estes, Carroll L. and Elizabeth A. Binney. "Toward a Transformation of Health and Aging Policy." *International Journal of Health Services* Vol. 18, No. 1 (1988): 69–82.

Etheredge, Lynn. "An Aging Society and the Federal Deficit." *Milbank Memorial Fund Quarterly* Vol. 62 (Fall 1984): 521–543.

Eustis, Nancy N., Jay N. Greenberg and Sharon K. Patten. *Long Term Care of Older Persons: A Policy Perspective.* Monterey, CA.: Brooks/Cole Publishing Co., 1984.

Fuchs, Victor R. "Though Much is Taken: Reflections on Aging, Health, and Medical Care." *Milbank Memorial Fund Quarterly* Vol. 62 (Spring 1984): 143–166.

Gill, Derek G. and Stanley R. Ingman. "Geriatric Care and Distributive Justice, Problems and

Prospects." *Social Science and Medicine* Vol. 23, No. 12 (1986): 1205–1215.

Ginzberg, Eli. "The Elderly: An International Policy Perspective." *Milbank Memorial Fund Quarterly* Vol. 61 (Summer 1983): 473–488.

Harrington, Charlene, Robert J. Newcomer, Carroll L. Estes and Associates. *Long Term Care of the Elderly: Public Policy Issues.* Beverly Hills, CA.: Sage Publications, 1985.

Justice, Diane. *State Long Term Care Reform: Development of Community Care Systems in Six States.* Washington, D.C.: National Governors' Association, April 1988.

Kane, Robert L. and Rosalie A. Kane. *A Will and a Way. What the United States Can Learn from Canada About Caring for the Elderly.* New York: Columbia University Press, 1985.

Kane, Rosalie A. and Robert L. Kane. "The Feasibility of Universal Long Term Care Benefits. Ideas from Canada." *New England Journal of Medicine* Vol. 312 (May 23, 1985) 1357–1363.

Kane, Rosalie A. and Robert L. Kane. *Long Term Care—Principles, Programs and Policies.* Philadelphia, Springer Publishing Co., 1987.

Katz, Michael B. "Poorhouses and the Origins of the Public Old Age Home." *Milbank Memorial Fund Quarterly* Vol. 62 (Winter 1984): 110–140.

Leutz, Walter. "Long Term Care for the Elderly: Public Dreams and Private Realities." *Inquiry* Vol. 23 (June 1986): 134–140.

Lipson, Debra J. *State Financing of Long Term Care Services for the Elderly.* Washington D.C.: Intergovernmental Health Policy Project, George Washington University, May 1988.

Lowe, Beverly F. "Future Directions for Community Based Long Term Care Research." *Milbank Memorial Fund Quarterly* Vol. 66, No. 3 (1988): 552–571.

Manard, Barbara Bolling. "Doing Research for Decision Makers: Nursing Home Reimbursement." In Marion Ein Lewin, ed., *From Research into Policy: Improving the Link for Health Services.* Washington, D.C.: American Enterprise Institute for Public Policy Research, 1986: 51–71.

Myles, John F. "Conflict, Crisis, and the Future of Old Age Security." *Milbank Memorial Fund Quarterly* Vol. 61 (Summer 1983): 462–472.

Plough, Alonzo L. *Borrowed Time: Artificial Organs and the Politics of Extending Lives.* Philadelphia: Temple University Press, 1986.

Quadagno, Jill S. "From Poor Laws to Pensions: The Evolution of Economic Support for the Aged in England and America." *Milbank Memorial Fund Quarterly* Vol. 62 (Summer 1984): 417–446.

Quadagno, Jill S. *The Transformation of Old Age Security Class and Politics in the American Welfare State.* Chicago: University of Chicago Press, 1988.

Rice, Dorothy P. and Carroll L. Estes. "Health of the Elderly: Policy Issues and Challenges." *Health Affairs* Vol. 3 (Winter 1984): 25–49.

Rowland, Diane. "Issues of Long Term Care." In Carl J. Schramm, ed., *Health Care and Its Costs. Can the U.S. Afford Adequate Health Care?* New York: W.W. Norton, 1987: 222–251.

Schaughnessy, Peter W. "Long-Term Care Research and Public Policy." *Health Services Research* Vol. 20 (October 1985): 489–499.

Smeeding, Timothy M. and LaVonne Straub. "Health Care Financing Among the Elderly: Who Really Pays the Bills?" *Journal of Health Politics, Policy and Law* Vol. 12 (Spring 1987): 35–52.

Ward, Russell and Sheldon S. Tobin, eds. *Health in Aging. Sociological Issues and Policy Directions.* New York: Springer Publishing Co., 1987.

Weissert, William G. "Hard Choices: Targeting Long Term Care to the 'At-Risk' Aged." *Journal of Health Politics, Policy and Law* Vol. 11 (Fall 1986): 463–481.

Influenza

Berliner, Howard S. and Warren J. Salmon. "Swine Flue, the Phantom Threat." *Nation* Vol. 223 (September 25, 1976): 269–272.

Neustadt, Richard E. and Harvey V. Fineberg. *The Swine Flue Affair: Decision-Making on a Slippery Disease.* Washington, D.C.: U.S. Government Printing Office, 1978.

Osborn, June. *Influenza in America, 1918–1976: History, Science and Politics.* New York: Prodist, Neale Watson Academic Publishers, 1977.

Silverstein, Arthur M. *Pure Politics and Impure Science. The Swine Flue Affair.* Baltimore, MD.: The Johns Hopkins University Press, 1981.

Viseltear, Arthur J. "Immunization and Public Policy: A Short Political History of the 1976 Swine Influenza Legislation." In June E. Osborn, ed., *Influenza in America, 1918–1976: History, Science and Politics.* New York: Prodist, Neal Watson Academic Publishers, 1977.

Medicine and the Medical Profession (Doctors and Politics)

Anderson, Odin W. "PSROs, The Medical Profession and the Public Interest." *Milbank Memorial Fund Quarterly/Health and Society* Vol. 54 (Summer 1976): 379–388.

Bonner, T.N. "Social and Political Attitudes of Midwestern Physicians." *Journal Hist. Med. and Allied Sciences* Vol. 8 (April 1953): 133–164.

Cain, Leonard D., Jr. "The AMA and the Gerontologists: Uses and Abuses of 'A Profile of the Aging: USA.' " in Gideon Sjoberg, ed., *Ethics, Politics, and Social Research.* Cambridge: Schenkman Publishing Co., 1967: 78–114.

Carter, Richard. *The Doctor Business.* New York: Doubleday & Co., 1958.

Chase, Edward T. "The Politics of Medicine." In Marion Sanders, ed., *The Crisis in American Medicine.* New York: Harpers, 1961: 1–19.

Colombotos, John. "Physicians and Medicare: A Before-After Study of the Effects of Legislation on Attitudes." *American Sociological Review* Vol. 34 (June 1969): 318–334.

Dodds, Richard W. "A Framework for Political Mapping of Conflict in Organized Medicine—Especially Pediatrics." *Medical Care Review* Vol. 27 (November 1970): 1035–1062.

Eckstein, Harry. *Pressure Groups Politics: The Case of the British Medical Association.* Palo Alto, Calif.: Stanford University Press, 1960.

Garceau, Oliver. *The Political Life of the American Medical Association.* Cambridge: Harvard University Press, 1941.

Ginzberg, Eli. *American Medicine: The Power Shift.* Totowa, N.J.: Rowman and Allanheld, 1985.

Glaser, William A. "Doctors and Politics." *American Journal of Sociology* Vol. 66 (November 1960): 230–245.

Gordon, Gerald and Selwyn Becker. "Changes in Medical Practice Bring Shifts in the Patterns of Power." *Modern Hospital* Vol. 102 (February 1964): 89–91.

Lewis, R. "New Power at the Polls: The Doctors." In H. Turner, ed., *Politics in the United States: Readings in Political Parties and Pressure Groups.* New York: McGraw-Hill, 1955: 180–185.

Marmor, Theodore R. and David Thomas. "Doctors, Politics and Pay Disputes: Pressure Group Politics Revisited." In Theodore R. Marmor. *Political Analysis and American Medical Care.* New York: Cambridge University Press, 1983: 107–130.

Means, James Howard. *Doctors, People, and Government.* Boston: Little, Brown & Co., 1953.

Mechanic, David. "The Transformation of Health Providers." *Health Affairs* Vol. 3 (Spring 1984): 65–72.

Melicke, Carl A. "The Saskatchewan Medical Care Dispute of 1962: An Analytic Social History." Unpublished doctoral dissertation, Microfilm No. 68-7435, University of Minnesota. 1967, Microfilm No. 68-7435

Millman, Michael L. *Politics and the Expanding Physician Supply.* Montclair, N.J.: Allanheld, Osmun and Co., 1980.

Stauffer, Robert B. *The Development of an Interest Group: The Phillippine Medical Association.* Quezon City: University of the Phillippines Press, 1966.

Stevenson, H. Michael and A. Paul Williams. "Physicians and Medicare: Professional Ideology and Canadian Health Care Policy." *Canadian Public Policy* Vol. 11 (September 3, 1985): 504–521.

Tollefson, E.A. *Bitter Medicine.* Toronto: University of Toronto Press, 1964.

Medicare and Medicaid: Government Health Insurance

Aaron, Henry J. Comment on "Alternative Medicare Financing Sources." *Milbank Memorial Fund Quarterly* Vol. 62 (Spring 1984): 349–355.

Adamache, Killard W. and Louis F. Rossiter. "The Entry of HMOs Into the Medicare Market: Implications for TEFRA's Mandate." *Inquiry* Vol. 23 (Winter 1986): 349–364.

Anderson, Maren D. and Peter D. Fox. "Lessons Learned from Medicaid Managed Care Approaches." *Health Affairs* Vol. 6 (Spring 1987): 71–86.

Anderson, Odin W. "Compulsory Medical Care Insurance, 1910–1950." In Eugene Feingold, ed., *Medicare: Policy and Politics.* San Francisco, CA.: Chandler Publishing Co., 1966: 85–156.

Anderson, Odin W. "The Medicare Act: The Public Policy Breakthrough, or Wheeling, Dealing and Healing." In Irving L. Webber, ed., *Medical Care Under Social Security—Potentials and Problems,* Institute of Gerontology Series. Gainsville, FL.: University of Florida Press, 1966: Vol. 15, 9–26.

Anderson, Odin W. *The Uneasy Equilibrium: Private and Public Financing of Health Services in the U.S., 1865–1975.* New Haven, CT.: College and University Press, 1968.

Bachman, Sara S., Stuart H. Altman and Dennis F. Beatrice. "What Influences a State's Approach to Medicaid Reform?" *Inquiry* Vol. 25 (Summer 1988): 243–250.

Bachman, Sara S., Dennis F. Beatrice and Stuart H. Altman. "Implementing Change: Lessons for Medicaid Reform." *Journal of Health Politics, Policy and Law* Vol. 12 (Summer 1987): 237–252.

Bayer, Ronald and Daniel Callahan. "Medicare Reform: Social and Ethical Perspectives." *Journal of Health Politics, Policy and Law* Vol. 10 (Fall 1985): 533–547.

Bernard, Sydney E. and Eugene Feingold. "The Impact of Medicaid." *Wisconsin Law Review* Vol. 1970, No. 3 (1970): 726–755.

Bernstein, Betty J. "The Politics of the New York State Medicaid Law of 1966: An Analysis." Unpublished doctoral dissertation, Microfilm No. 69–21, 237, New York University, 1969.

Bernstein, Betty J. "Public Health—Inside or Outside the Mainstream of the Political Process? Lessons from the Passage of Medicaid." *American Journal of Public Health* Vol. 60 (September 1970): 1690–1700.

Blumenthal, David, Mark Schlesinger and Pamela Brown Drumheller. *Renewing the Promise. Medicare and Its Reform.* New York: Oxford University Press, 1988.

Brewster, Agness W. *Health Insurance and Related Proposals for Financing Personal Health Services . . . A Digest of Major Legislation and Proposals for Federal Action, 1935–1957,* Division of Program Research, Social Security Administration. Washington, D.C.: U.S. Government Printing Office, 1958.

Brown, Lawrence D. "Technocratic Corporatism and Administrative Reform and Medicare." *Journal of Health Politics, Policy and Law* Vol. 10 (Fall 1985): 579–599.

Burney, Ira, Peter Hickman, Julia Paradise and George J. Schieber. "Medicare Physician Payment, Participation and Reform." *Health Affairs* Vol. 3 (Winter 1984): 5–24.

Cafferata, Gail Lee. "Private Health Insurance of the Medicare Population and the Baucus Legislation." *Medical Care* Vol. 23 (September 1985): 1086–1096.

Christensen, Sandra and Rick Kasten. "Covering Catastrophic Expenses under Medicare." *Health Affairs* Vol. 7 (Winter 1988): 79–93.

Christensen, Sandra, Stephen H. Long and Jack Rodgers. "Acute Health Care Costs for the Aged Medicare Population: Overview and Policy Options." *Milbank Memorial Fund Quarterly* Vol. 65, No. 3 (1987): 397–425.

Cohen, Wilbur. "Reflections on the Enactment of Medicare and Medicaid." *Health Care Financing Review,* 1985 Supplement, 3–11.

Corning, Peter A. *The Evolution of Medicare . . . From Idea to Law.* Office of Research and Statistics, Research Report No. 29, Social Security Administration. Washington, D.C.: U.S. Government Printing Office, 1969.

Cromwell, Jerry, Sylvia Hurdle and Rachel Schurman. "Defederalizing Medicaid: Fair to the Poor, Fair to the Taxpayers?" *Journal of Health Politics, Policy and Law* Vol. 12 (Spring 1987): 1–34.

Curtis, Richard and Ian Hill, eds. *Affording Access to Quality Care: Strategies for State Medicaid Cost Management.* Washington, D.C.: National Governors' Association Center for Policy Research, July 1986.

David, Sheri I. *With Dignity: The Search for Medi-*

care and Medicaid. Westport, CT.: Greenwood Press, 1985.

Davidson, Stephen M., Jerry Cromwell and Rachel Schurman. "Medicaid Myths: Trends in Medicaid Expenditures and the Prospects for Reform." *Journal of Health Politics, Policy and Law* Vol. 10 (Winter 1986): 699–728.

Davis, Feather Ann. "Medicare Hospice Benefit: Early Program Experiences." *Health Care Financing Review* Vol. 9 (Summer 1988): 99–111.

Davis, Karen. "Medicare Financing and Beneficiary Income." *Inquiry* Vol. 24 (Winter 1987): 309–323.

Davis, Karen and Diane Rowland. "Medicare Financing Reform: A New Medicare Premium." *Milbank Memorial Fund Quarterly* Vol. 62 (Spring 1984): 300–316.

Davis, Karen and Diane Rowland. *Medicare Policy: New Directions for Health and Long Term Care.* Baltimore, MD.: The Johns Hopkins University Press, 1985.

Demkovich, Linda E. "Medicaid for Welfare: A Controversial Swap." *National Journal* Vol. 14 (February 1982): 362–368.

Dobson, Allen, John C. Langenbrunner, Steven A. Pelovitz and Judith B. Willis. "The Future of Medicare Policy Reform: Priorities for Research and Demonstration." *Health Care Financing Review,* 1986 Annual Supplement (December 1986): 1–8.

Ehrenhaft, Polly M. and Marie Hackbarth. *Medicaid Reform: Four Studies of Case Management.* Washington, D.C.: American Enterprise Institute, 1984.

Feder, Judith M. *Medicare: The Politics of Federal Medical Insurance.* Lexington, MA.: D.C. Heath and Lexington Books, 1977.

Feder, Judith, Marilyn Moon and William Scanlon. "Medicare Reform: Nibbling at Catastrophic Costs." *Health Affairs* Vol. 6 (Winter 1987): 5–19.

Feingold, Eugene. *Medicare: Policy and Politics.* San Francisco, CA.: Chandler Publishing Co., 1966.

Feldman, Penny H. and Margaret Gerteis. "Private Insurance for Medicaid Recipients: The Texas Experience." *Journal of Health Politics, Policy and Law* Vol. 12 (Summer 1987): 271–298.

Filerman, Gary L. "The Legislative Campaign for the Passage of a Medical Care for the Aged Bill." Unpublished masters thesis, University of Minnesota, 1962.

Fisher, Charles R. "Impact of the Prospective Payment System on Physician Charges Under Medicare." *Health Care Financing Review* Vol. 8 (Summer 1987): 101–104.

Foltz, Anne-Marie. *An Ounce of Prevention. Child Health Politics Under Medicaid.* Cambridge: MIT Press, 1982.

Fraser, Irene, Theodore Koontz and William C. Moran. "Medicare Reimbursement for Hospice Care: An Approach for Analyzing Cost Consequences." *Inquiry* Vol. 23 (Summer 1986): 141–153.

Freund, Deborah A. with Polly M. Ehrenhaft and Marie Hackbarth. *Medicaid Reform: Four Studies of Case Management.* Washington, D.C.: American Enterprise Institute for Public Policy, 1984.

Gardiner, John A. and Theodore R. Lyman. *The Fraud Control Game: State Responses to Fraud and Abuse in the AFDC and Medicaid Programs.* Bloomington, IN.: Indiana University Press, 1984.

Garfinkel, Steven A., Arthur J. Bonito and Kenneth R. McLeroy. "Socioeconomic Factors and Medicare Supplemental Health Insurance." *Health Care Financing Review* Vol. 9 (Fall 1987): 21–30.

Gentry, John T. and Morris Schaefer. "The Impact of State and Federal Policy Planning Decisions on the Implementation and Functional Adequacy of Title XIX Health Care Programs." *Medical Care* Vol. 7 (January 1969): 92–104.

Ginsberg, Eli. Comment on "Medicare Benefits: A Reassessment." *Milbank Memorial Fund Quarterly* Vol. 62 (Spring 1984): 230–236.

Ginsburg, Paul B. and Marilyn Moon. "An Introduction to the Medicare Financing Problem." *Milbank Memorial Fund Quarterly* Vol. 62 (Spring 1984): 167–182.

Gornick, Marian, Jay N. Greenberg, Paul W. Eggers and Allen Dobson. "Twenty Years of Medicare and Medicaid: Covered Population, Use of Benefits, and Program Expenditures." *Health Care Financing Review,* 1985 Annual Supplement (December 1985): 13–59.

Gronfein, William. "Incentives and Intentions in Mental Health Policy: A Comparison of the

Medicaid and Community Mental Health Programs." *Journal of Health and Social Behavior* Vol. 26 (September 1985): 192–206.

Guterman, Stuart, Paul W. Eggers, Gerald Riley, Timothy F. Greene and Sherry A. Terrell. "The First Three Years of Medicare Prospective Payment: An Overview." *Health Care Financing Review* Vol. 9 (Spring 1988): 67–82.

Hadley, Jack. "How Should Medicare Pay Physicians?" *Milbank Memorial Fund Quarterly* Vol. 62 (Spring 1984): 279–299.

Hadley, Jack. "Medicare Spending and Mortality Rates of the Elderly." *Inquiry* Vol. 25 (Winter 1988): 485–493.

Harrington, Charlene, Carroll L. Estes, Philip R. Lee and Robert J. Newcomer. "Effects" of State Medicaid Policies on the Aged." *The Gerontologist* Vol. 26 (August 1986): 437–443.

Harrington, Charlene and James H. Swan. "The Impact of State Medicaid Nursing Home Policies on Utilization and Expenditures." *Inquiry* Vol. 24 (Summer 1987): 159–172.

Harris, Richard. "Annals of Legislation: Medicare—All Very Hegelian." *New Yorker* Vol. 42 (July 2, 1966): 29–62.

Harris, Richard. "Annals of Legislation: Medicare—We Do Not Compromise." *New Yorker* Vol. 42 (July 16, 1966): 35–91.

Harris, Richard. "Annals of Legislation: Medicare—A Sacred Trust." *New Yorker* Vol. 42 (July 23, 1966): 35–63.

Harris, Richard. *A Sacred Trust.* New York: New American Library, 1967.

Haynes, Pamela L. *Evaluating State Medicaid Reforms.* Washington, D.C.: American Enterprise Institute, 1985.

Hirshfield, Daniel S. *The Lost Reform: The Campaign for Compulsory Health Insurance in the United States from 1932–1943.* Cambridge: Harvard University Press, 1970.

Held, Philip J. and John Holahan. "Containing Medicaid Costs in an Era of Growing Physician Supply." *Health Care Financing Review* Vol. 7 (Fall 1985): 49–60.

Holahan, John. *The Effects of the 1981 Omnibus Budget Reconciliation Act on Medicaid.* Washington, D.C.: Urban Institute, 1985.

Holahan, John and Joel Cohen. *Medicaid: The Tradeoff Between Cost Containment and Access to Care.* Washington, D.C.: Urban Institute Press, 1986.

Holahan, John and Lynn Etheridge. *Medicare Physician Payment Reform.* Washington, D.C.: Urban Institute, 1986.

Holahan, John and John L. Palmer. "Medicare's Fiscal Problems: An Imperative for Reform." *Journal of Health Politics, Policy and Law* Vol. 13 (Spring 1988): 53–82.

Holahan, John and Stephen Zuckerman. "Medicare Mandatory Assignment: An Unnecessary Risk?" *Health Affairs* Vol. 8 (Spring 1989): 65–79.

Hsiao, William C. and Nancy L. Kelly. "Medicare Benefits: A Reassessment." *Milbank Memorial Fund Quarterly* Vol. 62 (Spring 1984): 207–229.

Iglehart, John K. "Payment of Physicians Under Medicare." *New England Journal of Medicine* Vol. 318 (March 31, 1988): 863–868.

Iglehart, John K. "Medicare's New Benefits: Catastrophic Health Insurance." *New England Journal of Medicine* Vol. 320 (February 2, 1989): 329–335.

Johns, Lucy and Gerald Alder. "Evaluation of Recent Changes in Medicaid." *Health Affairs* Vol. 8 (Spring 1989): 171–181.

Johns, Lucy, Maren D. Anderson and Robert A. Derzon. "Selective Contracting in California: Experience in the Second Year." *Inquiry* Vol. 22 (Winter 1985): 335–347.

Johns, Robert A. and Maren D. Anderson. "Selective Contracting in California: Early Effects and Policy Implications." *Inquiry* Vol. 22 (Spring 1985): 24–32.

Kalison, Michael J. and Richard F. Averill. "The Challenge of 'Real' Competition in Medicare." *Health Affairs* Vol. 5 (Fall 1986): 47–57.

Kern, Rosemary and Susan R. Windham. *Medicaid and Other Experiments in State Health Policy.* Washington, D.C.: American Enterprise Institute, 1986.

Kinkead, Brian M. "Medicare Payment and Hospital Capital: The Evolution of Policy." *Health Affairs* Vol. 3 (Fall 1984): 49–74.

Langwell, Kathryn M. and James P. Hadley. "Capitation and the Medicare Program: History, Issues and Evidence." *Health Care Financing Review,* 1986 Annual Supplement (December 1986): 9–20.

Lave, Judith R. "Hospital Reimbursement Under Medicare." *Milbank Memorial Fund Quarterly* Vol. 62 (Spring 1984): 251–268.

Lave, Judith R., Richard G. Frank, Carl Taube, Howard Goldman, and Agnes Rupp. "The Early Effects of Medicare's Prospective Payment System on Psychiatry." *Inquiry* Vol. 25 (Fall 1988): 354–363.

Long, Stephen H. and Russell F. Settle. "Medicare and the Disadvantaged Elderly: Objectives and Outcomes." *Milbank Memorial Fund Quarterly* Vol. 62 (Fall 1984): 609–656.

Long, Stephen H. and Timothy M. Smeedings. "Alternative Medicare Financing Sources." *Milbank Memorial Fund Quarterly* Vol. 26 (Spring 1984): 325–348.

Luft, Arnold S. "On the Use of Vouchers for Medicare." *Milbank Memorial Fund Quarterly* Vol. 62 (Spring 1984): 237–250.

Marmor, Theodore R. *The Politics of Medicare.* Chicago, IL.: Aldine Publishing Co., 1973, revised American edition.

McCall, Nelda, Thomas Rice and Arden Hall. "The Effect of State Regulations on the Quality and Sale of Insurance Policies to Medicare Beneficiaries." *Journal of Health Politics, Policy and Law* Vol. 12 (Spring 1987): 53–76.

McDevitt, Roland, William Buczko, Josephine Mauskopf. et al. "Medicaid Program Characteristics: Effects on Health Care Expenditures and Utilization." *Health Care Financing Review* Vol. 7 (Winter 1985): 1–29.

McMenamin, Peter. "Medicare's Part B Rising Assignment Rates: Rising Costs." *Inquiry* Vol. 24 (Winter 1987): 344–356.

McMenamin, Peter. "A Crime Story from Medicare Part B." *Health Affairs* Vol. 7 (Winter 1988): 94–101.

McMillan, Alma and James Lubitz. "Medicare Enrollment in Health Maintenance Organizations." *Health Care Financing Review* Vol. 8 (Spring 1987): 87–93.

Meyer, Jack A. Comment on "Medicare Financing Reform: A New Medicare Premium." *Milbank Memorial Fund Quarterly* Vol. 62 (Spring 1984): 317–324.

Mitchell, Janet B., et al. "Packaging Physician Services: Alternative Approaches to Medicare Part B Reimbursement. *Inquiry* Vol. 24 (Winter 1987): 324–343.

Mitchell, Janet B., Margo L. Rosenbach and Jerry Cromwell. "To Sign or Not to Sign: Physician Participation in Medicare, 1984." *Health Care Financing Review* Vol. 10 (Fall 1988): 17–26.

Mitchell, Janet B., Gerard Wedig and Jerry Cromwell. "The Medicare Physician Fee Freeze." *Health Affairs* Vol. 8 (Spring 1989): 21–33.

Munnell, Alicia H. "Paying for the Medicare Program." *Journal of Health Politics, Policy and Law* Vol. 10 (Fall 1985): 489–512.

Oberg, Charles N. and Cynthia L. Polich. "Medicaid: Entering the Third Decade." *Health Affairs* Vol. 7 (Fall 1988): 83–96.

Omenn, Gilbert S. "Lessons From a Fourteen-State Study of Medicaid." *Health Affairs* Vol. 6. (Spring 1987): 118–122.

Pauly, Mark V. and William B. Kissick, eds. *Lessons From the First Twenty Years of Medicare.* Philadelphia: University of Pennsylvania Press, 1988.

Pauly, Mark V. and Kathryn M. Langwell. "Physician Payment Reform—Who Shall Be Paid?" *Medical Care Review* Vol. 43 (Spring 1986): 101–132.

Perloff, Janet D., Phillip R. Kletke, and Kathryn M. Neckerman. "Physicians' Decision to Limit Medicaid Participation: Determinants and Policy Implications." *Journal of Health Politics, Policy and Law* Vol. 12 (Summer 1987): 221–236.

Poetz, Lisa and Thomas Buchberger. "Medicare's Transition to National Payment Rates: Effects on Hospitals." *Health Affairs* Vol. 4 (Winter 1985): 62–69.

Rettig, Paul C., Glenn R. Markus, James Bentley, et al. "Medicare's Prospective Payment System. The Expectations and the Realities." *Inquiry* Vol. 24 (Summer 1987): 173–188.

Rose, Arnold M. "The Passage of Legislation: The Politics of Financing Medical Care for the Aging." In Arnold M. Rose, ed., *The Power Structure.* New York: Oxford University Press, 1967: 400–455.

Rosenbaum, Sara and Kay Johnson. "Providing Health Care for Low- Income Children: Reconciling Child Health Goals with Child Health Financing Realities." *Milbank Memorial Fund Quarterly* Vol. 64, No. 3 (1986): 442–478.

Rosenblum, Robert W. "Medicare Reversed: A Look Through the Past to the Future." *Journal of Health, Politics, Policy and Law* Vol. 9 (Winter 1985): 669–682.

Rossiter, Louis F. and Kathryn Langwell. "Medicare's Two Systems for Paying Providers." *Health Affairs* Vol. 7 (Summer 1988): 120–132.

Ruby, Gloria, H. David Banta and Anne Kesselman Burns. "Medicare Coverage, Medicare Costs, and Medical Technology." *Journal of Health Politics, Policy and Law* Vol. 10 (Spring 1985): 141–156.

Russell, Louise B. and Carrie Lynn Manning. "The Effect of Prospective Payment on Medicare Expenditures." *New England Journal of Medicine* Vol. 320 (February 16, 1989): 439–443.

Rymer, Marilyn P. and Gerald S. Alder. "Children and Medicaid: The Experience in Four States." *Health Care Financing Review* Vol. 9 (Fall 1987): 1–20.

Sager, Mark A., Douglas V. Easterling, David Kindig and Odin W. Anderson. "Changes in the Location of Death After Passage of Medicare's Prospective Payment System: A National Study." *New England Journal of Medicine* Vol. 320 (February 16, 1989): 433–438.

Schneider, Saundra K. "Intergovernmental Influences on Medicaid Program Expenditures." *Public Administration Review* Vol. 48 (July-August 1988): 756–763.

Sheingold, Steven H. "Unintended Results of Medicare's National Prospective Payment Rates." *Health Affairs* Vol. 5 (Winter 1986): 5–21.

Sheingold, Steven H. and Thomas Buchberger. "Implications of Medicare's Prospective Payment System for the Provision of Uncompensated Hospital Care." *Inquiry* Vol. 23 (Winter 1986): 371–381.

Short, Pamela Farley, Joel C. Cantor and Alan C. Monheit. "The Dynamics of Medicaid Enrollment." *Inquiry* Vol. 25 (Winter 1988): 504–516.

Short, Pamela Farley and Alan C. Monheit. "Employers and Medicare as Partners in Financing Health Care for the Elderly." In Mark V. Pauly and William B. Kissick, eds., *Lessons from the First Twenty Years of Medicare*. University of Pennsylvania Press, 1988.

Sisk, Jane E., Peter McMenamin, Gloria Ruby and Ellen S. Smith. "An Analysis of Methods to Reform Medicare Payment for Physician Services." *Inquiry* Vol. 24 (Spring 1987): 36–47.

Skidmore, Max J. *Medicare and the American Rhetoric of Reconciliation.* Tuscaloosa, AL.: University of Alabama Press, 1970.

Sloan, Frank and Joel W. Hay. "Medicare Pricing Mechanisms for Physician Services: An Overview of Alternative Approaches." *Medical Care Review* Vol. 43 (Spring 1986): 59–100.

Spitz, Bruce. "A National Survey of Medicaid Case-Management Programs." *Health Affairs* Vol. 6 (Spring 1987): 61–70.

Stevens, Robert and Rosemary Stevens. *Welfare Medicine in America: A Case Study of Medicaid.* New York: The Free Press, 1974.

Stevens, Rosemary and Robert Stevens. "Medicaid: Anatomy of a Dilemma." *Law and Contemporary Problems* Vol. 1970 (Spring 1970): 348–425.

Stuart, Bruce, Edward Reutzel and Thomas Reutzel. "Medicaid Reform: Programming Solutions to the Equity Problem." *Journal of Health Politics, Policy and Law* Vol. 10 (Spring 1985): 93–118.

Swan, James H., Charlene Harrington and Leslie A. Grant. "State Medicaid Reimbursement for Nursing Homes, 1978–86." *Health Care Financing Review* Vol. 9 (Spring 1988): 33–50.

Taube, Carl A. and Agnes Rupp. "The Effect of Medicaid on Access to Ambulatory Mental Health Care for the Poor and Near Poor Under 65." *Medical Care* Vol. 24 (August 1986): 677–686.

Vladeck, Bruce C.. Comment on "Hospital Reimbursement Under Medicare," *Milbank Memorial Fund Quarterly* Vol. 62 (Spring 1984: 269–278.

Vladeck, Bruce C. "Reforming Medicare Provider Payment." *Journal of Health Politics, Policy and Law* Vol. 10 (Fall 1985): 513–532.

Vladeck, Bruce C. and Genrose J. Alfano, eds. *Medicare and Extended Care: Issues, Problems and Prospects.* Owings Mills, MD.: National Health Publishing (Rynd Communications), 1987.

Vuori, Hannu. "Ideology Versus Interest: The Case of Medicare." *Social Science & Medicine* Vol. 2 (September 1968): 355–363.

Walker, Georgia K. "Reforming Medicare: The Limited Framework of Political Discourse on Equity and Economy." *Social Science and Medicine* Vol. 23, No. 12 (1986): 1237–1250.

Weikel, M.K.. *A Decade of Medicaid. Some State and Federal Perspectives on Medicaid,* Special Report of Medicaid-Medicare Management Institute. Washington, D.C.: Health Care Financing Administration, 1979.

Wilensky, Gail R. and Marc L. Berk. "Health Care, the Poor, and the Role of Medicaid. Data Watch." *Health Affairs* Vol. 1 (Fall 1982): 93–100.

Wilensky, Gail R. and Louis F. Rossiter. "Alternative Units of Payment for Physician Services: An Overview of the Issues." *Medical Care Review* Vol. 43 (Spring 1986): 133–156.

Wing, Kenneth. "The Impact of Reagan-Era Politics on the Federal Medicaid Program." *Catholic University Law Review* Vol. 33 (Fall 1983): 1–93.

Wing, Kenneth. "Medicare and President Reagan's Second Term." *American Journal of Public Health* Vol. 75 (July 1985): 782–784.

Wolkstein, Irwin. "Medicare's Financial Status: How Did We Get Here?" *Milbank Memorial Fund Quarterly* Vol. 62 (Spring 1984): 183–206.

Zuckerman, Stephen. "Medicaid Hospital Spending: Effects of Reimbursement and Utilization Control Policies." *Health Care Financing Review* Vol. 9 (Winter 1987): 65–78.

Mental Health

Bardach, Eugene. *The Skill Factor in Politics: Repealing the Mental Commitment Laws in California.* Berkeley, CA.: University of California Press, 1972.

Brown, Phil, ed. *Mental Health Care and Social Policy.* Boston: Routledge and Kegan Paul, 1985.

Connery, Robert H. *The Politics of Mental Health.* New York: Columbia University Press, 1968.

Chu, Franklin D. and Sharland Trotter. *The Madness Establishment: Ralph Nader's Study Group* Report on the National Institute of Mental Health, New York: Grossman Publishers, 1974.

Falkson, Joseph L. "Minor Skirmish in a Monumental Struggle: HEW's Analysis of Mental Health Services." *Policy Analysis* Vol. 2 (Winter 1976): 93–119.

Felicetti, Daniel A. *Mental Health and Retardation Politics: The Mind Lobbies in Congress.* New York: Praeger Publishers, 1975.

Foley, Henry A. *Community Mental Health Legislation: The Formative Process.* Lexington, MA.: Lexington Books, 1975.

Foley, Henry A. *Madness and Government.* Washington, D.C.: American Psychiatric Press, 1983.

Freeman, Hugh L., Thomas Fryers, and John H. Henderson. *Mental Health Services in Europe: Ten Years On.* Copenhagen: World Health Organization, 1985.

Gilbert, Richard C. "Gramm—Rudman: What It Means to Mental Health and Domestic Spending." *Administration in Mental Health* Vol. 13 (Summer 1986): 249–259.

Goldman, Howard H. and Antoinette A. Gattozzi. "Balance of Powers: Social Security and the Mentally Disabled, 1980–1985." *Milbank Memorial Fund Quarterly* Vol. 66, No. 3 (1988): 531–551.

Goldman, Howard H. and Antoinette A. Gattozzi. "Murder in the Cathedral Revisited: President Reagan and the Mentally Disabled." *Hospital and Community Psychiatry* Vol. 39 (May 1988): 505–509.

Goldman, Howard and Joseph Morrissey. "The Alchemy of Mental Health Policy: Homelessness and the Fourth Cycle of Reform." *American Journal of Public Health* Vol. 75 (July 1985): 727–731.

Gronfein, William. "Incentives and Intentions in Mental Health Policy: A Comparison of the Medicaid and Community Mental Health Programs." *Journal of Health and Social Behavior* Vol. 26 (September 1985): 192–206.

Kiesler, Charles A. et al. "Federal Mental Health Policy Making: An Assessment of Deinstitutionalization." *American Psychologist* Vol. 38 (December 1983): 1292–1297.

Levine, Murray. *The History and Politics of Mental Health.* New York: Oxford University Press, 1981.

Logan, Bruce M., David A. Rochefort and Ernest W. Cook. "Block Grants for Mental Health: Elements of the State Responses." *Journal of Public Health Policy* Vol. 6 (December 1985): 476–492.

Mechanic, David. "Correcting Misconceptions in Mental Health Policy: Strategies for Improved Care of the Seriously Mentally Ill." *Milbank Memorial Fund Quarterly* Vol. 65, No. 2 (1987): 203–230.

Merwin, Mary R. and Frank M. Ochberg. "The Long Voyage: Policies for Progress in Mental Health." *Health Affairs* Vol. 2 (Winter 1983): 96–127.

Report on the National Institute of Mental Health. New York: Grossman Publishers, 1974.

Rochefort, David A. "The Political Context of Mental Health Care" in David Mechanic, ed. *Improving Mental Health Services: What the Social Sciences Can Tell Us. New Directions for Mental Health Services* No. 36. San Francisco: Jossey-Bass, 1987: 93–105.

Rochefort, David A. "Policymaking Cycles in Mental Health: Critical Evaluation of a Conceptual Model." *Journal of Health Politics, Policy and Law* Vol. 13 (Spring 1988): 129–152.

Rumer, Richard. "Community Mental Health Centers: Politics and Therapy." *Journal of Health Politics, Policy and Law* Vol. 2 (Winter 1978): 531–559.

Sardell, Alice. *The U.S. Experiment in Social Medicine. The Community Health Center Program, 1965–1986.* Pittsburgh: University of Pittsburgh Press, 1988.

Sundram, Clarence J. "Mental Illness and Health Care Policy." *Journal of Public Health Policy* Vol. 7 (Summer 1986): 174–182.

National Health Insurance

Anderson, Odin W. "Compulsory Medical Care Insurance, 1910–1950." In Eugene Feingold, ed., *Medicare: Policy and Politics.* San Francisco: Chandler Publishing Co., 1966: 85–156.

Anderson, Odin W. "The Politics of Universal Health Insurance in the United States: An Interpretation." *International Journal of Health Services* Vol. 2, No. 4 (1972): 577–582.

Anlyan, William G., Jr. and Joseph Lipscomb. "The National Health Care Trust Plan: A Blueprint for Market and Long Term Care Reform." *Health Affairs* Vol. 4 (Fall 1985): 5–31.

Cairl, Richard E. and Allen W. Imershein. "Na-

tional Health Insurance Policy in the United States—A Case of Non-Decision Making." *International Journal of Health Services* Vol. 7, No. 2 (1977): 167–178.

Enthoven, Alain and Richard Kronick. "A Consumer-Choice Health Plan for the 1990s: Universal Health Insurance in a System Designed to Promote Quality and Economy." *New England Journal of Medicine* Vol. 320 (January 5, 1989): 29–37; (January 12, 1989): 94–101.

Evang, Karl. "The Politics of Developing a National Health Policy." *International Journal of Health Services* Vol. 3, No. 3 (1973): 331–340.

Falk, I.S. "Proposals for National Health Insurance in the USA: Origins and Evolution, and Some Perceptions for the Future." *Milbank Memorial Fund Quarterly/Health and Society* Vol. 55 (Spring 1977): 161–192.

Goodman, Louis J. and Steven R. Steiber. "Public Support for National Health Insurance." *American Journal of Public Health* Vol. 71 (October 1981): 1105–1108.

Gordon, Jeoffry B. "The Politics of Community Medicine Projects: A Conflict Analysis." *Medical Care* Vol. 7 (November–December 1969): 419–428.

Himmelstein, David U. and Steffie Woolhandler. "Socialized Medicine: A Solution to the Cost Crisis in Health Care in the United States." *International Journal of Health Services* Vol. 16, No. 3 (1986): 339–354.

Himmelstein, David U., Steffie Woolhandler and the Writing Committee of the Working Group on Program Design. "A National Health Program for the United States: A Physicians' Proposal." *New England Journal of Medicine* Vol. 320 (January 12, 1989): 102–108.

Hirshfield, Daniel S. *The Lost Reform: The Campaign for Compulsory Health Insurance in the United States, 1932 to 1943.* Cambridge: Harvard University Press, 1970.

Lubove, Roy. "The New Deal and National Health." *Current History* Vol. 72 (May–June 1977): 198–199, 224–227.

Marmor, Theodore R. "Politics of National Health Insurance: Analysis and Prescription." *Policy Analysis* Vol. 3 (Winter 1977): 25–48.

Marmor, Theodore, R. "NHI in Crisis: Politics,

Predictions, Proposals." *Hospital Progress* Vol. 59 (January 1978): 68–72.

Morone, James A. and Andrew B. Dunham. "Slouching Toward National Health Insurance: The Unanticipated Politics of DRGs." *Bulletin of the New York Academy of Medicine* Vol. 62 (July/August, 1986): 646–662.

Navarro, Vicente. "The Arguments Against A National Health Program: Science or Ideology." *International Journal of Health Services* Vol. 18, No. 2 (1988): 179–189.

Navarro, Vicente. "Refuting Arguments Against a National Health Program." *Health/PAC Bulletin* (Summer 1988): 15–19.

Navarro, Vicente. "The Rediscovery of the National Health Program by the Democratic Party of the United States: A Chronicle of the Jesse Jackson 1988 Campaign." *International Journal of Health Services* Vol. 19, No. 1 (1989): 1–18.

Navarro, Vicente, David U. Himmelstein and Steffie Woolhandler. "The Jackson National Health Program." *International Journal of Health Services* Vol. 19, No. 1 (1989): 19–44.

Numbers, Ronald L. *Almost Persuaded: American Physicians and Compulsory Health Insurance, 1912–1920.* Baltimore, MD.: The Johns Hopkins University Press, 1978.

Numbers, Ronald L. *Compulsory Health Insurance, The Continuing Debate.* Westport, CT.: Greenwood Press, 1982.

Prussin, Jeffrey A. "National Health Insurance: Anatomy of a Political Issue." *Medical Group Management* Vol. 23 (March–April 1976): 22–25.

Relman, Arnold. "Universal Health Insurance: Its Time Has Come." *New England Journal of Medicine* Vol. 320 (January 12, 1989): 117–118.

Semmel, Herb. "National Health is Back on the Agenda." *Health/PAC Bulletin* (Fall 1987): 4–6.

Steiber, Steven R. and Leonard A. Ferber. "Support for National Health Insurance: Intercohort Differentials." *Public Opinion Quarterly* Vol. 45 (Summer 1981): 179–198.

Stern, Lawrence, Louis F. Rossiter and Gail R. Wilensky. "Ethics, Health Care, and the Enthoven Proposal." *Health Affairs* Vol. 1. (Summer 1982): 48–64.

Woolhandler, Steffie and David U. Himmelstein.

"Free Care: A Quantitative Analysis of Health and Cost Effects of a National Health Program in the United States." *International Journal of Health Services* Vol. 18, No. 3 (1988): 393–400.

The Poor

Blendon, Robert J., Linda H. Aiken, et al. "Uncompensated Care by Hospitals or Public Insurance for the Poor: Does is Make a Difference?" *New England Journal of Medicine* Vol. 314 (May 1, 1986): 1160–1163.

Brown, E. Richard and Michael R. Cousineau. "Effectiveness of State Mandates to Maintain Local Government Health Services for the Poor." *Journal of Health Politics, Policy and Law* Vol. 9 (Summer 1984): 223–236.

Coute, Richard A. *Poverty, Politics and Health Care: An Appalachian Experience.* New York: Praeger Publishers, 1975.

Cromwell, Jerry, Sylvia Hurdle and Rachel Schurman. "Defederalizing Medicaid: Fair to the Poor, Fair to Taxpayers?" *Journal of Health Politics, Policy and Law* Vol. 12 (Spring 1987): 1–34.

Dans, Peter E. and Samuel Johnson. "Politics in the Development of a Migrant Health Center." *New England Journal of Medicine* Vol. 292 (April 24, 1975) 890–895.

Davis, Karen. "A Decade of Policy Developments in Providing Health Care for Low-Income Families." In Robert H. Haveman, ed., *A Decade of Federal Antipoverty Programs: Achievements, Failures and Lessons.* New York: Academic Press, 1977: 197–231.

Desonia, Randolph and Kathleen M. King. *State Programs of Assistance for the Medically Indigent.* Washington, D.C.: Intergovernmental Health Policy Project, George Washington University, November 1985.

Kinzer, David M. "Care of the Poor Revisited." *Inquiry* Vol. 21 (Spring 1984): 5–16.

Lewin, Lawrence S. and Marion Ein Lewin. "Financing Charity Care in an Era of Competition." *Health Affairs* Vol. 6 (Spring 1987): 47–60.

Mundinger, Mary O'Neil. "Health Service Funding Cuts and the Declining Health of the

Poor." *New England Journal of Medicine* Vol. 313 (July 4, 1985): 44–47.

Rose, Marilyn G. "Federal Regulation of Services to the Poor Under the Hill-Burton Act: Realities and Pitfalls." *Northwestern University Law Review* Vol. 70 (March–April 1975): 168–201.

Shenkin, Budd N. *Health Care for Migrant Workers: Policies and Politics.* Cambridge: Ballinger Publishing Co., 1974.

Smith, Ellen M. "Health Care for Native Americans: Who Will Pay?" *Health Affairs* Vol. 6 (Spring 1987): 123–128.

Stevens, Robert and Rosemary Stevens. *Welfare Medicine in America: A Case Study of Medicaid.* New York: The Free Press, 1974.

Stone, Deborah A. "Diagnosis and the Dole: The Function of Illness in American Distributive Politics." *Journal of Health Politics, Policy and Law* Vol. 4 (Fall 1979): 507–521.

Turnquist, Trude Held. *An Examination of the Changing Nature of Charity Care in Hospitals: The Response of Minnesota Hospitals and Health Care Facilities to the Hill-Burton Uncompensated Care Obligation, 1980–1981.* Unpublished doctoral dissertation, University of Minnesota, 1987.

Wilensky, Gail R. "Solving Uncompensated Hospital Care: Targeting the Indigent and the Uninsured." *Health Affairs* Vol. 3 (Winter 1984): 50–62.

Public Health

Bellin, Lowell E. "Medicaid in New York: Utopianism and Bare Knuckles in Public Health, 3. Realpolitik in the Health Care Arena: Standard Setting of Professional Services." *American Journal of Public Health* Vol. 59 (May 1969): 820–825.

Bellin, Lowell E. "The New Left and American Public Health—Attempted Radicalization of the A.P.H.A. Through Dialectic." *American Journal of Public Health* Vol. 60 (June 1970): 973–981.

Bernstein, Betty J. "Public Health—Inside or Outside the Mainstream of the Political Process? Lessons from the Passage of Medicaid." *American Journal of Public Health* Vol. 60 (September 1970): 1690–1700.

Conant, Ralph W. *The Politics of Community Health.* Washington, D.C.: Public Affairs Press, 1968.

Courtwright, David T. "Public Health and Public Wealth: Social Cost as a Basis for Restrictive Policies." *Milbank Memorial Fund Quarterly/Health and Society* Vol. 58 (Spring 1980): 268–282.

Gilbert, Benjamin, Merry K. Moos, and C. Arden Miller. "State-Level Decision Making for Public Health: The Status of Boards of Health." *Journal of Public Health Policy* Vol. 3 (March 1982): 51–63.

Gordon, Jeoffry B. "The Politics of Community Medicine Projects: A Conflict Analysis." *Medical Care* Vol. 7 (November–December 1969): 419–428.

Greenberg, George D. "Reorganization- Reconsidered: The U.S. Public Health Service, 1960–1973." *Public Policy* Vol. 23 (Fall 1975): 483–522.

Institute of Medicine Committee to Study the Future of Public Health. *The Future of Public Health.* Washington, D.C.: National Academy Press, 1988

Kaufman, Herbert. "The Political Ingredient of Public Health Services: A Neglected Area of Research." *Milbank Memorial Fund Quarterly/Health and Society* Vol. 44 (October 1966): Part 2, 13–34.

Levine, Adeline G. *Love Canal. Science, Politics and People.* Lexington, MA.: Lexington Books, 1982.

Meyer, Jack A. and Marion Ein Lewin, eds. *Charting the Future of Health Care: Policy, Politics and Public Health.* Washington, D.C.: American Enterprise Institute for Public Policy Research, 1987.

Roemer, Milton I. "The Politics of Public Health in the United States." In Theodor J. Litman and Leonard Robins *Health Politics and Policy:* 261–273.

Russell, Louise B. *Is Prevention Better Than Cure?* Washington, D.C.: The Brookings Institution, 1985.

Snoke, Albert W. "What Good is Legislation—or Planning—If We Can't Make it Work? Need for Comprehensive Approach to Health and Welfare." *American Journal of Public Health* Vol. 72 (September 1982): 1028–1033.

Stone, Deborah A. "The Resistable Rise of Preventative Medicine." *Journal of Health Politics, Policy and Law* Vol. 11, No. 4 (1986): 671–695.

Rationing

Aaron, Henry J. and William B. Schwartz. *The Painful Prescription: Rationing Hospital Care.* Washington, D.C.: The Brookings Institution, 1984.

Blank, Robert H. *Rationing Medicine.* New York: Columbia University Press, 1988.

Blumstein, James F. "Rationing Medical Resources: A Constitutional, Legal and Policy Analysis." In President's Commission for the Study of Ethical Problems in Medical and Biomedical and Behavioral Research, *Securing Access to Health Care* Vol. 3. Washington, D.C.: United States Government Printing Office, 1983: 349–394.

Callahan, Daniel. *Setting Limits: Medical Goals in an Aging Society.* New York: Simon and Schuster, 1988.

Mechanic, David. "Cost Containment and the Quality of Medical Care: Rationing Strategies in an Era of Constrained Resources." *Milbank Memorial Fund Quarterly* Vol. 63 (Summer 1985): 453–475.

Merrill, Jeffrey C. and Alan B. Cohen. "The Emperor's New Clothes: Unraveling the Myths about Rationing." *Inquiry* Vol. 24 (Summer 1987): 105–109.

Reagan, Michael D. "Health Care Rationing: What Does it Mean?" *New England Journal of Medicine* Vol. 319 (October 27, 1988): 1149–1151.

Miscellaneous

Brumback, Clarence L. "The Politics of Smoking Prevention: A Report from the Field." *Journal of Public Health Policy* Vol. 2 (March 1980): 36–41.

Gordon, Linda. "The Politics of Birth Control, 1920–1940: The Impact of Professionals." *International Journal of Health Services* Vol. 5, No. 2 (1975): 253–278.

Kalisch, Beatrice J. and Philip A. Kalisch. "Discourse on the Politics of Nursing." *Journal of Nursing Administration* Vol. 6 (March–April 1976): 29–34.

Koplin, Allen N. "Anti-Smoking Legislation. The New Jersey Experience." *Journal of Public Health Policy* Vol. 2 (September 1981): 247–255.

Law, Sylvia and Stephen Polan. *Pain and Profit: The Politics of Malpractice.* New York: Harper and Row, 1978.

Littlewood, T.B. *The Politics of Population Control.* South Bend, IN.: University of Notre Dame Press, 1979.

Raphaelson, Arnold H. and Charles P. Hall. "Politics and Economics of Hospital Cost Containment." *Journal of Health Politics, Policy and Law* Vol. 3 (Spring 1978): 87–111.

Roth, William. *The Politics of Daycare. The Comprehensive Child Development Act of 1971,* Discussion Paper No. 369–76. Madison, WI.: University of Wisconsin, Institute for Research on Poverty, December 1976.

Steslicke, William E. *Politicization of Medical Malpractice in Michigan.* Ann Arbor, MI.: University of Michigan, Department of Medical Care Organization, April 18, 1977.

The Political Economy of Health

Alford, Robert R. "The Political Economy of Health Care Dynamics Without Change." *Politics and Society* Vol. 2 (Winter 1972): 126–164.

Bodenheimer, Thomas S. "The Fruits of Empire Rot on the Vine: United States Health Policy in the Austerity Era." *Social Science and Medicine* Vol. 28, No. 6 (1989): 531–538.

Bowler, M. Kenneth, Robert T. Kudrle and Theodore R. Marmor. "The Political Economy of National Health Insurance: Policy Analysis and Political Evaluation." In Kenneth M. Friedman and Stuart H. Rakoff, eds., *Toward a National Health Policy: Public Policy and the Control of Health Care Costs.* Lexington, MA.: Lexington Books, 1977.

Bowler, M. Kenneth, Robert T. Kudrle, Theodore R. Marmor and Amy Bridges. "Political Economy of National Health Insurance—Policy Analysis and Political Evaluation." *Journal of Health Politics, Policy and Law* Vol. 2 (Spring 1977): 100–133.

Brenner, M. Harvey. "Health Costs and Benefits of Economic Policy." *International Journal of Health Services* Vol. 7 No. 4 (1977): 581–623.

Campen, James T. *Benefit, Cost, and Beyond: The Political Economy of Benefit-Cost Analysis.* Cambridge, MA.: Ballinger Publishing Co., 1986.

Dowie, Jack. "The Political Economy of the NHS: Individualist Justifications of Collective Action." *Social Science and Medicine* Vol. 20, No. 10 (1985): 1041–1048.

Eyer, Joseph. "Does Unemployment Cause the Death Rate Peak in Each Business Cycle? A Multifactor Model of Death Rate Change." *International Journal of Health Services* Vol. 7 No. 4 (1977): 625–662.

Feldstein, Paul J. *Health Associations and the Demand for Legislation, The Political Economy of Health.* Cambridge: Ballinger Publishing Co., 1977.

Frech, H.E., III, ed. *Health Care in America: The Political Economy of Hospitals and Health Insurance.* San Francisco: Pacific Research Institute for Public Policy, 1988.

Fuchs, Victor R. *The Health Economy.* Cambridge, MA.: Harvard University Press, 1986.

Ginzberg, Eli. "The Political Economy of Health." *Bulletin New York Academy of Medicine* Vol. 41 (October 1965): 1015–1036.

Gritzer, Glenn and Arnold Arluke. *The Making of Rehabilitation: A Political Economy of Medical Specialization.* Berkeley: University of California Press, 1985.

Helt, Eric H. "Economic Determinism: A Model of the Political Economy of Medical Care." *International Journal of Health Services* Vol. 3, No. 3 (1973): 475–485.

Himmelstein, David U., Steffie Woolhandler and David H. Bor. "Will Cost Effectiveness Analysis Worsen the Cost Effectiveness of Health Care?" *International Journal of Health Services* Vol. 18, No. 1 (1988): 1–10.

Hollingsworth, J. Rogers. *A Political Economy of Medicine: Great Britain and the United States.* Baltimore, MD.: The Johns Hopkins Press, 1986.

Kelman, Sander. "Toward the Political Economy of Medical Care." *Inquiry* Vol. 8 (September 1971): 30–38.

Kelman, Sander. "Special Section on Political Economy of Health." *International Journal of Health Services* Vol. 5, No. 4 (1975): 535–693.

Kelman, Sander. "Introduction to the Theme: The Political Economy of Health." *International Journal of Health Services* Vol. 5, No. 4 (1975): 535–538.

Kelman, Sander. "Toward the Political Economy of Medical Care." In Lewis E. Weeks and Howard J. Berman, eds., *Economics in Health Care.* Germantown, MD.: Aspen Systems Corp., 1977: 39–48.

Klein, Rudolf. "The Political Economy of National Health: Report from London." *The Public Interest* Vol. 26 (Winter 1972): 112–125.

Krause, Elliott A. "Health and the Politics of Technology." *Inquiry* Vol. 8 (September 1971): 51–59.

Krause, Elliot A. *Power and Illness, The Political Sociology of Health and Medical Care.* New York: Elsevier North-Holland, 1977.

Lichtman, R. "The Political Economy of Medical Care." In Hans Peter Dreitzel, ed., *The Social Organization of Health.* New York: Macmillan, 1971: 265–290.

Markowitz, Gerald and David Rosner. "More Than Economism: The Politics of Worker's Safety and Health, 1932–1947." *Milbank Quarterly* Vol. 64, No. 3 (1986): 331–354.

Marmor, Theodore R. and Jon B. Christianson. *Health Care Policy. A Political Economy Approach.* Beverly Hills, CA.: Sage Publications, 1982.

Marmor, Theodore R., Amy Bridges and Wayne L. Hoffman. "Comparative Politics and Health Policies: Notes on Benefits, Costs and Limits." in Douglas E. Ashford, ed., *Company Public Policies: New Concepts and Methods* Vol. 4. Beverly Hills, CA.: Sage Publications, 1978: 59–80.

Maynard, Alan. "Public and Private Sector Interactions: An Economic Perspective." *Social Science and Medicine* Vol. 22. No. 11 (1986): 1161–1166.

McGuire, A. "Ethics and Resource Allocation: An Economist's View." *Social Science and Medicine* Vol. 22, No. 11 (1986): 1167–1174.

McKinlay, John B. *A Case for Refocussing Upstream: The Political Economy of Illness,*

Applying Behavioral Science to Cardiovascular Risk. Proceedings from the American Heart Association Conference, Seattle, Washington (June 17–19, 1974): 7–17.

McKinlay, John B. "A Case for Refocussing Upstream: The Political Economy of Illness." In E. Gartly Jaco, ed., *Patients, Physicians, and Illness.* New York: The Free Press, 1979, 3d ed.: 9–26.

McKinlay, John B., ed. *Issues in the Political Economy of Health Care.* New York: Tavistock Publications in association with Methuen, Inc., 1984.

Mendelson, Mary A. and David Hapgood. "Political Economy of Nursing Homes." *Annals of the American Academy of Political and Social Science* Vol. 415 (September 1974): 95–105.

Navarro, Vicente. "Political Economy of Medical Care, An Explanation of the Composition, Nature and Functions of the Present Health Sector of the United States." *International Journal of Health Services* Vol. 5, No. 1 (1975): 65–94.

Navarro, Vicente. "The Political and Economic Determinants of Health and Health Care in Rural America." *Inquiry* Vol. 13 (June 1976): 111–121.

Navarro, Vicente. "Social Class, Political Power, and the State and Their Implications in Medicine." *International Journal of Health Services* Vol. 7, No. 2 (1977): 255–292.

Navarro, Vicente. "The Crisis of the Western System of Medicine In Contemporary Capitalism." *International Journal of Health Services* Vol. 8, No. 2 (1978): 179–211.

Navarro, Vicente. "The 1980 and 1984 U.S. Elections and the New Deal: An Alternative Interpretation." *International Journal of Health Services* Vol. 15, No. 3 (1985): 359–394.

Navarro, Vicente. "U.S. Marxist Scholarship in the Analysis of Health and Medicine." *International Journal of Health Services* Vol. 15, No. 4 (1985): 525–546.

Renaud, Marc. "The Political Economy of the Quebec State Interventions in Health: Reform or Revolution?" Unpublished doctoral dissertation, University of Wisconsin, 1976, Microfilm No. 77–3421.

Rice, Dorothy P. and Douglas Wilson. "The American Medical Economy: Problems and Perspectives." *Journal of Health Politics, Policy and Law* Vol. 1 (Summer 1976): 150–172.

Russell, Louise B. and Carol S. Burke. "The Political Economy of Federal Health Programs in the United States: An Historical Review." *International Journal of Health Services* Vol. 8, No. 1 (1978): 55–77.

Schatzkin, Arthur. "Health and Labor-Power: A Theoretical Investigation." *International Journal of Health Services* Vol. 8, No. 2 (1978): 213–234.

Somers, Herman M. "Observations on Policy and Politics in the Health Care Economy." In Blue Cross Association, eds., *Health Care in the American Economy: Issues and Forecasts.* Chicago, IL.: Health Services Foundation, 1977.

Stevenson, Gelvin. "Profits in Medicine: A Context and an Accounting." *International Journal of Health Services* Vol. 8, No. 1 (1978): 41–54.

Waitzkin, Howard B. "How Capitalism Cares for our Coronaries: A Preliminary Exercise in Political Economy." In Eugene B. Gallagher, ed., *The Doctor-Patient Relationship in the Changing Health Scene,* DHEW Pub. No. (NIH) 78–183. Washington, D.C.: U.S. Government Printing Office, 1978: 317–332.

Windham, Susan R. "National Health Insurance as an Issue in Political Economy—The Implications of the Kennedy Health Security Act for Developing a Strategy to Effect Major Reorganization of Health Care Delivery in America." Unpublished Doctoral Dissertation, Brandeis University, 1977, Microfilm No. 77–15, 274.

Government and Health

Aday, Lu Ann, Ronald Andersen and Gretchen V. Fleming. *Health Care in the U.S.: Equitable for Whom?* Beverly Hills: Sage, 1980.

Amara, Roy, Gregory Schmid and J. Ian Morrison. *Looking Ahead at American Health Care.* Washington, D.C.: McGraw Hill, 1988.

Anderson, Odin W. *The Uneasy Equilibrium: Private and Public Financing of Health Services in the U.S., 1865–1975.* New Haven, CT.: College & University Press, 1968.

Anderson, Odin W. *The American Health Services: A Growth Enterprise Since 1875.* Health Administration Press, 1985.

American Nursing Home Association, Government Relations Department. *An Analysis and Partial Legislative History of Title II of Public Law: 92–603 (H.R.I.), The Social Security Amendments of 1972.* Washington, D.C.: American Nursing Home Association, February 1, 1973.

Bayer, Ronald and Jonathan D. Moreno. "Health Promotion: Ethical and Social Dilemmas of Government Policy." *Health Affairs* Vol. 5 (Summer 1986): 72–85.

Beauchamp, Dan E. *The Health of the Republic: Epidemic, Medicine, and Moralism as Challenges for Democracy.* Philadelphia: Temple University Press, 1988.

Becker, Dorothy D. and Ruth R. Johnson. *Chronology of Health Professions Legislation 1956–1979,* DHHS Publication No. (HRA) 80–69. Washington, D.C.: U.S. Government Printing Office, 1980.

Blumstein, James F. "Government's Role in Organ Transplantation Policy." *Journal of Health Politics, Policy and Law* Vol. 14 (Spring 1989): 5–40.

Blumstein, James F. and Michael Zubkoff. "Perspectives on Government Policy in the Health Sector." *Milbank Memorial Fund Quarterly/Health and Society* Vol. 51 (Summer 1973): 395–431.

Brian, Earl W., "Government Control of Hospital Utilization, A California Experience." *New England Journal of Medicine* Vol. 286 (June 22, 1972): 1340–1344.

Burger, Edward J., Jr. *Protecting the Nation's Health. The Problems of Regulation.* Lexington, MA.: Lexington Books, 1976.

Carey, Sarah C. "A Constitutional Right to Health Care: An Unlikely Development." *Catholic University of America Law Review* Vol. 23 (Spring 1974): 492–514.

Carleton, William G. "Government and Health Before the New Deal." *Current History* Vol. 72 (May–June 1977): 196–197, 223–226.

Carnegie Council on Policy Studies in Higher Education. *Progress and Problems in Medical and Dental Education: Federal Support Versus*

Federal Control. San Francisco: Jossey-Bass, 1976.

Chapman, Carleton B. and John M. Talmadge. "Historical and Political Background of Federal Health Care Legislation." *Law and Contemporary Problems* Vol. 35 (Spring 1970): 334–347.

Chapman Carleton B. and John M. Talmadge. "The Evolution of the Right to Health Concept in the United States." *Pharos* Vol. 34 (January 1971): 30–51.

Clark, Duncan W. "Politics and Health Services Research: A Cameo Study of Policy in the Health Services in the 1930's." E. Evelyn Flook and Paul J. Sanazaro, eds., *Health Services and R & D in Perspective,* Ann Arbor, MI.: Health Research Administration Press, 1973: 109–125.

Cohen, Elias S. "Integration of Health and Social Services in Federally Funded Programs." *Bulletin of the New York Academy of Medicine* Vol. 49 (December 1973): 1038–1050.

Cooper, Barbara S. and Nancy L. Worthington. *Comparison of Cost and Benefit Incidence of Government Medical Care Programs, Fiscal Years 1966 and 1969.* Office of Research and Statistics Staff Paper No. 18, DHEW Pub. No. (SSA) 75–11852. Washington, D.C.: U.S. Government Printing Office, September 1974.

Darling, Helen "The Role of the Federal Government in Assuring Access to Health Care." *Inquiry* Vol. 23 (Fall 1986): 286–295.

Davis, Karen, Marsha Lillie-Blanton, Barbara Lyons, Fitzhugh Mullan, Neil Powe and Diane Rowland. "Health Care for Black Americans: The Public Sector Role." *Milbank Memorial Fund Quarterly* Vol. 65, Supplement (1987): 213–247.

Densen, Paul M. "Public Accountability and Reporting Systems in Medicare and Other Health Programs." *New England Journal of Medicine* Vol. 289 (August 23, 1973): 401–406.

Detwiller, Lloyd F. "The Right to Health." *Hospitals* Vol. 45 (February 16, 1971): 63–66.

Detwiller, Lloyd F. *The Consequences of Health Care Through Government.* Research Publication No. 6, Sydney, Australia: The Office of Health Care Finance, October 1972.

Detwiller, Lloyd F. "Implications and Consequences of Government Involvement in Health and Health Care." In Theodor J. Litman and Leonard Robins, eds., *Health Politics and Policy*, New York: John Wiley and Sons, 1984: 81–96.

Dougherty, Charles J. *American Health Care: Realities, Rights, and Reforms*. New York: Oxford University Press, 1988.

Dowell, Michael A. "Hill-Burton: The Unfulfilled Promise." *Journal of Health Politics, Policy and Law* Vol. 12 (January 1987): 153–175.

Etheredge, Lynn. "Government and Health Care Costs: The Influences of Research on Policy." In Marion Ein Lewin, ed., *From Research into Policy. Improving the Link from Health Services*. Washington, D.C.: American Enterprise Institute for Public Policy Research, 1986: 7–19.

Evans, Robert G. *Illusions of Necessity: Evading Responsibility for Choice in Health Care*. University of British Columbia, Dept. of Economics, December 1984.

Evans, Robert G. "Illusions of Necessity: Evading Responsibility for Choice in Health Care," *Journal of Health Politics, Policy and Law* Vol. 10 (Fall 1985): 439–468.

Fenninger, Leonard D. "Health Manpower and the Education of Health Personnel." *Inquiry* Vol. 10 (March 1973, Supplement): 56–60. Comment: Malcolm C. Todd 61–65; Myron E. Wegman 66–68. Discussion 69–73.

Feshbach, Dan. "What's Inside the Black Box: A Case Study of Allocative Politics in the Hill-Burton Program." *International Journal of Health Services* Vol. 9, No. 2 (1979): 313–339.

Foley, Henry A. *Community Mental Health Legislation: The Formative Process*. Lexington, MA.: Lexington Books, 1975.

Fox, Peter D. "Access to Medical Care for the Poor: The Federal Perspective." *Medical Care* Vol. 10 (May–June 1972): 272–277.

Frank, Kenneth D. "Government Support of Nursing Home Care." *New England Journal of Medicine* Vol. 287 (September 14, 1972): 538–545.

Freedman, Benjamin and Francoise Baylis. "Purpose and Function in Government-Funded Health Coverage." *Journal of Health Politics, Policy and Law* Vol. 12 (Spring 1987): 97–112.

Friedman, Kenneth M. and Stuart H. Rakoff. *Toward a National Health Policy: Public Policy and the Control of Health Care Costs*, Lexington, MA.: D.C. Heath, 1977.

Ginzberg, Eli. "The Political Economy of Health." *Bulletin of the New York Academy of Medicine* Vol. 41 (October 1965): 1015–1036.

Ginzberg, Eli. "The Restructuring of U.S. Health Care." *Inquiry* Vol. 22 (Fall 1985): 272–281.

Ginzberg, Eli, ed. *The U.S. Health Care System: A Look to the 1990's*. Totowa, N.J.: Rowman and Allanheld, 1985.

Havighurst, Clark C. "Controlling Health Care Costs: Strengthening the Private Sector." *Journal of Health Politics, Policy and Law* Vol. 1 (Winter 1977): 471–498.

Health Resources Administration. *Health Resources Studies: Government Controls on the Health Care System: The Canadian Experience*, DHEW Pub. No. (HRA) 77–246. Washington, D.C.: U.S. Government Printing Office, 1977.

Himmelstein, David U. and Steffie Woolhandler. "Cost Without Benefit: Administrative Waste in U.S. Health Care." *New England Journal of Medicine* Vol. 314 (February 13) 1986, 441–445.

Iglehart, John K. "The Carter Administration's Health Budget: Charting New Priorities with Limited Dollars." *Milbank Memorial Fund Quarterly/Health and Society* Vol. 56 (Winter 1978): 53–77.

Jaeger, Boi Jon. "Government and Hospitals: A Perspective on Health Politics." *Hospital Administration* Vol. 17 (Winter 1972): 39–50.

Jonas, Steven, David Banta and Michael Enright. "Government in the Health Care Delivery System." In Steven Jonas, ed., *Health Care Delivery in the United States*. New York: Springer Publishing Co., 1977: 289–328.

Katz, Daniel, et al. *Bureaucratic Encounters: A Pilot Study in the Evaluation of Government Services*. Ann Arbor, MI.: University of Michigan, Institute for Social Research, 1975.

Kennedy, Edward M. "The Congress and National Health Policy." *American Journal of Public Health* Vol. 68 (March 1978): 241–244.

Kennedy, Virginia C. "Interpreting Legislative Voting Patterns on Health Issues: A Method and Rationale." *Journal of Community Health* Vol. 1 (Spring 1976): 188–195.

Kessel, Reuben A. *Ethical and Economic Aspects of Governmental Intervention in the Medical Care Market.* Washington, D.C.: American Enterprise Institute, Center for Health Policy Research, 1977.

Klarman, Herbert E. "Major Public Initiatives in Health Care." *The Public Interest* Vol. 34 (Winter 1974): 106–123.

Lally, John J. "Social Determinants of Differential Allocation of Resources to Disease Research: A Comparative Analysis of Crib Death and Cancer Research." *Journal of Health and Social Behavior* Vol. 18 (June 1977): 125–138.

Lashof, Joyce C. and Mark H. Lepper. "Federal-State Local Partnership in Health." In US-PHS, Health Resources Administration, eds., *Health in America: 1877–1976.* Washington, D.C.: U.S. Government Printing Office, 1976: 122–137.

Lave, Judith and Lester Lave. *The Hospital Construction Act: An Evaluation of the Hill-Burton Program, 1948–1973.* Washington, D.C.: American Enterprise Institute for Public Policy Research, 1974.

Leroy, Lauren and Philip R. Lee, eds. *Deliberations and Compromise, The Health Professions Educational Assistance Act of 1976.* Cambridge: Ballinger Publishing Co., 1977.

Lostetter. John O. and John E. Chapman. "The Participation of the United States Government in Providing Financial Support for Medical Education." *Health Policy and Education* Vol. 1, No. 1 (1979): 27–65.

Marmor, Theodore R. "Origins of the Government Health Insurance Issue." In David Kotelchuck, ed., *Prognosis Negative: Crisis in the Health Care System,* New York: Vintage Books, 1975: 293–303.

Marmor, T. and D. Thomas. "The Politics of Paying Physicians: The Determinants of Government Payment Methods in England, Sweden and the United States." *International Journal of Health Services* Vol. 1, No. 1 (1971): 71–78.

McEwan, E.D. "A Case for Government Sponsored Health Care Research and Development in the Formulation of Health Policy and an Account of Early Experience of Government-Sponsored Health Care Research in One Jurisdiction." *International Journal of Health Services* Vol. 3, No. 1 (1973): 45–58.

McNeil, Richard Jr. and Robert E. Schlenker. "HMOs, Competition and Government." *Milbank Memorial Fund Quarterly/Health and Society* Vol. 53 (Spring 1975): 195–224.

Meilicke, Carl A. "The Saskatchewan Medical Care Dispute of 1962: An Analytic Social History." Unpublished doctoral dissertation, University of Minnesota, 1967, Microfilm No. 68-7435.

Mooney, Anne. "The Great Society and Health: Policies for Narrowing the Gaps in Health Status Between the Poor and the Nonpoor." *Medical Care* Vol. 15 (August 1977): 611–619.

Morris, Jonas. *Searching for a Cure.* New York: Pica Press, 1984.

Naimark, Arnold. "Ethical Questions Posed by Community and Government Pressures on Medical Education in Canada." *Bulletin of the New York Academy of Medicine* Vol. 54 (July–August 1978): 687–696.

Neustadt, Richard E. and Harvey V. Fineberg. *The Swine Flu Affair: Decision-Making on a Slippery Disease.* Washington, D.C.: U.S. Government Printing Office, 1978.

Palley, Howard A. "Policy Formulation in Health, Some Considerations of Governmental Constraints on Pricing in the Health Delivery System." *American Behavioral Scientist* Vol. 7 (March–April 1974): 572–584.

Phelps, Charles E. "Public Sector Medicine: History and Analysis." In Institute for Contemporary Studies, eds., *New Directions in Public Health Care: An Evaluation of Proposals for National Health Insurance.* San Francisco: The Institute for Contemporary Studies, 1976.

Raffel, Marshall W. and Norma K. Raffel. *The U.S. Health System. Origins and Functions.* Media, PA.: Harwal Publishing Co., 1989.

Rakoff, Stuart H. and Kenneth M. Friedman, eds. "Health, Health Costs and the Role of Government." In Kenneth M. Friedman and Stuart H. Rakoff, eds. *Toward a National Health Policy: Public Policy and the Control of Health Care Costs.* Lexington, MA.: Lexington Books, 1977.

Renn, Steven. "The Structure and Financing of the Health Care Delivery System in the 1980's." In Carl J. Schramm, ed., *Health Care and Its Costs. Can the U.S. Afford Adequate Care?* New York: W.W. Norton, 1987: 8–48.

Rhein, Reginald W. and Larry Marion. *The Saccharin Controversy, A Guide for Consumers.* New York: Monarch Press, 1977.

Roemer, Milton I. and Mary H. McClanahan. "Impact of Government Programs on Voluntary Hospitals." *Public Health Reports* Vol. 75 (June 1960): 537–544.

Rohrer, James E. "The Political Development of the Hill-Burton Program: A Case Study in Distributive Policy." *Journal of Health Politics, Policy and Law* Vol. 12 (Spring 1977): 137–152.

Rudolf, Ronald J. "Physician Care and Government Programs: Analysis of the Distribution of Health and Health Services in New York City and the Nation." Unpublished doctoral dissertation, Rutgers University, 1976, Microfilm No. 77-7277.

Russell, Louise R. "Inflation and the Federal Role in Health." in Michael Zubkoff, ed., *Health: Victim or Cause of Inflation?* New York: Prodist, Neale Watson Academic Publishers, 1976: 225–244.

Sade, Robert M. "Medical Care as a Right: A Refutation." *New England Journal of Medicine* Vol. 285 (December 2, 1971): 1288–1292.

Schelling, Thomas C. "Government and Health." In Institute for Contemporary Studies, eds., *New Directions for Public Health Care: An Evaluation of Proposals for National Health Insurance.* San Francisco: The Institute for Contemporary Studies, 1976.

Schlesinger, Edward R. "The Impact of Federal Legislation on Maternal and Child Health Services in the United States." *Milbank Memorial Fund Quarterly/Health and Society* Vol. 52 (Winter 1974): 1–13.

Schlesinger, Edward R., Martha M. Skoner, Estelle D. Trooskin, Janet R. Markel and A. Frederick North. "The Effects of Anticipated Funding Changes on Maternal and Child Health Projects: A Case Study of Uncertainty." *American Journal of Public Health* Vol. 66 (April 1976): 385–388.

Schramm, Carl J., ed. *Health Care and Its Costs. Can the U.S. Afford Adequate Care?* New York: W.W. Norton, 1987.

Schwartz, Joshua I. *Public Health: Case Studies on the Origins of Government Responsibility for Health Services in the United States.* New York: Cornell University Program in Urban and Regional Studies, 1977.

Shuck, Peter H. "Government Funding for Organ Transplants." *Journal of Health Politics, Policy and Law* Vol. 14 (Spring 1989): 169–190.

Snoke, Albert W. "What Good is Legislation—or Planning—If We Can't Make It Work? The Need for a Comprehensive Approach to Health and Welfare." *American Journal of Public Health* Vol. 72 (September 1982): 1028–1033.

Sobel, Lester A. *Health Care: An American Crisis.* New York: Facts on File, 1976.

Somers, Herman M. "Health and Public Policy." *Inquiry* Vol. 12 (June 1975): 87–96.

Steiner, Gilbert Y. *The Children's Cause.* Washington, D.C.: The Brookings Institution, 1976.

Stevens, Robert and Rosemary Stevens. *Welfare Medicine in America, A Case Study of Medicaid.* New York: The Free Press, 1974.

Strickland, Stephen P. "Medical Research: Public Policy and Power Politics." In Douglass Cater and Philip R. Lee, eds., *Politics of Health.* New York: Medcom Press, 1972.

Strickland, Stephen P. *Research and the Health of Americans: Improving the Policy Process.* Lexington, MA.: Lexington Books, 1978.

Stuart, Bruce C. "Who Gains from Public Health Programs." *Annals of American Academy of Political and Social Science* Vol. 399 (January 1972): 145–150.

Walsh, Margaret E. *The Health Profession Educational Organization and the Governmental Process.* New York: National League for Nursing, 1974.

Wikler, Daniel I. "Persuasion and Coercion for Health: Ethical Issues in Government Efforts to Change Life-Styles." *Milbank Memorial Fund Quarterly/Health and Society* Vol. 56 (Summer 1978): 303–338.

Williams, A.P., Jr., et al. *Policy Analysis for Federal Biomedical Research.* Santa Monica, CA.: Rand Corp., March 1976, Rand Report No. R-1945-PBRPJRC.

Wilson, Florence and Duncan Neuhauser. *Health Services in the United States.* Cambridge, MA.: Ballinger Publishing Co., 1985.

Wilson, Walter A. "The Future Role of Government in Dental Practice and Education." *Journal of the American College of Dentists* Vol. 40 (April 1973): 111–116.

Wing, Kenneth R. *The Law and the Public's*

Health. St. Louis, MO.: C.V. Mosby Co., 1976.

Zubkoff, Michael and James Blumstein. *Framework for Government Intervention in the Health Sector.* Lexington, MA.: D.C. Health, 1976.

Some Foreign Comparisons

General

Abel-Smith, Brian. *Value for Money in Health Services: A Comparative Study.* New York: St. Martin's Press, 1976.

Abel-Smith, Brian. *Cost Containment in Health Care: A Study of 12 European Countries 1977–1983.* Occasional papers on Social Administration No. 73, Brookfield Publishing Co., Bedford, England.: London Square Press, 1984.

Abel-Smith, Brian. "Global Perspective on Health Service Financing." *Social Science and Medicine* Vol. 21, No. 9 (1985): 957–963.

Altenstetter, Christa. *Health Policy Making and Administration in West Germany and the United States.* Beverly Hills, CA.: Sage Publications, 1974.

Altenstetter, Christa. "Medical Interests and the Public Interest: A Comparison of West Germany and the United States." *International Journal of Health Services* Vol. 4 (Winter 1974): 29–48.

Barer, Morris, Amiram Gafni and Jonathan Lomas. "Accommodating Rapid Growth in Physician Supply: Lessons from Israel, Warnings for Canada." *International Journal of Health Services* Vol. 19, No. 1 (1989): 95–116.

Bates, Erica. *Health Systems and Public Scrutiny: Australia, Britain and the United States.* New York: St. Martin's Press, 1983.

Berlant, Jeffrey L. *Profession and Monopoly: A Study of Medicine in the United States and Great Britain.* Berkeley, CA.: University of California Press, 1975.

Blanpain, Jan. *National Health Insurance and Health Resources: The European Experience.* Cambridge, MA.: Harvard University Press, 1978.

Blendon, Robert J. "Three Systems: A Comparative Survey." *Health Management Quarterly* Vol. 11, No. 1 (1989): 2–10.

Crichton, Anne. *Health Policy Making.* Ann Arbor, MI.: Health Administration Press, 1980.

Culyer, A.J. and Bengt Jonsson, eds. *Public and Private Health Services.* London: Basil Blackwell, 1987.

deKervasdoue, Jean, John R. Kimberly and Victor Rodin, eds. *The End of an Illusion: The Future of Health Policy in Western Industrialized Nations.* Berkeley: University of California Press, 1984.

deSwaan, Abram. *In Care of the State: Health Care Education and Welfare in Europe and the U.S.A. in the Modern Era.* New York: Oxford University Press, 1989.

Elling, Ray H. *Cross-National Study of Health Systems: Political Economics and Health Care.* New Brunswick, N.J.: Transaction Books, 1980.

Elling, Ray H. *Cross-National Study of Health Systems: Concepts, Methods and Data Sources: A Guide to Information Sources.* Detroit, MI.: Gale Research Co., 1980.

Elling, Ray H. *Cross-National Study of Health Systems, Countries, World Regions and Special Problems: A Guide to Information Sources.* Detroit, MI.: Gale Research Co., 1980.

Fox, Daniel M. *Health Policies, Health Politics: The British and American Experience, 1911–1965.* Princeton: Princeton University Press, 1986.

Fry, John and W.A.J. Farndale, ed. *International Medical Care: A Comparison and Evaluation of Medical Care Services Throughout the World.* Wallingsford, PA.: Washington Square East Publishers, 1972.

Glaser, William A. "Paying the Hospital: Foreign Lessons for the United States." *Health Care Financing Review* Vol. 4 (Summer 1983): 99–110.

Glaser, William. "Health Politics: Lessons from Abroad." In Theodor J. Litman and Leonard Robins *Health Politics and Policy.* New York: John Wiley and Sons, 1984: 305–340.

Glaser, A. William A. "Hospital Rate Regulation: American and Foreign Comparisons." *Journal of Health Politics, Policy and Law* Vol. 8 (Winter 1984): 702–731.

Glaser, William A. "Juggling Multiple Payers: American Problems and Foreign Solutions." *Inquiry* Vol. 21 (Summer 1984): 178–188.

Godt, Paul J. "Confrontation, Consent and Corporatism: State Strategies and the Medical Profession in France, Great Britain and West Germany." *Journal of Health Politics, Policy and Law* Vol. 12 (Fall 1987): 459–480.

Hollingsworth, J. Rogers. *A Political Economy of Medicine: Great Britain and the United States.* Baltimore, MD.: Johns Hopkins University Press, 1986.

Kleczkowski, B.M., M.I. Roemer and A. Vander Werf. *National Health Systems and Their Reorientation Toward Health for all Guidance for Policy Making.* Public Health Papers, No. 77, Geneva: World Health Organization, 1984.

Kohn, Robert and Susan Radius. "Two Roads to Health Care: U.S. and Canadian Policies, 1945–1975." *Medical Care* Vol. 12 (March 1974): 189–201.

Leichter, Howard M. *Comparative Approach to Policy Analysis: Health Care Policy in Four Nations.* New York: Cambridge University Press, 1979.

Litman, Theodor J. "National Health Care Systems." In Theodor J. Litman *The Sociology of Medicine and Health Care: A Bibliography.* San Francisco: Boyd and Fraser Publications, 1976, Chapter 10: 556–581.

Litman, Theodor J. and Leonard Robins. "Comparative Analysis of Health Care Systems— A Socio-Political Approach." *Social Science and Medicine* Vol. 5 (December 1971): 573–581.

Marmor, Theodore R., Amy Bridges and Wayne L. Hoffman. "Comparative Politics and Health Policies: Notes on Benefits, Costs, Limits." In Theodore R. Marmor *Political Analysis and American Medical Care.* New York: Cambridge University Press, 1983: 45–60.

Maxwell, Robert J. *Health and Wealth: An International Study of Health Care Spending.* Lexington, MA.: Lexington Books, D.C. Heath and Co., 1981.

Navarro, Vicente. "The Public/Private Mix in the Funding and Delivery of Health Services: An International Survey." *American Journal of Public Health* Vol. 75 (November 1985): 1318–1320.

Pescosolido, Bernice, Carol A. Boyer and Wai-Ying Tsui. "Medical Care in the Welfare State: A Cross-National Study of Public Evaluations." *Journal of Health and Social Behavior* Vol. 26 (December 1985): 276–297.

Raffel, Marshall W. *Comparative Health Systems: Descriptive Analyses of Fourteen National Health Systems.* University Park, PA.: Pennsylvania State University Press, 1984.

Rodwin, Victor G. *The Health Planning Predicament: France, Quebec, England, and the United States.* Berkeley, CA.: University of California Press, 1984.

Rodwin, Victor G. "American Exceptionalism in the Health Sector: The Advantages of 'Backwardness' in Learning from Abroad." *Medical Care Review* Vol. 44 (Spring 1987): 119–154.

Roemer, Milton I. *Comparative National Policies on Health Care.* New York: Marcel Dekker, 1977.

Roemer, Milton I. *National Strategies for Health Care Organization: A World Overview.* Ann Arbor, MI.: Health Administration Press, 1985.

Roemer, Milton I., ed. *Health Care Systems in World Perspective.* Ann Arbor, MI.: Health Administration Press, 1976.

Roemer, Milton I. and Ruth J. Roemer. *Health Care Systems and Comparative Manpower Policies.* New York: Marcel Dekker, 1981.

Ron, Aviva "Sharing in the Financing of Health Care: Government, Insurance and the Patient." *Health Policy* Vol. 6, No., 1 (1986): 87–101.

Rosenthal, Marilynn M. *Dealing with Medical Malpractice: The British and Swedish Experience.* Durham, N.C.: Duke University Press, 1988.

Rosenthal, Marilynn and Deborah Frederick. "Physician Maldistribution in Cross-Cultural Perspective: United States, United Kingdom, and Sweden." *Inquiry* Vol. 21 (Spring 1984): 60–74.

Sass, Hans-Martin and Robert U. Massey, eds. *Health Care Systems: Moral Conflicts in European and American Public Policy.* Hingham, MA.: Kluwer Academic Publishers, 1988.

Schieber, George J. and Jean-Pierre Poullier. "Recent Trends in International Health Care Spending." *Health Affairs* Vol. 6 (Fall 1987): 105–112.

Van Atteveld, Lettie, Corine Broeders and Ruud

Lapré. "International Comparative Research in Health Care. A Study of the Literature." *Health Policy* Vol. 8, No. 1 (1987): 105–136.

Weiner, Jonathan P. "Primary Care Delivery in the United States and Four Northwest European Countries: Comparing the 'Corporatized' with the 'Socialized.' " *Milbank Quarterly* Vol. 65, No. 3 (1987): 426–461.

Weller, Geoffry R. and Pranal Manga. "The Push for Reprivatization of Health Care in Canada, Britain and the United States." *Journal of Health Politics, Policy and Law* Vol. 8 (Fall 1983): 495–517.

Welsh, William W. "Modeling Budgetary Strategies in Health Policy, East and West." *Journal of Health Politics, Policy and Law* Vol. 8 (Fall 1983): 519–553.

Wilsford, David. "The Cohesion and Fragmentation of Organized Medicine in France and the United States." *Journal of Health Politics, Policy and Law* Vol. 12 (Fall 1987): 481–503.

Canada

Andrepolous Spyros. *National Health Insurance: Can We Learn from Canada?* New York: John Wiley and Sons, 1975.

Atkinson, Michael A. and Marsha A. Chandler, eds. *The Politics of Canadian Public Policy.* Toronto, University of Toronto Press, 1983.

Barer, Morris, L. "Regulating Physician Supply: The Evolution of British Columbia's Bill 41." *Journal of Health Politics, Policy and Law* Vol. 13 (Spring 1988) 1–26.

Bryant, Bertha E. "Issues on the Distribution of Health Care: Some Lessons from Canada." *Public Health Reports* Vol. 96 (September-October 1981): 442–447.

Coburn, David B., George M. Torrance and Joseph M. Kaufert. "Medical Dominance in Canada in Historical Perspective: The Rise and Fall of Canadian Medicine?" *International Journal of Health Services* Vol. 13, No. 3 (1983): 407–432.

Contandriopoulos, André-Pierre. "Cost Containment Through Payment Mechanisms: The Quebec Experience." *Journal of Public Health Policy* Vol. 7 (Summer 1986): 224–238.

Crighton, Anne. "The Shift from Entrepreneurial to Political Power in the Canadian Health System." *Social Science and Medicine* Vol. 10 (January 1976): 59–66.

Culyer, A.J. *Health Expenditures in Canada: Myth and Reality, Past and Future.* Toronto: Canadian Tax Foundation, 1988.

Evans, Robert G. "Health Care in Canada: Patterns of Funding and Regulation." *Journal of Health Politics, Policy and Law* Vol. 8 (Spring 1983): 1–43.

Evans, Robert G. *Strained Mercy: The Economics of Canadian Health Care.* Toronto: Butterworths, 1984.

Evans, Robert G. "Finding the Levers, Finding the Courage: Lessons from Cost Containment in North America." *Journal of Health Politics, Policy and Law* Vol. 11, No. 4 (1986): 585–615.

Evans, Robert G., et al. "Controlling Health Expenditures—The Canadian Reality." *New England Journal of Medicine* Vol. 320 (March 2, 1989): 571–577.

Evans, Robert G. and Greg L. Stoddart eds. *Medicare at Maturity: Achievements, Lessons and Challenges.* Calgary Alberta: University of Calgary Press, 1986.

Fried, Bruce J., Raisa B. Deber and Peggy Leatt. "Corporatization and Deprivatization of Health Services in Canada." *International Journal of Health Services* Vol. 17, No. 4 (1987): 567–584.

Hamowy, Ronald. *Canadian Medicine: A Study of Restricted Entry.* Vancouver, B.C.: The Fraser Institute, 1984.

Heiber, S. and R. Deber. "Banning Extra-Billing in Canada: Just What the Doctor Didn't Order." *Canadian Public Policy* Vol. 13 (March 1987) 62–74.

Iglehart, John K. "Canada's Health Care Systems." *New England Journal of Medicine* Vol. 315 (July 17, 1986) 202–208; (September 18, 1986) 778–784; (December 18, 1986): 1623–1628.

Kane, Robert L. and Rosalie A. Kane. *A Will and a Way: What the United States Can Learn from Canada About Caring for the Elderly.* New York: Columbia University Press, 1985.

Kohn, Robert and Susan Radius. "Two Roads to Health Care: U.S. and Canadian Policies; 1945–1975." *Medical Care* Vol. 12 (March 1974): 189–199.

Lomas, Jonathan, Catherine Fooks, Thomas Rice, and Roberta J. LaBelle. "Paying Physicians in Canada: Minding our Ps and Qs." *Health Affairs* Vol. 8 (Spring 1989): 80–102.

Marmor, Theodore R. "Canada's Path, America's Choices: Lessons from the Canadian Experience with National Health Insurance." In Peter Conrad and Rochelle Kern *Sociology of Health and Illness, Critical Perspectives.* New York: St. Martin's Press, 1985, 2d ed.: 443–467.

Naylor, C. David. *Private Practice, Public Payment: Canadian Medicine and the Politics of Health Insurance, 1911–1966.* Kingston and Montreal: McGill-Queen's University Press, 1986.

Palley, Howard A. "Canadian Federalism and the Canadian Health Care Program: A Comparison of Ontario and Quebec." *International Journal of Health Services* Vol. 17, No. 4 (1987): 595–616.

Pineault, Raynald, Andre-Pierre Contandriopoulos and Richard Lessard. "The Quebec Health System: Care Objectives or Health Objectives." *Journal of Public Health Policy* Vol. 6 (September 1985): 394–409.

Stevenson, H. Michael and A. Paul Williams. "Physicians and Medicare: Professional Ideology and Canadian Health Care Policy." *Canadian Public Policy* Vol. 11 (September 1985): 504–521.

Stevenson, H. Michael, A. Paul Williams and Eugene Vayda. "Medical Politics and Canadian Medicare: Professional Response to the Canada Health Act." *Milbank Quarterly* Vol. 66, No. 1 (1988): 65–104.

Taylor, Malcolm G. *Health Insurance and Canadian Public Policy: The Seven Decisions that Created the Canadian Health Insurance System and Their Outcomes.* Montreal: McGill-Queen's University Press, 1978.

Touhy, C.J. "Medical Politics After Medicare: The Ontario Case." *Canadian Public Policy* Vol. 2, No. 2 (1976): 192–210.

Vayda, Eugene. "Aspects of Medical Manpower under National Health Insurance in Canada." *Journal of Public Health Policy* Vol. 4 (December 1983): 504–513.

Vayda, Eugene and Deber B. Raiser. "The Canadian Health Care System: An Overview." *Social Science and Medicine* Vol. 18, No. 3 (1984): 191–197.

Weller, Geoffrey R. "Common Problems, Alternative Solutions: A Comparison of the Canadian and American Health Systems." *Policy Studies Journal* Vol. 14 (June 1986): 604–620.

Weller, Geoffrey R. and Pranal Manga. "The Development of Health Policy in Canada." In Michael A. Atkinson and Marsha A. Chandler, eds., *The Politics of Canadian Public Policy.* Toronto: University of Toronto Press, 1983: 223–246.

Weller, Geoffrey R. and Pranal Manga. "The Push for Reprivatization of Health Care Services in Canada, Britain, and the United States." *Journal of Health Politics, Policy, and Law* Vol. 8 (Fall 1983): 495–517.

Wolfe, Samuel and Robin Badgley. "How Much is Enough? The Payment of Doctors—Implications for Health Policy in Canada." *International Journal of Health Services* Vol. 4 (Spring 1974): 245–264.

Wolfe, Samuel and Robin Badgley. "Immigration, Emigration and Opting Out by Canadian Physicians under National Medicare." *Journal of Public Health Policy* Vol. 2, No. 1 (1981): 80–86.

Great Britain and the United Kingdom

Allen, David. "Perspectives in NHS Management: Are There Lessons from Abroad for the NHS?" *British Medical Journal* Vol. 289 (July 28, 1984): 265–268.

Barnard Keith and Kenneth Lee, eds. *Conflicts in the National Health Service.* New York: Prodist: Neale Watson Academic Publication, 1977.

Birch, Stephen. "DRGs U.K. Style: A Comparison of U.K. and U.S. Policies for Hospital Cost Containment and their Implications for Health Status." *Health Policy* Vol. 10, No. 2 (1988): 143–154.

Butler, John R. and Michael S.B Vaile. *Health and Health Services: An Introduction to Health Care in Britain.* Boston: Routledge and Kegan Paul, 1984.

Draper, Peter and Tony Smart. "Social Science and Health Policy in the United Kingdom: Some Contributions of the Social Sciences to the Bureaucratization of the National Health Service." *International Journal of Health Services.* Vol. 4 (Summer 1974): 453–470.

Enthoven, Alain C. *Reflections on the Management of the National Health Service,* Occasional Paper No. 5. London: The Nuffield Provincial Hospitals Trust, 1985.

Halper, Thomas. "Life and Death in a Welfare State: End-Stage Renal Disease in the United Kingdom." *Milbank Memorial Fund Quarterly* Vol. 63 (Winter 1985): 52–93.

Ham, Christopher. *Health Policy in Britain: The Politics and Organization of the National Health Service.* London: MacMillan Press, 1985.

Hollingsworth, J. Rogers. *A Political Economy of Medicine: Great Britain and the United States.* Baltimore, MD.: Johns Hopkins University Press, 1986.

Iglehart, John. "The British National Health Service under the Conservatives." *New England Journal of Medicine* Part I., Vol. 309 (November 17, 1983): 1264–68; Part II., Vol. 310 (January 5, 1984): 63–67.

Jonas, Steven and David Banta. "The 1974 Reorganization of the British National Health Service: An Analysis." *Journal of Community Health* Vol. 1 (Winter 1975): 91–105.

Klein, Rudolf. "The Rise and Decline of Policy Analysis: The Strange Case of Health Policymaking in Britain." *Policy Analysis* Vol. 2 (Summer 1976): 459–475.

Klein, Rudolf. "Ideology, Class and the National Health Service." *Journal of Health Politics, Policy and Law* Vol. 4 (Fall 1979): 464–490.

Klein, Rudolf. *The Politics of the National Health Service.* London; New York: Longman, 1983.

Klein, Rudolf. "The Politics of Ideology Vs the Reality of Politics: The Case of Britain's National Health Service in the 1980's." *Milbank Memorial Fund Quarterly* Vol. 62 (Winter 1984): 82–109.

Klein, Rudolf. "Why Britain's Conservatives Support a Socialist Health Care System." *Health Affairs* Vol. 4 (Spring 1985): 41–58.

Kushnick, Louis. "Racism, The National Health Service, and the Health of Black People." *International Journal of Health Services* Vol. 18, No. 3 (1988): 457–470.

Levitt, Ruth and Andrew Hall. *The Reorganized National Health Service.* London: Croom-Helm, 1984, 3d ed.

Lister, John. "The Politics of Medicine in Britain and the United States." *New England Journal of Medicine* Vol. 315 (July 17, 1986): 168–173.

Lister, John. "Proposals for Reform of the British National Health Service." *New England Journal of Medicine* Vol. 320 (March 30, 1989): 877–880.

MacKenzie, W.J.M. *Power and Responsibility in Health Care: The National Health Service as a Political Institution.* New York: Oxford University Press, 1979.

MacMillan, Donald, et al., eds. *NHS Reorganization: Issues and Prospects.* Leeds: Nuffield Centre for Health Services Studies, 1975.

Maynard, Alan. "Financing the U.K. National Health Services." *Health Policy* Vol. 6, No. 4 (1986): 329–340.

Mohan, John and Kevin J. Woods. "Restructuring Health Care: The Social Geography of Public and Private Health Care under the British Conservative Government." *International Journal of Health Services* Vol. 15, No. 2 (1985): 197–216.

Rayner, Geoffrey. "Lessons from America? Commercialization and Growth of Private Medicine in Britain." *International Journal of Health Services* Vol. 17, No. 2 (1987): 197–216.

Schulz, Rockwell and Steve Harrison. "Consensus Management in the British National Health Service: Implications for the United States?" *Milbank Memorial Fund Quarterly* Vol. 62 (Fall 1984): 657–681.

Schwartz, William B. and Henry J. Aaron. "Rationing Hospital Care: Lessons from Britain." *New England Journal of Medicine* Vol. 310 (January 5, 1984): 52–56.

Germany

Altenstetter, Christa. *Health Policy Making and Administration in West Germany and the United States.* Beverly Hills, CA.: Sage Publications, 1974.

Altenstetter, Christa. "Medical Interests and the Public Interest: A Comparison of West Germany and the United States." *International Journal of Health Services* Vol. 4 (Winter 1974): 29–48.

Altenstetter, Christa. "An End to a Consensus on Health Care in the Federal Republic of Germany?" *Journal of Health Politics, Policy and Law* Vol. 12 (Fall 1987): 505–536.

Glaser, William. "Lessons from Germany: Some Reflections Occasioned by Schulenberg's Report." *Journal of Health Politics, Policy and Law* Vol. 8 (Summer 1983): 352–365.

Henke, Klaus-Dirk. "A 'Concerted' Approach to Health Care Financing in the Federal Republic of Germany." *Health Policy* Vol. 6, No. 4 (1986): 341–351.

LaBisch, Alfons. "The Role of the Hospital in the Health Policy of the German Social Democratic Movement Before World War I." *International Journal of Health Services* Vol. 17, No. 2 (1987): 279–294.

Light, Donald W. "Comparing Health Care Systems: Lessons from East and West Germany." In Peter Conrad and Rochelle Kern, eds., *Sociology of Health and Illness: Critical Perspectives,* 2d ed. New York: St. Martin's Press, 1985: 429–443.

Light, Donald W. "Values and Structure in the German Health Care Systems." *Milbank Memorial Fund Quarterly* Vol. 63 (Fall 1985): 615–647.

Light, Donald W. and Alexander Schuller. *The Impact of Political Values and Health Care: The German Experience.* Cambridge, MA: MIT Press, 1986.

Light, Donald W., Stephan Liebfried and Florian Tennstedt. "Social Medicine vs. Professional Dominance: The German Experience." *American Journal of Public Health* Vol. 76 (January 1986): 78–83.

Schulenburg, J-Matthias Graf. "Report from Germany: Current Conditions and Controversies in Health Care Systems." *Journal of Health Politics, Policy and Law* Vol. 8 (Summer 1983): 320–351.

Stone, Deborah A. *The Limits of Professional Power: National Health Care in the Federal Republic of Germany.* Chicago: University of Chicago Press, 1980.

Sweden

Gustafsson, Rolf A. "Origins of Authority: The Organization of Medical Care in Sweden." *International Journal of Health Services* Vol. 19, No. 1 (1989): 121–133.

Heidenheimer, Arnold J. and Nils Elvander, eds. *The Shaping of the Swedish Health System.* New York: St. Martin's Press, 1980.

Heidenheimer, Arnold and Lars N. Johansen. "Organized Medicine and Scandinavian Professional Unionism: Hospital Policies and Exit Options in Denmark and Sweden." *Journal of Health Politics, Policy and Law* Vol. 10 (Summer 1985): 347–370.

Hessler, Richard M. and Andrew C. Twaddle. "Sweden's Crisis in Medical Care: Political and Legal Changes." *Journal of Health Politics, Policy and Law* Vol. 7 (Summer 1982): 440–459.

Rosenthal, Marilynn M. "Beyond Equity: Swedish Health Policy and the Private Sector." *Milbank Quarterly* Vol. 64, No. 4 (1986): 592–621.

Shenkin, Budd N. "Politics and Medical Care in Sweden: The Seven Crowns Reform." *New England Journal of Medicine* Vol. 288 (March 15, 1973): 555–559.

Twaddle, Andrew C. and Richard M. Hessler. "Power and Change: The Case of the Swedish Commission of Inquiry on Health and Sickness Care." *Journal of Health Politics, Policy and Law* Vol. 11 (Spring 1986): 19–40.

Federalism, the Federal Government, and Health and Health Care

Altenstetter, Christa and James W. Bjorkman. "The Rediscovery of Federalism: The Impact of Federal Child Health Programs in Connecticut State Health Policy Formation and Service Delivery." In R. Thomas and C. O. Jones, eds., *Public Policy-Making in a Federal System.* Beverly Hills, CA.: Sage Publications, 1976: 217–237.

Altenstetter, Christa and James W. Bjorkman. "Policy, Politics and Child Health, Four Decades of Federal Initiative and State Response." *Journal of Health Politics, Policy and Law* Vol. 3 (Summer 1978): 196–234.

Altman, Stuart H. and Harvey M. Sapolsky, eds. *Federal Health Programs. Problems and Prospects.* Cambridge: Lexington Books, 1981.

Banta, David. "The Federal Legislative Process and Health Care." In Steven Jonas, ed., *Health Care Delivery in the United States.* New York: Springer Publishing Co., 1977: 329–345.

Barfield, Claude. "New Federalism and Long Term Care of the Elderly." *Update. Health Affairs* Vol. 2 (Spring 1983): 113–125.

Baydin, Lynda D. "The End-Stage Renal Disease Networks: An Attempt Through Federal Regulation to Regionalize Health Care Delivery." *Medical Care* Vol. 15 (July 1977): 586–598.

Berkowitz, Edward D. "Rehabilitation: The Federal Government's Response to Disability, 1935–1954." Unpublished doctoral dissertation, Northwestern University, 1976. Also, New York: Arno Press, 1980.

Bloom, Bernard S. and Samuel P. Martin. "The Role of the Federal Government in Financing Health and Medical Services." *Journal of Medical Education* Vol. 51 (March 1976): 161–169.

Blumenthal, David. "Federal Policy Toward Health Care Technology: The Case of the National Center." *Milbank Memorial Fund Quarterly* Vol. 61 (Fall 1983): 584–613.

Blumstein, James F. "Foundations of Federal Fertility Policy." *Milbank Memorial Fund Quarterly/Health and Society* Vol. 52 (Spring 1974): 131–168.

Bonnen, James T. "Federal Statistical Coordination Today: A Disaster or a Disgrace?" *Milbank Memorial Fund Quarterly* Vol. 62 (Winter 1984): 1–41; Elliot L. Richardson, Comment: "The Democracy of Facts," 42–47; John T. Dunlop, Comment: "Federal Statistical Coordination," 48–52.

Brown, Lawrence D. "The Formulation of Federal Health Care Policy." *Bulletin of the New York Academy of Medicine* Vol. 54 (January 1978): 45–58.

Brown, Lawrence D. "The Politics of Devolution in Nixon's New Federalism." In Lawrence D. Brown, James W. Fossett and Kenneth T. Palmer, *The Changing Politics of Federal Grants.* Washington, D.C.: Brookings Institution, 1984: 54–107.

Bryant, John H., Myron E. Wegman, Reuel A. Stallones, Lester Breslow and Cecil G. Sheps. "The Impact of the New Federalism on Schools of Public Health." *Milbank Memorial Fund Quarterly/Health and Society* .Vol. 51 (Fall 1973): 435–472.

Budetti, Peter P., John Butler and Peggy McManus. "Federal Health Program Reform: Implications for Child Health." *Milbank Memorial Fund Quarterly/Health and Society* Vol. 60, No. 1 (Winter 1982): 155–181.

Buntz, C. Gregory, Theodore F. Macaluso and Jay A. Azarow. "Federal Influence on State Health Policy." *Journal of Health Politics, Policy and Law* Vol. 3 (Spring 1978): 71–86.

Carter, G.M., D. Schu, J.E. Koehler, R.L. Slighton and A.P. Williams, Jr. *Federal Manpower Legislation and the Academic Health Centers: An Interim Report.* Santa Monica, CA.: Rand Corp., April 1974, Rand Report No. 4-1464-HEW.

Chapman, Carleton B. and John M. Talmadge. "Historical and Political Background of Federal Health Care Legislation." *Law and Contemporary Problems* Vol. 35 (Spring 1970): 334–347.

Darling, Helen. "The Role of the Federal Government in Assuring Access to Health Care." *Inquiry* Vol. 23 (Fall 1986): 286–295.

Decker, Barry. "Federal Strategies and the Quality of Local Health Care." In Arthur Levin, ed., *Health Services: The Local Perspective, Proceedings of the Academy of Political Science* Vol. 32, No. 3. New York: The Academy of Political Science, 1977: 200–214.

Derzon, Robert A. *A Legitimate Role of Government in the Private Health Services System,* 1979, Michael M. Davis Lecture. Chicago: University of Chicago Center for Health Administration Studies, Graduate School of Business, 1979.

Drew, David E., John G. Wirt, F.W. Finnegan, M.C. Fujisaki and A.L. Laniear. *The Effects of Federal Funds Upon Selected Health- Related Disciplines.* Santa Monica, CA.: Rand Corp., March 1976, Rand Report No. R-1944-PBRP.

Dunham, Andrew B. and Theodore Marmor. "Federal Policy and Health: Recent Trends and Different Perspectives." In Theodore J. Lowi and Alan Stone, eds., *Nationalizing Government: Public Policies in America.* Beverly Hills, CA.: Sage Publications, 1978.

Edwards, Charles C. "The Federal Involvement in Health, A Personal View of Current Problems and Future Needs." *New England Journal of Medicine* Vol. 292 (March 13, 1975): 559–562.

Etheredge, Lynn. "An Aging Society and the Federal Deficit." *Milbank Memorial Fund Quarterly* Vol. 62 (Fall 1984): 521–543.

Feingold, Eugene and George D. Greenberg. "Health Policy and the Federal Executive." In Theodor J. Litman and Leonard Robins *Health Politics and Policy.* New York: John Wiley and Sons, 1984, 1st ed.: 114–125.

Foltz, Anne-Marie. "The Development of Ambiguous Federal Policy: Early and Periodic Screening, Diagnosis and Treatment (EPSDT)." *Milbank Memorial Fund Quarterly/ Health and Society* Vol. 53 (Winter 1975): 35–64.

Foltz, Anne-Marie. *Uncertainties of Federal Child Health Politics: Impact in Two States,* DHEW Pub. No. (PHS) 78-3190. Hyattsville, MD.: National Center for Health Services Research, 1978.

Fox, Peter D. "Access to Medical Care for the Poor: The Federal Perspective." *Medical Care* Vol. 10 (May–June 1972): 272–277.

Fritschler, A. Lee. *Smoking and Politics: Policymaking and the Federal Bureaucracy.* Englewood Cliffs, N.J.: Prentice-Hall, 1975.

Glaser, William A. *Federalism in Canadian Health Services—Lessons for the United States,* Preprint Series. New York: Center for the Social Sciences, Columbia University, December 1977.

Gold, Byron D. "Role of the Federal Government in the Provision of Social Services to Older Persons." *Annals of the American Academy of Political and Social Science* Vol. 415 (September 1974): 55–69.

Hageboeck, Helen E. "An Analysis of the Impact of Federal Legislation on Community Based Health Services to Functionally Dependent Adults." Unpublished doctoral dissertation, University of Iowa, 1978, Microfilm No. 79-02, 907.

Jaeger, Boi Jon. "Hospitals and the Federal Government: A Study of the Development and Outcomes of Public Policy." Unpublished doctoral dissertation, Duke University, 1971, Microfilm No. 72-10, 887.

Jones, E. Terrence. "The Impact of Federal Aid on the Quality of Life: The Case of Infant Health." *Social Indicators Research* Vol. 1 (September 1974): 209–216.

Judd, Leda R. "Federal Involvement in Health Care After 1945." *Current History* Vol. 12 (May–June 1977): 201–206, 277–228.

Klerman, Lorraine V. "Intergovernmental Relationships: A Delicate Balance," (editorial). *American Journal of Public Health* Vol. 74 (September 1984): 965–967.

Koleda, Michael, Carol Burke and Jane S. Willems. *The Federal Health Dollar: 1969–1976, A Chartbook Analysis of Activities Supported and Strategies Pursued in Federal Expenditures for Health.* Washington, D.C.: Center for Health Policy Studies, National Planning Association, February 1977.

Komaroff, Anthony L. and Paul J. Duffell. "An Evaluation of Selected Federal Categorical Health Programs for the Poor." *American Journal of Public Health* Vol. 66 (March 1976): 255–261.

Lee, Philip R. and Caroll L. Estes. "New Federalism and Health Policy." *The Annals of the American Academy of Political and Social Science* Vol. 468 (July 1983): 88–102.

Lockett, Betty A. "Setting the Federal Agenda in Health Research: The Case of the National Institute on Aging." *Journal of Health Politics, Policy and Law* Vol. 9 (Spring 1984): 63–79.

Logan, Bruce M., David A. Rochefort and Ernest W. Cook. "Block Grants for Mental Health: Elements of the State Response." *Journal of Public Health Policy* Vol. 6 (December 1985): 476–492.

Lostetter, John O. and John E. Chapman. "The Participation of the United States Government in Providing Financial Support for Medical Education." *Health Policy and Education* Vol. 1, No. 1 (1979): 27–65.

Martin, Edward D. "Federal Initiative in Rural Health." *Public Health Reports* Vol. 90 (July–August 1975): 291–297.

Mooney, Anne. "The Great Society and Health: Policies for Narrowing the Gaps in Health Status Between the Poor and the Nonpoor." *Medical Care* Vol. 15 (August 1977): 611–619.

National Planning Association. *Chartbook of Fed-*

eral Health Spending, 1969–1974. Washington, D.C.: National Planning Association, Center for Health Policy Studies, August 1974.

National Planning Association. The Federal Health Dollar: 1969–1974. Washington, D.C.: National Planning Association, Center for Health Policy Studies, 1977.

Navarro, Vicente. "Federal Health Policies in the United States: An Alternative Explanation." Milbank Memorial Fund Quarterly Vol. 65, No. 1 (1987): 81–111.

Penchansky, Roy and Elizabeth Axelson. "Old Values, New Federalism and Program Evaluation." Medical Care Vol. 12 (November 1974): 893–905.

Perkoff, Gerald. "The Impact of Federal Programs, Long-Term Dialysis Programs: New Selection Criteria, New Problems." The Hastings Center Report Vol. 6 (June 1976): 8–13.

Prussin, Jeffrey A. "The Nursing Home Administrator as an Effective Political Advocate: An Overview of the Federal Arena." Journal of Long Term Care Administration Vol. 4, No. 4 (1976): 1–13.

Rabe, Barry G. "The Refederalization of American Health Care." Medical Care Review Vol. 44 (Spring 1987): 37–63.

Raskin, Ira E. "Conceptual Framework for Research on the Cost-Effective Allocation of Federal Resources." Socio-Economic Planning Sciences Vol. 9 (February 1975): 1–10.

Rich, Robert F. "Selective Utilization of Social Sciences Related Information by Federal Policy-Makers." Inquiry Vol. 12 (September 1975): 239–245.

Roemer, Milton I. and Mary H. McClanahan. "Impact of Government Programs on Voluntary Hospitals." Public Health Reports Vol. 75 (June 1960): 537–544.

Russell, Louise B. "Effects of Inflation on Federal Health Spending." Medical Care Vol. 13 (September 1975): 713–721.

Russell, Louise B. "Inflation and the Federal Role in Health." In Michael Zubkoff, ed., Health: A Victim or Cause of Inflation? New York: Prodist, Neale Watson Academic Publishers, 1976: 225–244.

Russell, Louise B. and Carol S. Burke. "The Political Economy of Federal Health Programs in the United States: An Historical Review." International Journal of Health Services Vol. 8, No. 1 (1978): 55–77.

Russell, Louise B., Blair Bourque, Daniel Bourque and Carol Burke. Federal Health Spending, 1969–1974. Washington, D.C.: Center for Health Policy Studies, National Planning Association, August 1974.

Schlesinger, Edward R. "The Impact of Federal Legislation on Maternal and Child Health Services in the United States." Milbank Memorial Fund Quarterly/Health and Society Vol. 52 (Winter 1974): 1–14.

Scotch, Richard K. From Good Will to Civil Rights: Transforming Federal Disability Policy. Philadelphia: Temple University Press, 1984.

Shannon, James A. "Federal Support of Biomedical Sciences, Development and Academic Impact." Journal of Medical Education Vol. 51 (July 1976): Supplement, 1–98.

Smith, David G. "Emerging Patterns of Federalism: The Case of Public Health." In Marv F. Arnold, L. Vaughn Blankenship and John M. Hess, eds., Administering Health Systems, Issues and Perspectives. Chicago, IL: Aldine Publishing Co., 1971: 131–142.

Stone, Deborah. "The Problem of Monopoly Power in Federal Health Policy." Milbank Memorial Fund Quarterly/Health and Society Vol. 58 (Winter 1980): 50–53.

Thompson, Frank J. "New Federalism and Health Care Policy: States and the Old Questions." Journal of Health Politics, Policy and Law Vol. 11, No. 1 (1986): 647–669.

Vladeck, Bruce C. "The Design of Failure. Health Policy and the Structure of Federalism." Journal of Health Politics, Policy and Law Vol. 4 (Fall 1979): 522–535.

Warner, Judith S. "Trends in the Federal Regulation of Physicians' Fees." Inquiry Vol. 13 (December 1976): 364–370.

Warren, B.S. "Coordination and Expansion of Federal Health Activities." Public Health Reports Vol. 9 (May–June 1975): 270–277.

White, Ben B. Falling Arches: The Case Against Federal Intervention in the Practice of Medicine. Hicksville, N.Y.: Exposition Press, 1977.

Williams, A. P., et al. "The Effect of Federal Biomedical Research Programs on Academic Medical Centers." Santa Monica, CA.: Rand Corp., March 1976, Rand Report No. R-1943-PBRP.

Wilson, Florence A. and Duncan Neuhauser. "The Federal Government and Health." In Florence A. Wilson and Duncan Neuhauser, eds., *Health Services in the United States.* Cambridge, MA.: Ballinger Publishing Co., 1985, 2d ed.: 130–225.

Zwick, Daniel I. and Clyde J. Behney. "Federal Health Services Grants, 1965–1975." *Public Health Reports* Vol. 91 (November–December 1976): 493–495.

Congress and the Legislative Process

Bradley, John P. "Shaping Administrative Policy with the Aid of Congressional Oversight: The Senate Finance Committee and Medicare." *Western Political Quarterly* Vol. 33 (December 1980: 492–501.

Davis, Raymond G. "Congress and the Emergence of Public Health Policy." *Health Care Management Review* Vol. 10 (Winter 1985): 61–74.

Feldstein, Paul J. *The Politics of Health Legislation: An Economic Perspective.* Ann Arbor, MI.: Health Administration Press, 1988.

Fuchs, Beth C. and John F. Hoadley. "Reflections from Inside the Beltway: How Congress and the President Grapple with Health Policy." *PS* Vol. 20 (Spring 1987): 212–220.

Ginsburg, Paul B. "Physician Payment Policy in the 101st Congress." *Health Affairs* Vol. 8 (Spring 1989): 5–20.

Jones, Woodrow, Jr. and K. Robert Keiser. "U.S. Senate Voting on Health and Safety Regulation: The Effects of Ideology and Interest-Group Orientations." *Health Policy* Vol. 6, No. 1 (1986): 33–44.

Mueller, Keith J. "An Analysis of Congressional Health Policy Voting in the 1970's." *Journal of Health Politics, Policy and Law* Vol. 11 (Spring 1986): 117–135.

Nexon, David, "The Politics of Congressional Health Policy in the Second Half of the 1980's." *Medical Care Review* Vol. 44 (Spring 1987) 65–88.

Whiteman, David. "What Do They Know and When Do They Know It? Health Staff on the Hill." *PS* Vol. 20 (Spring 1987): 221–225.

Federal Bureaucracy

Chu, Franklin D. and Sharland Trotter. *The Madness Establishment, Ralph Nader's Study Group Report on the National Institute of Mental Health.* New York: Grossman Publishers, 1974.

Falkson, Joseph L. "Minor Skirmish in a Monumental Struggle: HEW's Analysis of Mental Health Services." *Policy Analysis* Vol. 2 (Winter 1976): 93–119.

Feder, Judith M. "The Social Security Administration and Medicare: A Strategy of Implementation." In Kenneth M. Friedman and Stuart H. Rakoff, eds., *Toward a National Health Policy: Public Policy and the Control of Health Care Cost.* Lexington, MA.: Lexington Books, 1976.

Fredrickson, Donald S. "The National Institute of Health: Yesterday, Today and Tomorrow," *Public Health Report* Vol. 93 (November–December 1978): 642–647.

Greenberg, George D. "Reorganization Reconsidered: The U.S. Public Health Service 1960–1973." *Public Policy* Vol. 23 (Fall 1975): 483–522.

Greenberg, George D. "Constraints on Management and Secretarial Behavior at HEW." *Polity* Vol. 13 (Fall 1980): 57–79.

Harden, Victoria A. *Inventing the NIH: Federal Biomedical Research Policy, 1887–1937.* Baltimore, MD.: Johns Hopkins University, 1986.

Miles, Rufus E., Jr. *The Department of Health, Education and Welfare.* New York: Praeger Publishers, 1974: 168–243.

Sherman, John F. "The Organization and Structure of the National Institutes of Health." *New England Journal of Medicine* Vol. 297 (July 1977): 18–26.

Thompson, Frank J. *Health Policy and the Bureaucracy Politics and Implementation.* Cambridge: MIT Press, 1981.

Federal—State Relations in Health and Health Care

Altenstetter, Christa and James Bjorkman. *Federal Impacts on State Health Policy: Lessons from Connecticut and Vermont.* New Haven, Conn.: Yale Health Policy Project, 1975.

Altenstetter, Christa and James W. Bjorkman. "The Impact of Federal Child Health Programs in Connecticut State Health Policy Formation and Service Delivery: The Rediscovery of Federalism." In R. Thomas and C.O. Jones, ed., *Public Policy Making in a Federal System,* Sage Yearbooks in Politics and Public Policy. Beverly-Hills, CA.: Sage Publications, 1976, Vol. 111: 217–237.

Altenstetter, Christa and James W. Bjorkman. *Federal-State Health Policies and Impacts: The Politics of Implementation.* Washington, D.C.: University Press of America, 1978.

Buntz, C. Gregory, Theodore F. Macaluso and Jay A. Azarow. "Federal Influence on State Health Policy." *Journal of Health Politics, Policy and Law* Vol. 3 (Spring 1978): 71–86.

Foltz, Anne-Marie. *Uncertainties of Federal Child Health Politics: Impact in Two States,* DHEW Pub. No. (PHS) 78–3190. Washington, D.C.: National Center for Health Services Research, April 1978.

Foltz, Anne-Marie and Donna Brown. "State Response to Federal Policy: Children, EPSDT and the Medicaid Muddle." *Medical Care* Vol. 13 (August 1975): 630–642.

Lashof, Joyce C. and Mark H. Lepper. "Federal-State-Local Partnership in Health." In United States Public Health Service, Health Resources Administration, eds., *Health in America, 1776–1976,* DHEW Pub. No. (HRA) 76–616. Washington, D.C.: U.S. Government Printing Office, 1976: 122–137.

Passel, Petter and Leonard Ross. *State Policies and Federal Programs: Priorities and Constraints.* New York: Praeger Publishers, 1978.

Price, Isabel. "What's Happening to Federally Aided Health Programs Under State Departments of Human Resources." *Public Health Reports* Vol. 93 (May–June 1978): 221–231.

Robins, Leonard. "The Impact of Decategorizing Federal Programs: Before and After 314 (d)." *American Journal of Public Health* Vol. 62 (January 1972): 24–29.

Robins, Leonard. "The Impact of Converting Categorical into Block Grants: The Lessons from the 314 (d) Block Grant in the Partnership for Health Act." *Publius* Vol. 6 (Winters 1975): 49–70.

Scherr, Lawrence. "Coping with Intrusions by State and Federal Government Agencies." *Federal Bulletin* Vol. 65, No. 3 (1978): 69–80.

Schneider, Saundra K. "Intergovernmental Influences on Medicaid Program Expenditures." *Public Administration Review* Vol. 48 (July–August 1988): 756–763.

Snoke, Albert W. and Parnie S. Snoke. "Linking Private, Public Energies in Health and Welfare Planning." *Hospitals* Vol. 50 (August 16, 1976): 53–58.

Webb, Bruce J. "Impact of Revenue Sharing on Local Health Centers." *The Black Scholar* Vol. 5 (May 1974): 10–15.

Role of the States in Health and Health Care

Altenstetter, Christa and James W. Bjorkman. *Federal- State Health Policies and Impacts: The Politics of Implementation.* Washington, D.C.: University Press of America, 1978.

Altman, Drew E. and Douglas H. Morgan. "The Role of State and Local Government in Health." *Health Affairs* Vol. 2 (Winter 1983): 7–31.

Bachman, Sara, Stuart H. Altman and Dennis F. Beatrice. "What Influences a State's Approach to Medicaid Reform?" *Inquiry* Vol. 25 (Summer 1988): 243–250.

Bentak, J.M., ed. *A Digest of State Laws Affecting Prepayment of Medical Care, Group Practice and HMO's.* Rockville, MD.: Health Law Center, Germantown, MD.: Aspen Systems Corporation, 1973.

Blendon, Robert J. "The Prospects for State and Local Governments Playing a Broader Role in Health Care in the 1980's." *American Journal of Public Health* Vol. 71 (January 1981):Supplement, 9–14.

Bovbjerg, Randall R. and Christopher F. Koller. "State Health Insurance Pools: Current Performance, Future Prospects." *Inquiry* Vol. 23 (Summer 1986): 111–121.

Bovbjerg, Randall R. and Barbara A. Davis. "State's Responses to Federal Health Care 'Block Grants:' The First Year." *Milbank Me-*

morial Fund Quarterly Vol. 61 (Fall 1983): 523–560.

Brown, E. Richard and Michael R. Cousineau. "Effectiveness of State Mandates to Maintain Local Government Health Services for the Poor." *Journal of Health Politics, Policy and Law* Vol. 9 (Summer 1984): 223–236.

Brown, Ray E. "Health Facilities and Health Services." *Inquiry* Vol. 10 (March 1973):Supplement, 17–22. Comment: Melvin A. Glasser 23–25; J.D. Wallace 26–28. Discussion: 29–39.

Butter, Irene H. and Bonnie J. Kay. "State Laws and the Practice of Midwifery." *American Journal of Public Health* Vol. 78 (September 1988): 1161–1169.

Chirikos, Thomas N. "State Health Manpower Policy: An Appraisal." *Journal of Community Health* Vol. 2 (Spring 1977): 163–177.

Christianson, Jon B. and Diane G. Hillman. *Health Care for the Indigent and Competitive Contracts: The Arizona Experience.* Ann Arbor, MI.: Health Administration Press, 1986.

Christianson, Jon B., Diane G. Hillman and Kenneth R. Smith. "The Arizona Experience: Competitive Bidding for Indigent Medical Care." *Health Affairs* Vol. 2 (Fall 1983): 87–103.

Clarke Gary J. *Health Programs in the States, A Survey.* New Brunswick, N.J.: Rutgers—The State University, Eagleton Institute of Politics, 1975.

Clarke, Gary J. *Health Expenditures by State Governments.* Washington, D.C.: Georgetown University Health Policy Center, 1976.

Clarke, Gary J. "The Role of the State in the Delivery of Health Services." *American Journal of Public Health* Vol. 71 (January 1981):Supplement, 59–61.

Colner, Alan N. "The Impact of State Government Rate Setting on Hospital Management." *Health Care Management Review* Vol. 2 (Winter 1977): 37–49.

Connor, Gerald R. "State Government Financing of Health Planning." *American Journal of Health Planning* Vol. 1 (October 1976): 48–49 51.

Cromwell, Jerry, "Impact of State Hospital Rate Setting on Capital Formation," *Health Care Financing Review* Vol. 8 (Spring 1987): 57–67.

Curtis, Rick. "The Role of State Governments in Assuring Access to Care." *Inquiry* Vol. 23 (Fall 1986): 277–285.

Davidson, Stephen M. "Variations in State Medicaid Programs." *Journal of Health Politics, Policy and Law* Vol. 3 (Spring 1978): 54–70.

Desonia, Randolph and Kathleen M. King. *State Programs of Assistance for the Medically Indigent.* Washington, D.C.: Intergovernmental Health Policy Project, George Washington University, November 1985.

Dranove, David and Kenneth Kone. "Do States' Rate Setting Regulations Really Lower Hospital Expenses?" *Journal of Health Economics* Vol. 4 (June 1985): 159–165.

Ellet, T. Van. *State Comprehensive and Catastrophic Health Insurance Plans: An Overview.* Washington, D.C.: George Washington University, Intergovernmental Health Project, 1980.

Ellet, T. Van. *Medigap: State Responses to Problems with the Sale of Health Insurance to the Elderly.* Washington, D.C.: George Washington University, Intergovernmental Health Policy Project, 1980.

Finkler, Merton D. "State Rate Setting Revisited." *Health Affairs* Vol. 6 (Winter 1987): 82–89.

Freedman, Ben. "Cost of Fragmentation of State Government Operated Health Services." *Inquiry* Vol. 12 (September 1975): 216–227.

Gardiner, John A. and Theodore R. Lyman. *The Fraud Control Game: State Responses to Fraud and Abuse in the AFDC and Medicaid Programs.* Bloomington, IN.: Indiana University Press, 1984.

Gilbert, Benjamin, Merry-K Moos and C. Arden Miller. "State Level Decision Making for Public Health: The Status of Boards of Health." *Journal of Public Health Policy* Vol. 3 (March 1982): 51–63.

Ginzberg, Eli, Edith Davis and Miriam Ostow. *Local Health Policy in Action. The Municipal Health Services Program.* Savage, MD.: Rowman and Littlefield Publishers, Inc., 1985.

Glantz, Leonard H. "Mandating Health Insurance Benefits in the Private Sector: A Decision for State Legislatures." *American Journal of Public Health* Vol. 75 (November 1985): 1344–1346.

Goggin, Malcolm L. *Policy Design and the Politics*

of Implementation: The Case of Child Health Care in the American States. Knoxville, TN.: University of Tennessee Press, 1987.

Harrington, Charlene, et al . "Effects of State Medicaid Policies on the Aged." The Gerontologist Vol. 26 (September 1986): 437–443.

Harrington, Charlene and James H. Swan. "The Impact of State Medicaid Nursing Home Policies on Utilization and Expectations." Inquiry Vol. 24 (Summer 1987): 157–172.

Haynes, Pamela L. Evaluating State Medicaid Reforms. Washington, D.C.: American Enterprise Institute, 1985.

Hillman, Diane G. and Jon B. Christianson. "Health Care Expenditure Containment in the United States: Strategies at the State and Local Levels." Social Science and Medicine Vol. 20, No. 12 (1985): 1319–1330.

Holahan, John. "State Rate Setting and Its Effects on the Cost of Nursing Home Care." Journal of Health Politics, Policy and Law Vol. 9 (Winter 1985): 647–668.

Jain, Sager, ed. "Role of State and Local Governments in Relation to Personal Health Services." American Journal of Public Health Vol. 71 (January 1981):Supplement.

Jain, Sager, ed. "Role of State and Local Governments in Relation to Personal Health Services. Washington, D.C.: American Public Health Association, 1981.

Justice, Diane. State Long Term Care and Reform: Development of Community Care Systems in Six States. Washington, D.C.: National Governors' Association, April 1988.

Kennedy, Virginia C., Stephen H. Linder and William D. Spears. "Estimating the Impact of State Manpower Policy: A Case Study of Reducing Medical School Enrollments." Journal of Health Politics, Policy and Law Vol. 12 (Summer 1987): 299–312.

Kern, Rosemary Gibson and Susan R. Windham. Medicaid and Other Experiments in State Health Policy. Washington, D.C.: American Enterprise Institute, 1986.

Kovner, Anthony R. and Edward J. Lusk. "State Regulation of Health Care Costs." Medical Care Vol. 13 (August 1975): 619–629.

Laird, Maureen. "State Roles in Financing Medical Education." Journal of Medical Education Vol. 51 (March 1976) 206–209.

Laumann, Edward O., David Knoke and Yong-Hak Kim. "An Organizational Approach to State Policy Formation: A Comparative Study of Energy and Health Domains." American Sociological Review Vol. 50 (February 1985): 1–19.

Lavin, John H. "How Would You Fare Under States Health Insurance?" Medical Economics Vol. 53 (September 6, 1976): 77–81.

Levine, Peter. "An Overview of the State Role in the United States Health Scene." In Theodor J. Litman and Leonard Robins Health Politics and Policy. New York: John Wiley and Sons, 1984, 1st edition: 194–220.

Levit, Katherine R. "Personal Health Care Expenditures, by State: 1966–1982." Health Care Financing Review Vol. 6 (Summer 1985): 1–49.

Lewin, Lawrence S. and Robert A. Derzon. "Health Professions Education: State Responsibilities under the New Federalism." Health Affairs Vol. 1 (Spring 1982): 69–85.

Lipson, Debra J. Major Changes in State Medicaid and Independent Care Programs. Washington, D.C.: Intergovernmental Health Policy Project, George Washington University, 1988.

Lipson, Debra J. "Massachusetts Legislation: A Model for Other States or a Costly Mistake?" Business and Health Vol. 5 (August 1988): 48–49.

Lipson, Debra J. and Elizabeth Donohoe. State Financing of Long Term Care Services for the Elderly. Washington, D.C.: Intergovernmental Health Policy Project, George Washington University, May 1988.

Logan, Bruce M., David A. Rochefort and Ernest W. Cook. "Block Grants for Mental Health: Elements of the State Response." Journal of Public Health Policy Vol. 6 (December 1985): 476–492.

Lutterman, Theodore, Noel Mazade, Cecil Wurster and Robert Glover. "Trends in Revenues and Expenditures of State Mental Health Agencies: Fiscal Years 1981, 1983 and 1985." State Health Reports, No. 34, Washington, D.C.: Intergovernmental Health Policy Project, George Washington University, September/October 1987.

Manning, Bayless and Bruce C. Vladeck. "The Role of State and Local Government in Health. Update." Health Affairs Vol. 2 (Winter 1983): 134–140.

McCall, Nelda. *Medigap—Study of Comparative Effectiveness of Various State Regulations,* Menlo Park, CA.: SRI International, 1983.

McCall, Nelda, Thomas Rice and Arden Hall. "The Effect of State Regulations on the Quality and Sale of Insurance Policies to Medicare Beneficiaries." *Journal of Health Politics, Policy and Law* Vol. 12 (Spring 1987): 53–76.

McCombs, Jeffrey S. and Jon B. Christianson. "Applying Competitive Bidding to Health Care." *Journal of Health Politics, Policy and Law* Vol. 12 (Winter 1987): 703–722.

Merritt, Richard and Susan Mertes. *State Innovations in Health.* Washington, D.C.: George Washington University, Intergovernmental Health Policy Project, 1980.

Miller and Byrne Inc. *Annotated Bibliography: The Impact of Public Health Service Programs and State Government.* Rockville, MD.: Miller and Byrne. April 1977.

Morrisey, Michael A., Frank A. Sloan and Samuel A. Mitchell. "State Rate Setting: An Analysis of Some Unresolved Issues." *Health Affairs* Vol. 2 (Summer 1983): 36–47.

Moscovice, Ira. "Health Services Research and the Policy Making Process: State Response to Federal Cutbacks in Programs Affecting Child Health." In Marion Ein Lewin, ed., *From Research into Policy. Improving the Link for Health Services.* Washington, D.C.: American Enterprise Institute for Public Policy Research, 1986: 34–50.

O'Kane, Margaret. "State Implementation of Health Block Grants." *Focus On . . .* No. 5. Washington, D.C.: Intergovernmental Health Policy Project, George Washington University, August 1984.

Omenn, Gilbert S. "Lessons From a Fourteen State Study of Medicaid." *Health Affairs* Vol. 6 (Spring 1987): 118–122.

Peterson, George E., Randall R. Bovbjerg and Barbara A. Davis. *The Reagan Block Grants: What Have We Learned?* Washington, D.C.: Urban Institute Press, 1986.

Polich, Cynthia L. and Laura H. Iversen. "State Preadmission Screening Programs for Controlling Utilization of Long Term Care." *Health Care Financing Review* Vol. 8 (Fall 1987) 43–48.

Renaud, Marc. "On the Structural Constraints to State Intervention in Health." *International Journal of Health Services* Vol. 5, No. 4 (1975): 559–572.

Rosenbaum, Sara and Kay Johnson. "Providing Health Care for Low Income Children: Reconciling Child Health Goals with Child Health Financing Realities." *Milbank Quarterly* Vol. 64, No. 3 (1986): 442–478.

Rosenkrantz, Barbara G. *Public Health and the State: Changing Views in Massachusetts, 1842–1936.* Cambridge: Harvard University Press, 1972.

Schramm, Carl J. "Regulatory Hospital Labor Costs: A Case Study in the Politics of State Rate Commissions" *Journal of Health Politics, Policy and Law* Vol. 3 (Fall 1978): 364–374.

Schramm, Carl J. "State Hospital Cost Containment: An Analysis of Legislative Initiatives." *Indiana Law Review* Vol. 19 No. 4 (1986): 919–954.

Schwartz, Jerome L. "Strategies for Monitoring the Effects of Proposition 13 on Health Services." *Journal of Health Politics, Policy and Law* Vol. 4 (Summer 1979): 142–154.

Shultz James M., Michael E. Moen, Terry F. Pechacek, *et al.* "The Minnesota Plan for Nonsmoking and Health: The Legislative Experience." *Journal of Public Health Policy* Vol. 7 (Autumn 1986): 300–313.

Sloan, Frank A. "State Responses to the Malpractice Insurance 'Crises' of the 1970's: An Empirical Assessment." *Journal of Health Politics, Policy and Law* Vol. 9 (Winter 1985): 629–646.

Snoke, Parnie S. and Albert W. Snoke. "State Role in the Regulation of the Health Delivery System." *University of Toledo Law Review* Vol. 6 (Spring 1975): 617–646.

Swan, James H., Charlene Harrington and Leslie A. Grant. "State Medicaid Reimbursement for Nursing Homes, 1978–1986." *Health Care Financing Review* Vol. 9 (Spring 1988): 33–50.

Ziegler, Andrew. "States Address Shortage, Distribution of Health Professionals." *State Health Notes,* No. 75. Washington, D.C.: Intergovernmental Health Policy Project, George Washington University, July/August 1987.

State—Local Relationships

Berger, Stephen. "The Interplay of State and Local Government in Health Care." In Arthur Levin, ed., *Health Services: The Local Perspective, Proceedings of the Academy of Political Science,* Vol. 32, No. 3. New York: The Academy of Political Science, 1977: 63–67.

Fowinkle, Eugene. "The State Role in the Delivery of Local Health Services." In Arthur Levin, ed., *Health Services: The Local Perspective,* Proceedings of the Academy of Political Science Vol. 32, No. 3. New York: The Academy of Political Science, 1977: 53–62.

Gayer, David. "The Effects of Medicaid on State and Local Government Finances." *National Tax Journal* Vol. 25 (December 1972): 511–519.

Local Government

Bellin, Lowell E. "Local Health Departments: A Prescription Against Obsolescence." In Arthur Levin, ed., *Health Services: The Local Perspective,* Proceedings of the Academy of Political Science Vol. 32, No. 3. New York: The Academy of Political Science, 1977: 42–52.

Koppel, J. and J. Clark. *The Role of Country Government in Medicaid.* Washington, D.C.: National Association of Counties, July 1976.

Ingraham, Norman R. "Formulation of Public Policy in Medical Care: Dynamics of Community Action at Local Level." *American Journal of Public Health* Vol. 51 (August 1961): 1144–1151.

Levin, Arthur, ed. *Health Services: The Local Perspective* Proceedings of the Academy of Political Science, Vol. 32, No. 3. New York: The Academy of Political Science, 1977.

Miller, C. Arden "Issues of Health Policy: Local Government and the Public's Health." *American Journal of Public Health* Vol. 65 (December 1975): 1330–1334.

Millman, Michael. "The Role of City Government in Personal Health Services." *American Journal of Public Health* Vol. 71 (January 1981):Supplement, 47–57.

Mytinger, Robert E. "Barriers to Adoption of New Programs as Perceived by Local Health Officers." *Public Health Reports* Vol. 82 (February 1967): 108–114.

Piore, Nora, Purlaine Lieberman ani James Linnane. "Financing Local Health Services." In Arthur Levin, ed., *Health Services: The Local Perspective,* Proceedings of the Academy of Political Science, Vol. 32, No. 3. New York: The Academy of Political Science, 1977: 15–28.

Piore, Nora, Purlaine Lieberman and James Linnane. "Public Expenditures and Private Control? Health Care Dilemma in New York City." *Milbank Memorial Fund Quarterly/Health and Society* Vol. 55 (Winter 1977): 79–116.

Robins, Leonard. "Controlling Health Care Costs." In Arthur Levin, ed., *Health Services: The Local Perspective, Proceedings of the Academy of Political Science, Vol. 32, No. 3. New York: The Academy of Political Science, 1977: 215–226.*

Schwartz, Jerome L. "Strategies for Monitoring the Effects of Proposition 13 on Health Services." Journal of Health Politics, Policy and Law Vol. 4 (Summer 1979): 142–154.

Shonick, William and Walter Price. "Reorganizations of Health Agencies by Local Government in American 'Urban Centers: What Do They Portend for "Public Health." *Milbank Memorial Fund Quarterly/Health and Society* Vol. 55 (Spring 1977): 233–271.

Shonick, William and Walter Price. "Organizational Milieus of Local Public Health Units: Analysis of Response to Questionnaire." *Public Health Reports* Vol. 93 (November–December 1978): 648–665.

Participatory Democracy

Public Opinion

Blendon, Robert J. "The Public's View of the Future of Health Care." *Journal of the American*

Medical Association Vol. 259 (June 24, 1988): 3587–3593.

Blendon, Robert J. and Drew E. Altman. "Public Attitudes Above Health Care Costs: A Lesson in National Schizophrenia." *New England Journal of Medicine* Vol. 311 (August 30, 1984): 613–616.

Blendon, Robert J. and Drew E. Altman. "Public Opinion and Health Care Costs." In Carl J. Schramm, ed. *Health Care and Its Cost. Can the U.S. Afford Adequate Care ?"* New York: W.W. Norton, 1987: 49–63.

Blendon, Robert J. and Humphrey Taylor. "Views on Health Care: Public Opinion in Three Nations." *Health Affairs* Vol. 8 (Spring 1989): 149–157.

Erskine, Hazel. "The Polls: Health Insurance." *Public Opinion Quarterly* Vol. 39 (Spring 1975): 128–143.

Gabel, Jon, Howard Cohen and Stephen Fink. "Americans' Views on Health Care." *Health Affairs* Vol. 8 (Spring 1989): 103–118.

Harvey, Lynn and Stephanie Shubat. *AMA Surveys of Physician and* Public Opinion: 1986. Chicago, American Medical Association, October 1986.

Iglehart, John R. "Opinion Polls on Health Care." *New England Journal of Medicine* Vol. 310 (June 14, 1984): 1616–1620.

Jeffe, Douglas and Sherry Bebitch Jeffe. "Losing Patience with Doctors: Physicians Versus the Public On Health Care Costs." *Public Opinion* Vol. 7 (February—March 1984): 45–55.

Mick, Stephen S. and John D. Thompson. "Public Attitudes Towards Health Planning under the Health Systems Agencies." *Journal of Health Politics, Policy and Law* Vol. 8 (Winter 1984): 782–800.

Perlstadt, Harry and Russell E. Holmes. "The Role of Public Opinion Polling in Health Legislation." *American Journal of Public Health* Vol. 77 (May 1987): 612–614.

Rochefort, David A. and Carol A. Boyer. "Use of Public Opinion Data in Public Administration: Health Care Polls." *Public Administration Review* Vol. 48 (March/April 1988): 649–660.

Shapiro, Robert Y. and John T. Young. "The Polls: Medical Care in the United States." *Public Opinion Quarterly* Vol. 50 (Fall 1986): 418–428.

Singer, Eleanor, Theresa F. Rogers and Mary Corcoran. "The Polls—A Report: AIDS." *Public Opinion Quarterly* Vol. 51 (Winter 1987): 580–595.

Steiber, Steven R. and Leonard A. Ferber. "Support for National Health Insurance: Intercohort Differentials." *Public Opinion Quarterly* Vol. 45 (Summer 1981): 179–198.

Taylor, Humphrey. "Healing the Health Care System." *Public Opinion* Vol. 8 (August–September 1985): 16–20, 60.

Political Parties and Health

Goldsmith, Seth B. "Political Party Platform Planks: A Mechanism for Participation and Prediction?" *American Journal of Public Health* Vol. 63 (July 1973): 594–601.

Silver, George A. "Medical Politics, Health Policy, Party Health Platforms, Promise and Performance." *International Journal of Health Services* Vol. 6, No. 2 (1976): 331–343.

Interest Group Politics and Health

Alford, Robert R. *Health Care Politics: Ideological and Interest Group Barriers to Reform.* Chicago, IL.: University of Chicago Press, 1975.

Binstock, Robert H. "Interest-Group Liberalism and the Politics of Aging." *Gerontologist* Vol. 12 (Autumn 1972): Part 1, 265–280.

Congressional Quarterly. *Legislators and Lobbyists: Medicare Over the Years.* Washington, D.C.: *Congressional Quarterly*, May 1968, 2d ed.

Drew, Elizabeth. "The Health Syndicate—Washington's Noble Conspirators." *Atlantic Monthly* Vol. 220 (December 1967): 75–82.

Feldstein, Paul J. *Health Associations and the Demand for Legislation, The Political Economy of Health.* Cambridge: Ballinger Publishing Co., 1977.

Feldstein, Paul J. "Health Associations and the Legislative Process." University of Michigan, 1982.

Feldstein, Paul J. *The Politics of Health Legislation. An Economic Perspective.* Ann Arbor, MI.: Health Administration Press, 1988.

Felicetti, Daniel A. *Mental Health and Retardation Politics: The Mind Lobbies in Congress.* New York: Praeger Publishers, 1975.

Flash, William, Milton Roemer and Sander Kelman. "Stalking the Politics of Health Care Reform: Three Critical Perspectives on Robert Alford's 'Health Care Politics Ideological and Interest Group Barriers to Reform.'" *Journal of Health Politics, Policy and Law* Vol. 1 (Spring 1976): 112–129.

Hoffman, Lily M. *The Politics of Knowledge. Activist Movements in Medicine and Planning.* Ithaca, N.Y.: State University of New York Press, 1989.

Jones, Woodrow, Jr. and K. Robert Keiser. "U.S. Senate Voting on Health and Safety Regulations: The Effects of Ideology and Interest-Group Orientations." *Health Policy* Vol. 6, No. 1 (1986): 33–44.

Marmor, Theodore R. and D. Thomas. "Doctors, Politics and Pay Disputes: Pressure Group Politics Revisited." *British Journal of Political Science* Vol. 2 (October 1972): 421–442.

Marmor, Theodore R. and David Thomas. "Doctors, Politics and Pay Disputes: Pressure Group Politics Revisited." In Theodore Marmor *Political Analysis and American Medical Care.* New York: Cambridge University Press, 1983: 107–130.

Novello, Dorothy J. "People, Power and Politics for Health Care." In National League for Nursing, eds., *People, Power, Politics for Health Care.* New York: National League for Nursing, 1976: 1–8.

Poen, Monte M. *Harry S. Truman versus the Medical Lobby: The Genesis of Medicare.* Columbia, MO.: University of Missouri Press, 1979.

Pond, M. Allen. "Politics of Social Change: Abortion Reform, The Role of Health Professionals in the Legislative Process." *American Journal of Public Health* Vol. 61 (May 1971): 904–909.

Rosen, George. "The Committee of One Hundred on National Health and the Campaign for a National Health Department, 1906–1912." *American Journal of Public Health* Vol. 62 (February 1972): 261–263.

Tierney, John T. "Organized Interests in Health Politics and Policy Making." *Medical Care* Vol. 44 (Spring 1987): 89–118.

"Health Lobbies: Vested Interests and Pressure Politic." In Douglass Cater and Philip R. Lee, eds., *Politics of Health.* New York: Medcom Press, 1972.

Weller, G.R. "From 'Pressure Group Politics' to 'Medical-Industrial Complex': The Development of Approaches to the Politics of Health." *Journal of Health Politics, Policy, and Law* Vol. 1 (Winter 1977): 444–470.

Wier, Richard A. "Patterns of Interaction Between, Interest Groups and the Canadian Political System: The Case of the Canadian Medical Association." Unpublished doctoral dissertation, Georgetown University, 1970, Microfilm No. 70–23, 874.

Wilsford, David. "The Cohesion and Fragmentation of Organized Medicine in France and the United States." *Journal of Health Politics, Policy and Law* Vol. 12 (Fall 1987): 481–503.

Community Power Structure and Health

Arnold, Mary F. and Isabel M. Welsh. "Community Politics and Health Planning." In Mary F. Arnold, L. Vaughn Blankenship and John M. Hess, eds., *Administering Health Systems: Issues and Perspectives.* Chicago: Aldine-Atherton, 1971: 154–175.

Belknap, Ivan and John G. Steinle. *The Community and Its Hospitals: A Comparative Analysis.* Syracuse, N.Y.: Syracuse University Press, 1963.

Berg, Robert L. "Movers' and 'Statics' Refine Political Strategies in HSAs." *Hospital Progress* Vol. 58 (September 1977): 64–69.

Blankenship, L. Vaughn. "Organizational Support and Community Leadership in Two New York State Communities." Unpublished doctoral dissertation, Cornell University, 1962.

Blankenship, L. Vaughn and Ray H. Elling. "Organizational Support and Community Power Structure: The Hospital." *Journal of Health and Human Behavior* Vol. 3 (Winter 1962): 257–269.

Blankenship, L. Vaughn and Ray H. Elling. "Effects of Community Power on Hospital Organization." In Mary F. Arnold, L. Vaughn Blankenship and John M. Hess, eds., *Administering Health Systems: Issues and Perspectives.* Chicago: Aldine Publishing Co., 1971: 176–196.

Elling, Ray H. "The Hospital Support Game in Urban Center." In Eliot Friedson, ed. *The Hospital in Modern Society.* New York: The Free Press, 1963: 73–111.

Elling, Ray H. "The Shifting Power Structure in Health." *Milbank Memorial Fund Quarterly* Vol. 46 (January 1968): Part 2, 119–144.

Elling, Ray H. and Sandor Halebsky. "Organizational Differentiation and Support: A Conceptual Framework." *Administrative Science Quarterly* Vol. 6 (September 1961): 185–209. Also in W. Richard Scott and Edmund Volkart, eds., *Readings in the Sociology of Medical Institutions.* New York: John Wiley & Sons, 1966: 543–557.

Elling, Ray H. and Ollie J. Lee. "Formal Connections of Community Leadership to the Health System." *Milbank Memorial Fund Quarterly* Vol. 44 (July 1966): Part I, 294–306.

Elling, Ray H. and Milton I. Roemer. "Determinants of Community Support." *Hospital Administration* Vol. 6, (Summer 1961): 17–34.

Freeborn, Donald K. and Benjamin J. Darsky. "A Study of the Power Structure of the Medical Community." *Medical Care* Vol. 12 (January 1974): 1–12.

Gossert, Daniel J. and C. Arden Miller. "State Boards of Health, Their Members and Commitments." *American Journal of Public Health* Vol. 63 (June 1973): 486–493.

Hanson, Robert C. "The Systemic Linkage Hypothesis and Role Consensus Patterns in Hospital-Community Relations." *American Sociological Review* Vol. 27 (June 1962): 304–313.

Holloway, Robert G., Jay H. Artis, and Walter E. Freeman. "The Participation Patterns of 'Economic Influentials' and Their Control of a Hospital Board of Trustees." *Journal of Health and Human Behavior* Vol. 4 (Summer 1963): 88–98.

Hunter, Floyd, Ruth C. Schaffer, and Cecil G. Sheps. *Community Organization: Action and Inaction.* Chapel Hill: University of North Carolina Press, 1956.

Kupst, Mary Jo, Phil Reidda and Thomas F. McGee. "Community Mental Health Boards: A Comparison of Their Development, Functions, and Powers by Board Members and Mental Health Center Staff." *Community Mental Health Journal* Vol. 11 (Fall 1975): 249–256.

Laur, Robert J. "A Study of the Extramural Sector of Governing Board Responsibility in Non-Profit General Hospitals: Trustee Interest in Interorganizational Relations." Unpublished doctoral dissertation, University of Minnesota, 1969, Microfilm No. 69–20, 032.

Miller, Paul A. "The Process of Decision-Making Within the Context of Community Organization." *Rural Sociology* Vol. 17 (June 1952): 153–161.

Perrow, Charles. "Organizational Prestige: Some Functions and Dysfunctions." *American Journal of Sociology* Vol. 66 (January 1961): 335–341.

Saunders, J.V.D. and J.H. Bruehing. "Hospital-Community Relations in Mississippi." *Rural Sociology* Vol. 24 (March 1959): 48–51.

Smith, David B. and Carl G. Homer. "The Hospital Support Group Revisited." *Journal of Health Politics, Policy and Law* Vol. 2 (Summer 1977): 257–265.

Smith, Richard A. "Community Power and Decision Making: A Replication and Extension of Hawley." *American Sociological Review* Vol. 41 (August 1976): 691–705.

Thacker, Stephen B., Carolee Osborne and Eva J. Salber. "Health Care Decision Making in a Southern County." *Journal of Community Health* Vol. 3 (Summer 1978): 347–356.

Warnecke, Richard B., Saxon Graham, William Mosher and Erwin B. Montgomery. "Health Guides as Influentials in Central Buffalo." *Journal of Health and Social Behavior* Vol. 17 (March 1976): 22–34.

White, Marjorie A. "Attitudes of Influentials Toward Health and Illness Care Delivery." Unpublished doctoral dissertation, Case Western Review University, 1976, Microfilm No. 76–28, 428.

Community Participation

Anderson, Donna M. and Markay Kerr. "Citizen Influence in Health Service Programs." *American Journal of Public Health* Vol. 61 (August 1971): 1518–1523.

Anderson, John B. "Associations Between Participation in Community Mental Health Planning and Adherence to Community Mental

Health Ideology: A Study of Citizen Participation in Two Community Mental Health Center Planning Projects." Unpublished doctoral dissertation, Ohio State University, 1973, Microfilm No. 73–26, 760.

Andrejewski, Norman S., Carl G. Homer and Richard H. Schlesinger. "Consumer Participation in Health Planning." *Health Education Monographs* No. 32 (1972): 23–36.

Arnold, Mary F. and Isabel M. Welsh. "Community Politics and Health Planning." In Mary F. Arnold, L. Vaughn Blankenship and John M. Hess, eds., *Administrating Health Systems: Issues and Perspectives.* Chicago: Aldine Publishing Co., 1971: 154–175.

Bazell, R.J. "Health Radicals: Crusade to Shift Medical Power to the People." *Science* Vol. 173 (August 6; 1971): 506–509.

Bellin, Lowell E., Florence Kavaler, and Al Schwarz. "Phase One of Consumer Participation in Policies of 22 Voluntary Hospitals in New York City." *American Journal of Public Health* Vol. 62 (October 1972): 1370–1378.

Brandon, William. "Politics, Administration and Conflict in Neighborhood Health Centers." *Journal of Health Politics, Policy and Law* Vol. 2 (Spring 1977): 79–99.

Burlage, Robb K. "Confrontation: Consumer Forces will Liberate Systems." *Modern Hospital* Vol. 3 (December 1968) 81 + .

Cornely, Paul B. "Community Participation and Control: A Possible Answer to Racism in Health." *Milbank Memorial Fund Quarterly/ Health and Society* Vol. 48 (April 1970):Part 2, 347–362.

Dana, Bess. "Consumer Health Education." In Arthur Levin, ed., *Health Services: The Local Perspective,* Proceedings of the Academy of Political Science, Vol. 32, No. 3. New York: The Academy of Political Science, 1977: 182–191.

Danaceau, Paul. *Consumer Participation in Health Care: How it's Working.* Arlington, VA.: Human Services Institute for Children and Families, 1975. Also available from Springfield, VA.: National Technical Information Service, 1975.

Doong, Jean. Consumer Participation in Health Planning: An Annotated *Bibliography.* Health Planning Bibliography Series No. 2, DHEW Pub. No. (HRA) 77–14551, Rockville, MD.:

National Health Planning Information Center, 1976.

Douglass, Chester W. "Effect of Provider Attitudes in Community Health Decision-Making." *Medical Care* Vol. 11 (March–April 1973): 135–144.

Douglass, Chester W. "Representation Patterns in Community Health Decision-Making." *Journal of Health and Social Behavior* Vol. 14 (March 1973): 80–86.

Douglass, Chester W. "Consumer Influence in Health Planning in the Urban Ghetto." *Inquiry* Vol. 12 (June 1975) 157–163.

Duvall, Wallace, L. "Consumer Participation in Health Planning." *Hospital Administration* Vol. 16 (Fall 1971): 35–49.

Falkson, Joseph L. "Review Article: An Evaluation of Policy-Related Research on Citizen Participation in Municipal Health Service Systems." *Medical Care Review* Vol. 33 (February 1976): 156–221.

Feingold, Eugene. *Citizen Participation: A Review of the Issues, The Citizenry and the Hospital,* 1973 National Forum on the Citizenry and the Hospital. Durham, N.C.: Duke University, Program in Hospital Administration, 1973.

Fox, Daniel M. and Jean W. Wofford. "Citizen Participation: A Substitute for Action." *Health Education Monographs* No. 32 (1972): 37–40.

Glogow, Eli. "Community Participation and Sharing in Control of Public Health Services." *Health Service Reports* Vol. 88 (May 1973): 442–448.

Gordon, Jeffrey B. "The Politics of Community Medicine Projects: A Conflict Analysis." *Medical Care* Vol. 7 (November–December 1969): 419–428.

Gosfield, Alice. *PSRO's: The Law and the Health Consumer.* Cambridge: Ballinger Publishing Co., 1975.

Gosfield, Alice. "Consumer Accountability in PSRO's." *University of Toledo Review* Vol. 6 (Spring 1975): 764–803.

Gosfield, Alice. "Approaches of Nine Federal Health Agencies to Patients' Rights and Consumer Participation: An Overview of Responses of Agency Representatives to an Interview Survey." *Public Health Reports* Vol. 91 (September—October 1976): 403–405.

Greer, Ann L. "Training Board Members for

Health Planning Agencies: A Review of the Literature." *Public Health Reports* Vol. 91 (January–February 1976): 56–61.

Grossman, Randolph M. "Voting Behavior of HSA Interest Groups: A Case Study." *American Journal of Public Health* Vol. 68 (December 1978): 1191–1194.

Hersch, Charles. "Social History, Mental Health and Community Control." *American Psychologist* Vol. 27 (August 1972): 749–754.

Hessler, Richard M. "Consumer Participation, Social Organization and Culture: a Neighborhood Health Center for Chicanos." *Human Organization* Vol. 36 (Summer 1977): 124–134.

Hollister, Robert M. "From Consumer Participation to Community Control of Neighborhood Health Centers." Unpublished doctoral dissertation, Massachusetts Institute of Technology, 1971.

Holton, Wilfred E., Peter K. New, and Richard M. Hessler. "Citizen Participation and Conflict." *Administration in Mental Health* Vol. 1 (Fall 1973): 96–103.

Jonas, Steven. "A Theoretical Approach to the Question of 'Community Control' of Health Services Facilities." *American Journal of Public Health* Vol. 61 (May 1971): 916–921.

Jonas, Steven. "Limitations of Community Control of Health Facilities and Services." *American Journal of Public Health* Vol. 68 (June 1978): 541–543.

Kane, Daniel. "Community Participation in the Health Services System." *Hospital Administration* Vol. 16 (Winter 1971): 36–43.

Kane, Thomas J. "Citizen Participation in Decision-Making: Myth or Strategy." *Administration on Mental Health* Vol. 3 (Spring 1975): 29–45.

Kelman, Howard R. "Evaluation of Health Care Quality by Consumers." *International Journal of Health Services* Vol. 6, No. 3 (1976): 431–441.

Klein, Rudolf and Janet Lewis. *The Politics of Consumer Representation: A Study of Community Health Councils.* London: Center for Studies in Social Policy, 1976.

Koseki, L.K. and J. Hayakawa. "Consumer Participation and Community Organization Practice—Implications of National Health Legislation," *Medical Care* Vol. 17, No. 3 (March 1979): 244–254.

Kramer, Marlene. "Consumer's Influence on Health Care." *Nursing Outlook* Vol. 20 (September 1972): 574–578.

Lavery, Thomas J. "Consumer Participation at a Neighborhood Health Center." Unpublished doctoral dissertation, University of Iowa, 1978, Microfilm No. 70–01, 899.

Lipsky, Michael and Morris Lounds. "Citizen Participation and Health Care: Problems of Government Induced Participation." *Journal of Health Politics, Policy and Law* Vol. 1 (Spring 1976): 85–111.

Marmor, Theodore R. and James A. Morone. "Representing Consumer Interests: Imbalanced Markets, Health Planning and the HSAs." *Milbank Memorial Fund Quarterly/Health and Society* Vol. 58 (Winter 1980): 125–165.

McNamara, John J. "Communities and Control of Health Services." *Inquiry* Vol. 9 (September 1972): 64–69.

MacStravic, Robin E. "Community Participation and Influences in Health Care Delivery: Expectations, Performance and Satisfaction." Unpublished doctoral dissertation, University of Minnesota, 1973, Microfilm No. 74-10, 539.

MacStravic, Robin E. "Scalability of Community Participation in Health Program Decisions." *Health Services Research* Vol. 10 (Spring 1975): 76–81.

Metsch, Jonathan M. and James E. Veney. "Measuring the Outcome of Consumer Participation." *Journal of Health and Social Behavior* Vol. 14 (December 1973): 368–374.

Metsch, Jonathan M. and James E Veney. "A Model of the Adaptive Behavior of Hospital Administrators to the Mandate to Implement Consumer Participation." *Medical Care* Vol. 12 (April 1974): 338–350.

Metsch, Jonathan M. and James E. Veney. "Consumer Participation and Social Accountability." *Medical Care* Vol. 14 (April 1976): 283–293.

Metsch, Jonathan, Martin Weitzner and Ann Berson. "Impact of Training on Consumer Participation in the Delivery of Health Services." *Health Education Monographs* Vol. 3 (Fall 1975): 251–261.

Meyerhoff, Allen S. and David A. Crozier. "Health Care Coalitions: The Evaluation of a Movement: Datawatch." *Health Affairs* Vol. 3 (Spring 1984): 120–128.

Milio, Nancy. "Dimensions of Consumer Participation and National Health Legislation." *American Journal of Public Health* Vol. 64 (April 1974): 357–363.

Millis, John S. "The Future of Medicine: The Role of the Consumer." *Journal of the American Medical Association* Vol. 210 (October 20, 1969): 498–501.

Moore, Mary L. "The Role of Hostility and Militancy in Indigenous Community Health Advisory Groups." *American Journal of Public Health* Vol. 61 (May 1971): 922–930.

Mushkin, Selma J., ed. *Consumer Incentives for Health Care.* New York: Prodist, 1974.

New, Peter Kong-Ming, Richard M. Hessler and Phyllis B. Carter. "Consumer Control and Public Accountability." *Anthropological Quarterly* Vol. 46 (July 1973): 196–213.

Newman, Ian Mount, ed. *Consumer Behavior in the Health Marketplace, A Symposium Proceedings, 1976.* Lincoln, NE.: University of Nebraska, Nebraska Center for Health Education, 1976.

Nutt, Paul C. "Merits of Using Experts or Consumers as Members of Planning Groups: A Field Experiment in Health Planning." *Academy of Management Journal* Vol. 19 (September 1976): 378–394.

Oakes, Charles G. *The Walking Patient and the Health Crisis.* Columbia: University of South Carolina Press, 1973.

Office of Consumer Education and Information, Health Maintenance Organization Service. *Selected Papers on Consumerism in the HMO Movement,* DHEW Pub. No. (HSM) 73-13012. Washington, D.C.: U.S. Government Printing Office, 1973.

Padgett, Edward R. "The Political Effects of Consumer Participation—A Political Scientist's View." *Health Education Monographs* No. 32 (1972): 67–78.

Padilla, Elena. "Community Participation in Health Affairs." In Arthur Levin, ed., *Health Services: The Local Perspective,* Proceedings of the Academy of Political Science, Vol. 32, No. 3. New York: The Academy of Political Science, 1977: 227–237.

Palmer, Boyd Z., Roger L. Sisson, Lorrinne Kyle and Adele Hebb. "Community Participation in the Planning Process." *Health Education Monographs* No. 32 (1972): 5–22.

Papp, Warren, R. "Consumer-Based Boards of Health Centers: Structural Problems in Achieving Effective Control." *American Journal of Public Health* Vol. 68 (June 1978): 578–582.

Partridge, Kay B. "Community and Professional Participation in Decision-Making at a Health Center." *Health Services Reports* Vol. 88 (June–July 1973): 527–534.

Partridge, Kay B. and Paul E. White. "Community and Professional Participation in Decision-Making at a Health Center: A Methodology for Analysis." *Health Services Reports* Vol. 87 (April 1972): 336–342.

Pecarchik, Robert, Edmund Ricci and Bardin Nelson Jr. "Potential Contribution of Consumers to an Integrated Health Care System." *Public Health Reports* Vol. 91 (January-February 1976): 72–76.

Ready, William E. "The Consumer's Role in the Politics of Health Planning." *Health Education Monographs* No. 32 (1972): 51–58.

Riska, Elianne and James A. Taylor. "Consumer and Provider Views on Health Policy and Health Legislation." In E. Gartly Jaco, ed., *Patients, Physicians and Illness.* New York: The Free Press, 1979: 356–359, 3d ed.

Rivkin, M.O. and P.J. Bush. "The Satisfaction Continuum in Health Care: Consumer and Provider Preferences." In Selma J. Mushkin, ed., *Consumer Incentives for Health Care.* New York: Prodist, 1974.

Rogatz, Peter and Marge Rogatz. "Role for the Consumer." *Social Policy* Vol. 2 (January–February 1971): 52–56.

Rosen, Harry, Jonathan Metsch and Samuel Levey, eds. *The Consumer and the Health Care System: Social and Managerial Perspectives.* Health Systems Management Series No. 9. New York: Halsted Press (Spectrum Publishers), 1977.

Salber, Eva J. *Caring and Curing, Community Participation in Health Services.* New York: Prodist, 1975.

Sanders, Irwin T. and Ann Brownlee. "Health in the Community." In Howard E. Freeman, Sol Levine and Leo G. Reeder, eds., *Handbook of Medical Sociology.* Englewood Cliffs, N.J.: Prentice-Hall, 1979, 3d ed.: 412–436.

Sheps, Cecil G. "The Influence of Consumer Sponsorship on Medical Services." *Milbank Memorial Fund Quarterly/Health and Society* Vol. 50 (October 1972): Part II, 41–72.

Silver, George A. "Community Participation in Health Resource Allocation." *International Journal of Health Services* Vol. 3, No. 2 (1973): 117–131.

Smith, Richard A. "Community-Power and Decision Making: A Replication and Extension of Hawley." *American Sociological Review* Vol. 41 (August 1976): 691–705.

Stamps, Paula L., Thomas E. Duston, Edward J. Rising, Donald Allen and Marcia Bondy-Levy. "How Consumers Exercise Control Through Their Bill-Paying Patterns." *Inquiry* Vol. 15 (June 1978): 151–159.

Steinberg, Marcia K. "Consumer Participation in a Health Care Organization—The Case of the Health Insurance Plan of Greater New York." Unpublished doctoral dissertation, City University of New York, 1977, Microfilm No. 77–14, 590.

Stokes, Ann, David Banta and Samuel Putnam. "The Columbia Point Health Association: Evaluation of a Community Health Board." *American Journal of Public Health* Vol. 62 (September 1972): 1229–1234.

Stoller, Eleanor Palo. "New Roles for Health Care Consumers—A Study of Role Transformation." *Journal of Community Health* Vol. 3 (Winter 1977): 171–177.

Strauss, Marvin D. "Bibliography on Consumer Participation." *Health Education Monographs* No. 32 (1972): 79–86.

Strauss, Marvin D. "Consumer Participation in Health Planning." *Health Education Monographs* No. 32 (1972): (entire issue). Also Thorofare, N.J.: Charles B. Slack, 1972.

Taylor, Rex. "The Local Health System: An Ethnography of Interest Groups and Decision-Making." *Social Science and Medicine* Vol. 11 (September 1977): 583–592.

Thompson, Theodis. "Consumer Involvement in Health: A Conceptual Approach to Evaluating the Consumer Participation Process in Neighborhood Health Centers." Unpublished doctoral dissertation, University of Michigan, 1973, Microfilm No. 74–15, 907.

Thompson, Theodis. *The Politics of Pacification: The Case of Consumer Participation in Community Health Organizations.* Washington, D.C.: Institute for Urban Affairs and Research, Howard University, 1974.

Thompson, Ruth. "The Whys and Why Nots of Consumer Participation." *Community Mental Health Journal* Vol. 9 (Summer 1973): 143–150.

Tichy, Noel M. and June Irmiger Taylor. "Community Control of Health Services." *Health Education Monographs* Vol. 4 (Summer 1976): 108–131.

Tranquada, Robert E. "Participation of the Poverty Community in Health Care Planning." *Social Science and Medicine* Vol. 7 (September 1973): 719–728.

Vladeck, Bruce C. "Interest Group Representation and the HSA's: Health Planning and Political Theory." *American Journal of Public Health* Vol. 67 (January 1977): 23–29.

Young, T. Kue. "Lay-Professional Conflict in a Canadian Community Community Health Center: A Case Report." *Medical Care* Vol. 13 (November 1975): 897–904.

Westermeyer, Joseph. "Absentee Health Workers and Community Participation." *American Journal of Public Health* Vol. 62 (October 1972): 1364–1369.

Politics of Public Referenda on Health: Fluoridation Controversy

Abelson, Robert P., and Alex Bernstein. "A Computer Simulation Model of Community Referendum Controversies." *Public Opinion Quarterly* Vol. 27 (Spring 1963): 93–122.

Burns, James MacGregor. "The Crazy Politics of Fluorine." *New Republic* Vol. 128 (July 13, 1953): 14–15.

Burt, B.A., P.D. Bristow and T.B. Dowell. "Influencing Community Decisions on Fluoridation." *British Dental Journal* Vol. 135 (July 1973): 75–77.

Christoffel, Tom. "Fluorides, Facts and Fanatics: Public Health Advocacy Shouldn't Stop at the Court House Door." *American Journal of Public Health* Vol. 75 (August 1985): 888–891.

Conant, Ralph W. "Bibliography of Social-Scientific Studies in the Fluoridation Controversy." *Journal of Oral Therapeutics & Pharmacology* Vol. 3 (November 1966): 203–211.

Crain, Robert L. "Fluoridation: The Diffusion of an Innovation Among Cities." *Social Forces* Vol. 44 (June 1966): 467–476.

Crain, Robert L. Elihu Katz and Donald B. Rosenthal. *The Politics of Community Conflict: The Fluoridation Decision.* Indianapolis: Bobbs-Merrill Co., 1969.

Dalzell-Ward, A.J. "Fluoridation and Public Opinion." *Health Education Journal* Vol. 17 (November 1959): 247–258.

Davis, Morris. "Community Attitudes Toward Fluoridation." *Public Opinion Quarterly* Vol. 23 (Winter 1960): 474–482.

Dickson, S. "Class Attitudes to Fluoridation." *Health Education Journal* Vol. 28 (September 1969): 139–149.

Douglass, Chester W. and Dennis C. Stacey. "Demographical Characteristics and Social Factors Related to Public Opinion on Fluoridation." *Journal of Public Health Dentistry* Vol. 32 (Spring 1972): 128–134.

Dwore, Richard B. "A Case Study of the 1976 Referendum in Utah on Fluoridation." *Public Health Reports* Vol. 93 (January–February 1978): 73–78.

Evans, Caswell A., Jr. and Tomm Pickles. "Statewide Antifluoridation Initiatives: A New Challenge to Health Workers." *American Journal of Public Health* Vol. 68 (January 1978): 59–62.

Eveland, Charles L. "The Political Significance of Dental Health Orientations in the Fluoridation Controversy: A Post-Referendum Assessment." Unpublished doctoral dissertation, University of Michigan, 1969, Microfilm No. 70–4076.

Fish, D.G., E.S. Hirabayashi and G.K. Hirabayashi. "Voting Turnout on a Fluoridation Plebiscite." *Journal of the Canadian Medical Association* Vol. 31 (February 1965): 88–93.

Flanders, Raymond A. "The Denturism Initiative." *Public Health Reports* Vol. 96 (September–October 1981): 410–418.

Frankel, John M. and Myron Allukian. "Sixteen Referenda on Fluoridation in Massachusetts: An Analysis." *Journal of Public Health Dentistry* Vol. 33 (Spring 1973): 96–103.

Gamson, William A. "Public Information in a Fluoridation Referendum: A Summary of Research." *Health Education Journal* Vol. 19 (March 1961): 47–54.

Gamson, William A. "Social Science Aspects of Fluoridation: A Summary of Research." *Health Education Journal* Vol. 19 (September 1961): 159–169.

Gamson, William A. "The Fluoridation Dialogue: Is It An Ideological Conflict?" *Public Opinion Quarterly* Vol. 25 (Winter 1961): 526–537.

Gamson, William A. "Social Science Aspects of Fluoridation: A Supplement." *Health Education Journal* Vol. 24 (September 1965): 135–43.

Gamson, William A. and Peter H. Orons. "Community Characteristics and Fluoridation Outcome." *Journal of Social Issues* Vol. 17, No. 4 (1961): 66–74.

Gamson, William A. and Carolyn G. Lindberg. "An Annotated Bibliography of Social Science Aspects of Fluoridation." *Health Education Journal* Vol. 19 (November 1961): 209–230.

Green, Arnold L. "The Ideology of Anti-Fluoridation Leaders." *Journal of Social Issues* Vol. 17 No. 4 (1961): 13–25.

Grossman, J. "Problems in the Translation of Social Science Theory to Field Action: An Example in the Case of Fluoridation." *Journal of Dental Research* Vol. 45 (November–December 1966) Supplement, pp. 1595–1601.

Hahn, Harlan. "Voting Behavior on Fluoridation Referendums: A Reevaluation." *Journal of American Dental Association* Vol. 71 (November 1965): 1138–1144.

Hahn, Harlan. "Health Concerns and Attitudes Regarding Fluoridation." *Public Health Reports* Vol. 84 (July 1969): 655–659.

Hutchison, John A. "A Small-Town Fluoridation Fight." *Scientific Monthly* Vol. 77, No. 5 (1953): 240–243.

Isman, Robert. "Fluoridation: Strategies for Success." *American Journal of Public Health* Vol. 71 (July 1981): 717–721.

Jackson, D. "Attitudes to Fluoridation: A Survey of British Housewives." *British Dental Journal* Vol. 132 (March 21, 1972): 219–222.

Kegeles, S. Stephen. "Some Unanswered Questions and Action Implications of Social Research in Fluoridation." *Journal of Social Issues* Vol. 17, No. 4 (1961): 75–81.

Kegeles, S. Stephen and Gloria Latter. "Population Characteristics and Fluoridation Referendums." U.S. Public Health Service, Division of Dental Health. Unpublished paper, 1962.

Kimball, Solon T. and Marion Pearsall. "The Health Inventory at Work: The Fluoridation Project." In Solon T. Kimball and Marion Pearsall, eds., *The Talladega Story: A Study in Community Process.* Tuscaloosa: University of Alabama Press, 1954: 100–115.

Kirscht, John P. "Attitude Research on the Fluoridation Controversy." *Health Education Monographs* No. 10 (1961): 16–28.

Kirscht, John P. and Andie L. Knutson. "Science and Fluoridation: An Attitude Study." *Journal of Social Issues* Vol. 17, No. 4 (1961): 37–44.

Kirscht, John P. and Andie L. Knutson. "Fluoridation and the 'Threat' of Science." *Journal of Health and Human Behavior* Vol. 4 (Summer 1963): 129–135.

Lantos, Joseph, Lois A. Marsh and Ronald P. Schultz. "Small Communities and Fluoridation; Three Case-Studies." *Journal of Public Health Dentistry* Vol. 33 (Summer 1973): 149–159.

Linn, E.L. "Effect of Community Leaders and Organizations on Public Attitudes Toward Fluoridation." *Journal of Public Health Dentistry* Vol. 29 (Spring 1969): 108–117.

Linn, E.L. "An Appraisal of Sociological Research on the Public's Attitudes Toward Fluoridation." *Journal of Public Health Dentistry* Vol. 29 (Winter 1969): 36–45.

MacRae, P., C.R. Castaldi and W. Zacherl. "Dental Health, Socioeconomic Level, Interest Response to Polio Vaccination Program, and Voting in a Fluoridation Plebiscite." *Journal of Dental Research* Vol. 43 (October 1964):Supplement, 898–899.

Markle, Gerald E., James C. Petersen and Morton O. Wagenfeld. "Notes from the Cancer Underground: Participation in the Laetrile Movement." *Social Science and Medicine* Vol. 12 No. 1 (1978): 31–37.

Marmor, Judd, Viola W. Bernard and Perry Ottenberg. "Psychodynamics of Group Opposition to Health Programs." *American Journal of Orthopsychiatry* Vol. 30 (April 1960): 330–345.

Masterton, G. "A Study of Responses to a Questionnaire on Fluoridation." *American Journal of Public Health* Vol. 53 (August 1963): 1243–1251.

Mausner, Bernard. "The Fluoridation Controversy: A Study in the Acceptance of Scientific Authority." *Journal of American College of Dentists* Vol. 24 (September 1957): 202–205.

Mausner, Bernard and J. Mausner. "A Study of the Anti-Scientific Attitude." *Scientific American* Vol. 192 (February 1955): 35–39.

Mazur, Allan. *The Dynamics of Technical Controversy.* Washington, D.C.: Communication Press, 1981.

McNeil, Donald R. *The Fight For Fluoridation.* New York: Oxford University Press, 1957.

McNeil, Donald R. "Political Aspects of Fluoridation." *Journal of the American Dental Association* Vol. 65 (November 1962): 659–662.

Metz, A. Stafford. "Research Directions in Fluoridation." In *Social Science Research Opportunities in Dental Health,* U.S. Public Health Service, Division of Dental Health. Washington, D.C.: U.S. Government Printing Office, 1965: 31–35.

Metzner, Charles A. "Referenda for Fluoridation." *Health Education Journal* Vol. 15 (September 1957): 168–177.

Metzner, Charles A. "Planning a Survey to Secure an Objective Understanding of the Public's Reactions to Fluoridation." in *Proceedings of the Fourth Workshop on Dental Public Health,* Continued Education Papers No. 69. Ann Arbor, MI.: University of Michigan, 1965: 134–142.

Mitchell, Austin. "Fluoridation in Dunedin: A Study of Pressure Groups and Public Opinion." *Political Science* (New Zealand) Vol. 12 (March 1960): 71–93.

Mueller, John E. "The Politics of Fluoridation in Seven California Cities." *Western Political Quarterly* Vol. 19 (March 1966): 54–67.

Mueller, John E. "Fluoridation Attitude Change." *American Journal of Public Health* Vol. 58 (October 1968): 1876–1882.

Murray, J.J. "Water Fluoridation: A Choice for the Community." *Community Health* (England) Vol. 6 (September–October 1974): 75–83.

O'Meara, B.J. "Observations on a Fluoridation Plebiscite." *Canadian Journal of Public Health* Vol. 51 (May 1960): 207–209.

O'Shea, Robert M. and Lois K. Cohen. "Social Science and Dentistry: Public Opinions on Fluoridation, 1968." *Journal of Public Health Dentistry* Vol. 29 (Winter 1969): 57–58.

O'Shea, Robert J. and S. Stephen Kegeles. "An Analysis of Anti-Fluoridation Letters." *Journal of Health and Human Behavior* Vol. 4 (Summer 1963): 135–140.

Paul, Benjamin D. "Synopsis of Report on Fluoridation." *Massachusetts Dental Society Journal* Vol. 8 (January 1959): 19–21.

Paul, Benjamin D. "Fluoridation and the Social Scientists: A Review." *Journal of Social Issues* Vol. 17, No. 4 (1961): 1–12.

Paul, Benjamin D., William A. Gamson, S. Stephen Kegeles, et al. "Trigger for Community Conflict: The Case of Fluoridation." *Journal of Social Issues* Vol. 17, No. 4 (1961): entire issue. Benjamin D. Paul, "Fluoridation and the Social Scientists—A Review," 1–12; Arnold Green, "The Ideology of Anti-Fluoridation Leaders," 13–25; Arnold Simmel, "A Signpost for Research on Fluoridation Conflicts: The Concept of Relative Deprivation," 26–36; John P. Kirscht and Andie L. Knutson, "Science and Fluoridation: An Attitude Study," 37–44; Harry M. Raulet, "The Health Professional and the Fluoridation Issue: A Case Study of Role Conflict," 45–54; Irwin T. Sanders, "The Stages of a Community Controversy: The Case of Fluoridation," 55–65; William A. Gamson and Peter Irons, "Community Characteristics and Fluoridation Outcome," 66–74; S. Stephen Kegeles: "Some Unanswered Questions and Implications of Social Research in Fluoridation," 75–81.

Petersen, James C. and Gerald E. Markle. "The Laetrile Controversy." In Dorothy Nelkin, ed., *Controversy: Politics of Technical Decisions*. Beverly Hills, CA.: Sage Publications, 1979,: 159–179.

Petterson, Elof O. "Abolition of the Right of Local Swedish Authorities to Fluoridate Drinking Water." *Journal of Public Health Dentistry* Vol. 32 (Fall 1972): 243–247.

Pinard, Maurice. "Structural Attachments and Political Support in Urban Politics: The Case of Fluoridation Referendums." *American Journal of Sociology* Vol. 68 (March 1963): 513–526.

Plaut, Thomas F.A. "Analysis of Voting Behavior on a Fluoridation Referendum." *Public Opinion Quarterly* Vol. 23 (Summer 1958): 213–222.

Ramirez, A., R.B. Connor, R.M. Gibbs, H.G. Griggs, J.O. Neilsen and O.W. Reeder. *Anomie and Political Powerlessness. Their Relationship to Attitudes and Knowledge Concerning Fluoridation*. Birmingham, AL.: University of Alabama, School of Dentistry, 1969.

Raulet, Harry M. "The Health Professional and the Fluoridation Issue: A Case of Role Conflict." *Journal of Social Issues* Vol. 17, No. 4 (1961): 45–53.

Roemer, Ruth. "Water Fluoridation: Public Health Responsibility and Democratic Process." *American Journal of Public Health* Vol. 55 (September 1965): 1337–1348.

Rosenstein, David I., Robert Isman, Tomm Pickles and Craig Benben. "Fighting the Latest Challenge to Fluoridation in Oregon." *Public Health Reports* Vol. 93 (January–February 1978) 69–72.

Rosenthal, Donald B. and Robert L. Crain. "Executive Leadership and Community Innovation: The Fluoridation Experience." *Urban Affairs Quarterly* Vol. 1 (March 1966): 39–57.

Sanders, Irwin T. *The Physician and Fluoridation: A Summary of Research Findings*. Cambridge: Harvard University School of Public Health, August 1960, Document No. 16-S, Social Science Program.

Sanders, Irwin T. "The Stages of a Community Controversy: The Case of Fluoridation." *Journal of Social Issues* Vol. 17, No. 4 (1961): 55–65.

Sanders, Irwin T. "The Involvement of Health Professionals and Local Officials in Fluoridation Controversies." *American Journal of Public Health* Vol. 52 (August 1962): 1274–1287.

Sapolsky, Harvey M. "Science, Voters, and the Fluoridation Controversy." *Science* Vol. 62 (October 1968): 427–433.

Sapolsky, Harvey M. "The Fluoridation Controversy: An Alternative Explanation." *Public Opinion Quarterly* Vol. 33 (Summer 1969): 240–248.

Scism, Thomas E. "Fluoridation in Local Politics: Study of the Failure of a Proposed Ordinance in One American City." *American Journal of Public Health* Vol. 62 (October 1972): 1340–1345.

Shaw, C.T. "Characteristics of Supporters and Rejecters of a Fluoridation Referendum and a Guide for Other Community Programs." *Journal of the American Dental Association* Vol. 78 (February 1969): 339–341.

Simmel, Arnold G. "A Signpost on Fluoridation Conflicts: The Concept of Relative Deprivation." *Journal of Social Issues* Vol. 17, No. 4 (1961): 23–36.

Simmel, Arnold G. "The Structuring of Opinion on a Controversial Topic: Studies and Explanations of Fluoridation Conflicts." Unpublished doctoral dissertation, Columbia University, 1969, Microfilm No. 70-17, 047.

Smith, Richard A. "Community Power and Decision Making: A Replication and Extension of Hawley." *American Sociological Review* Vol. 41 (August 1976): 691–705.

Stephens, Douglas W. "Why Fluoridation Was Defeated in Long Beach, California." *Oral Hygiene* Vol. 48 (May 1958): 30–34.

Sturgeon, L.W.C. "A Plebiscite on Continuing Fluoridation in Thorold, Ontario." *Canadian Journal of Public Health* Vol. 49 (October 1958): 425–429.

Thomas, C.R. "The Press and Fluoridation Referenda in Selected Wisconsin Cities." Unpublished master's thesis, University of Wisconsin, 1966.

Turk, Herman. *Organizations in Modern Life: Cities and Other Large Networks.* San Francisco, CA.: Jossey-Bass, 1977.

Walsh, Diana C. "Fluoridation: Slow Diffusion of a Proven Preventive Measure." *New England Journal of Medicine* Vol. 296 (May 12, 1977): 1118–1120.

Warner, Morton. "Communication Overkill in a Fluoridation Campaign." *Canadian Journal of Public Health* Vol. 63 (May–June 1972): 219–227.

Wilson, Robert N. *Community Structure and Health Action.* Washington, D.C.: Public Affairs Press, 1968.

San Francisco, CA.: Boyd & Fraser Publication Co., Vol. I, 1976; Vol. II, 1983 (tentative).

Congressional Quarterly, Inc. *Congressional Quarterly's Guide to Congress.* Washington, D.C.: Congressional Quarterly, Inc., 1976, 2d ed.

Cirn, John T. *A Guide to Doing Library Research in American Health, Policy and Politics.* University of Iowa, Graduate Program in Hospital and Health Administration, 1979 (mimeo).

Vose, Clement. *A Guide to Library Sources in Political Science: American Government.* Washington, D.C.: American Political Science Association, 1975.

REFERENCES

Litman, Theodor J. *The Sociology of Medicine and Health Care: A Research Bibliography.*

Index